BICARBONATE IV, IO — 1mEq/kg — Q10min — 1.5mEq — 3mEq — 5mEq — 10mEq — 15mEq — 20mEq — 30mEq — 50mEq — 70mEq

Metabolic acidosis	
with good	**Newborn:**
ventilation	0.5mEq/kg
Hyperkalemia	(=2mL/kg)
Tricyclic	**Adult:**
antidepressant	1mEq/mL
overdose	(=1mL/kg)

*ETT size (mm) = [16 + Age (yr)]/4.

†Approx. distance of insertion = Internal diameter (ID)...

‡'LANE' drugs may be given by ETT: lidocaine, atropi...

§Beware: Standard drug concentrations may vary.

‖Use 1:10,000 concentration of epinephrine via ET tu... gh-dose (1:1000) epinephrine for ET tube dosing beyond the neonatal period.

¶Low-dose epinephrine (1:10,000) 0.1–0.3mL/kg pr... ...ses and all routes.

NARCAN: 0.1mg/kg/dose IM/ET/IV/SC to **ma**...

May repeat Q2–3min.

OXYGEN: 100%.

GLUCOSE: If hypoglycemic: 2–4mL/kg bolus of D$_{25}$W, then constant infusion of
glucose at 8mg/kg/min. See Chapter 20 for infusion calculation.

CALCIUM: If hypocalcemic, hyperkalemic, or Ca channel blocker toxic: 100mg/kg
10% Ca gluconate, or 20mg/kg 10% Ca chloride.

DEFIBRILLATION: 2J/kg. May double and repeat.

CARDIOVERSION: Initial: 0.5J/kg. May double and repeat.

ADENOSINE: 0.1–0.2mg/kg rapid IV push. May double and repeat.
Max. total dose: 12mg.

LIDOCAINE: 1mg/kg IV. If successful, begin lidocaine infusion.

Dilute medication with normal saline to minimum volume of 3–5mL. Follow with positive pressure ventilation...

IV INFUSIONS

$$6 \times \frac{\text{Desired dose (mcg/kg/min)}}{\text{Desired rate (ml/hr)}} \times \text{Wt (kg)} = \frac{\text{mg drug}}{100mL \text{ fluid}}$$

Medication	Usual Dose (mcg/kg/min)	Dilution in 100mL D$_5$W	IV infusion rate
Dopamine	2–20	6mg/kg	1mL/hr = 1mcg/kg/min
Dobutamine	2.5–15	6mg/kg	1mL/hr = 1mcg/kg/min
Epinephrine	0.1–1	0.6mg/kg	1mL/hr = 0.1mcg/kg/min
Isoproterenol	0.1–2	0.6mg/kg	1mL/hr = 0.1mcg/kg/min
Lidocaine	20–50	6mg/kg	1mL/hr = 1mcg/kg/min
Prostaglandin E$_1$	0.05–0.1	0.3mg/kg	1mL/hr = 0.05mcg/kg/min
Terbutaline	0.1–0.4	0.6mg/kg	1mL/hr = 0.1mcg/kg/min

D102040I6

THE HARRIET LANE HANDBOOK

A Manual for Pediatric House Officers

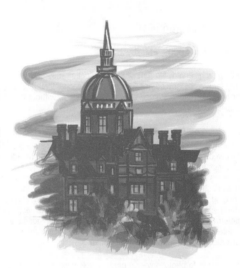

fifteenth
EDITION

with 151 illustrations and 24 color plates

The Harriet Lane Service
Children's Medical and Surgical Center of
The Johns Hopkins Hospital

EDITORS

GEORGE K. SIBERRY, MD, MPH
ROBERT IANNONE, MD

 Mosby

St. Louis Baltimore Boston Carlsbad Chicago Minneapolis New York Philadelphia Portland
London Milan Sydney Tokyo Toronto

LIBRARY
ARAPAHOE COMMUNITY COLLEGE
5900 S. SANTA FE DRIVE
P.O. BOX 9002
LITTLETON, CO 80160-9002

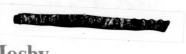

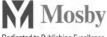 **Mosby**

Dedicated to Publishing Excellence

*12/02 there is a more recent
ed (2002), but demand
does not warrant*

FIFTEENTH EDITION

Copyright © 2000 by Mosby, Inc.

All rights reserved. No part of this publication may be reproduced or transmitted in any form or by any means, electronic or mechanical, including photocopy, recording, or any information storage and retrieval system, without permission in writing from the publisher.

NOTICE

Pharmacology is an ever-changing field. Standard safety precautions must be followed, but as new research and clinical experience broaden our knowledge, changes in treatment and drug therapy may become necessary or appropriate. Readers are advised to check the most current product information provided by the manufacturer of each drug to be administered to verify the recommended dose, the method and duration of administration, and contraindications. It is the responsibility of the treating physician, relying on experience and knowledge of the patient, to determine dosages and the best treatment for each individual patient. Neither the publisher nor the editor assumes any liability for any injury and/or damage to persons or property arising from this publication.

Permission to photocopy or reproduce solely for internal or personal use is permitted for libraries or other users registered with the Copyright Clearance Center, provided that the base fee of $4.00 per chapter plus $.10 per page is paid directly to the Copyright Clearance Center, 222 Rosewood Drive, Danvers, Massachusetts 01923. This consent does not extend to other kinds of copying, such as copying for general distribution, for advertising or promotional purposes, for creating new collected works, or for resale.

Mosby, Inc.
A Harcourt Health Sciences Company
11830 Westline Industrial Drive
St. Louis, Missouri 63146

Printed in the United States

International Standard Book Number 0-323-00812-7

00 01 02 03 TG/FF 9 8 7 6 5

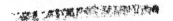

To our parents

Patricia K. Siberry and George Siberry, Jr.
For giving me guidance and independence in loving balance

Emma V. Iannone and Matthew M. Iannone (in memoriam)
Their personal sacrifices have privileged me with opportunity
that comes from a quality education.

To our families

Uma M. Reddy, Vikram G. Siberry, and Vinod W. Siberry
They make every day special

Peg Iannone
Her enduring support for all of my endeavors brings out the best in me.

To our mentor in pediatrics

Julia A. McMillan

We are grateful to Dr. McMillan as our role model. Her example has
inspired us to be both students and teachers of pediatrics. She reminds
us that our principal commitment is to our patients, the children whose
illnesses we work to cure, whose pain we want to lessen, and whose
suffering motivates us to seek better methods.

MAR 2 3 2001

FOREWORD

The Harriet Lane Handbook will celebrate its fiftieth year during the printing of the fifteenth edition. Please permit us to share with you a part of our heritage.

A SHORT HISTORY OF HARRIET LANE

Until 1964, The Harriet Lane Home for Invalid Children housed The Department of Pediatrics at Johns Hopkins. Harriet Lane Johnston and her husband Henry Johnston were the donors. Harriet Lane, who was born in Lancaster County, Pennsylvania, lost both of her parents while a child. She was raised with a cousin, also parentless, by their Uncle James Buchanan. Buchanan, a lawyer, was successively a member of the U.S. House of Representatives, a member of the U.S. Senate, Ambassador to Russia, and finally Ambassador to Great Britain. Harriet went to England with her uncle and there is said to have greatly impressed Queen Victoria, who urged her to stay in England and marry into the aristocracy. But in 1857, this possibility had to be tabled because her uncle was elected president of the United States and Harriet returned with him to fulfill the role of first lady. This she did with flair and confidence.

Buchanan's term in office was beset by the turmoil leading up to the War Between The States, and in the end, Abraham Lincoln was elected to replace him. Sadly, he and Harriet retreated to Lancaster, but before many years had passed, she married Henry Johnston, a Baltimore banker. The Johnstons had two children, both boys, and both died as teenagers of rheumatic fever. It was this loss that caused the Johnstons to set aside the money for a children's hospital to be called, at Mr. Johnston's wish, The Harriet Lane Home for Invalid Children. Mr. Johnston died in his fifties, after which Harriet moved back to Washington, the scene of her long ago social triumphs. She died in 1902 at 73, and 10 years later the Harriet Lane Home opened its doors as a part of The Johns Hopkins Hospital.

Barton Childs, MD

THE HARRIET LANE HANDBOOK

A Manual for Pediatric
House Officers

This book is dedicated to those who do and
to those who suffer in the doing

The Harriet Lane Home
Johns Hopkins Hospital
Baltimore Maryland

19 50 53

Cover of the first *Harriet Lane Handbook*. Dr. Henry Seidel, editor. 1950-1953.

A SHORT HISTORY OF *The Harriet Lane Handbook*

Harrison Spencer, chief resident in 1950-1951, suggested that residents develop a pocket-sized "pearl book." Six of us began without funds and without the supervision of our elders, meeting sporadically around a table in the library of The Harriet Lane Home. We were busy. The work dragged on. The residents changed but not our fervor. Helen Taussig provided diagrams for interpreting fluoroscopy of the heart. Drug doses appeared without substantial pharmacologic advice, developed in large part by rampant empiricism. Rhesa Penn, a resident, drew four marvelous cartoons (see p. ix). Without obvious financial support for mimeographing and looseleafs, our *Handbook* slipped into the pockets of our residents in 1953. Succeeding residents kept revising, updating, improving. Robert Cooke, Department Chief from 1956 to1974, realized the potential, and the fifth edition was published widely by Year Book. Jerry Winkelstein and Herbert Swick led that effort, since, happily, Dr. Cooke kept the residents in charge. *The Handbook* is theirs, and it now fills pockets too numerous to count.

Henry M. Seidel, MD

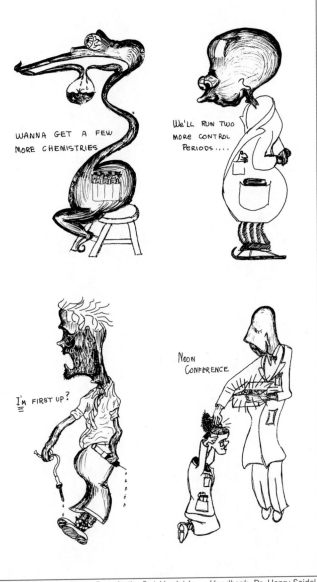

Original cartoons by Rhesa Penn in the first *Harriet Lane Handbook*. Dr. Henry Seidel, editor. 1950-1953.

PREFACE

It is on this inspiring historical backdrop that other chief residents updated our pediatric practice manual. We are greatly indebted to all the prior editors of *The Harriet Lane Handbook*: Drs. Harrison Spencer, Henry Seidel, Herbert Swick, William Friedman, Robert Haslam, Jerry Winkelstein, Dennis Headings, Kenneth Schuberth, Basil Zitelli, Jeffrey Biller, Andrew Yeager, Cynthia Cole, Mary Greene, Peter Rowe, Kevin Johnson, and Michael Barone. The current revision process occurs every 3 years. Under the direction of the chief residents, senior residents review, modify, and develop material for each chapter, always with the guidance of our pediatric faculty. Over the years, new chapters have been added when deemed necessary. We are excited to include new sections on surgery, oncology, psychiatry, and biostatistics. We are confident that those who use this manual will greatly benefit from the efforts of these individuals:

Chapter	Resident	Chapter Title	Advisor
1	Michele R. McKee, MD	Emergency Management	Allen R. Walker, MD
2	Sheila M. Hofert, MD	Poisonings	Erica Liebelt, MD
			Wendy Klein-Schwartz, PhD
			Cecilia Davoli, MD
3	Wendy Burk Roberts, MD	Procedures	Allen R. Walker, MD
4	Adrianna Maria Bravo, MD	Trauma and Burns	Charles Paidas, MD
5	Diane M. Straub, MD, MPH	Adolescent Medicine	Alain Joffe, MD, MPH
6	Mary K. Choukair, MD	Blood Chemistries/ Body Fluids	John Andrews, MD
7	Lydia Ko Chiang, MD	Cardiology	W. Reid Thompson, MD
	Alison Ensor Dunn, MD		
8	George K. Siberry, MD, MPH	Conversion Formulas and Biostatistics	Harold Lehmann, MD
			Marie Diener-West, PhD
9	Adrianna Maria Bravo, MD	Development	Peter Blasco, MD
10	Jeffrey Renn Keefer, MD, PhD	Endocrinology	David Cooke, MD
11	Mary K. Choukair, MD	Fluids and Electrolytes	John S. Andrews, MD
			Fred J. Heldrich, MD
			Mathuram Santosham, MD
12	B. Kelly Gleason, MD	Gastroenterology	José Saavedra, MD
13	Amy B. Hirshfeld, MD	Genetics	Ada Hamosh, MD
14	George K. Siberry, MD, MPH	Growth Charts	Ada Hamosh, MD
15	Beth E. Ebel, MD, MSc	Hematology	James F. Casella, MD
	Leslie Raffini, MD		
16	Pamela C. Schamber, MD	Immunology	Jerry Winkelstein, MD
17	Beth E. Ebel, MD, MSc	Immunoprophylaxis	Neal A. Halsey, MD
	Amy B. Hirshfeld, MD		
18	Aklil Getachew, MD	Infectious Diseases	Rodney Willoughby, MD
	Beth D. Kaufman, MD		
19	Beth D. Kaufman, MD	Microbiology	Julia A. McMillan, MD
	Aklil Getachew, MD		James Dick, PhD

Continued

For many, the formulary is the most often referenced section. Credit for this concise, yet comprehensive pediatric dosage resource is owed in large part to Carlton K.K. Lee, PharmD. The reader will notice substantial changes in the fomulary. Modern typesetting has allowed us to use the portrait layout to list brand names, standard preparations, dosage, and important remarks. We have also added important information on safety in breast-feeding, pregnancy, and renal failure, flagging these drugs with easily recognizable icons.

We would also like to thank the many other persons who contributed their expertise to the fifteenth edition: Jeanne Cox, MS, RD, for her work on the nutrition section; Dr. William Zinkham for providing the hematology color plates; and Josie Pirro, RN, for providing the illustrations in Chapter 3 (Procedures). We thank the following faculty who reviewed specific sections of chapters in areas of their expertise: Drs. Barbara Fivush (hypertension), Claude Migeon (steroids), Allen Chen (chemotherapy), Bernard Cohen (acne), Judy Vogelhut (breastfeeding), Beryl Rosenstein (cystic fibrosis), Leslie Plotnick (DKA), Charles Paidas (pediatric surgery), Dave Rodeberg (pediatric surgery), Steve Docimo (pediatric urology), Russell Faust (pediatric otolaryngology), John Graybeal, DDS (dentistry/oral surgery), Paul Sponseller (pediatric orthopedics), and Laura Sterni (pulmonary). The artwork at the section headings is the work of the late Aaron Sopher, whose timeless illustrations of the Harriet Lane Home were made some 30 years ago.

Please allow us also to thank those with whom we have worked daily over the past year and whose support we could not have done without:

Kenneth Judd, Francine Cheese, Kathy Miller, and Leslie Burke. We would like to give special thanks to Monica Casella, who coordinated our collective efforts in putting the manuscript together.

We would especially like to thank Dr. George Dover, Chairman of the Department of Pediatrics at Johns Hopkins. Dr. Dover has supported us in all aspects of our job as chief residents, especially in issues related to Harriet Lane residents and resident life.

Finally, thanks to all of the residents. Learning from you and assisting in your professional growth has been the most enjoyable part of our jobs.

Assistant Residents	Interns
Gail Addlestone	Sanjay Aggarwal
Henry "Kip" Baggett	Hans Agrawal
Elizabeth Cristofalo	Kamal Bharucha
David Fleischer	Patrick Brown
Ruchira Garg	Colleen Clendenin
Julia Arana	Angela Ellison
Lisa Gesualdo	Dana Erikson
Jeffrey Gossett	Jeffrey Fadrowski
Veronica Gunn	Michael Fields
Alex Huang	Allison Koenig
Paul Law	Karen Lewis
Anuj "Steve" Narang	Manisha Makker
Christian Nechyba	Deborah McWilliams
Declan O'Riordan	Namrata Pai
Tyler Reimschisel	Hardin Pantle
Mark Rigby	Genevieve Parsons
Brian Sard	Stacie Peddy
Susan Scherer	Kristina Powell
Julie Snell	Erica Reed
Jennifer Tucker	Kerry VanVoorhis
Sandhya Vasan	Tong-Yi Yao
Anne-Lise Yohay	
Kaleb Yohay	

George K. Siberry
Robert Iannone

ABBREVIATIONS

A-a	alveolar-arterial	DSM-IV	Diagnostic and Statistical Manual-IV
ABG	arterial blood gas	DTaP	diphtheria–tetanus–acellular pertussis
ACE	angiotensin converting enzyme	DTP	diphtheria-tetanus-pertussis
ACTH	adrenocorticotropic hormone	DTR	deep tendon reflex
ADH	antidiuretic hormone	DVT	deep vein thrombosis
AD(H)D	attention deficit (hyperactivity) disorder	EBV	Epstein-Barr virus
AFP	alpha fetoprotein	ECF	extracellular fluid
AGA	average (weight) for gestational age	ECG	electrocardiogram
AIDS	acquired immunodeficiency syndrome	ECMO	extracorporeal membrane oxygenation
ALL	acute lymphocytic leukemia	EEG	electroencephalogram
ALT	alanine aminotransferase	ELISA	enzyme-linked immunosorbent assay
ALTE	apparent life-threatening event	ESR	erythrocyte sedimentation rate
AML	acute myelocytic leukemia	ETT	endotracheal tube
ANC	absolute neutrophil count	FDP	fibrin degradation products
AP	anteroposterior	FFP	fresh frozen plasma
aPTT	activated partial thromboplastin time	FISH	fluorescent in situ hybridization
ASD	atrial septal defect	FTT	failure to thrive
ASO	antistreptolysin O	FW	free water
AST	aspartate aminotransferase	GBS	group B streptococcus; Guillain-Barré syndrome
AXR	abdominal x-ray	GER(D)	gastroesophageal reflux (disease)
BAER	brainstem auditory evoked responses	GFR	glomerular filtration rate
BCG	bacille Calmette-Guérin	GI	gastrointestinal
BID	bis in die (twice a day)	HBIG	hepatitis B immune globulin
BMI	body mass index	HBV	hepatitis B virus
BP	blood pressure	HCG, β-HCG	human chorionic gonadotropin
BPD	bronchopulmonary dysplasia	Hct	hematocrit
BSA	body surface area	Hib	Haemophilus influenzae type b
BUN	blood urea nitrogen	HIE	hypoxic-ischemic encephalopathy
BVH	biventricular hypertrophy	HIV	human immunodeficiency virus
BW	birthweight	HSP	Henoch-Schönlein purpura
CBC	complete blood count	HSV	herpes simplex virus
CDC	Centers for Disease Control and Prevention	HUS	hemolytic-uremic syndrome
CGD	chronic granulomatous disease	IBD	inflammatory bowel disease
CHF	congestive heart failure	ICF	intracellular fluid
CHO	carbohydrate	ICP	intracranial pressure
CLD	chronic lung disease	Ig	immunoglobulin
CMV	cytomegalovirus	IM	intramuscular(ly)
CNS	central nervous system	IMV	intermittent mandatory ventilation
CO	carbon monoxide	INH	isoniazid
CO_2	carbon dioxide	IO	intraosseous(ly)
CP	cerebral palsy	IPV	inactivated polio virus vaccine
CPAP	continuous positive airway pressure	ITP	idiopathic thrombocytopenic purpura
Cr	creatinine	IUGR	intrauterine growth retardation
CRP	C-reactive protein	IV	intravenous(ly)
CSF	cerebrospinal fluid	IVC	inferior vena cava
CT	computed tomography	IVH	intraventricular hemorrhage
CXR	chest x-ray	IVIG	intravenous immune globulin
DIC	disseminated intravascular coagulation		
DKA	diabetic ketoacidosis		
DMSA	dimercaptosuccinic acid		
DPL	diagnostic peritoneal lavage		
DQ	developmental quotient		

IVP	intravenous pyelogram	PS	pulmonic stenosis
JRA	juvenile rheumatoid arthritis	PT	prothrombin time
LAE	left atrial enlargement	PTT	*See aPTT*
LBBB	left bundle branch block	PTH	parathyroid hormone
LFT	liver function tests	PV	pulmonic valve
LGA	large (weight) for gestational age	PVC	premature ventricular contraction
LSD	lysergic acid diethylamide	QD	*quaque die* (every day)
LV	left ventricle	QID	*quater in die* (four times a day)
LVH	left ventricular hypertrophy		
LVOT	left ventricular outflow tract	RAE	right atrial enlargement
MAOI	monoamine oxidase inhibitor	RBBB	right bundle branch block
MAP	mean arterial pressure; mean airway pressure	RBC	red blood cell
		RDA	recommended dietary allowance
MBC	mean bactericidal concentration	RDS	respiratory distress syndrome
MCV	mean corpuscular volume	RDW	red cell distribution width
MIC	mean inhibitory concentration	RF	rheumatoid factor
		ROP	retinopathy of prematurity
MMR	measles–mumps–rubella	RPR	rapid plasma reagin
MMSE	Mini-Mental State Examination	RSV	respiratory syncytial virus
		RTA	renal tubular acidosis
MR	mental retardation; mitral regurgitation	RV	right ventricle
		RVH	right ventricular hypertrophy
MRI	magnetic resonance imaging	RVOT	right ventricular outflow tract
MS	mitral stenosis; multiple sclerosis	SBE	subacute bacterial endocarditis
MV	mitral valve	SC	subcutaneous(ly)
NEC	necrotizing enterocolitis	SGA	small (weight) for gestational age
NG	nasogastric		
NPO	*nil per os* (nothing by mouth)	SIDS	sudden infant death syndrome
NSAID	nonsteroidal antiinflammatory drug	SSRI	selective serotonin reuptake inhibitor
OCP	oral contraceptive pill	STD	sexually transmitted disease
OGTT	oral glucose tolerance test	STS	serologic test for syphilis
OPV	oral polio virus vaccine	SVC	superior vena cava
ORS	oral rehydration solution	SVT	supraventricular tachycardia
ORT	oral rehydration therapy	TB	tuberculosis
PA	posteroanterior; pulmonary artery	TCA	tricyclic antidepressant
		TGA	transposition of the great arteries
PAC	premature atrial contraction	TID	*ter in die* (three times a day)
PCA	patient-controlled analgesia	TSH	thyroid-stimulating hormone
PCP	*Pneumocystis carinii* pneumonia; phenylcyclohexyl piperidine or phencyclidine	TTP	thrombotic thrombocytopenic purpura
		TV	tricuspid valve
PCR	polymerase chain reaction	UA	urinalysis
PD	peritoneal dialysis	UAC	umbilical artery catheter
PDA	patent ductus arteriosus	UGI	upper gastrointestinal (series)
PEEP	positive end-expiratory pressure	UTI	urinary tract infection
PEFR	peak expiratory flow rate	UVC	umbilical vein catheter
PEG	percutaneous endoscopic gastrostomy	VBG	venous blood gas
		VCUG	voiding cystourethrogram
PEM	protein energy malnutrition	VDRL	Veneral Disease Research Laboratory
PFT	pulmonary function tests		
PID	pelvic inflammatory disease	VSD	ventricular septal defect
PIP	peak inspiratory pressure	VUR	vesicoureteral reflux
PMN	polymorphonuclear leukocyte	VZIG	varicella-zoster immune globulin
PO	*per os* (by mouth)		
PR	per rectum	VZV	varicella-zoster virus
PRP	phosphylribosopyro-phosphate	WB	Western blot
		WPW	Wolff–Parkinson–White

CONTENTS

THE HARRIET LANE HANDBOOK

A Manual for Pediatric House Officers

fifteenth
EDITION

PART I

Pediatric Acute Care

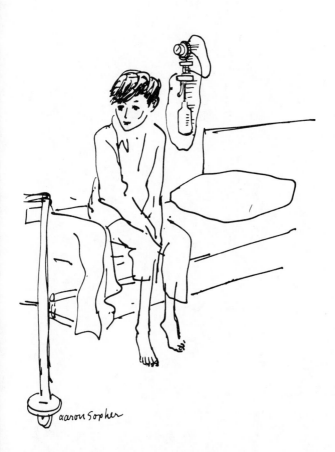

aaron sopher

EMERGENCY MANAGEMENT

Michele R. McKee, MD

I. AIRWAY

A. ASSESSMENT

1. **Open airway:** Establish open airway with head-tilt/chin-lift maneuver. If neck injury is suspected, jaw-thrust should be used.
2. **Obstruction:** Rule out foreign body, anatomic or other obstruction.

B. MANAGEMENT

1. **Equipment**
a. Oral airway
   1) Poorly tolerated in conscious patient.
   2) Size: With flange at teeth, tip reaches angle of jaw.
   3) Length ranges from 4–10cm.
b. Nasopharyngeal airway
   1) Relatively well tolerated in conscious patient. Rarely provokes vomiting or laryngospasm.
   2) Size: Length = tip of nose to angle of jaw.
   3) Diameter: 12–36 French.
2. **Intubation:** Sedation and paralysis recommended unless patient is unconscious or a newborn.
a. Indications: Obstruction (functional or anatomic), prolonged ventilatory assistance or control, respiratory insufficiency, loss of protective airway reflexes, or route for approved medications.
b. Equipment (See table on inside front cover.)
   1) Endotracheal tube (ETT): Size = (Age + 16)/4 = Internal diameter. Uncuffed ETT in patients <8 years old. Depth of insertion (in cm; at the teeth or lips) is approximately $3 \times$ ETT size.
   2) Laryngoscope blade: Generally, a straight blade can be used in all patients. A curved blade may be easier in patients >2 years old.
   3) Bag and mask attached to 100% oxygen.
   4) ETT stylets: Not to extend beyond the distal end of the ETT.
   5) Suction: Large-bore (Yankauer) suction catheter or 14–18 French suction catheter.
   6) Nasogastric (or orogastric) tube: Size from nose to angle of jaw to xyphoid process.
   7) Monitoring equipment: For electrocardiogram (ECG), pulse oximetry, blood pressure.
c. Procedure
   1) Preoxygenate with 100% O_2 via bag and mask.
   2) Administer intubation medications (Table 1.1 and Fig. 1.1).
   3) Ask assistant to apply cricoid pressure to prevent aspiration (Sellick maneuver).
   4) With patient lying supine on a firm surface, head midline and slightly extended, open mouth with right thumb and index finger.

1

3

5) Hold laryngoscope blade in left hand. Insert blade into right side of mouth, sweeping tongue to the left out of line of vision.

6) Advance blade to epiglottis. With straight blade, lift laryngoscope straight up, directly lifting the epiglottis until vocal cords are visible. With curved blade, the tip of blade rests in the vallecula (between the base of the tongue and epiglottis). Lift straight up to elevate the epiglottis and visualize the vocal cords.

7) While maintaining direct visualization, pass the ETT from the right corner of the mouth through the cords.

8) Verify ETT placement by end-tidal CO_2 detection (false negative if no effective pulmonary circulation), auscultation, view chest rise, and/or chest radiograph.

9) Securely tape ETT in place, noting depth of insertion (cm) at teeth or lips.

C. RAPID SEQUENCE INTUBATION MEDICATIONS

Note: Titrate drug doses to achieve desired effect (Fig. 1.1 and Table 1.1).

II. BREATHING

A. ASSESSMENT: Once the airway is established, evaluate air exchange. Examine for evidence of abnormal chest wall dynamics, such as tension pneumothorax, or central problems such as apnea.

B. MANAGEMENT: Positive pressure ventilation (application of 100% oxygen is never contraindicated in resuscitation situations).

1. **Mouth-to-mouth or nose-to-mouth breathing:** This is used in situations where no supplies are available. Provide two slow breaths (1–1.5 sec/breath) initially, then 20 breaths/min. One breath every fifth chest compression in cardiopulmonary resuscitation (CPR).

2. **Bag–mask ventilation:** This is used at a rate of 20 breaths/min. Assess chest expansion and breath sounds.

3. **Endotracheal intubation:** See p. 3.

4. **Laryngeal mask airway:** This is an option for a secure airway that does not require laryngoscopy or tracheal intubation. It allows spontaneous or assisted respiration, but does not prevent aspiration.

III. CIRCULATION

A. ASSESSMENT

1. **Rate:** Assess for bradycardia, tachycardia, or absent heart rate. Generally, bradycardia is <100 beats/min in a newborn and <60 beats/min in an infant or child; tachycardia of >240 beats/min suggests primary cardiac disease.

2. **Assess pulse (central and peripheral) and capillary refill (assuming extremity is warm):** <2 sec is normal, 2–5 sec is delayed, and >5 sec is markedly delayed, suggesting shock. Decreased mental status may be a sign of inadequate perfusion.

3. **Blood pressure (BP):** This is one of the least sensitive measures of adequate circulation in children.

Hypotension = Systolic BP <[70 + (2 × Age in years)]

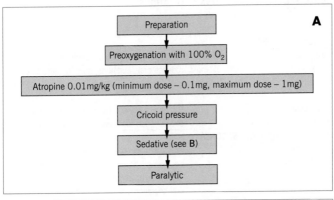

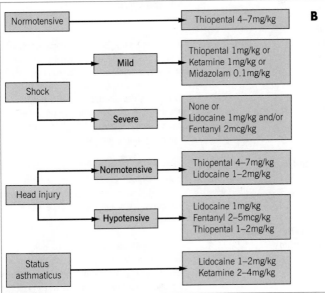

FIG. 1.1

A, Treatment algorithm for intubation. B, Sedation options. (Adapted from Nichols[1].)

B. MANAGEMENT

1. **Chest compressions** (Table 1.2)
2. **Fluid resuscitation**
a. If peripheral intravenous access is not obtained in 90 sec or three attempts, then place an intraosseous (IO) needle (see p. 49). If still unsuccessful, consider central venous access.

TABLE 1.1

RAPID SEQUENCE INTUBATION MEDICATIONS

Drug	Dose (IV) (mg/kg)	Comments
ADJUNCTS (FIRST)		
Atropine *(vagolytic)*	0.01–0.02 min. 0.1mg max. 1.0mg	Vagolytic, prevents bradycardia and reduces oral secretions, may increase HR
Lidocaine *(optional anesthetic)*	1–2	Blunts ICP spike, cough reflex, and CV effects of intubation; controls ventricular dysrhythmias
SEDATIVE/HYPNOTIC (SECOND)		
Thiopental *(barbiturate)*	1–7	May cause hypotension; myocardial depression decreases ICP and cerebral blood flow; use low dose in hypovolemia (1–2mg/kg); may increase oral secretions, cause bronchospasm and laryngospasm; contraindicated in status asthmaticus
OR		
Ketamine *(general anesthetic)*	1–4	May increase ICP, BP, HR, and oral secretions; causes bronchodilation, emergence delirium; give with atropine; contraindicated in eye injuries
OR		
Midazolam *(benzodiazepine)*	0.05–0.1	May cause decreased BP and HR, and respiratory depression; amnestic properties; benzodiazepines reversible with flumazenil (seizure warning applies)
OR		
Fentanyl *(opiate)*	2–5mcg/kg	Fewest hemodynamic effects of all opiates; chest wall rigidity with high dose or rapid administration; opiates reversible with naloxone (seizure warning applies); don't use with MAO inhibitors
PARALYTICS (THIRD)*		
Rocuronium	0.6–1.2	Onset 30–60 sec, duration 30–60 min; coadministration with sedative; may reverse in 30 min with atropine and neostigmine; minimal effect on HR or BP; precipitates when in contact with other drugs, so flush line before and after use
OR		
Pancuronium	0.1–0.2	Onset 70–120 sec, duration 45–90 min; contraindicated in renal failure, tricyclic antidepressant use; may reverse in 45 min with atropine and neostigmine

BP, blood pressure; CV, cardiovascular; HR, heart rate; ICP, intracranial pressure; MAO, monoamine.
*Nondepolarizing neuromuscular blockers, except succinylcholine, which is depolarizing.

TABLE 1.1

RAPID SEQUENCE INTUBATION MEDICATIONS—cont'd

Drug	Dose (IV) (mg/kg)	Comments
PARALYTICS (THIRD)* (Continued)		
OR		
Vecuronium	0.1–0.2	Onset 70–120 sec, duration 30–90 min; minimal effect on BP or HR; may reverse in 30–45 min with atropine and edrophonium
OR		
Succinylcholine	1–2	Onset 30–60 sec, duration 3–10 min; increases ICP, irreversible; contraindicated in burns, massive trauma, neuromuscular disease, eye injuries, malignant hyperthermia, and pseudocholinesterase deficiency. Risk: Lethal hyperkalemia in undiagnosed muscular dystrophy

TABLE 1.2

MANAGEMENT OF CIRCULATION

	Location	Depth (in)	Rate (per min)	Compressions: Ventilation
Infants	1 finger-breadth below intermammary line	0.5–1	>100	5:1
Children	2 finger-breadths below intermammary line	1–1.5	100	5:1

b. Initial fluid should be lactated Ringer's (LR) or normal saline (NS). Bolus with 20mL/kg over 5–15 minutes. Reassess. If no improvement, consider repeat bolus with 20mL/kg of same fluid. Reassess. If replacement requires >40mL/kg or if acute blood loss, consider 5% albumin, plasma, or packed red blood cells at 10mL/kg.

c. If cardiogenic etiology is suspected, fluid resuscitation may worsen clinical status.

3. **Pharmacotherapy:** See inside front and back covers for arrest drug guidelines.

Note: Consider early administration of antibiotics or corticosteroids if clinically indicated.

IV. ALLERGIC EMERGENCIES (ANAPHYLAXIS)

A. **DEFINITION:** Anaphylaxis is the clinical syndrome of immediate hypersensitivity. It is characterized by cardiovascular collapse and respiratory compromise, as well as cutaneous and gastrointestinal symptoms (e.g., urticaria, emesis).

B. **INITIAL MANAGEMENT**

1. **ABCs:** Establish airway (A) if necessary. Supply with 100% oxygen

with respiratory support (B) as needed. Assess circulation (C) and establish IV access. Place on cardiac monitor.

2. **Epinephrine:** Give epinephrine 0.01mL/kg (1:1000) subcutaneously (SC) (max. 0.3mL). Repeat Q15 min as needed.
3. **Albuterol:** Give nebulized albuterol 0.05–0.15mg/kg in 3mL NS (quick estimate: 2.5mg for <30kg, 5.0mg for >30kg) Q15 min as needed.
4. **H_1-receptor antihistamine:** Diphenhydramine 1–2mg/kg IM/IV/PO (max. 50mg).
5. **Corticosteroids:** These help prevent late phase of the allergic response. Methylprednisolone 2mg/kg IV bolus, then 2mg/kg per day ÷ Q6hr IV/IM or prednisone 2mg/kg PO bolus and once daily.

C. **HYPOTENSION**

1. **Trendelenburg position:** Head 30° below feet.
2. **Normal saline:** Administer 20mL/kg IV NS rapidly. Repeat bolus as necessary.
3. **Epinephrine:** Epinephrine 0.1mL/kg (1:10,000) may be given IV over 2–5 minutes while an epinephrine or dopamine infusion is being prepared. (See Infusion table on front cover for details of preparation and dosages.)

V. RESPIRATORY EMERGENCIES

The hallmark of upper airway obstruction is inspiratory stridor, whereas lower airway obstruction is characterized by cough, wheeze, and a prolonged expiratory phase.

A. **ASTHMA**

1. **Assessment:** Assess heart rate (HR), respiratory rate (RR), O_2 saturation, peak expiratory flow rate, use of accessory muscles, pulsus paradoxus (>20mmHg difference in systolic BP for inspiratory vs expiratory), dyspnea, alertness, color.
2. **Initial management**
   a. Oxygen to keep saturation ≥95%.
   b. Inhaled β-agonists: Nebulized albuterol 0.05–0.15mg/kg per dose every 20 min for three doses.
   c. If very poor air movement or if unable to cooperate with a nebulizer, give epinephrine 0.01mL/kg SC (1:1000; max. 0.3mL) Q15min up to 3 doses or terbutaline 0.01mg/kg SC (max dose 0.4mg) Q15min up to 3 doses.
   d. Start corticosteroids if no response after one nebulizer or if steroid dependent. Prednisone 2mg/kg PO Q24hr; or methylprednisolone 2 mg/kg IV then 2mg/kg per day divided Q6hr, if severe.
3. **Further management if incomplete or poor response**
   a. Continue nebulization therapy Q20–30 min and space interval as tolerated.
   b. Additional nebulized bronchodilators include ipratropium bromide 0.5 mg nebulized with albuterol (as above).

c. Aminophylline 6mg/kg IV bolus, then continuous infusion (dosages in formulary).

d. Terbutaline 2–10mcg/kg IV load followed by continuous infusion at 0.1–0.4mcg/kg per min titrated for effect.

e. Magnesium 25–50mg/kg/dose IV/IM (2g max.) Q4–6hr up to 3–4 doses.

4. **Intubation:** Intubation of those with acute asthma is dangerous and should be reserved for impending respiratory arrest.

B. **UPPER AIRWAY OBSTRUCTION:** This is most commonly caused by foreign body aspiration or infection.

1. **Epiglottitis:** This is a true emergency requiring immediate intubation. Any manipulation, including aggressive physical examination, attempt to visualize the epiglottis, venipuncture, or IV placement may precipitate complete obstruction. If epiglottitis is suspected, definitive airway placement should precede all diagnostic procedures. A prototypic 'epiglottitis protocol' may include the following:

a. Unobtrusively give O_2 (blow-by). Make patient NPO.

b. Have parent accompany child to allay anxiety.

c. Have physician accompany patient at all times.

d. Summon predetermined 'epiglottitis team' (most senior pediatrician, anesthesiologist, and otolaryngologist in hospital).

e. Management options

   1) If unstable (unresponsive, cyanotic, bradycardic), emergently intubate.

   2) If stable with high suspicion, escort patient with team to operating room for endoscopy and intubation under general anesthesia.

   3) If stable with moderate or low suspicion, obtain lateral radiographic examination to confirm. Epiglottitis team must accompany patient at all times.

f. After airway is secured, obtain cultures of blood and epiglottis surface. Begin antibiotics to cover *Haemophilus influenzae* type b (Hib), *Streptococcus pneumoniae*, and group A streptococci.

2. **Croup**

a. Mild (no stridor at rest): Cool mist therapy, minimal disturbance, hydration, and antipyresis.

b. Moderate to severe

   1) Mist tent or humidified oxygen mask near the child's face.

   2) Racemic epinephrine (2.25%) 0.05mL/kg per dose (max dose 0.5mL) in 3mL NS, no more than Q1–2hr; or nebulized epinephrine 0.5mL/kg of 1:1000 (1 mg/mL) in 3mL NS (max. dose 2.5mL for ≤4-year-old, 5.0mL for ≥4-year-old). Hospitalize if more than one nebulization is required. Observe for 4–6hr if discharge is planned.

   3) Dexamethasone 0.6mg/kg IM once. Oral steroids may be adequate.

   4) Nebulized steroids have been shown to be effective in mild-to-moderate croup where available. Budesonide 2mg/4mL NS via nebulization.

1

EMERGENCY MANAGEMENT

     5) A helium–oxygen mixture may decrease work of breathing by decreased resistance to turbulent gas flow through narrowed airway. Inspired He concentration must be >70% to be effective.

c. If child fails to respond as expected to therapy, consider airway films and evaluation by otolaryngology or anesthesiology. Consider retropharyngeal abscess, bacterial tracheitis, subglottic stenosis, epiglottitis, or foreign body.

3. Foreign body aspiration: Occurs most often in children <5 years old. Involves hot dogs, candy, peanuts, grapes, balloons, small toys, and other objects.

a. If patient is stable (i.e., forcefully coughing, well oxygenated), removal of the foreign body by bronchoscopy or laryngoscopy should be attempted in a controlled environment.

b. If patient is unable to speak, moves air poorly, or is cyanotic, intervene immediately.

     1) (i) Infant: Place infant over arm or rest on lap. Give five back blows between the scapulae. If unsuccessful, turn infant over and give five

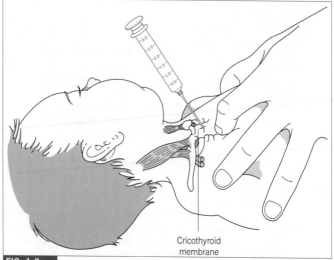

FIG. 1.2

Percutaneous (needle) cricothyrotomy. Extend neck, attach a 3ml syringe to a 14–18 gauge IV catheter and introduce catheter through the cricothyroid membrane (inferior to the thyroid cartilage, superior to the cricoid cartilage). Aspirate to confirm position. Remove the syringe and needle, attach the catheter to an adaptor from a 3.0mm ETT, which can then be used for positive-pressure oxygenation. (Adapted from Dieckmann[2].)

chest thrusts (in the same location as external chest compressions). Use tongue–jaw lift to open mouth. Remove object *only if visualized.* Attempt to ventilate if unconscious. Repeat sequence as often as necessary.

(ii) Child: Perform five abdominal thrusts (Heimlich maneuver) from behind a sitting or standing child or straddled over a child lying supine. Direct thrusts upward in the midline and not to either side of the abdomen.

2) If back, chest, and/or abdominal thrusts have failed, open mouth and remove foreign body if visualized. Blind finger sweeps are not recommended. Magill forceps may allow removal of foreign bodies in the posterior pharynx.

3) If the patient is unconscious, remove foreign body using Magill forceps if needed after direct visualization or laryngoscopy. If complete airway obstruction, consider percutaneous (needle) cricothyrotomy (Fig. 1.2), if attempts to ventilate via bag-valve-mask or ETT are unsuccessful.

VI. CARDIOVASCULAR EMERGENCIES

A. SEE INSIDE BACK COVER FOR ALGORITHMS OF ASYSTOLE AND PULSELESS ARREST, BRADYCARDIA, AND TACHYCARDIA.

B. ACUTE HYPERTENSION

1. Assessment

a. Width of bladder in blood pressure cuff should be at least two thirds the length of the upper arm and completely encircle the upper arm. Inadequate bladder size can result in a falsely elevated reading.

b. Patients with BP >95th percentile require further evaluation.

c. Hypertensive urgency, much more common in children, is significant evaluation in BP without accompanying end-organ damage. Symptoms include headache, blurred vision, and nausea. Hypertensive emergency is defined as elevation of both systolic and diastolic BP with acute end-organ damage (e.g., cerebral infarction, pulmonary edema, hypertensive encephalopathy, and cerebral hemorrhage).

d. Evaluate for underlying etiology: Medication/ingestion, cardiovascular, renovascular, renal parenchymal, endocrine, and CNS. **Rule out hypertension secondary to elevated intracranial pressure (ICP) before lowering BP.**

e. Physical examination should include four-extremity BP, fundoscopy (papilledema, hemorrhage, exudate), visual acuity, thyroid examination, evidence of congestive heart failure (tachycardia, gallop rhythm, hepatomegaly, edema), abdominal examination (mass, bruit), thorough neurologic examination, evidence of virilization, or cushingoid effect.

f. Initial diagnostic evaluation should include urinalysis, blood urea nitrogen (BUN), creatinine, electrolytes, chest radiograph, ECG. Consider obtaining renin level before antihypertensive therapy.

1

EMERGENCY MANAGEMENT

TABLE 1.3

MEDICATIONS FOR HYPERTENSIVE EMERGENCY

Drug	Onset (route)	Duration	Interval to repeat or increase dose	Comments
Diazoxide (arteriole vasodilator)	1–5 min (IV)	Variable (2–12 hr)	15–30 min	May cause edema, hyperglycemia
Hydralazine (IV) (arteriole vasodilator)	10–20 min (IV)	3–6 hr	10 min	Reflex tachycardia
Infusions				
Nitroprusside (arteriolar and venous vasodilator)	<30 sec (IV)	Very short	30–60 min	Requires ICU setting Follow thiocyanate level
Labetalol (α-, β-blocker)	1–5 min (IV)	Variable, about 6 hr	10 min	May require ICU setting
Nicardipine (calcium channel blocker)	1 min (IV)	3 hr	15 min	May cause edema, headache, nausea/vomiting

TABLE 1.4

MEDICATIONS FOR HYPERTENSIVE URGENCY

Drug (route)	Onset	Duration	Interval to repeat	Comments
Nifedipine (PO, SL)	15–30 min	6 hr	15 min	May cause headache
Enalaprilat (IV)	15 min	12–24 hr	8–24 hr	May cause hyperkalemia, hypoglycemia
Minoxidil (PO)	30 min	2–5 days	4–8 hr	Contraindicated in pheochromocytoma

PO, per os; SL, sublingual.

2. **Management**

a. Hypertensive emergency: IV line, monitor, possible arterial line for continuous BP. Consultation with nephrologist or cardiologist. Goal is to lower BP promptly but gradually in order to preserve cerebral autoregulation. Mean arterial pressure (MAP) where

$$MAP = \frac{1}{3} SBP + \frac{2}{3} DBP$$

should be lowered by one third of planned reduction over 6hr, an additional third over next 24–36hr and the final third over next 48hr.

After elevated ICP is ruled out, **do not delay treatment** because of diagnostic evaluation (Table 1.3).

b. Hypertensive urgency: Aim to lower MAP by 20% over 1hr. Oral or sublingual routes may be adequate. Observe in emergency room for 4–6hr. Close follow-up is mandatory. Many other medications are available; the three listed have been used with success (Table 1.4).

VII. NEUROLOGIC EMERGENCIES

A. INCREASED INTRACRANIAL PRESSURE (See also pp. 474–475 for evaluation and management of hydrocephalus.)

1. Assessment

a. History: Trauma, vomiting, fever, headache, neck pain, unsteadiness, seizure or other neurologic conditions, visual change, gaze preference, and change in mental status. In infants: irritability, poor feeding, lethargy, and bulging fontanel.

b. Examination: Assess for Cushing's response (hypertension, bradycardia, abnormal respiratory pattern), neck stiffness, photophobia, pupillary response, cranial nerve dysfunction (especially paralysis of upward gaze or of abduction), papilledema, absence of venous pulsations on eye grounds, neurologic deficit, abnormal posturing, and mental status examination.

2. Management: Do not lower BP if elevated ICP is suspected. C-spine immobilization necessary if trauma suspected.

a. Stable child (not comatose, stable vital signs, no focal findings): Cardiac monitor. Elevate head of bed 30°. Obtain complete blood count (CBC), electrolytes, glucose, and blood culture. Urgent head CT and neurosurgical consultation. Give antibiotics early if meningitis is suspected.

b. Unstable child: Emergent involvement of neurosurgery.
   1) Elevate head of bed 30°.
   2) Avoid hypoosmolar IV solutions.
   3) Mannitol 0.25–1g/kg IV and/or furosemide 1mg/kg IV for temporary reduction of ICP.
   4) Reserve hyperventilation for acute management, keep Pco_2 at 30–35mmHg. Controlled intubation as outlined on pp. 5–7. (Consider lidocaine, atropine, thiopental, pancuronium; avoid ketamine.) Continue paralysis and sedation.
   5) Emergent head CT. Shunt series if prior VP shunt (see p. 475).
   6) Treat hyperthermia.
   7) Avoid hypotension or hypovolemia.

B. COMA

1. Assessment

a. History: Trauma, ingestion, infection, fasting, drug use, diabetes, seizure or other neurologic disorder.

b. Examination: HR, BP, respiratory pattern, temperature, pupillary response, fundoscopy, rash, abnormal posturing, focal neurologic signs.

EMERGENCY MANAGEMENT

1

2. **Management: 'ABC DON'T'**
a. **A**irway (with C-spine immobilization), **B**reathing, **C**irculation, **D**extrostick, **O**xygen, **N**aloxone, **T**hiamine.
   1) Naloxone 0.1mg/kg IV/IM/SC/ETT (max. 2mg/dose). May repeat as necessary.
   2) Thiamine 50mg IV and 50mg IM (before starting glucose). Consider in adolescents for deficiencies secondary to alcoholism or eating disorders.
   3) $D_{25}W$ 2–4mL/kg IV bolus if hypoglycemia present.
b. Laboratory tests: CBC, electrolytes, liver function tests (LFTs), NH_3, lactate, toxicology screen (serum and urine), blood gas, blood culture. If infant or toddler, plasma amino acids and urine organic acids.
c. If meningitis or encephalitis is suspected, consider lumbar puncture and consider antibiotics/acylovir.
d. Emergent head CT, neurosurgical consultation, electroencephalogram (EEG).
e. If ingestion is suspected, airway must be protected before gastrointestinal (GI) decontamination (see p. 19).
f. Monitor Glasgow Coma Scale (Table 1.5).

TABLE 1.5

COMA SCALES

Glasgow Coma Scale		Modified coma scale for infants	
Activity	Best response	Activity	Best response
EYE OPENING			
Spontaneous	4	Spontaneous	4
To speech	3	To speech	3
To pain	2	To pain	2
None	1	None	1
VERBAL			
Oriented	5	Coos, babbles	5
Confused	4	Irritable	4
Inappropriate words	3	Cries to pain	3
Nonspecific sounds	2	Moans to pain	2
None	1	None	1
MOTOR			
Follows commands	6	Normal spontaneous movements	6
Localizes pain	5	Withdraws to touch	5
Withdraws to pain	4	Withdraws to pain	4
Abnormal flexion	3	Abnormal flexion	3
Abnormal extension	2	Abnormal extension	2
None	1	None	1

From Jennet[3] and James[4].

C. **STATUS EPILEPTICUS:** See also pp. 466–474 for nonacute evaluation and management of seizures.
1. **Assessment:** Common causes of childhood seizures include fever, subtherapeutic anticonvulsant levels, CNS infections, trauma, toxic ingestion, and metabolic abnormalities. Less common causes include vascular, neoplastic, and endocrinologic diseases.
2. **Acute management of seizures** (Table 1.6)

TABLE 1.6

ACUTE MANAGEMENT OF SEIZURES

Time (min)	Intervention
0–5	Stabilize the patient
	Assess airway, breathing, circulation, and vital signs
	Administer oxygen
	Obtain intravenous access or intraosseus access
	Correct hypoglycemia if present
	Obtain labs: **glucose,** electrolytes, calcium, magnesium, BUN, creatinine, LFTs, CBC, toxicology screen, anticonvulsant levels, blood culture (if infection is suspected)
	Initial screening history and physical examination
5–15	Begin pharmacotherapy
	Lorazepam (Ativan), 0.05–0.1mg/kg IV, up to 4–6mg
	OR
	Diazepam (Valium), 0.3mg/kg IV (0.5mg/kg rectally) up to 6–10mg
	May repeat lorazepam or diazepam 5–10min after initial dose
15–35	If seizure persists, load with:
	Phenytoin[a] load 15–20mg/kg IV at rate not to exceed 1mg/kg/min
	OR
	Fosphenytoin[b] load 15–20mg PE/kg IV/IM at 3mg PE/kg/min (max. 150mg PE/min). If given IM may require multiple dosing sites
	OR
	Phenobarbital load 15–20mg/kg IV at rate not to exceed 1mg/kg/min
45	If seizure persists:
	Load with phenobarbital if phenytoin was previously used
	Additional phenytoin or fosphenytoin 5mg/kg over 12hr for goal serum level of 20mg/L
	Additional phenobarbital 5mg/kg per dose Q15–30min (max. total dose at 30mg/kg; be prepared to support respirations)
60	If seizure persists[c], consider pentobarbital or general anesthesia in intensive care unit

Modified from Fischer[5].
BUN, blood urea nitrogen; CBC, complete blood count; CT, computed tomography; EEG, electroencephalogram.
[a]Phenytoin may be ineffective for seizures secondary to alcohol withdrawal or ingestion of theophylline or imipramine or carbamazepine.
[b]Fosphenytoin dosed as phenytoin equivalent (PE).
[c]Pyridoxine 100mg IV in infant with persistent initial seizure.

3. **Diagnostic workup:** When stable, may include CT, EEG, lumbar puncture.

VIII. REFERENCES

1. Nichols DG, Yaster M, Lappe DG, Haller JA Jr, eds. *Golden hour: the handbook of advanced pediatric life support*. St Louis: Mosby; 1996.
2. Dieckmann RA, Fiser DH, Selbst SM. *Illustrated textbook of pediatric emergency & critical care procedures*. St Louis: Mosby; 1997.
3. Jennet B, Teasdale G. Aspects of coma after severe head injury. *Lancet* 1977; 1:878.
4. James HE. Neurologic evaluation and support in the child with an acute brain insult. *Pediatr Ann* 1986; 15:16.
5. Fischer P. Seizure disorders. *Child Adol Psychiatr Clin North Am* 1995; 4:461.

POISONINGS

Sheila M. Hofert, MD

The importance of local poison control centers must be emphasized. Early consultation with these centers allows physicians access to resources not normally found in emergency departments, as well as guidance from expert personnel trained in the management of toxic exposure.

I. HISTORY[1]

1. **Corroboration:** Corroborate histories from different family members to help in confirming the type and dose of the exposure.
2. **High suspicion for toxic exposure**
   a. Abrupt onset of symptoms.
   b. Inconsistent history.
   c. Previous history of ingestion.
3. **Identification of toxin:** Obtain the bottle or container of the ingestant; access the police if necessary. Obtain all medicines from the household if there is any doubt as to which agent(s) have been ingested. Ask specifically about herbal or folk remedies, medications that the patient is on and that are present in the home, as well as over-the-counter (OTC) medications.
4. **Details of drug ingested or chemical exposure:** The following should be noted:
   a. Exact name of the drug or chemical exposure.
   b. Preparation and concentration of the drug or chemical.
   c. Probable dose (by history) of drug ingested in milligrams per kilogram, as well as the maximum possible dose.
   d. Time since ingestion/exposure.

II. SIGNS AND SYMPTOMS OF POISONING[1]

A. VITAL SIGNS

1. **Pulse**
   a. Bradycardia: β-blockers, calcium channel blockers (diltiazem, verapamil), carbamates, clonidine, digoxin, opiates, organophosphates, phenylpropanolamine, plants (lily of the valley, foxglove, oleander).
   b. Tachycardia: Sympathomimetics (amphetamine, cocaine, OTC cough and cold medications), phencyclidine, synthroid, theophylline, tricyclic antidepressants, anticholinergics, antihistamines, ethanol withdrawal.
2. **Respiration**
   a. Bradypnea: Alcohols and ethanol, barbiturates (late), clonidine, opiates, sedative/hypnotics.
   b. Tachypnea: Amphetamines, barbiturates (early), caffeine, cocaine, ethylene glycol, methanol, salicylates.

3. **Blood pressure**
a. Hypotension: Antihypertensives, barbiturates, β-blockers and calcium channel blockers, clonidine, cyanide, methemoglobinemia (nitrates, nitrites), opiates, phenothiazines, tricyclic antidepressants (late).
b. Hypertension: Amphetamines/sympathomimetics (especially pseudoephedrine, phenylpropanolamine in OTC cold remedies, diet pills), antihistamines, anticholinergics, clonidine (short-term effect at high doses), ethanol withdrawal, marijuana, phencyclidine.
4. **Temperature**
a. Hypothermia: Antidepressants, barbiturates, clonidine, ethanol, hypoglycemic agents, opiates, phenothiazines, sedative/hypnotics.
b. Hyperthermia: Amphetamines, anticholinergic agents, antipsychotic agents, cocaine, monoamine oxidase inhibitors, phenothiazines, salicylates, theophylline, tricyclic antidepressants.

B. **NEUROMUSCULAR**
1. **Ataxia:** Alcohol, barbiturates, phenytoin, sedatives/hypnotics (including benzodiazepines), carbon monoxide, heavy metals, organic solvents.
2. **Delirium/psychosis:** Antihistamines, drugs of abuse (phencyclidine, lysergic acid diethylamide [LSD], peyote, mescaline, marijuana, cocaine), ethanol, heavy metals (lead), phenothiazines, steroids, sympathomimetics and anticholinergics (including prescription and OTC cold remedies), theophylline.
3. **Convulsions:** Amphetamines, antihistamines, boric acid, caffeine, camphor, carbamazepine, cocaine, ethanol withdrawal, isoniazid, lead, lidocaine, lindane, nicotine, organophosphates, phenothiazines, phencyclidine, plants (water hemlock), salicylates, strychnine, theophylline, tricyclic antidepressants.
4. **Paralysis:** Botulinum toxin, heavy metals, organophosphates, plants (poison hemlock).
5. **Coma:** Alcohols, anticholinergics, anticonvulsants, antihistamines, barbiturates, carbon monoxide, clonidine, opiates, organophosphate insecticides, OTC sleep preparations, PCP, phenothiazines, salicylates, sedatives/hypnotics, sulfonylureas, tricyclic antidepressants, γ-hydroxybutyrate.

C. **OPHTHALMOLOGIC**
1. **Pupils**
a. Miosis (constricted pupils): barbiturates, clonidine, ethanol, mushrooms of the muscarinic type, nicotine, opiates, organophosphates, phencyclidine, phenothiazines.
b. Mydriasis (dilated pupils): Amphetamines, anticholinergics, carbamazepine, cocaine, diphenhydramine, LSD, marijuana.
2. **Nystagmus:** Barbiturates, carbamazepine, ethanol, glutethimide, phencyclidine (both vertical and horizontal), phenytoin, sedatives/hypnotics.

D. SKIN

1. **Jaundice:** Acetaminophen, carbon tetrachloride, cyclopeptide mushrooms, fava beans, heavy metals (phosphorus, arsenic), naphthalene.
2. **Cyanosis** (unresponsive to oxygen as a result of methemoglobinemia): Aniline dyes, benzocaine, dapsone, nitrates, nitrites, nitrobenzene, phenacetin, phenazopyridine, pyridium.
3. **Pink to red:** Alcohol, anticholinergics and antihistamines, boric acid, carbon monoxide, cyanide.
4. **Dry:** Anticholinergics, antihistamines.
5. **Needle tracks:** Substance abuse.
6. **Urticaria:** Reaction to any medication.

E. ODORS

1. **Acetone:** Acetone, isopropyl alcohol, salicylates.
2. **Alcohol:** Ethanol, isopropyl alcohol.
3. **Bitter almond:** Cyanide.
4. **Garlic:** Heavy metals (arsenic, phosphorus, and thallium), organophosphates.
5. **Oil of wintergreen:** Methyl salicylates.
6. **Pears:** Chloral hydrate.
7. **Carrots:** Water hemlock.

III. MANAGEMENT OF ACUTE POISONING

A. GASTROINTESTINAL DECONTAMINATION

Note: Airway protection is the major concern with gastrointestinal (GI) decontamination procedures because aspiration of charcoal may cause a severe and potentially fatal pneumonitis. Insertion of an endotracheal tube (ETT) is important in patients who have a depressed gag reflex or altered mental status, especially in those undergoing gastric lavage.

1. **Activated charcoal:** Activated charcoal is the treatment of choice for GI decontamination in the emergency department for substances that can adsorb onto charcoal. Numerous studies fail to show a clear benefit of treatment with ipecac or lavage plus activated charcoal over treatment with charcoal administered alone.
a. Mechanism of action: Effectively adsorbs toxins and prevents their systemic absorption.
b. Initial dose (if patient vomits dose within one hour, it should be repeated). (Premixed charcoal with sorbitol may be used for initial dose.)
   1) Children: 1g/kg body weight activated charcoal PO or NG, or more ideally 10g charcoal/g ingested drug.
   2) Adults: 50–60g PO or NG.

   c. Contraindications
     1) Increased risk of aspiration: Ileus, intestinal obstruction, hydrocarbons, absent gag reflex.
     2) Alcohols, iron, boric acid, caustics, lithium, electrolyte solutions.
   d. Multiple-dose activated charcoal
     1) Consider multiple-dose charcoal regimen (cathartic only in first dose) for severe intoxication with salicylates, theophylline, phenobarbital, digoxin, carbamazepine, sustained-release preparations.
     2) Give half the initial dose every 2–4 hours. End point is nontoxic blood levels or lack of signs or symptoms of clinical toxicity after 12–24 hours. Check for bowel sounds and abdominal distention.
     3) Tolerance can be improved using metoclopramide or ondansetron.

2. Cathartics
   a. Indications: May be used in conjunction with activated charcoal therapy (with the first dose only). Give sorbitol administered as a 70% solution with appropriate dose of charcoal (preferred) or magnesium citrate (4mL/kg [max. dose of 200mL in adults]).
   b. Dosage: The dose for sorbitol is 1–2mL/kg, and for magnesium citrate it is 4–6mL/kg (max. 200mL).
   c. Contraindications: Caustic ingestions, absent bowel sounds, recent bowel surgery. Avoid magnesium-containing cathartics in patients with compromised renal function.

3. Gastric lavage
   a. Indications: Orogastric lavage with a large-bore tube may still be useful in patients who arrive soon (within 1 hour) after a life-threatening ingestion and/or are obtunded. **The decision to lavage should be made in consultation with a toxicologist or poison control center.**
   b. Contraindications: Caustic or hydrocarbon ingestions, co-ingestion of sharp objects.
   c. Airway protection: In the patient with altered mental status or a depressed gag reflex, insertion and inflation of an ETT before gastric lavage may protect against aspiration of gastric contents.
   d. Method
     1) Position patient on left side, with the head slightly lower than the body. Insert large-bore orogastric tube (18–20 French in children, 36–40 French in adults).
     2) Lavage with normal saline (NS), 15mL/kg per cycle, to maximum of 200mL/cycle in adults, until gastric contents are clear. This may require several liters. Save initial return for toxicologic examination.

4. Ipecac
   a. Indications: Ipecac remains the drug of choice for home GI decontamination of selected ingestions within 30 minutes of onset (under the guidance of a health care provider or poison control center). It is rarely indicated for emergency department use.

b. Dosage:
  aged 6–12 months: 10mL with 15mL clear fluid/kg PO
  aged 1–5 years: 15mL with 120mL clear fluid
  >5 years old: 30mL with 240–480mL clear fluid.

Note: If no emesis occurs in 20 minutes, repeat dose with more fluids only once. Note also that ipecac can cause drowsiness and that children who have taken ipecac should be laid prone or on their side when falling asleep to avoid aspiration after emesis.

c. Contraindications: Ingestions with a potential for decreased or fluctuating level of consciousness (e.g., tricyclic antidepressant ingestions), caustic ingestions, hydrogen ingestion, hematemesis, prior vomiting, seizure, and age ≤6 months.

d. Relative contraindications: Severe cardiorespiratory disease, late-stage pregnancy, uncontrolled hypertension, and bleeding diathesis.

5. Whole bowel irrigation

a. Indications: Polyethylene glycol solution via continuous NG infusion has been shown to be useful in certain ingestions when charcoal is not effective. Examples include toxic iron or lithium ingestion, ingestion of vials or whole packets of illicit substances (cocaine and heroin), and ingestion of lead chips. May also be useful in delayed therapy of enteric-coated or sustained-release preparations such as salicylates, calcium channel blockers, and β-blockers.

b. Contraindications: GI hemorrhage or obstruction, ileus, obtunded or comatose patient who is not intubated.

c. Method
  1) Children: Use polyethylene glycol electrolyte lavage solution (GOLYTELY, Colyte) at a rate of 500mL/hr NG for 4–6hr or until rectal effluent is clear.
  2) Adults: Same solution at a rate of 1–2L/hr NG for 4–6hr or until rectal effluent is clear.

B. ENHANCED ELIMINATION[2,3]

1. pH alteration

a. Urinary alkalinization
  1) Indications: Elimination of weak acids such as salicylates, barbiturates, and methotrexate.
  2) Method: Intravenous bolus of $NaHCO_3$ 1–2mEq/kg is recommended, followed by continuous infusion of D_5W with $NaHCO_3$ 132mEq/L (3 ampoules of $NaHCO_3$ added to D_5W to make 1L, with each ampoule containing 44mEq $NaHCO_3$) at 1.5–2 times maintenance. Goal is urinary pH of 7–8.

2. Hemodialysis: Useful for low-molecular-weight substances that have a low volume of distribution and low binding to plasma proteins, such as aspirin, theophylline, lithium, phenobarbital, and alcohols.

IV. SPECIFIC POISONINGS

A. ACETAMINOPHEN POISONING[4-7]

1. **Signs and symptoms:** Nausea, vomiting, and malaise for 24 hours, improvement over the next 48 hours, followed by clinical or laboratory evidence of hepatic dysfunction. Aspartate transaminase (AST) is the earliest and most sensitive laboratory test of hepatotoxicity, usually being elevated by 24–36 hours. Death can occur from fulminant hepatic failure.

2. **Management:** A single dose of 150mg/kg in an otherwise healthy child requires intervention.

a. Ipecac: Doses of >150mg/kg, but <200mg/kg, may be managed with ipecac-induced emesis alone; consult your local poison control center for assistance.

b. Plasma level: Draw level at 4 hours after ingestion and plot on nomogram.

Note: For extended-release acetaminophen, obtain levels at 4 and 8 hours after ingestion. Initiate NAC if either level is above the lower line on the nomogram (Fig. 2.1).

c. Charcoal: Use as described on p. 19 if less than 4 hours from the time of ingestion.

d. *N*-Acetylcysteine (NAC): This is most effective if administered within 8 hours of ingestion. However, it should be administered within 24 hours and greater than 24 hours after ingestion if evidence of hepatotoxicity is present.

   1) Dosage

     a) Oral NAC regimen PO or NG (may be given as a slow bolus or continuous infusion): Give 20% NAC diluted 1:4 in a carbonated beverage as a loading dose of 140mg/kg, then 70mg/kg Q4hr for 17 doses. Metoclopramide droperidol or ondansetron can be used as an antiemetic.

Note: Although charcoal adsorbs oral NAC and ideally simultaneous administration should be avoided (an interval of 1 hour between doses is recommended), NAC and charcoal can be given together without any measurable difference in NAC's efficacy.

     b) Intravenous NAC regimen is indicated for the following: oral NAC not tolerated despite adequate antiemetic therapy, GI bleeding or obstruction, neonatal acetaminophen toxicity from maternal overdose. Protocol: Dilute 20% NAC solution to 3% solution with D_5W. Administer 140mg/kg loading dose over 1 hour using an in-line 0.2 micromillipore filter. Then administer maintenance dose of 70mg/kg per dose over 1 hour every 4 hours for 12 doses (Smilkstein[7]). Check plasma acetaminophen level at 24 hours. Small risk of anaphylaxis with IV NAC.

Note: Oral preparation of NAC is not pyrogen free and should be used only as an IV preparation under the guidance of the hospital pharmacy.

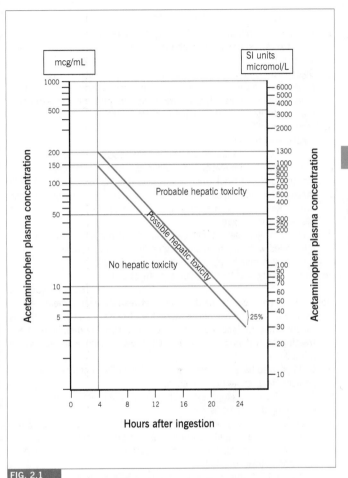

FIG. 2.1

Semilogarithmic plot of plasma acetaminophen levels vs time. (From Jones[4].)
Note: This nomogram is valid for use after acute single ingestions of
acetaminophen. The need for treatment cannot be extrapolated based on a level
before 4 hours. In chronic overdose, toxicity can be seen with much lower plasma
levels.

B. **ALCOHOLS**[8]
1. **Agents:** Ethanol (often >50% in mouthwashes, colognes, aftershaves), isopropanol, methanol (windshield wiper fluid), ethylene glycol (antifreeze).
2. **Signs and symptoms:** Blindness (methanol), inebriation, CNS depression, seizures, coma, hypoglycemia, metabolic acidosis, and renal failure (ethylene glycol). Toxic effects are primarily the result of the metabolites of methanol and ethylene glycol.
3. **Management**
a. Measure anion gap.

$$\text{Anion gap} = Na - (Cl + HCO_3)$$

b. A high anion gap metabolic acidosis is common in significant ingestions of methanol and ethylene glycol and is usually caused by its metabolites. Sometimes the acidosis is the result of accumulated lactic acid or ketones. A high anion gap is considered $\geq 14\text{mEq/L}$.
c. Measure osmolar gap.
d. An osmolar gap may be increased with the alcohols but must be interpreted with caution depending on time from ingestions. The osmolar gap may be normal late in course of toxicity.

$$\text{Serum osmolarity} = 2\,[Na^+] + [\text{Glucose (mg/dL)}/18] + [\text{BUN (mg/dL)}/2.8]$$

Note: The osmolar gap is the difference between the actual measured osmolality and the calculated value from the Na^+, glucose, and BUN. Be sure that the laboratory measures the osmolality directly by the freezing point depression method. Otherwise, a significant gap will be missed.

c. Children who have ingested a significant quantity of ethanol are particularly prone to hypoglycemia.
d. Blood volatile toxicology testing and specific levels are useful in confirming the diagnosis.
e. Charcoal is generally not useful because it adsorbs alcohols poorly, and most alcohols are rapidly absorbed through the GI tract.
f. Ethanol: Support blood glucose as necessary with IV dextrose.
g. Methanol, ethylene glycol:
   1) Give 5–10% ethanol at 800mg/kg IV or 50% ethanol at 800mg/kg PO for a loading dose, then give 130mg/kg per hr. The goal is to attain a blood alcohol level of 100–150mg/dL. Maintain adequate urine output. Commercially available ethanol can be used, but always consider the absolute ethanol content of each product (i.e., 80 proof = 40% ethanol). Monitor blood alcohol and blood glucose level.
   2) Fomepizole is an antidote for methanol and ethylene glycol poisoning. Indications for use are for levels $\geq 20\text{mg/dL}$ or high anion gap metabolic acidosis. Loading dose of 15mg/kg followed by doses of 10mg/kg every 12 hours for 4 doses, then 15mg/kg every 12

hours until levels are below 20mg/dL. A separate dosing schedule is recommended for patients requiring hemodialysis.

3) Consider hemodialysis in severe cases, i.e., level >50mg/dL, renal failure, blindness, and severe metabolic acidosis refractory to bicarbonate therapy.

C. ANTICHOLINERGIC TOXICITY[8]

1. **Agents:** Antihistamines, antiparkinsonian agents, scopolamine, belladonna alkaloids, plants (Jimson weed, deadly nightshade, selected mushrooms), ophthalmic mydriatics, diphenoxylate/atropine (e.g., Lomotil), phenothiazines, glycopyrrolate, antispasmodics, muscle relaxants, tricyclic antidepressants, and carbamazepine.

2. **Signs and symptoms:** 'Mad as a hatter, red as a beet, blind as a bat, hot as a hare, dry as a bone:' Oral dryness and burning, speech and swallowing difficulties, decreased GI motility, thirst, blurred vision, photophobia, mydriasis, skin flushing, tachycardia, fever, urinary retention, delirium, hallucinations, cardiovascular collapse.

3. **Management**

a. Activated charcoal and cathartic: see pp. 19 and 20.

b. Supportive care is all that is necessary in mild cases.

c. Benzodiazepines should be used to control agitation.

d. In life-threatening emergencies secondary to pure anticholinergic poisoning unresponsive to standard therapy (dysrhythmias, hypertension, seizures, severe hallucinations), physostigmine may reverse symptoms.

Note: Do not use physostigmine simply to maintain an alert state in an otherwise stable comatose patient. Do not use physostigmine for tricyclic-related anticholinergic toxicity (see p. 40). Do not use phenytoin for seizures.

1) Dose: Physostigmine 0.02mg/kg per dose (up to 0.5mg) IV every 5 min until a therapeutic effect is seen (max. total dose 2mg).

Note: Each dose should be given over 5 minutes.

2) Atropine should be available to reverse excess cholinergic side effects. Give 0.5mg for every milligram of physostigmine just given.

D. BARBITURATES[1]

1. **Agents:** Pentobarbital, phenobarbital, secobarbital, amobarbital.

2. **Signs and symptoms**

a. CNS: Ataxia, lethargy, headache, vertigo, coma, hypothermia.

b. Respiratory: Pulmonary edema, respiratory depression.

c. Cardiovascular: Hypotension.

d. Skin: Bullae.

e. Electroencephalogram (EEG) may correlate with progression of coma.

3. **Management**

a. Ensure ventilation and oxygenation.

b. Give 10 times ingested dose or 1g/kg body weight of charcoal followed by a cathartic. May use multiple doses of activated charcoal for phenobarbital (see p. 20).

c. Urinary alkalinization can increase phenobarbital excretion; consider hemodialysis or hemoperfusion in severe phenobarbital toxicity (e.g., level >100mg/L).

E. BENZODIAZEPINES[8]

1. **Agents:** Alprazolam, chlorazepate, chlordiazepoxide, clonazepam, diazepam, flurazepam, lorazepam, midazolam, oxazepam, temazepam, triazolam.

2. **Signs and symptoms:** Dizziness, ataxia, slurred speech, respiratory depression, coma, hypotension.

3. **Management**

a. Ensure ventilation oxygenation, and circulation if airway and breathing are secured, there is rarely any need for other interventions.

b. Activated charcoal as on p. 19.

c. Flumazenil may be used as a diagnostic tool in pure benzodiazepine toxicity, in 0.1–0.2mg increments up to 1mg. Resedation occurs within 20–120 minutes.

Note: Flumazenil may precipitate seizures that are difficult to control; it is therefore contraindicated in patients who have a seizure disorder, in those who have chronically been taking benzodiazepines, or in those who may have co-ingested any substances that can cause seizures (including tricyclic antidepressants, theophylline, chloral hydrate, isoniazid, and carbamazepine).

F. β-BLOCKERS[9]

1. **Agents:** Atenolol, esmolol, labetalol, metoprolol, nadolol, propranolol, timolol.

2. **Signs and symptoms:** Bronchospasm (in those with preexisting bronchospastic disease), respiratory depression, bradydysrhythmias (such as atrioventricular [AV] block), hypotension, hypoglycemia, altered mental status, hallucinations, seizures, and coma.

3. **Management**

a. Establish airway, ensure ventilation, and support circulation with isotonic fluids.

b. Give activated charcoal; consider whole bowel irrigation for sustained-release preparations (see p. 21). Consider lavage in very serious intoxication.

c. Glucagon: Pediatric dose—0.05–0.1mg/kg per bolus, followed by 0.1 mg/kg per hr infusion. Adult dose—3–5mg bolus, followed by 1–5mg/hr infusion. Is useful in reversing bradycardia and hypotension in β-blocker overdoses.

Note: Atropine, isoproterenol, and amrinone can be used if bradycardia or hypotension persists after using glucagon. May consider pacing for severe bradycardia.

d. In cases of cardiac arrest, may need to give massive doses of epinephrine, titrating to clinical effect (sometimes 10–20 times the standard dose).

G. CALCIUM CHANNEL BLOCKERS[8]

1. **Agents:** Amlodipine, bepridil, diltiazem, felodipine, isradipine, nicardipine, nifedipine, nimodipine, verapamil.

2. Signs and symptoms
a. Hypotension, bradycardia, altered mental status, seizures, hyperglycemia.
b. ECG can show atrioventricular conduction abnormalities such as AV block, as well as sinoatrial node abnormalities, idioventricular rhythms, or asystole.

3. Management
a. Establish airway, assure ventilation, and support circulation with isotonic fluids.
b. Give activated charcoal. Consider whole bowel irrigation for sustained-release preparations (see p. 21).
c. Use calcium chloride (20mg/kg of 10% CaCl) or calcium gluconate (100mg/kg of 10% calcium gluconate) for hypotension and bradydysrhythmias. Give glucagon (see p. 26), amrinone, isoproterenol, atropine, and dopamine for hypotension unresponsive to fluids and calcium. Consider pacing for dysrhythmias.

H. CARBAMAZEPINE[8–10]

1. **Signs and symptoms:** Ataxia, mydriasis, nystagmus, tachycardia, altered mental status, coma, seizures, nausea, vomiting, respiratory depression, hypotension or hypertension, dystonic posturing, and abnormal DTRs. Chronic toxicity may lead to AV block and SIADH.

2. Management
a. Serum levels poorly correlate with toxicity; treatment should proceed based on clinical status with respiratory depression, coma, and seizures being the most problematic.
b. ECG may show prolonged PR, QRS, or QT intervals, but malignant dysrhythmias are rare.
c. Maintain airway and cardiovascular status.
d. Activated charcoal and cathartics for significant ingestions; multiple doses of charcoal can be used for serious intoxications (see pp. 19–20).
e. Seizures should be treated with benzodiazepines and phenobarbital. Phenytoin should not be used.

I. CARBON MONOXIDE POISONING[8,10,11]

1. **Sources:** Fire, automobile exhaust, gasoline or propane engines operating in enclosed spaces, faulty furnaces or gas stoves, charcoal burners, paint remover with methylene chloride.

2. **Signs and symptoms:** Mild-to-moderate exposures can cause headache, dizziness, nausea, confusion, chest pain, dyspnea, gastroenteritis, and weakness. Severe exposures can cause syncope, seizures, coma, myocardial ischemia, dysrhythmias, pulmonary edema, skin bullae, and myoglobinuria.

Note: Pulse oximetry may be misleadingly normal.

3. **Management**

a. Obtain COHgb level; however, toxicity does not necessarily correlate with levels.

b. In fires, consider the possibility of concomitant cyanide poisoning.

c. Chest radiographs should be obtained to rule out pneumonitis, atelectasis, and pulmonary edema.

d. An ECG should be obtained to rule out cardiac dysrhythmias and myocardial ischemia.

e. Administer 100% O_2.

f. Ensure adequate airway; prevent hypercapnia.

g. Consider hyperbaric O_2 therapy if the COHgb level is >25%, there is evidence of myocardial ischemia or dysrhythmias, the patient has any serious neurologic or neuropsychiatric impairment, the patient is pregnant with a COHgb >15% or shows evidence of fetal distress, or the patient has persistent symptoms after 4 hours of 100% O_2.

h. If hyperbaric O_2 is unavailable, administer 100% O_2 until COHgb level decreases <10%.

J. CAUSTIC INGESTIONS[8,12–14]

1. **Strong acids and alkalis:** Hair relaxers, drain and oven cleaners, dishwater detergent crystals. Have the potential for airway swelling or esophageal perforation, even if there are no symptoms initially or no oropharyngeal burns.

2. **Signs and symptoms:** Stridor, hoarseness, dyspnea, aphonia, chest pain, abdominal pain, vomiting (often with blood or tissue), drooling, persistent salivation.

3. **Management**

a. Asymptomatic patients who have ingested substances that are GI irritants but not caustic (e.g., household bleaches) and who can demonstrate good oral intake should be given PO fluids as a diluent (10–15mL/kg of water, milk, etc.). These patients may be followed as outpatients.

b. Symptomatic patients

1) Stabilize airway: Flexible fiberoptic intubation over an endoscope is preferable to a standard orotracheal intubation. Intubation may further traumatize damaged areas or perforate the pharynx; therefore blind nasotracheal intubation is contraindicated. Emergent cricothyrotomy may be necessary.

2) Obtain IV access and start isotonic fluids. Obtain blood count, chest radiographic examination, blood type, and crossmatch. Chest radiographic examination may demonstrate esophageal perforation or free intraperitoneal air.

3) Provide tetanus as needed.

4) Maintain NPO status. Attempts to neutralize the caustic are ineffective and obscure and delay endoscopy. Ipecac or lavage is contraindicated.

5) Obtain surgical consultation; proceed to endoscopy. Do **not** pass nasogastric tube. Discontinue endoscopy immediately if esophageal burn identified.

6) Consider IV steroid therapy (methylprednisolone at 2mg/kg per 24hr divided Q6hr or Q8hr); may be beneficial for some patients, although this is controversial.

Note: Ingestion of alkaline button batteries can lead to esophageal and gastric burns. If initial radiographic examination shows battery to be lodged in esophagus, immediate endoscopic retrieval is indicated. If the battery is beyond the esophagus, the patient can be discharged and follow-up radiographic examinations performed only if battery has not passed in 4–7 days. For batteries >23mm diameter a 48-hour radiographic examination should be performed to exclude persistent gastric position, hence need for endoscopic retrieval.

K. DIGOXIN[8]

1. **Signs and symptoms:** Major manifestations include the following:
a. Cardiac: Any new rhythm, especially those exhibiting induction of ectopic pacemakers and impaired conduction, atrial tachycardias with 2:1 block, PVCs, and junctional tachycardia.
b. GI: Anorexia, nausea, and vomiting.
c. CNS: Headache, disorientation, somnolence, seizures.
d. Other: Fatigue, weakness, blurry vision, and aberrations of color vision such as yellow halos around light.

2. **Management**
a. Determine serum digoxin level. Therapeutic level is between 0.5 and 2ng/mL. Toxic symptoms predict a serum level >2ng/mL, but toxicity can develop in initially asymptomatic patients and can occur at therapeutic levels, especially in chronic users. Quinidine, amiodarone, or poor renal function increases the digoxin level.
b. Determine electrolytes: Low potassium (K^+), magnesium (Mg^{2+}), or thyroxine (T_4) will increase digoxin toxicity at a given level, as will high calcium (Ca^{2+}). Initial hyperkalemia results from release of intracellular K^+ and indicates serious acute toxicity.
c. Continuous ECG monitoring.
d. Give charcoal (even several hours after ingestion) and cathartic.
e. Correct electrolyte abnormalities:
1) Hypokalemia: If any dysrhythmias are present, then give potassium IV at 0.5–1mEq/min.
2) Hyperkalemia: If $[K^+]$ >5mEq/L, then give insulin and dextrose, sodium bicarbonate, and Kayexalate. **Do not give calcium chloride or calcium gluconate because these can potentiate ventricular dysrhythmias.**
3) Hypomagnesemia: May result in refractory hypokalemia if not treated. Give Mg^{2+} cautiously because high levels can cause AV block.

f. Digoxin-specific Fab: Indicated for ventricular dysrhythmias, supraventricular bradydysrhythmias unresponsive to atropine, hyperkalemia (K^+ >5mEq/L), hypotension, second- and third-degree heart block, and ingestion of ≥10mg of digoxin by adults or more than 4mg of digoxin by children. Dose (based on total body load of digoxin): Digoxin-immune Fab (Digibind) is available in 40mg vial. Each vial will bind approximately 0.6mg digoxin. Estimate total body load in milligrams using either of the following methods:

1) Use the known acutely given dose in milligrams for IV doses, as well as liquid filled capsules. For PO tablets or elixir, multiply dose by 0.8 to correct for incomplete absorption.

2) Calculate total body load based on the following formula: Total body load (TBL) = serum digoxin concentration (ng/mL) × volume of distribution × weight of patient in kg ÷ 1000 (volume of distribution in this case is 5.6). Then, number of vials to be given equals the total body load (mg)/0.6mg of digoxin neutralized per vial. Administer IV over 30 minutes. If cardiac arrest is imminent, give as bolus injection.

Note: If ingested dose is unknown, and level is not available, and patient is symptomatic, then give 10 vials of Fab (i.e., 400mg).

g. Cardiac rhythm disturbances:

1) Bradydysrhythmias: Atropine alone 0.01–0.02mg/kg IV may reverse sinus bradycardia or AV block and may be used before digoxin Fab. Phenytoin improves AV conduction. If atropine, digoxin Fab, and phenytoin fail, may use external pacing first, followed by transvenous ventricular pacing if external pacing fails. Avoid propranolol, quinidine, procainamide, isoproterenol, or disopyramide if AV block is present.

2) Tachydysrhythmias: Phenytoin and lidocaine are effective for ventricular dysrhythmias; propranolol is useful for both ventricular and supraventricular tachydysrhythmias. Cardioversion is indicated when pharmacotherapy fails in the hemodynamically unstable patient.

L. HYDROCARBON INGESTIONS[15,16,]

1. Agents

a. Aliphatic: Gasoline, kerosene, mineral seal oil, lighter fluid, tar mineral oil, lubricating oils.

b. Aromatic: Benzene, toluene, camphor, turpentine.

c. Halogenated: Carbon tetrachloride, methylene chloride, trichloroethane, perchloroethylene.

2. Signs and symptoms

a. Pulmonary: Tachypnea, dyspnea, tachycardia, cyanosis, grunting, cough.

b. CNS: Lethargy, seizures, coma.

c. Hepatic toxicity: Acute liver failure.
d. Cardiac toxicity: Dysrhythmias.

Note: Aliphatic hydrocarbons have the greatest risk for aspiration and pulmonary toxicity. Aromatic hydrocarbons have systemic toxicity.

3. **Management**
a. Decontamination
    1) Avoid emesis or lavage because of the risk of aspiration.
    2) If the hydrocarbon contains a potentially toxic substance (e.g., insecticide, heavy metal, camphor) and a toxic amount has been ingested, consider intubation with a cuffed ETT followed by lavage.
    3) Avoid charcoal unless there is co-ingestion. It does not bind aliphatics and will increase the risk of aspiration.
b. Obtain chest radiograph and arterial blood gases on patients with pulmonary symptoms.
c. Observe patient for 6 hours.
    1) If child is asymptomatic for 6 hours and chest radiograph is normal, discharge home.
    2) If child becomes symptomatic in 6-hour period, admit.
    3) If asymptomatic but chest radiograph abnormal, consider admission for further observation. Discharge only if close follow-up can be ensured.
d. Treat pneumonitis with oxygen and positive end-expiratory pressure (PEEP). Routine administration of antibiotics and steroids are not warranted.

M. IRON POISONING[17–19]

1. **Signs and symptoms**
a. First stage: GI toxicity (30 minutes to 6 hours after ingestion). Nausea, vomiting, diarrhea, abdominal pain, hematemesis, and melena. Rarely, this phase may progress to shock, seizures, and coma.
b. Second stage: Latent period (6–24 hours after ingestion). Improvement and sometimes resolution of clinical symptoms.
c. Third stage: Systemic toxicity (6–48 hours after ingestion). Hepatic injury or failure, hypoglycemia, metabolic acidosis, bleeding, shock, coma, convulsions, and death.
d. Fourth stage: Late complications (4–8 weeks after ingestion). Pyloric or antral stenosis.

2. **Management**
a. Determine serum iron concentration 2–6 hours after ingestion (time of peak concentration varies with iron product ingested). A level >350mcg/dL is frequently associated with systemic toxicity.
b. Abdominal radiograph is helpful in decision about whether or not to lavage because most iron tablets are radio-opaque (except chewable vitamins and children's liquid).

Note: Iron is rapidly cleared from plasma and distributed; thus serum iron levels obtained after the peak do not accurately reflect the severity of intoxication. Treatment should be determined by clinical symptoms.

c. If dose of elemental iron <20mg/kg, no treatment is needed.

d. For all ingestions of unknown amount or those between 20–60mg/kg, consider gastric emptying. If the patient does not develop symptoms in the first 6 hours, then no further treatment is needed.

e. Consider gastric lavage if dose ingested ≥60 mg/kg and/or presence of large amount of pills on radiograph. If iron tablets are present in the stomach despite lavage, begin whole bowel irrigation (see p. 21), especially if abdominal radiograph reveals iron tablets distal to the pylorus.

f. Give deferoxamine IV at 15mg/kg per hr via continuous infusion in all cases of serious poisoning (e.g., presence of significant clinical symptoms, positive abdominal radiograph with significant number of pills, or serum iron level >500mcg/dL). Give continuous infusion until all symptoms and signs of toxicity have resolved and 24 hours after vinrose urine color disappears.

g. Supportive care is the most important therapy. Large IV fluid volumes may be needed in the first 24 hours to avoid hypovolemic shock and acidemia. Urine output should be maintained at >2mL/kg per hr. Additionally, metabolic acidosis should be corrected with sodium bicarbonate.

N. LEAD POISONING[20–24]

1. Signs and symptoms

Note: Most children with lead poisoning are asymptomatic. A blood test is the only way to determine the lead level.

a. Gastrointestinal: Anorexia, constipation, abdominal pain, colic, vomiting, failure to thrive, and diarrhea. Abdominal radiograph may show opacities in the GI tract.

b. Neurologic: Irritability, overactivity, lethargy, decreased play, increased sleep, ataxia, incoordination, headache, decreased nerve conduction velocity, encephalopathy, cranial nerve paralysis, papilledema, seizures, coma, death.

c. Hematologic: Microcytic anemia, basophilic stippling, increased free erythrocyte protoporphyrin (FEP).

d. Skeletal: Lead lines may be seen in the metaphyseal regions of long bones of leg and arm.

2. Environmental exposures

a. Residence (primary, secondary, daycare, etc.) built before 1960, with lead-based paint.

b. Recent or ongoing renovation.

c. Nearby industry, such as battery plants, smelters.

d. Old furniture, vinyl mini-blinds, ceramics, leaded crystal, imported food cans, leaded toys, art supplies, cosmetics.

e. Presence of lead in water pipes, lead solder in connecting pipes, and brass or bronze plumbing fittings.

f. Use of lead-based insecticides and folk remedies such as azarcon, greta, surma.

3. **Screening:** All children below the age of 6 years should be screened at least once. Start screening at age 9–12 months. However, children with high-risk factors, such as the previous environmental exposures, should be screened at age 6 months. Subsequent screens are determined by the blood lead level (Table 2.1).

4. **Prevention**

a. Nutrition: Balanced diet, more frequent meals high in iron, vitamin C, and calcium and low in added fat.

b. Hygiene: Wash hands regularly, avoid hand-to-mouth behavior.

c. House cleaning: Damp-cleaning methods; use high-phosphate detergent such as powdered dishwasher detergent; special vacuum cleaner called HEPA-VAC is capable of picking up microscopic lead particles.

d. Abatement: It must be performed by trained workers.

TABLE 2.1
INTERVENTIONS IN LEAD POISONING

Class	Blood lead level (mcg/dL)	Intervention
I	≤9	Rescreen annually, unless high risk.
IIA	10–14	If large number of children in community in this range, community-wide prevention should be started. Individual children in this range should be tested every 3–4mo, until two consecutive measurements are <10; then retest in 1yr.
IIB	15–19	Education on environment, cleaning, and nutrition should be started; Health Department should be notified. Patient should be tested for iron deficiency. Rescreen Q3–4mo until two consecutive levels are <10. Consider abatement.
III	20–44	Conduct a complete medical evaluation. Identify and eliminate environmental sources of lead. These children require close follow-up. Chelation may be considered in selected children.
IV	45–69	Begin both medical and environmental intervention. Chelation treatment (either oral or IV/IM) should begin within 48hr with close follow-up.
V	≥70	This is a medical emergency requiring immediate intervention, which includes hospitalization. In addition, environmental remediation should be started.

2

POISONINGS

5. Management (Table 2.1)

a. Patient with venous lead levels ≥15mcg/dL

   1) Obtain comprehensive environmental history.

   2) Remove child from the lead source.

   3) Alert local health department.

   4) Refer to lead poisoning specialist.

   5) If iron deficient, may begin iron (unless British Anti-Lewisite [BAL] is to be used).

b. Chelation: Patient with venous lead levels ≥45mcg/dL.

Note: Chelation is a process to bind lead chemically in a form that is easily excreted. Most agents bind lead so it is soluble in water and excreted through the kidneys. Examples of agents are: BAL, $CaNa_2EDTA$, succimer (DMSA), D-penicillamine. Before starting chelation administer two pediatric Fleet enemas to clear the GI tract. Obtain baseline laboratory results: Venous lead level, CBC with differential, FEP, chemistry panel (including electrolytes, BUN and creatinine, hepatic function test), reticulocyte count, urinalysis.

   1) Oral chelation: This is used for children with blood lead levels between 45 and 69mcg/dL. Chelation must occur in an environment free of lead, which may be the hospital.

   a) Succimer (dimercaptosuccinic acid [DMSA])

   - First 5 days $1050mg/m^2$ per day or 30 mg/kg per day divided every 8 hours.
   - Next 14 days $700mg/m^2$ per day or 20mg/kg per day divided every 12 hours.
   - Mix capsule contents in warm ginger ale and administer within 5 minutes. Give on empty stomach to improve GI absorption.
   - Weekly CBC with differential, chemistry panel, and lead level to ensure response to treatment and monitor for possible drug side effects (decreased absolute neutrophil count and elevated liver function tests).

   b) D-Penicillamine

   - Currently it is not labeled for use in lead toxicity. However, it has been used successfully in selected cases of low-level lead poisoning.

   2) Parenteral chelation (blood lead levels >45 mcg/dL)

   a) $CaNa_2EDTA$

   - First begin multivitamin to replenish copper and zinc.
   - Start $1000mg/m^2$ per day IM Q12hr for 5 days.
   - 12 hours after the 10th injection, obtain CBC with differential, chemistry panel, venous lead level, FEP; if this lead level is still >45mcg/dL, start the second 5-day therapy with $CaNa_2EDTA$ after a 3-day break from chelation therapy.
   - For pain control use EMLA (eutectic mixture of local anesthetics) cream and mix $CaNa_2EDTA$ with 0.5% procaine.

Note: It is important to use CaNa$_2$EDTA, not Na$_2$EDTA because the latter may cause tetany and life-threatening hypocalcemia.

b) BAL: This agent is recommended only for levels ≥70mcg/dL.

- Initial dose of 75mg/m^2 is given as deep IM injection.
- Establish adequate urine output.
- 4 hours later start CaNa$_2$EDTA 1500mg/m^2 per day via continuous IV infusion for 48 hours. If there is risk of cerebral edema, dose may be given IM every 4 hours to decrease IV fluids.
- BAL is then continued simultaneously at 75mg/m^2 per dose IM every 4 hours for 48 hours.
- Use of EMLA cream and 0.5% procaine is recommended for the IM doses.
- After 48 hours obtain serum lead level to determine whether to continue chelation.

Note: Side effects of BAL include fever, tachycardia, hypertension, salivation, tingling around the mouth, anaphylaxis (BAL is suspended in peanut oil, which may cause severe allergic reaction), hemolysis (in patients with G6PD deficiency), and toxicity if given with iron.

6. Follow-up
a. Repeat venous lead level, CBC, and FEP 2 weeks after completion of chelation therapy. Venous lead level may rebound to 50–75% of pretreatment value.
b. Repeat chelation with DMSA for levels >45mcg/dL may be indicated.
c. Neuropsychologic evaluation, speech evaluation, and monitoring of school progress.

O. OPIATES[25–27]

1. **Agents:** Codeine, fentanyl, heroin, hydromorphone, meperidine, methadone, morphine, oxycodone, proproxyphene.

2. **Signs and symptoms:** Depressed mental status; pinpoint pupils, respiratory depression, and hypotension.

3. **Management**
a. Administer naloxone 2mg IV (regardless of weight or age) if there is respiratory or CNS depression. Repeat every 2 minutes as needed to improve respiratory and mental status. Dose = 0.1mg/kg.
b. Careful inpatient monitoring is required because of the short half-life of naloxone compared with most opiates. Indications for continuous naloxone infusion include the following:
   1) Repetitive bolus doses.
   2) Ingestion of large amount of opiate or long-acting opiate, e.g., methadone, or poorly antagonized opiates, e.g., proproxyphene.
c. Suggested regimen is as follows:
   1) Repeat the previously successful bolus as a loading dose.

2) Administer two thirds of the above loading dose as an hourly infusion dose.

3) Wean naloxone drip in 50% decrements as tolerated over 6–12 hours depending on the half-life of the opiate ingested. For methadone, may require infusion for up to 48 hours.

Note: Naloxone can potentiate acute withdrawal in patients with opiate addiction. Monitor for nausea, vomiting, hyperactive bowel sounds, yawning, piloerection, and pupillary dilatation.

P. PHENOTHIAZINE AND BUTYROPHENONE INTOXICATION[3,8]

1. **Agents:** Chlorpromazine, fluphenazine, haloperidol, perphenazine, prochlorperazine, promethazine, thioridazine, trifluoperazine.

2. **Signs and symptoms**

a. Symptoms (may be delayed 6–24 hours after ingestion): Depressed neurologic status, lethargy, coma, miosis, hypotension, dysrhythmias (including prolonged QT_C intervals and occasional QRS interval), extrapyramidal signs (oculogyric crisis, dysphagia, tremor, rigidity, torticollis, opisthotonus, trismus), neuroleptic malignant syndrome (fever, diaphoresis, rigidity, tachycardia, coma), anticholinergic symptoms.

3. **Management**

a. Activated charcoal.

b. Support and monitoring of respiratory and cardiovascular status.

c. Obtain ECG.

d. Extrapyramidal signs

1) Intravenous diphenhydramine: 1mg/kg for children (up to 50mg) slowly over 2–5 minutes; 25–50mg for adults; give every 6 hours for 48 hours.

2) Intravenous benztropine: for children >3 years 0.02–0.05mg/kg per dose (1–2 doses per day), for children <3 years should not be used except in severe life-threatening situations. For adults the dose is 1–2mg IM or IV.

e. Dysrhythmias

1) Ventricular: Lidocaine (1mg/kg IV push); sodium bicarbonate (1mEq/kg per bolus) for QRS widening. Procainamide and disopyramide are contraindicated. Cardioversion is indicated if hemodynamically unstable.

2) Supraventricular: If hemodynamically stable and tachycardic, use adenosine; however, if hemodynamically unstable, proceed to cardioversion.

f. Neuroleptic malignant syndrome: Hyperthermia, muscle rigidity, autonomic disturbances of heart rate and blood pressure, and altered consciousness.

1) Reduce hyperthermia with cooling blankets, external sponging, fanning, and gastric/colonic lavage. Antipyretics are not helpful.

2) Support respiratory and cardiovascular status; monitor neurologic and fluid status.

    3) Neuromuscular paralysis for severe hyperthermia and rigidity.
    4) Benzodiazepines may be adjunct in reducing muscle rigidity.
    5) Dantrolene and bromocriptine should be used in selected cases of severe toxicity.

Q. PHENYTOIN[28]

1. **Signs and symptoms:** Ataxia, dysarthria, drowsiness, tremor, nystagmus, seizures, and hyperglycemic nonketotic coma. Intravenous preparations may cause bradycardia, dysrythmia, and hypotension. (Above symptoms seen with serum levels >20mg/L.)

2. **Management**

a. Supportive care: If seizures, discontinue phenytoin and use benzodiazepines and/or phenobarbital. Use insulin for hyperglycemic nonketotic coma. Give fluids and monitor glucose.

b. Activated charcoal: Consider multiple dose activated charcoal (see p. 20) for selected cases to enhance elimination.

R. SALICYLATE[10,29]

1. **Preparations** (milligrams of aspirin or aspirin equivalent).

a. Children's aspirin: 80mg tablets (36 tablets per bottle).

b. Adult aspirin: 325mg tablets.

c. Methyl salicylate, e.g., oil of wintergreen (98%).

d. Pepto Bismol: 236mg of nonaspirin salicylate/15mL.

2. **Signs and symptoms**

a. Acute: Vomiting, hyperpnea, tinnitus, lethargy, hyperthermia, seizures, coma.

b. Chronic: Confusion, dehydration, metabolic acidosis, cerebral edema, pulmonary edema.

3. **Management**

a. Establish severity of ingestion: Acute toxicity can occur at doses of 150mg/kg, whereas chronic overdose can produce toxicity at much lower doses.

b. Serum salicylate level

    1) Toxicity of salicylates correlates poorly with serum levels, and levels are less useful in chronic toxicity. Serial salicylate levels (every 2–4 hours) are mandatory after ingestion to monitor for peak levels. In seriously ill patients, frequent determination of salicylate concentration is necessary to monitor efficacy of treatment and possible need for hemodialysis. Signs and symptoms of acute toxicity can occur at levels >30mg/dL.

Note: 6-hour serum salicylate level of ≥100mg/dL is considered potentially lethal and is an indication for hemodialysis. Be cautious of different laboratories using different units (10mg/L = 1.0mg/dL).

c. Consider multiple doses of activated charcoal if serum salicylate levels continue to increase after 6 hours (see p. 20). Consider whole bowel irrigation in ingestions of enteric-coated preparations (see p. 21).

2

POISONINGS

   d. Monitor serum electrolytes, calcium, arterial blood gases, glucose, urine pH and specific gravity, and coagulation studies as needed.

   e. Treat fluid and solute deficits; alkalinization is important in increasing the excretion of salicylate, as well as decreasing the entry of salicylate into the CNS.

     1) Replenish intravascular volume with D_5 lactated Ringer's (LR) at 20mL/kg per hr for 1–2 hours until adequate urine output is established.

     2) Begin alkalinization by initial bolus of $NaHCO_3$ (1–2mEq/kg). Then begin infusing D_5W with 132mEq $NaHCO_3$/L (3 ampules of 44mEq $NaHCO_3$ each) and 20–40mEq K^+/L at rates of 2–3L/m^2 per 24hr (i.e., 1.5–2 times maintenance fluids). Aim for a urine output of 2mL/kg per hr. Adjust concentrations of the electrolytes as needed to correct serum electrolyte abnormalities (especially hypokalemia, which inhibits salicylate excretion), and to maintain a urinary pH >7.5.

     3) Note that CNS glucose levels can be low despite normal serum glucose levels; thus increasing glucose delivery is indicated in the presence of hypoglycemic symptoms.

   f. Administer parenteral vitamin K as indicated by abnormalities in coagulation studies (especially in chronic intoxications).

   g. Continue fluid therapy until the patient is asymptomatic for several hours, regardless of the serum salicylate level.

   h. Proceed to hemodialysis in the presence of metabolic acidosis or electrolyte abnormality unresponsive to appropriate therapy, renal or hepatic failure, persistent CNS impairment, pulmonary edema, progressive clinical deterioration despite adequate therapy, or salicylate level >100mg/dL at 6 hours after ingestion.

S. THEOPHYLLINE[8]

1. Signs and symptoms of acute toxicity

   a. GI: Vomiting, hematemesis, abdominal pain, bloody diarrhea.

   b. Cardiovascular: Tachycardia, dysrhythmias, hypotension, cardiac arrest.

   c. CNS: Seizures, agitation, coma, hallucinations.

   d. Metabolic: acidosis, hyopkalemia, hyperglycemia, leukocytosis.

2. Management

   a. Obtain a theophylline level immediately and again in 1–4 hours to determine the pattern of absorption. Peak absorption has been reported to be delayed as long as 13–17 hours after ingestion. Serial theophylline levels should be obtained to assess for persistent increase, monitor efficacy of treatment and determine need for hemodialysis.

     1) Levels >20mcg/mL are associated with clinical symptoms of toxicity.

     2) Levels >40mcg/mL or patients with neurotoxicity require admission and careful monitoring.

   b. Obtain serum electrolytes, glucose, and blood gas.

c. Charcoal followed by a cathartic, regardless of the length of time after ingestion. For severe intoxication consider multiple-dose charcoal. If there is persistent vomiting, give metoclopramide or ondansetron, and instill charcoal by nasogastric tube (see p. 19).

d. Establish IV access and treat dehydration.

e. Cardiac monitor until level falls below 20mcg/mL. Treat dysrhythmias by correcting electrolytes and administering appropriate antidysrhythmics.

f. Monitor serum K^+, Mg^{2+}, PO_4^{3-}, Ca^{2+}, acid–base balance in moderate-to-severe intoxication until trends are reassuring.

g. Treat seizures aggressively with benzodiazepines and phenobarbital. **Do not use phenytoin.**

h. Extracorporeal methods
  1) Hemodialysis is just as effective as charcoal hemoperfusion, more readily available, and lower risk. Indications are as follows:
  i = Theophylline level ≥90mg/mL at any time.
  ii = Theophylline level ≥70mcg/mL 4 hours after ingestion of sustained-release preparation.
  iii = Theophylline level ≥40mcg/mL and seizures, dysrythmias, and protracted vomiting unresponsive to antiemetics.
  2) Exchange transfusion may be indicated in neonate with severe toxicity.

T. TRICYCLIC ANTIDEPRESSANTS[30–33]

1. **Agents:** Amitriptyline, desipramine, doxepin, imipramine, nortriptyline.

2. **Signs and symptoms**

a. CNS: Agitation, delirium, psychosis, seizures, myoclonus, lethargy, coma.

b. Cardiovascular: Conduction abnormalities, dysrhythmias, hypotension.

c. Anticholinergic symptoms (see p. 25).

3. **Management**

a. Signs of toxicity usually appear within 4 hours of ingestion. Any ingestion should be observed for at least 6 hours.

b. ECG (acute overdose): QRS duration >0.10 second and R wave in lead aVR ≥3mm are associated with increased risk of seizures and ventricular dysrhythmias. ECG must be monitored for at least 12–24 hours if these conduction abnormalities are present in the first 6 hours.

c. Serum drug levels do not necessarily predict outcome.

d. Ensure adequate airway, ventilation, and circulation. Establish IV access, and start continuous ECG monitoring, even in the patient who is asymptomatic at presentation. If the patient remains asymptomatic, has normal bowel sounds, and has no ECG abnormalities in the 6-hour period after the ingestion, then no further medical intervention is necessary.

2

POISONINGS

e. If altered mental status, stabilize with dextrose, oxygen, and naloxone.

f. Treat seizures with benzodiazepines, then phenobarbital if seizures persist. Phenytoin is not indicated because it may precipitate ventricular dysrrhythmias.

g. For cardiac conduction abnormalities, dysrrhythmias, and hypotension:
    1) Give hypertonic NaHCO₃ (1mEq/kg) bolus until desired clinical effect or pH between 7.45–7.5.
    2) Then give continuous infusion of D₅W with 132mEq/L of NaHCO₃ at 1.5–2 times maintenance.
    3) May also give fluid boluses with isotonic saline as needed for hypotension.
    4) High-dose dopamine and norepinephrine for hypotension unresponsive to fluids may be used.

h. Give charcoal and cathartic.

i. Physostigmine is **contraindicated** for anticholinergic toxicity in tricyclic antidepressant ingestions; its use can cause serious complications, including death.

j. Admit if any signs of major toxicity, such as change in mental status, conduction delays on ECG, dysrrhythmias, seizures, or hypotension; place patient on cardiac monitor until symptom-free for 24 hours.

The author would like to thank Maryland Poison Control Center for providing information critical to the development of this chapter.

V. REFERENCES

1. Ellenhorn MJ. *Ellenhorn's medical toxicology*. New York: William & Wilkins; 1997.

2. Kulig K. Initial management of ingestions of toxic substances. *N Engl J Med* 1992; **326**:1677.

3. Olson KR. *Poisoning and drug overdose*. Norwalk, CT: Appleton & Lange; 1994.

4. Jones AL. Mechanism of action and value of *N*-acetylcysteine in the treatment of early and late acetaminophen poisoning: a critical review. *J Toxicol Clin Toxicol* 1998; **36**:277–285.

5. Anker AL, Smilkstein MJ. Acetaminophen concepts and controversies. *Emerg Med Clin North Am* 1994; **12**:335.

6. Smilkstein MJ, Bronstein AC, Linden C, Augenstein WL, Kulig KW, Rumack BH. Acetaminophen overdose: a 48 hour intervenous, *N*-acetylcysteine treatment protocol. *Ann Emerg Med* 1991; 20:1058–1063.

7. Yip L, Dart RC, Hurlbut KM. Intravenous administration of oral *N*-acetylcysteine. *Crit Care Med* 1998; **26**:40–43.

8. Goldfrank LR. *Toxicologic emergencies*. Norwalk, CT: Appleton & Lange; 1998.

9. Weaver DF, Camfield P, Fraser A. Massive carbamazepine overdose: clinical and pharmacological observation in five episodes. *Neurology* 1988; **38**:755.

10. Woolf AD. Poisoning in children and adolescents. *Pediatr Rev* 1993; **14**:472.

11. Walker AR. Emergency department management of house fire burns and carbon monoxide poisoning in children. *Curr Opin Pediatr* 1996; **8**:239–242.

12. Rothstein FC. Caustic injuries to the esophagus in children. *Pediatr Clin North Am* 1986; **33**:665.

13. Moore WR. Caustic ingestion: pathophysiology, diagnosis, and treatment. *Clin Pediatr* 1986; **25**:192.

14. Wason S. The emergency management of caustic ingestion. *Emerg Med* 1985; **2**:175.

15. Tenenbein M. Pediatric toxicology: current controversies and recent advances. *Curr Probl Pediatr* 1986; **16**:185.

16. Klein BL. Hydrocarbon poisonings. *Pediatr Clin North Am* 1986; **33**:411.

17. Schauben JL, Augenstein WL, Cox J, Sato R. Iron poisoning: report of three cases and a review of therapeutic interventions. *J Emerg Med* 1990; **8**:309.

18. Mills KC, Curry SC. Acute iron poisoning. *Emerg Med Clin North Am* 1994; **12**:397.

19. Lovejoy FH, Nizet V, Priebe CJ. Common etiologies and new approaches to management of poisoning in pediatric practice. *Curr Opin Pediatr* 1993; **5**:524–530.

20. Personal communication. Dr Cecilia T. Davoli, Lead poisoning prevention program, Kennedy Krieger Institute.

21. Schonfeld DJ, Needham D. Lead: a practical perspective. *Contemp Pediatr* 1994; **11**:64–96.

22. Committee on Drugs. Treatment guidelines for lead exposure in children. *Pediatrics* 1995; **96**:155–160.

23. Centers for Disease Control and Prevention. *Guidelines for lead poisoning prevention*. Atlanta, GA: CDC; 1997.

24. Liebelt EL, Shannon MW. Oral chelators for childhood lead poisoning. *Pediatr Ann* 1994; **23**:616–626.

25. Moore R, Rumack BH, Conner CS, Peterson RG. Naloxone: under dosage after narcotic poisoning. *Am J Dis Child* 1980; **134**:156.

26. Tenenbein M. Continuous naloxone infusion for opiate poisoning in infancy. *J Pediatr* 1984; **105**:645.

27. Berlin CM. Advances in pediatric pharmacology and toxicology. *Adv Pediatr* 1993; **40**:404–439.

28. Larsen LS, Sterrett JR, Whitehead B, Marcus SM. Adjunctive therapy of phenytoin overdose: a case report using plasmaphoresis. *Clin Toxicol* 1986; **24**:37.

2

POISONINGS

29. Yip L, Dart RC, Gabow PA. Concepts and controversies in salicylate toxicity. *Emerg Med Clin North Am* 1994; **12:**351.

30. Boehnert MT, Lovejoy FH. Value of the QRS duration versus the serum drug level in predicting seizures and ventricular arrhythmias after an acute overdose of tricyclic antidepressant. *N Engl J Med* 1985; **313:**474.

31. Pimentel L, Trommer L. Cyclic antidepressant overdoses: a review. *Emerg Med Clin North Am* 1994; **12:**533.

32. Shannon M, Liebelt EL. Toxicology reviews: targeted management strategies for cardiovascular toxicity from tricyclic antidepressant overdose—the pivotal role for alkanization and sodium loading. *Pediatr Emerg Care* 1998; **14:**293–298.

33. Liebelt EL, Francis PD, Woolf AD. ECG lead aVR versus QRS interval in predicting seizures and arrythmias in acute tricyclic antidepressant toxicity. *Ann Emerg Med* 1995; **26:**195–201.

PROCEDURES

'See one, do one, teach one'

Wendy Burk Roberts, MD

I. INFORMED CONSENT AND PREPARATION OF CHILD

Before performing any procedure, it is crucial to obtain informed consent by explaining the procedure, the indications, and any risks involved, as well as alternatives. The child must also be prepared for the procedure, including discussing the procedure, explaining what the child can expect, and ensuring that a parent or another adult is present to provide support. Never lie to a child. Preparation may also include sedation (see ch. 30) or restraining the patient to ensure proper immobilization during the procedure. Those trained to work with children, such as Child Life personnel, can be instrumental in helping to prepare a child and provide support during a procedure.

II. BLOOD SAMPLING AND VASCULAR ACCESS

A. HEELSTICK/FINGERSTICK

1. **Indications:** Blood sampling in infants for laboratory studies unaffected by hemolysis.
2. **Complications**
   a. Infection.
   b. Osteomyelitis.
3. **Procedure**
   a. Warm heel or finger.
   b. Clean with alcohol.
      1) Puncture heel using a lancet on lateral part of heel, avoiding posterior area.
      2) Puncture finger using a lancet on the ventral lateral surface of finger near tip.
   c. Wipe away first drop of blood, then collect using capillary tube or container.
   d. Alternate between squeezing blood from the leg toward the heel (or from the hand toward the finger) and then releasing the pressure for several seconds.

B. INTRAVENOUS PLACEMENT AND ACCESS SITES

1. **Indications:** To obtain access to peripheral venous circulation; to deliver fluid, medications, or blood products.
2. **Complications**
   a. Thrombosis.
   b. Infection.
3. **Procedure**
   a. Choose IV placement site and prepare with alcohol (Fig. 3.1).

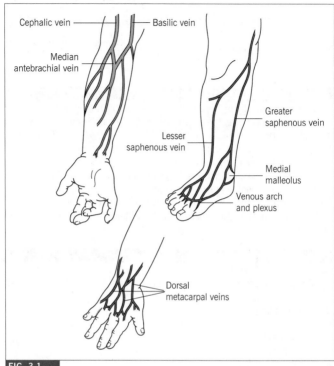

FIG. 3.1
Venous access sites. (Original drawing courtesy Josie Pirro, RN, Johns Hopkins Children's Center.)

b. Apply tourniquet and then insert IV catheter, bevel up, at angle almost parallel to the skin, advancing until 'flash' of blood is seen in the catheter hub. Advance the plastic catheter only, remove the needle, and secure the catheter.

c. Attach T connector filled with saline to the catheter, flush with several mL of normal saline (NS) to ensure patency of the IV line.

C. EXTERNAL JUGULAR PUNCTURE

1. **Indications:** Blood sampling in patients with inadequate peripheral vascular access or during resuscitation.

2. **Complications**

a. Hematoma.

b. Pneumothorax.

c. Infection.

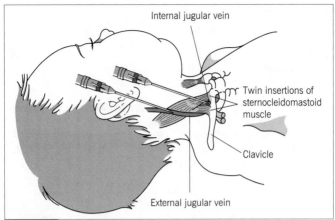

FIG. 3.2

Approach for external and internal jugular puncture. (Original drawing courtesy Josie Pirro, RN, Johns Hopkins Children's Center.)

3. **Procedure** (Fig. 3.2)

a. Restrain infant securely.

b. Place infant with head turned away from side of blood sampling. Position with towel roll under shoulders or with head over side of bed to extend neck and accentuate the posterior margin of sternocleidomastoid muscle on the side of the venipuncture.

c. Prep area carefully with povidone–iodine and alcohol.

d. To distend the external jugular vein, occlude its most proximal segment, or provoke child to cry. The vein runs from angle of mandible to posterior border of lower third of sternocleidomastoid muscle.

e. With continuous negative suction on the syringe, insert the needle at about a 30° angle to the skin. Continue as with any peripheral venipuncture.

f. Apply sterile dressing and pressure on site for 5 minutes.

D. FEMORAL ARTERY AND FEMORAL VEIN PUNCTURE

1. **Indications:** Venous or arterial blood sampling of patients with inadequate vascular access or during resuscitation.

2. **Contraindications:** Femoral puncture is particularly hazardous in neonates and is not recommended in this age group. It is also discouraged in children because of the risk of trauma to the femoral head and joint capsule. Avoid femoral punctures in children who have thrombocytopenia or coagulation disorders or who are scheduled for cardiac catheterization.

3. Complications

a. Hematoma at femoral triangle.

b. Thrombosis of vessel.

c. Infection.

d. Osteomyelitis.

e. Septic arthritis of femur or hip.

4. Procedure (Fig. 3.3)

a. Hold child securely in frog leg position with the hips flexed and abducted.

b. Prepare area with povidone–iodine and alcohol.

c. Locate femoral pulse just distal to inguinal crease, then insert needle 2cm distal to inguinal ligament and 0.5–0.75cm into the groin. Note that vein is medial to pulse. Aspirate while maneuvering the needle until blood is obtained.

d. Apply direct pressure for minimum of 5 minutes.

E. RADIAL ARTERY PUNCTURE AND CATHETERIZATION

1. Indications: Arterial blood sampling or for frequent blood gases and blood pressure monitoring in an intensive care setting.

2. Complications

a. Occlusion of artery by hematoma or thrombosis.

b. Infection, thrombophlebitis.

c. Ischemia if ulnar circulation inadequate.

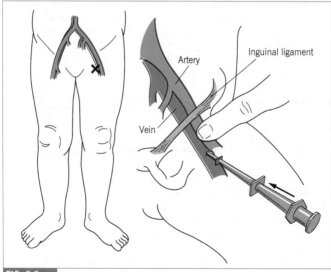

FIG. 3.3

Femoral puncture technique. (Adapted from Nichols[1].)

3. **Procedure**
a. Before procedure, test adequacy of ulnar blood flow with the Allen test. Clench the hand while simultaneously compressing ulnar and radial arteries. The hand will blanch. Release pressure from the ulnar artery and observe the flushing response. Procedure is safe to perform if entire hand flushes.
b. Secure the hand to an arm board with the wrist extended. Leave the fingers exposed to observe any color changes.
c. Locate the radial pulse. It is optional to infiltrate area over point of maximal impulse with lidocaine. Cleanse site with povidone–iodine.
   1) Puncture: Insert butterfly needle attached to a syringe at a 30–60° angle over point of maximal impulse; blood should flow freely into syringe in pulsatile fashion; suction may be required for plastic tubes. Once sample is obtained, apply firm, constant pressure for 5 minutes and then place pressure dressing.
   2) Catheter placement: Secure hand to arm board. Prep wrist with sterile technique and infiltrate over point of maximal impulse with 1% lidocaine. Make a small skin puncture over point of maximal impulse with a needle, then discard needle. Insert IV catheter with needle through the puncture site at a 30° angle to the horizontal; pass the needle and catheter through the artery to transfix it, then withdraw the needle. Very slowly withdraw the catheter until free flow of blood is noted. Then advance the catheter and secure in place via sutures or tape. Apply antibiotic ointment dressing. Infuse isotonic heparinized saline (1 unit heparin/mL saline) at 1mL/hr. A pressure transducer may be attached to monitor blood pressure.
   Note: Do not infuse any medications, blood products, or hypertonic solutions through arterial line.

F. **POSTERIOR TIBIAL AND DORSALIS PEDIS ARTERY PUNCTURE**
1. **Indications:** Arterial blood sampling when radial artery puncture unsuccessful or inaccessible.
2. **Complications:** See p. 46.
3. **Procedure**
a. Posterior tibial artery: Puncture the artery posterior to the medial malleolus while holding the foot in dorsiflexion.
b. Dorsalis pedis artery: Puncture the artery at dorsal midfoot between the first and second toe while holding the foot in plantar flexion.

G. **CENTRAL VENOUS CATHETER PLACEMENT**
1. **Indications:** To obtain emergency access to central venous circulation, to monitor central venous pressure, to deliver high-concentration parenteral nutrition or prolonged IV therapy, to infuse blood products or large volumes of fluid.

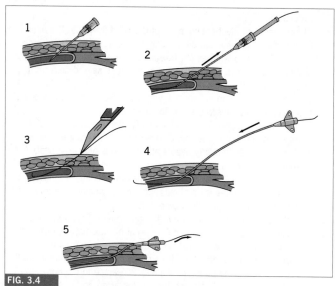

FIG. 3.4
The Seldinger technique for central venous catheter placement. (Original drawing
courtesy Josie Pirro, RN, Johns Hopkins Children's Center.)

2. **Complications**
a. Arterial or venous laceration.
b. Infection.
c. Pneumothorax, hemothorax.
d. Catheter fragment in circulation.
e. Air embolism.
f. Atrioventricular fistula.
g. Hematoma.
h. Thrombosis.
3. **Access sites**
a. External jugular vein.
b. Internal jugular vein.
c. Subclavian vein.
d. Femoral vein.
   **Note: Femoral vein catheterization is contraindicated in severe
   abdominal trauma, and the internal jugular is contraindicated in
   patients with elevated intracranial pressure (ICP).**
4. **Procedure:** The Seldinger technique (Fig. 3.4)
a. Secure patient, choose vessel for catheterization, prep, and drape in
   sterile fashion.
b. Insert needle, applying negative pressure to locate vessel.

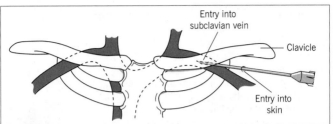

FIG. 3.5

Approach for catheterization of subclavian vein. (Original drawing courtesy Josie Pirro, RN, Johns Hopkins Children's Center.)

c. When there is blood return, insert a guidewire through needle into vein to about a fourth to a third the length of wire.

d. Remove needle, holding guidewire firmly.

e. Slip catheter that has been preflushed with sterile saline over wire into vein in a twisting motion. Entry site may be enlarged with a small skin incision or dilator. Pass entire catheter over wire until hub is at skin surface. Slowly remove wire and secure catheter by suture and attach IV infusion.

f. Apply sterile dressing over site.

g. For neck vessels, obtain chest radiograph results to rule out pneumothorax.

5. **Approach**

a. External jugular (see Fig. 3.2): Place patient in 15–20° Trendelenburg. Turn head 45° to contralateral side. Enter vein at point where vein crosses sternocleidomastoid.

b. Internal jugular (see Fig. 3.2): Place patient in 15–20° Trendelenburg. Hyperextend the neck to tense the sternocleido-mastoid muscle and turn head away from site of line placement. Palpate sternal and clavicular heads of the muscle and enter at the apex of the triangle formed. Insert needle at a 30° angle to the skin and aim toward the ipsilateral nipple. When blood flow is obtained, continue with Seldinger technique.

c. Subclavian vein (Fig. 3.5): Position child in Trendelenburg position with towel roll under thoracic spine to hyperextend the back. Aim needle under the distal third of clavicle toward sternal notch. When blood flow is obtained, continue with Seldinger technique.
Note: This is the least common site for central lines because of the increased risk of complications.

d. Femoral vein (see Fig. 3.3).

H. INTRAOSSEOUS (IO) INFUSION

1. **Indications:** Obtain emergency access in children <6 years old. This is very useful during circulatory collapse and/or cardiac arrest. Optimally

the needle should be removed after 3–4 hours once adequate vascular access has been established.

2. **Complications**
a. Osteomyelitis.
b. Fat embolism.
c. Extravasation of fluid into subcutaneous tissue.
d. Subcutaneous abscess.
e. Fracture, epiphyseal injury.
3. **Sites of entry** (in order of preference)
a. Anteromedial surface of proximal tibia, 2cm below and 1–2cm medial to the tibial tuberosity on the flat part of bone (Fig. 3.6).
b. Distal femur 3cm above lateral condyle in the midline.

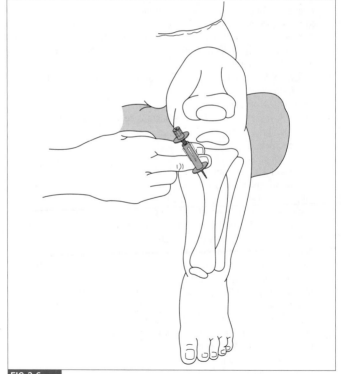

FIG 3.6
Intraosseous insertion (anterior tibia). (Original drawing courtesy Jose Pirro, RN, Johns Hopkins Children's Center.)

c.   Medial surface of the distal tibia 1–2cm above the medial malleolus.

4. Procedure

a.   Prep and drape the patient for a sterile procedure.

b.   Anesthetize the puncture site down to the periosteum with 1% lidocaine (optional in emergency situations).

c.   Insert 15G IO needle perpendicular to the skin and advance to the periosteum. Then, with a boring rotary motion, penetrate through cortex until there is a decrease in resistance, indicating that you have reached the marrow. Needle should stand firm without support. Secure needle carefully.

d.   Remove stylet and attempt to aspirate marrow if samples are needed, then flush saline. Observe for fluid extravasation. (Note that it is not necessary to aspirate marrow.) Marrow can be sent for electrolytes, glucose, blood urea nitrogen (BUN), creatinine, type and crossmatch, but not complete blood count (CBC).

e.   Attach standard IV tubing. Any crystalloid, blood product, or drug that may be infused into a peripheral vein may also be infused into the IO space, but a higher pressure (via pressure bag or push) is needed for infusion.

I.   UMBILICAL ARTERY (UA) CATHETERIZATION

1. Indications: Vascular access, blood pressure, and blood gas monitoring in critically ill neonates.

2. Complications

a.   Hemorrhage from displacement of line or perforation of artery.

b.   Thrombosis.

c.   Infection.

d.   Ischemia/infarction of lower extremities, bowel, kidney.

e.   Arrhythmias.

3. Caution: UA catheterization should never be performed if omphalitis is present; it is contraindicated in the presence of possible necrotizing enterocolitis or intestinal hypoperfusion.

4. Line placement

a.   Low line vs high line

   1) Low line: Tip of the catheter should lie just above the aortic bifurcation between L3 and L5. This avoids renal and mesenteric arteries near L1, perhaps decreasing the incidence of thrombosis.

   2) High line: Tip of the catheter should be above the diaphragm between T6 and T9. A high line may be recommended in infants less than 750g when a low line could easily slip out.

b.   Catheter length: Determine the length of catheter required using either a standardized graph or the regression formula. Add length for the height of the umbilical stump.

   1) Standardized graph: Determine the shoulder–umbilical length by measuring the perpendicular line dropped from the tip of the

shoulder to the level of the umbilicus. Use the graph in Fig. 3.7 to determine the catheter length.

2) Birth weight (BW) regression formula:

Low line: UA catheter length (cm) $\approx$ BW (kg) + 7.

High line: UA catheter length (cm) = [3 × BW (kg)] + 9.

Note: Formula may not be appropriate for small-for-gestational-age (SGA) or large-for-gestational-age (LGA) infants.

5. **Procedure** (see Fig. 3.9)

a. Determine the length of catheter to be inserted for either high (T6–T9) or low (L3–L5) position.

b. Restrain infant. Prep and drape umbilical cord and adjacent skin using sterile technique. Infant's warmth is critical.

c. Flush catheter with sterile saline solution before insertion.

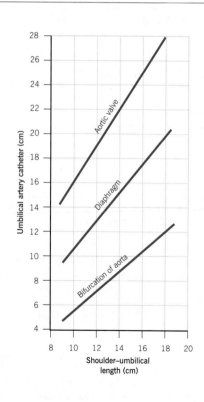

FIG. 3.7

Umbilical artery catheter length.

d. Place sterile umbilical tape around base of cord. Cut through cord horizontally about 1.5–2.0cm from skin; tighten umbilical tape to prevent bleeding.

e. Identify the one large, thin-walled umbilical vein and two smaller, thick-walled arteries. Use one tip of open, curved forceps to probe and dilate one artery gently; use both points of closed forceps and dilate artery by allowing forceps to open gently.

f. Grasp catheter 1cm from tip with toothless forceps and insert catheter into lumen of artery. Aim the tip toward the feet, and gently advance catheter to desired distance. **Do not force.** If resistance is encountered, try loosening umbilical tape, applying steady gentle pressure, or manipulating angle of umbilical cord to skin. Often catheter cannot be advanced because of creation of a 'false luminal tract'.

g. Secure catheter with a suture through the cord, a marker tape and a tape bridge. Confirm the position of the catheter tip radiologically. Line may be pulled back but not advanced once sterile field broken.

h. Observe for complications: Blanching or cyanosis of lower extremities; perforation; thrombosis; embolism; or infection. If any complications occur, line should be removed.
Note: Infants remain NPO until 24 hours after catheter removed. Never run hypoosmolar fluids through UA line. Isotonic fluids should contain 0.5 unit heparin/mL.

J. UMBILICAL VEIN (UV) CATHETERIZATION

1. Indications: Vascular access in critically ill neonate.

2. Complications

a. Hemorrhage from displacement of line or perforation of vessel.

b. Infection.

c. Air embolism.

d. Arrhythmias.

3. Line placement: UV catheters should be placed in the inferior vena cava above the level of the ductus venosus and the hepatic veins and below the level of the left atrium.

a. Catheter length: Determine the length of the catheter required using either a standardized graph or the regression formula. Add length for the height of the umbilical stump.

1) Standardized graph: Determine the shoulder-umbilical length by measuring the perpendicular line dropped from the tip of the shoulder to the level of the umbilicus. Use the graph in Fig. 3.8 to determine the catheter length needed to place the tip between the diaphragm and left atrium.

2) Regression formula:
UV catheter length (cm) = $[0.5 \times UA\ (cm)] + 1$
(see pp. 51–52 for UA length determination).
Note: May not be appropriate for SGA or LGA infants.

PROCEDURES 3

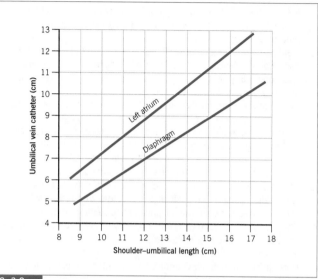

FIG. 3.8
Umbilical vein catheter length.

4. **Procedure** (Fig. 3.9)
a. Follow procedure steps a–d for UA catheter placement. However, determine length via Fig. 3.8.
b. Isolate thin-walled umbilical vein, clear thrombi with forceps, and insert catheter, aiming the tip toward the right shoulder. Gently advance catheter to desired distance. **Do not force.** If resistance is encountered, try loosening umbilical tape, applying steady gentle pressure, or manipulating angle of umbilical cord to skin.
c. Secure catheter as described on p. 53. Confirm position of the catheter tip radiologically.

III. BODY FLUID SAMPLING
A. LUMBAR PUNCTURE
1. **Indications:** Examination of spinal fluid for suspected infection or malignancy, instillation of intrathecal chemotherapy, or measurement of opening pressure.
2. **Complications**
a. Headache.
b. Acquired epidermal spinal cord tumor caused by implantation of epidermal material into spinal canal if no stylet used on skin entry.
c. Local back pain.

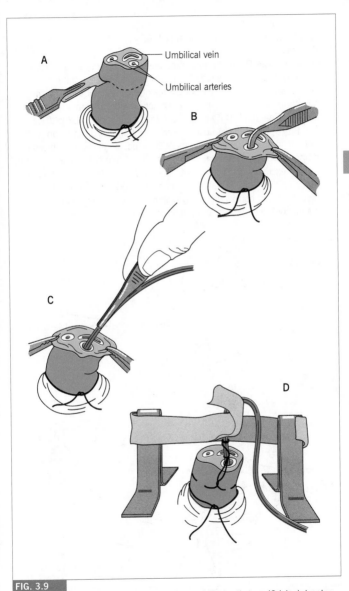

A
Umbilical vein
Umbilical arteries

B

C

D

FIG. 3.9
A four-step technique for placing and securing umbilical catheters. (Original drawing courtesy Josie Pirro, RN, Johns Hopkins Children's Center.)

d. Infection or bleeding.

e. Herniation associated with increased ICP.

3. Cautions

a. Increased ICP: Before lumbar puncture (LP), perform fundoscopic examination. The presence of papilledema, retinal hemorrhage, or clinical suspicion of increased ICP may be contraindications to the procedure. A sudden drop in intraspinal pressure by rapid release of cerebrospinal fluid (CSF) may cause fatal herniation. If LP is to be performed, proceed with extreme caution. Computed tomography (CT) may be indicated before LP if there is suspected intracranial bleeding or increased ICP. A normal CT scan does not rule out increased ICP but usually excludes conditions that may put patient at risk of herniation.

b. Bleeding diathesis: A platelet count of $>50,000/mm^3$ is desirable before LP, and correction of any clotting factor deficiencies prevents spinal cord hemorrhage and potential paralysis.

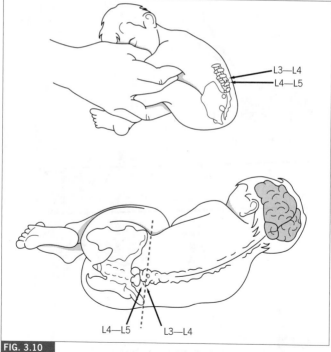

FIG. 3.10

Lumbar puncture. (Original drawing courtesy Josie Pirro, RN, Johns Hopkins Children's Center.)

c. Overlying skin infection: May result in inoculation of CSF with organisms.

4. **Procedure** (Fig. 3.10)

a. Prepare the child for the procedure (see section I) and apply eutectic mixture of local anesthetics (EMLA).

b. Position the child in either the sitting position or lateral recumbent position with hips, knees, and neck flexed. Do not compromise small infants' cardiorespiratory status by positioning.

c. Locate the desired interspace (either L3–L4 or L4–L5) by drawing an imaginary line between the top of the iliac crests.

d. Clean the skin with povidone–iodine and 70% alcohol. Drape conservatively so it is possible to monitor the infant. Use a 20–22G 1½-inch spinal needle with stylet (3½-inches for children >12 years).

e. Anesthetize overlying skin and subcutaneous tissue with lidocaine.

f. Puncture skin in midline just caudad to palpated spinous process, angling slightly cephalad toward umbilicus. Advance several millimeters at a time and withdraw stylet frequently to check for CSF flow. The needle may be advanced without the stylet once through the skin completely. In small infants, one may not feel a change in resistance or 'pop' as the dura is penetrated.

g. If resistance is met initially (you hit bone), withdraw needle to skin surface and redirect angle slightly.

h. Send CSF for appropriate studies (see p. 128 for normal values). Send first tube for culture and Gram stain, second tube for glucose and protein, and last tube for cell count and differential.

i. Accurate measurement of CSF pressure can be made only with the patient lying quietly on the side in an unflexed position. Once free flow of spinal fluid is obtained, attach the manometer and measure CSF pressure.

B. BONE MARROW ASPIRATION

1. **Indications:** Examination of bone marrow in a hematologic or oncologic workup.

2. **Complications**

a. Bleeding/hematoma.

b. Infection.

c. Bone spur formation (if biopsy is performed).

3. **Procedure**

a. Prepare child for procedure (see p. 43).

b. Identify site for aspiration. For most children the posterior iliac crest is preferred, although the anterior iliac crest may be used. For some children <3 months of age the tibia can be used.

c. Position patient in prone position with pillow elevating pelvis (for posterior iliac crest).

d. Prep the site with povidone–iodine and anesthetize skin, soft tissue, and periosteum with 1% lidocaine.

e. Insert needle (16 or 18G) with steady pressure in a boring motion. Needle should be directed perpendicular to the surface of the bone. Enter the ileum at the posterior superior iliac spine, which is a visible and palpable bony prominence superior and lateral to the intergluteal cleft. Needle will enter cortex and 'pop' into marrow space; needle should be firmly anchored in the bone.

f. Remove stylet and aspirate marrow with at least 20mL syringe. **Note: In young infants and those with infiltrated leukemia, marrow aspiration may be impossible; bone marrow biopsy thus may be necessary.**

C. CHEST TUBE PLACEMENT AND THORACENTESIS

1. **Indications:** Evacuation of a pneumothorax, hemothorax, chylothorax, large pleural effusion, or empyema for diagnostic or therapeutic purposes.

2. **Complications**

a. Pneumothorax or hemothorax.

b. Bleeding or infection.

c. Pulmonary contusion or laceration.

d. Puncture of diaphragm, liver, or spleen.

3. **Procedure:** Needle decompression

a. For tension pneumothoraces it may be possible to decompress quickly by sterilely inserting a 23G butterfly or 22G angiocatheter at the anterior second intercostal space in the midclavicular line.

b. Attach to three-way stopcock and syringe, and aspirate air.

c. Chest tube may still be necessary.

4. **Procedure:** Chest tube insertion (see inside front cover and Fig. 3.11)

a. Position child supine or with affected side up.

b. Point of entry is the third to fifth intercostal space in the mid to anterior axillary line, usually at level of nipple (avoid breast tissue).

c. Prep and drape sterilely with povidone–iodine and alcohol.

d. Patient may require sedation (see ch. 30). Locally anesthetize skin, subcutaneous tissue, periosteum of rib, chest wall muscles, and pleura with lidocaine.

e. Make sterile incision one intercostal space below desired insertion point, and bluntly dissect through tissue layers until the superior portion of the rib is reached, avoiding neurovascular bundle on the inferior portion of the rib.

f. Push hemostat over top of rib, through the pleura, and into the pleural space. Enter pleural space cautiously, not >1cm. Spread hemostat to open, place chest tube in clamp, and guide through entry site to desired distance.

g. For a pneumothorax, insert the tube anteriorly toward the apex. For a pleural effusion, direct the tube inferiorly and posteriorly.

h. Secure tube with purse-string sutures in which the suture is first tied at the skin, then wrapped around tube once and tied at tube.

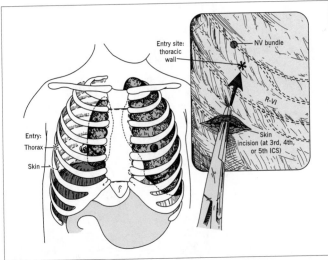

FIG. 3.11
Technique for insertion of chest tube. NV, Neurovascular; R-VI, sixth rib; ICS, intercostal space. (Adapted from Fleisher[2].)

i.   Attach to drainage system with −20 to −30cm H_2O pressure.
j.   Apply sterile occlusive dressing.
k.   Confirm position and function with chest radiograph.

5. **Procedure:** Thoracentesis (Fig. 3.12)

a.   Confirm fluid in pleural space via clinical examination, radiographs, or sonography.
b.   If possible, place child in sitting position leaning over table; otherwise place supine.
c.   Point of entry usually in the seventh intercostal space and posterior axillary line.
d.   Sterilely prep and drape area.
e.   Anesthetize skin, subcutaneous tissue, rib periosteum, chest wall, and pleura with lidocaine.
f.   Advance an 18–22G IV catheter or large-bore needle attached to a syringe onto rib and then 'walk' over superior aspect into pleural space while providing steady negative pressure; often a 'popping' sensation is generated. Be careful not to advance too far into the pleural cavity. If an IV catheter is used, the soft catheter may be advanced into the pleural space aiming downward.
g.   Attach syringe and stopcock device to remove fluid for diagnostic studies and symptomatic relief. (See p. 128 for evaluation of pleural fluid.)

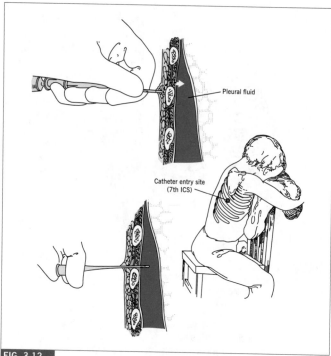

FIG. 3.12

Thoracentesis. ICS, Intercostal space. (Adapted from Fleisher[2].)

h. After removing needle or catheter, place occlusive dressing and obtain chest radiograph results to rule out pneumothorax.

D. PERICARDIOCENTESIS

1. **Indications:** To obtain pericardial fluid emergently for diagnostic or therapeutic purposes.

2. **Complications**

a. Puncture of cardiac chamber.

b. Hemopericardium/pneumopericardium.

c. Cardiac dysrhythmias.

d. Pneumothorax.

3. **Procedure** (Fig. 3.13)

a. Unless contraindicated, sedate the patient. Monitor ECG.

b. Place patient at a 30° angle (reverse Trendelenburg). Have patient secured.

c. Prep and drape puncture site. A drape across the upper chest is unnecessary and may obscure important landmarks.

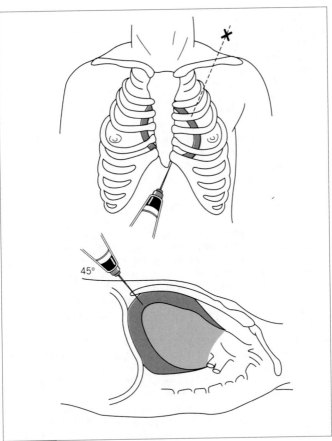

FIG. 3.13
Pericardiocentesis. (Adapted from Nichols[1].)

d. Anesthetize the puncture site with 1% lidocaine.
e. Insert an 18 or 20G needle just to the left of the xiphoid process, 1cm inferior to the bottom rib at about a 45° angle to the skin.
f. While gently aspirating, advance needle toward the patient's left shoulder until pericardial fluid is obtained.
g. Upon entering the pericardial space, clamp the needle at the skin edge to prevent further penetration. Attach a 30mL syringe with a stopcock.
h. Gently and slowly remove the fluid. Rapid withdrawal of the pericardial fluid can result in shock or myocardial insufficiency.
i. Send fluid for appropriate laboratory studies (see p. 127).

E. **PARACENTESIS**

1. **Indications:** Removal of intraperitoneal fluid for diagnostic or therapeutic purposes.
2. **Complications**
   a. Bleeding or infection.
   b. Puncture of internal organs.
3. **Cautions**
   a. Do not remove a large amount of fluid too rapidly because hypovolemia and hypotension may result from rapid fluid shifts.
   b. Avoid scars from previous surgery; localized bowel adhesions increase the chances of entering a viscus in these areas.
   c. The bladder should be empty to avoid perforation.
   d. Never perform paracentesis through an area of cellulitis.
4. **Procedure**
   a. Prep and drape the abdomen as for a surgical procedure. Anesthetize puncture site.
   b. With patient in semisupine, sitting, or lateral decubitus position, insert 16–22G IV catheter attached to a syringe in midline 2cm below the umbilicus; in neonates, just lateral to the rectus muscle in the right or left lower quadrants, a few centimeters above the inguinal ligament.
   c. Aiming cephalad, insert needle at 45° angle while one hand pulls skin caudally until entering the peritoneal cavity. This creates a 'Z' tract when the skin is released and needle removed. Apply continuous negative pressure.
   d. Once fluid appears in the syringe, remove introducer needle and leave catheter in place. Attach a stopcock and aspirate slowly until an adequate amount of fluid has been obtained for studies.
   e. If, on entering the peritoneal cavity, air is aspirated, withdraw the needle immediately. Aspirated air indicates entrance into a hollow viscus. (In general, penetration of a hollow viscus during paracentesis does not lead to complications.) Then repeat paracentesis with sterile equipment.
   f. Send fluid for appropriate laboratory studies (see p. 127).

F. **URINARY BLADDER CATHETERIZATION**

1. **Indications:** To obtain urine for urinalysis and culture sterilely and to monitor hydration status.
2. **Complications**
   a. Trauma to urethra or bladder.
   b. Vaginal catheterization.
   c. Infection.
   d. Intravesical knot of catheter (rarely occurs).
   Note: Infant/child should not have voided within 1 hour of technique. Catheterization is contraindicated in pelvic fractures.
3. **Procedure**
   a. Prepare the urethral opening using sterile technique.
   b. In boys, apply gentle traction to the penis to straighten the urethra.

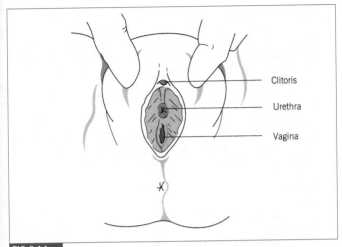

FIG 3.14
Female urethra. (Original drawing courtes Jose Pirro, RN, Johns Hopkins Children's Center.)

c. Gently insert a lubricated catheter into the urethra. Slowly advance the catheter until resistance is met at the external sphincter. Continued pressure will overcome this resistance, and the catheter will enter the bladder. In girls, the urethral orifice may be difficult to visualize, but it is usually immediately anterior to the vaginal orifice (Fig. 3.14). Only a few centimeters of advancement is required to reach the bladder in girls. In boys, insert a few centimeters longer than the shaft of the penis.
d. Carefully remove the catheter once the specimen is obtained.
e. Cleanse skin of povidone–iodine.

G. SUPRAPUBIC BLADDER ASPIRATION

1. **Indications:** To obtain urine for urinalysis and culture sterilely in children aged <2 years (avoid in children with genitourinary tract anomalies).

2. **Complications**
a. Hematuria, usually microscopic.
b. Intestinal perforation.
c. Infection of abdominal wall.
d. Bleeding.

3. **Procedure**
a. Anterior rectal pressure in girls or gentle penile pressure in boys may be used to prevent urination during the procedure. Child should not have voided within 1 hour of procedure.

b. Restrain the infant in the supine, frog leg position. Clean the suprapubic area with povidone–iodine and alcohol.

c. The site for puncture is 1–2cm above the symphysis pubis in the midline. Use a syringe with a 22G, 1-inch needle and puncture at 10–20° angle to the perpendicular, aiming slightly caudad.

d. Exert suction gently as the needle is advanced until urine enters syringe. The needle should not be advanced more than 1 inch. Aspirate the urine with gentle suction.

H. KNEE JOINT ASPIRATION

1. Indications: Removal of joint effusion causing severe pain or limitations of function and to obtain fluid for diagnosis of systemic illness (collagen vascular disease) or septic arthritis.

2. Complications

a. Bleeding.

b. Infection.

c. Damage to articular cartilage.

3. Procedure (Fig. 3.15)

a. Secure the child with knee actively extended.

b. Prep and drape for a sterile procedure.

c. Anesthetize the aspiration site with 1% lidocaine/bicarbonate (see p. 895). Anesthetize the subcutaneous tissue down to the joint capsule.

d. Localize the undersurface of patella. Extend the knee as much as possible. Insert an 18G or larger-bore needle into the joint space lateral to the patella at its posterior margin.

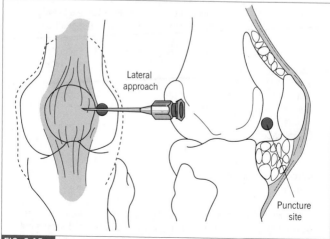

Lateral approach

Puncture site

FIG. 3.15

Knee joint aspiration. (Adapted from Fleischer[2].)

e. Aspiration of joint contents confirms an intraarticular placement.

f. Collect fluid for appropriate studies (see p. 129).

g. Place a dry, sterile dressing over aspiration site when finished.

I. TYMPANOCENTESIS (Fig. 3.16)

1. **Indications:** Removal of middle ear fluid for diagnostic or therapeutic purposes.

2. **Complications**

a. Bleeding.

b. Persistent perforation.

c. Tympanic membrane scar.

d. Very rare: incostapedius joint dislocation; facial nerve injury, puncture of exposed jugular bulb.

3. **Procedure**[4]

a. Prepare patient for the procedure. Consider input from Child Life specialist. Consider use of anxiolytic, such as midazolam (see p. 902). Restrain patient securely; a papoose board is recommended.

b. Remove all cerumen from canal (e.g., with No. 0 Buck cure). Then gently swab ear canal with alcohol-soaked applicator as a "wet mop" (e.g., 5mm Farrell applicator tip wrapped with alcohol-soaked cotton).

c. Attach 18–22G, 2½–3-inch spinal needle, bevel upward, to the Luer-Lok adaptor of a disposable tympanocentesis aspirator (Xomed Surgical Products, Jacksonville, FL). Alternatively, attach needle to a 1mL tuberculin syringe and bend needle 30–45° (to allow for visualization during puncture).

d. Visualize the point of maximal bulge in the inferior portion (posteriorly or anteriorly) of the tympanic membrane through an otoscope fitted with an operating head.

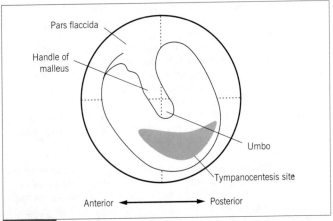

FIG. 3.16

Tympanocentesis in the left ear. (Adapted from Dieckmann[3].)

e. Perforate the tympanic membrane and then apply negative pressure to remove fluid in 1–2 seconds. Remove needle, avoiding contamination in the canal.

f. Send fluid for appropriate cultures and Gram stain.

g. Place a small cotton pledget in the outer portion of the external auditory canal to absorb extra blood and discharge. Perforation usually heals in 3–5 days.

IV. IMMUNIZATION AND MEDICATION ADMINISTRATION

A. SUBCUTANEOUS INJECTIONS

1. **Indications:** Immunizations and other medications.

2. **Complications**

a. Allergic reaction.

b. Formation of subcutaneous nodules after repeated injections.

3. **Procedure**

a. Locate injection site: Upper outer arm or outer aspect of upper thigh.

b. Clean skin with alcohol.

c. Insert 0.5-inch, 25 or 27G needle into subcutaneous layer at angle of 45° to skin. Aspirate for blood, then inject medication.

B. INTRAMUSCULAR INJECTIONS

1. **Indications:** Immunizations, antibiotics, and other medications.

2. **Complications**

a. Allergic reaction.

b. Bleeding, hematoma.

c. Nerve injury.

d. Infection.

3. **Cautions**

a. Avoid in child with bleeding disorder.

b. Maximum volume to be injected is 0.5mL in small infant, 1mL in older infant, 2mL in school-age child, and 3mL in adolescent.

4. **Procedure**

a. Locate injection site: Anterolateral upper thigh (vastus lateralis muscle) in smaller child or outer aspect of upper arm (deltoid) in older one. The dorsal gluteal region is less commonly used because of risk of nerve or vascular injury. To find the ventral gluteal site, form a triangle by placing your index finger on the anterior iliac spine and your middle finger on the most superior aspect of the iliac crest. The injection should occur in the middle of the triangle formed by the two fingers and the iliac crest.

b. Clean skin with alcohol.

c. Pinch muscle with free hand and insert 1-inch, 23 or 25G needle until hub is flush with the skin surface. For deltoid and ventral gluteal, the needle should be perpendicular to the skin. For the anterolateral thigh, needle should be 45° to the long axis of the thigh. Aspirate for blood, then inject medication.

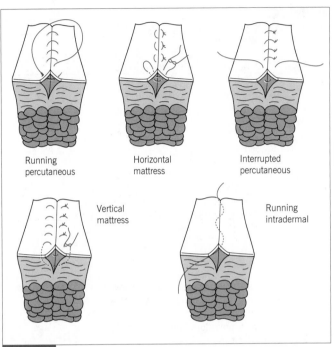

Running
percutaneous

Horizontal
mattress

Interrupted
percutaneous

Vertical
mattress

Running
intradermal

FIG 3.17

Basic skin closure techniques. (Original drawing courtesy Jose Pirro, RN, Johns Hopkins Children's Center.)

V. BASIC LACERATION REPAIR

A. SUTURING

1. **Techniques** (Fig. 3.17)
a. Simple interrupted.
b. Horizontal mattress: Provides eversion of wound edges.
c. Vertical mattress: For added strength in areas of thick skin or areas of skin movement; provides eversion of wound edges.
d. Running intradermal: For cosmetic closures.
2. **Procedure**
Note: Lacerations of the face, lips, hands, genitalia, mouth, or periorbital area may require consultation with a specialist. Lacerations to be sutured must be <6 hours old (12 hours on face). In general, bite wounds should not be sutured and, the longer sutures are left in place, the greater the scarring and potential for infection. Sutures in

TABLE 3.1

GUIDELINES FOR SUTURE MATERIAL, SIZE, AND REMOVAL

Body region	Monofilament[a] (for superficial lacerations)	Absorbable[b] (for deep lacerations)	Duration (days)
Scalp	5–0 or 4–0	4–0	5–7
Face	6–0	5–0	3–5
Eyelid	7–0 or 6–0	—	3–5
Eyebrow	6–0 or 5–0	5–0	3–5
Trunk	5–0 or 4–0	3–0	5–7
Extremities	5–0 or 4–0	4–0	7
Joint surface	4–0	—	10–14
Hand	5–0	5–0	7
Foot sole	4–0 or 3–0	4–0	7–10

[a]Examples of monofilament nonabsorbable sutures: Nylon, polypropylene.
[b]Examples of absorbable sutures: Polyglycolic acid and polyglactin 910 (Vicryl).

cosmetically sensitive areas should be removed as soon as possible, whereas sutures in high-tension areas, such as exterior surfaces, should stay in longer.

a. Prepare child for procedure (see p. 43).
b. Securely restrain child.
c. Forcefully irrigate wound with copious amounts of sterile NS. Use at least 250mL for smaller, superficial wounds and more for larger wounds. This is the most important step in preventing infection.
d. Prep and drape the patient for a sterile procedure.
e. Anesthetize the wound with topical anesthetic or with lidocaine/bicarbonate by infusing the anesthetic into the subcutaneous tissues (see p. 895).
f. Debride the wound and probe for foreign bodies. Consider radiograph if a foreign body was involved in injury.
g. Select suture type for percutaneous closure (Table 3.1).
h. When suturing is complete, apply topical antibiotic and sterile dressing. Splinting of the affected arm to limit mobility often speeds healing.
i. Check wounds at 48–72 hours where wounds are of questionable viability, if wound was packed, or for patients prescribed prophylactic antibiotics. Change dressing at check.
j. For hand lacerations, close skin only; do not use subcutaneous stitches. Elevate and immobilize the hand.
k. Consider the child's need for tetanus prophylaxis.

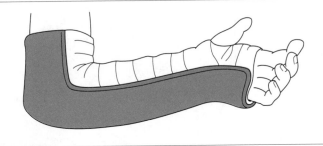

FIG. 3.18
Long arm posterior splint.

VI. MUSCULOSKELETAL

A. BASIC SPLINTING
1. **Indications:** To provide short-term stabilization of limb injuries.
2. **Complications**
a. Pressure sores.
b. Dermatitis.
c. Neurovascular impairment.
3. **Procedure**
a. Determine style of splint needed.
b. Measure and cut plaster to appropriate length, noting that upper extremity splints require 8–10 layers and lower extremity splints require 12–14 layers.
c. Pad extremity with cotton webril, taking care to overlap each turn by 50%. Place cotton in between digits if they are in splint.
d. Immerse plaster slab into room-temperature water.
   Warning: Plaster becomes hot upon drying.
e. Smooth out wet plaster slab, avoiding any wrinkles.
f. Position splint over extremity and wrap externally with gauze. When dry, an elastic wrap can be added.
g. Use crutches or slings as indicated.

B. LONG ARM POSTERIOR SPLINT (Fig. 3.18)
1. **Indications:** Immobilization of elbow and forearm injuries.

C. SUGAR TONG FOREARM SPLINT (Fig. 3.19)
1. **Indications:** For distal radius and wrist fractures, to immobilize the elbow and minimize pronation and supination.

D. POSTERIOR ANKLE SPLINT
1. **Indications:** Immobilization of ankle sprains and fractures of the foot, ankle, and distal fibula.

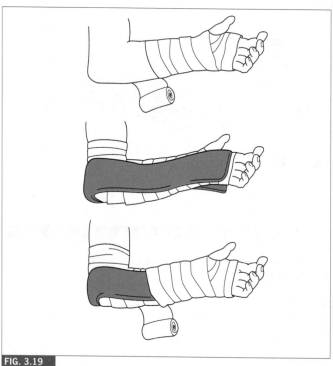

FIG. 3.19

Sugar tong forearm splint.

2. **Procedure:** Measure leg for appropriate length of plaster. The splint should extend to base of toes and the upper portion of calf. A sugar tong splint can be added to increase stability for ankle fractures.

E. **RADIAL HEAD DISLOCATION REDUCTION (NURSEMAID'S ELBOW)**

1. **Presentation:** Commonly occurs in children ages 1–4 years with a history of inability to use an arm after it was pulled. The child presents with the affected arm held at the side in pronation, with elbow slightly flexed.

2. **Caution:** Rule out a fracture clinically (generally by history) or radiographically before doing procedure.

3. **Procedure**

a. Support the elbow with one hand and place your thumb laterally over the radial head at the elbow. With your other hand, grasp the child's hand in a handshake position.

b. Quickly and deliberately supinate the forearm and flex the elbow. Alternatively, hyperpronation alone may be used. You may feel a click as reduction occurs.

c. Most children will begin to use the arm within 15 minutes, some immediately after reduction. If reduction occurs after prolonged period, it may take the child longer to recover use of the arm. In this case, the arm should be immobilized with a posterior splint.

d. Maneuver may be repeated if needed.

VII. REFERENCES

1. Nichols DG, Yaster M, Lappe D, Haller JA. *Golden hour: the handbook of advanced pediatric life support,* St Louis: Mosby; 1996.
2. Fleisher G, Ludwig S. *Pediatric emergency medicine,* 3rd edn. Baltimore: Williams & Wilkins; 1993.
3. Dieckmann R, Fiser D, Selbst S. *Illustrated textbook of pediatric emergency and critical care procedures,* St Louis: Mosby; 1997.
4. Hoberman A, Paradise JL, Wald ER. Tympanocentesis technique revisited. *Pediatr Infect Dis J* 1997; **16(2):**S25–S26

TRAUMA AND BURNS

Adrianna Maria Bravo, MD

I. BASIC TRAUMA PRINCIPLES

A. AIRWAY

1. Immobilize cervical spine with semirigid cervical collar. Consider placing firm padding beneath shoulder to facilitate neutral position of head; a child's prominent occiput predisposes the neck to slight flexion when on a completely flat board. Do not remove collar until cervical spine injury ruled out by radiographs and physical examination (see p. 77).
2. Inspect for foreign body, blood, mucus, or broken teeth.
3. Suction secretions with large-bore (Yankauer) suction catheter.
4. Jaw thrust/spinal stabilization maneuver: Head-tilt/chin-lift contraindicated because of risk of converting an incomplete spinal cord injury to a complete spinal cord injury.
5. Consider oral airway in unconscious child.
6. Intubate if indicated: Respiratory arrest, respiratory failure (hypoventilation, arterial hypoxemia despite supplemental oxygen, and/or respiratory acidosis), airway obstruction, coma (GCS<8), need for prolonged ventilatory support (e.g., thoracic injuries or need for diagnostic studies), airway protection, or inability to ventilate with BVM.
7. Cricothyrotomy may be required when severe orofacial trauma present and occasionally for patient with unstable cervical spine injury. Remember, this maneuver allows for oxygenation but not ventilation (removal of CO_2). See p. 10.

B. BREATHING

1. If airway is patent and respiratory effort effective, administer 100% oxygen by nonrebreather.
2. If respiratory effort is ineffective, administer BVM ventilatory assistance. Hyperventilation will eliminate excess CO_2 (hypocapnia), which can buffer metabolic acidosis associated with shock and hypovolemia, and reduce excessive cerebral blood flow (CBF) after closed head trauma. Overventilation may reduce CBF to ischemic levels, so avoid in situations where CBF may be diminished.
3. Consider orogastric tube for gastric decompression. Distention may compromise ventilation and increase risk of vomiting and aspiration.
4. Inspect chest for open wounds, abrasions, contusions, and overall color.
5. Note abnormal breathing pattern; assess adequacy of ventilation using endtidal CO_2. During arrest/resuscitation, end-tidal CO_2 should be 15–20, otherwise CPR is ineffective.
6. Evaluate for pneumothorax.
   a. Tension pneumothorax presents as severe respiratory distress, distended neck veins, contralateral tracheal deviation, diminished breath sounds, and compromised systemic perfusion by obstruction

of venous return. Treatment: Needle decompression followed by chest tube placement directed toward the lung apex. See p. 58.

b. Open pneumothorax, or sucking chest wound, is rare but allows free flow of air between atmosphere and hemithorax. Treatment: Cover defect with an occlusive dressing (e.g., petroleum jelly gauze), give positive pressure ventilation, and insert a chest tube.

c. Hemothorax treatment: Fluid resuscitation followed by placement of a thoracostomy tube directed posteriorly and inferiorly.

C. CIRCULATION

1. Direct pressure to external bleeding with thin sterile gauze dressings. Avoid tourniquets except in cases of traumatic amputation associated with uncontrolled bleeding from a large vessel.

2. Hypotension not present until 25–30% of the child's blood volume is lost acutely. Heart rate is always a better indicator of circulatory status.

3. Intravenous catheter access with two large-bore catheters. Allow three attempts or 90 seconds.

4. Consider intraosseous needle (patient <8 years old) if access delayed. Then consider percutaneous cannulation of femoral vein or, lastly, resort to saphenous vein cutdown.

5. Fluid therapy

a. Rapid volume replacement with warmed isotonic crystalloid (e.g., lactated Ringer's [LR] solution or NS). Initial treatment of shock should include hemostasis and 20mL/kg bolus of fluid. Assess response by monitoring urine output, skin perfusion, heart rate, capillary refill, central and peripheral pulses, and blood pressure. Another 20mL/kg bolus may be given, and systemic perfusion should be reassessed. After giving three 20mL/kg boluses of fluids, if systemic perfusion remains poor, consider giving colloid, and obtain surgical consultation.

b. If signs of shock persist, resuscitate with 10mL/kg packed RBCs or 20mL/kg whole blood. If type-specific crossmatched blood is not readily available, give O-negative blood. If shock persists despite fluid resuscitation and hemostasis, internal bleeding is likely and emergency surgical consultation is indicated. Medical antishock trousers (MAST) have not been shown to be efficacious in pediatric hemorrhagic shock except in unstable pelvic fractures without associated head injury.

c. When patient is hemodynamically stable, begin maintenance fluids.

6. If increased intracranial pressure (ICP) is suspected, see p. 13.

D. SECONDARY SURVEY
   See Table 4.1.

E. LABORATORY EVALUATION

1. **Hemoglobin/hematocrit**

2. **Liver function enzymes** if suspicious of hepatic injury.

TABLE 4.1

SECONDARY SURVEY

Remove all patient's clothing, and perform thorough head-to-toe examination, with special emphasis on the following. Remember to keep the child warm throughout the examination.

Organ system	Secondary survey
Head	Scalp/skull injury.
	Raccoon eyes: Periorbital ecchymosis, which suggests orbital roof fracture.
	Battle's sign: Ecchymosis behind pinna, which suggests mastoid fracture.
	Cerebrospinal fluid (CSF) leak from ears/nose or hemotympanum suggests basilar skull fracture.
	Pupil size, symmetry, and reactivity: Unilateral dilatation of one pupil suggests compression of cranial nerve III (CNIII) and possibly impending herniation; bilateral dilatation of pupils is ominous and suggests bilateral CNIII compression or severe anoxia and ischemia.
	Corneal reflex.
	Fundoscopic examination for papilledema as evidence of increased ICP.
	Hyphema.
Neck	Cervical spine tenderness, deformity, injury.
	Trachea midline.
	Subcutaneous emphysema.
Chest	Clavicle deformity, tenderness.
	Breath sounds, heart sounds.
	Chest wall symmetry, paradoxical movement, rib deformity/fracture.
	Petechiae over chest/head suggest traumatic asphyxia.

Continued

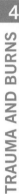

4

TRAUMA AND BURNS

TABLE 4.1

SECONDARY SURVEY—cont'd

Organ system	Secondary survey
Abdomen	Serial examinations to evaluate tenderness, distention, ecchymosis.
	Shoulder pain suggests referred subdiaphragmatic process.
	Orogastric aspirates with blood or bile suggest intraabdominal injury.
	Splenic laceration suggested by left upper quadrant rib tenderness, flank pain, and/or flank ecchymosis.
Pelvis	Tenderness, symmetry, deformity, stability.
Genitourinary	Laceration, ecchymosis, hematoma, bleeding.
	Rectal tone, blood, displaced prostate.
	Blood at urinary meatus suggests urethral injury; do not catheterize.
Back	Step-off along spinal column.
	Tenderness.
	Open or penetrating wound.
Extremities	Neurovascular status: Pulse, perfusion, pallor, paresthesias, paralysis, pain.
	Deformity, crepitus, pain.
	Motor/sensory examination.
	Compartment syndrome: Pain out of proportion to expected; distal pallor/pulselessness. See pp. 587–588.
Neurologic	See p. 461 for thorough examination.
Skin	Capillary refill, perfusion.
	Lacerations, abrasions.
	Contusion:
	Blue-purple: ≤1 day old. Brown: 10–14 days old.
	Green: 5–7 day old. Resolution: 2–4 weeks old.
	Yellow: 7–10 days old.

3. Blood type and crossmatch
4. **Urinalysis:** Assess for microscopic or gross hematuria (see p. 79).
5. Consider toxicology screen
6. **Review tetanus status** (see p. 353)
F. **BASIC RADIOLOGIC EVALUATION**
1. Cervical spine (C spine)
a. Obtain PA view, lateral view to include 7th cervical vertebra, and odontoid view. Additional flexion and extension views of the C spine should be obtained if point tenderness or symptoms on palpation or any suspicion of abnormality on PA or lateral view. Flexion and extension views may be contraindicated if an unstable C-spine injury is suspected.
b. Cervical spine injury is more likely to occur in children with an acceleration–deceleration injury such as a motor vehicle accident or fall. Assume cervical spine injury in the child with multiple injuries of any cause. Neurologic recovery after acute spinal cord injury is improved with prompt administration of methylprednisolone 30mg/kg IV loading dose, followed by 5.4mg/kg/hr IV infusion[1].
c. Common patterns of injury
   1) Infants and toddlers: Subluxation of atlantoocciptal joint (skull base–C1) or atlantoaxial joint (C1–C2).
   2) School-age children: Lower cervical spine involvement (C5–C6).
d. SCIWORA: **S**pinal **C**ord **I**njury **W**ith **O**ut **R**adiographic **A**bnormality; a functional cervical spine injury that cannot be excluded by abnormality on a radiograph; thought to be attributable to the increased mobility of a child's spine. Suspect in the setting of normal C-spine images, when clinical signs or symptoms (e.g., point tenderness or focal neurologic symptoms) suggest C-spine injury. If neurologic symptoms persist despite normal C-spine and flexion/extension views, MRI is indicated to rule out swelling or intramedullary hemorrhage of the spinal cord.
e. Reading C-spine films: The following **ABCD's** mnemonic is useful:
   1) **A**lignment: The anterior vertebral body line, posterior vertebral body line, facet line, and spinous process line should each form a straight line with smooth contour and no step-offs.
   2) **B**ones: Assess each bone looking for chips or fractures.
   3) **C**ount: Must see C7 body in its entirety.
   4) **D**ens: Examine for chips or fractures.
   5) **D**isc spaces: Should see consistent distance between each vertebral body.
   6) **S**oft tissue: Assess for swelling, especially in the prevertebral area.
f. Clinically clear the C spine: Patient must be awake; examiner must palpate posterior neck for localized tenderness. If no pain, assess active and passive range of motion. If any direct pain over bone, C collar should be maintained until further evaluation can definitively rule out injury.
2. **Chest radiograph:** Evaluate lung fields, cardiac silhouette, and bony structures; rib fractures indicate severe chest trauma and are associated with visceral injury.

4

TRAUMA AND BURNS

3. **Pelvic films**
4. **Abdominal film:** Consider based on history and examination.
5. **Facial films:** Consider based on history and examination.
a. Le Fort classification of facial fractures (Fig. 4.1).
6. **Extremity film:** Consider if fracture is suspected.
a. Fracture patterns unique to children (Fig. 4.2).
b. Ligaments are stronger than bone or growth plates in children; thus dislocations and sprains are relatively uncommon, whereas growth plate disruption and bone avulsion are more common.
c. Growth plate injuries are classified by the Salter–Harris classification (Table 4.2)
G. **SPECIAL STUDIES**
1. **Head CT:** Indicated for loss of consciousness, change in mental status, seizures, amnesia, focal neurologic deficit, severe headache, or persistent emesis.
2. **Abdominal CT:** If suspected abdominal trauma; oral contrast should be avoided if bowel perforation suspected. Evidence of microscopic or gross hematuria warrants CT scan with IV contrast to rule out renal trauma. Any localizing abdominal signs or symptoms warrant CT scan

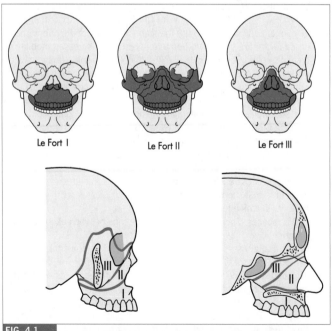

Le Fort I   Le Fort II   Le Fort III

FIG. 4.1

Le Fort fractures. (Redrawn from May[2].)

with IV contrast to rule out laceration to liver or spleen or damage to other abdominal viscera.

3. **Retrograde cystourethrogram:** If CT scan normal and gross hematuria persists; to rule out bladder and/or urethral injury. Foley catheter should not be inserted if there is gross blood at the urethral meatus.

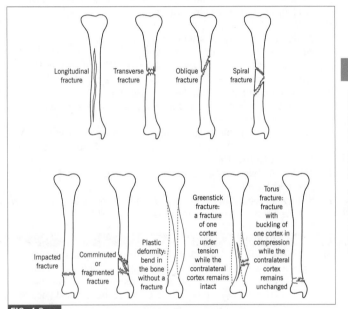

FIG. 4.2

Fracture patterns unique to children. (Modified from Ogden[3].)

4

TRAUMA AND BURNS

TABLE 4.2

SALTER-HARRIS CLASSIFICATION OF GROWTH PLATE INJURY

Class I	Class II	Class III	Class IV	Class V
Fracture along growth plate	Fracture along growth plate with metaphyseal extension	Fracture along growth plate with epiphyseal extension	Fracture across growth plate, including metaphysis and epiphysis	Crush injury to growth plate without obvious fracture

4. **Compartment pressure measurement:** If increased compartment pressure suspected. See p. 587.
5. **Echocardiography:** Indicated to detect cardiac contusion or wall motion abnormality.
6. **Diagnostic peritoneal lavage (DPL):** Useful to rule out blood or intestinal contents in the abdomen; indicated in patient with severe head injury requiring emergent surgery.

H. MONITORING
1. **Cardiac monitor, oxygen saturation monitor**
2. **Vital signs,** including body temperature
   a. Cushing's response of bradycardia, increased BP, and abnormal respiratory pattern may be late findings in increased ICP.
3. **Glasgow Coma Scale (GCS):** Serial assessment; p. 14.
4. **Follow urine output;** recommend Foley catheter unless blood at meatus or displaced prostate.
5. **Orogastric tube for decompression;** consider nonparticulate antacid or IV H_2 blocker to reduce pulmonary consequence if aspiration occurs.

I. AMPLE AND HISTORY
1. **AMPLE:** **A**llergies, **M**edications, **P**ast illnesses, **L**ast meal, **E**vents preceding the injury.
2. **History of events:** Get a history of events surrounding traumatic injury and the history of present complaints.

II. MINOR CLOSED HEAD TRAUMA (CHT)

A. INTRODUCTION: Injury to the brain parenchyma or vasculature can be caused by a variety of mechanisms including direct laceration, blunt force, rotational acceleration, or acceleration–deceleration injury. CHT may result in depressed or nondepressed skull fracture, epidural hematoma, subdural hematoma, brain edema, deep shearing injuries of nerve fibers (diffuse axonal injury, DAI), altered CBF with resultant ischemic injury, increased ICP, brain herniation, and/or concussion. The term 'concussion' can be applied to a clinical syndrome resulting from traumatic forces; it is characterized by immediate and transient impairment of neural function, such as alteration of consciousness, amnesia, or disturbance of vision or equilibrium. CHT not warranting intensive care or surgical management can be termed 'minor CHT' and should be managed according to the following principles.

B. EVALUATION
1. **Initial assessment:** Follow basic trauma principles.
2. **Physical examination:** Including careful neurologic evaluation.
3. **Associated symptoms:** Loss of consciousness (LOC), amnesia (before, during, or after the event), mental status change, behavior change, seizure activity, vomiting, headache, gait disturbance, visual change, level of consciousness and activity since time of event.

4. **Mechanism of injury**
a. Linear forces are less likely to cause LOC; they more commonly lead to skull fractures, intracranial hematoma, or cerebral contusion.
b. Rotational forces commonly cause LOC associated with/without DAI.
c. If mechanism of injury is not consistent with sustained injuries, suspect abuse.
5. **Medications and illicit drug use:** These are helpful in determining complete etiology of mental status changes in a patient.
6. **Assess for wounds**

C. **MANAGEMENT**
1. **Initial management:** According to basic trauma principles with attention to ABCs, secondary survey, C-spine immobilization, and basic radiologic evaluation. Apply basic wound management to any lacerations sustained to the scalp or face.
2. **CT scan of head:** This is warranted in the child with documented LOC. In the child with an unwitnessed event, unknown LOC, or no documented LOC, the decision to perform head CT must be based on the mechanism of injury, severity of known injuries, and persistence of complaints or deficits. Confusion and amnesia can occur without loss of consciousness and may not always warrant head CT when present without other concerns or complaints.
3. **Observation:** In all children with minor CHT, observation under medical supervision for at least 4 hours allows for detection of delayed signs or symptoms of intracranial injury. Delayed signs and symptoms more commonly occur with epidural bleeds in which a symptom-free lucid period can precede variable degrees of acute-onset mental status change. The patient should also be observed carefully for at least 4–48 hours after any CHT. The decision of where (home vs hospital) to continue this observation period can be based on the degree of identified injury or associated injuries, reliable follow-up and care by the parent/guardian, and persistence of symptoms.
4. **Indications for hospitalization**[2]
a. Depressed or declining level of consciousness or prolonged unconsciousness.
b. Neurologic deficit.
c. Increasing headache or persistent vomiting.
d. Seizures.
e. CSF otorrhea or rhinorrhea; hemotympanum.
f. Linear skull fracture crossing the groove of the middle meningeal artery, a venous sinus of the dura, or the foramen magnum.
g. Compound skull fracture or fracture into the frontal sinus.
h. Depressed skull fracture.
i. Bleeding disorder or patient receiving anticoagulation therapy.
j. Intoxication or illness obscuring neurologic state.
k. Suspected child abuse.

4

TRAUMA AND BURNS

5. **For observation at home:** Indications for reevaluation include excessive sleepiness, more than two episodes of emesis, gait disturbance, severe headache not relieved with standard doses of acetaminophen or ibuprofen, drainage of blood or liquid from nose or ears, visual change, unequal pupil size, and/or seizure activity.

6. **For information on concussions,** when sustained in the setting of sports activity and for recommendations on return to play, see *Guidelines for the Management of Concussion in Sports*[4].

III. BITES

A. **INTRODUCTION:** Characteristics of the bite wound, location, offending species, and wound management will determine the outcome of bite injuries. The spectrum of injury ranges from scratches, abrasions, crushing, and contusions, to punctures, tears, lacerations, and those complicated by superinfection. Oral aerobic and anaerobic species are inoculated into the wound at the time of the bite. In addition, super-infection can occur with an even broader range of organisms. It is always important to identify and isolate the offending animal whenever possible.

B. **WOUND CONSIDERATIONS**

1. **Wound location:** Consider the potential for damage or infection of underlying structures including tendon sheaths, bones, vessels, and nerves. Radiographs should be considered for deep bite wounds in which there is the possibility of foreign body, bone disruption, or fracture, especially when involving the scalp or hand. For bites in the periorbital area, ophthamologic evaluation is suggested to rule out corneal abrasion, lacrimal duct involvement, and/or ocular damage. Bites of the hand are prone to infection because tendons, vessels, compartments, and bones all occupy a small and compact area. Osteomyelitis is common in hand infections secondary to bites. Bites to the nose must be evaluated for tears or disturbances of cartilage.

2. **Animal species**

a. Dog bite: Usually crush injury resulting in infection-prone devitalized tissue. Common organisms include *Staphylococcus aureus* and *Pasteurella multocida*.

b. Cat bite: Typically deep puncture wound; wound hygiene difficult; increased risk of infection. *Pasteurella multocida* is the most common organism inoculated; may present in a fulminant manner with rapid development of erythema, swelling, and pain in 12–24 hours. These infections respond slowly to drainage and appropriate antibiotics. Cat scratches are common and have increased risk of superinfection compared with scratches from other domestic animals; the complication of cat scratch disease should be considered in anyone presenting with regional lymphadenitis and/or fever and malaise 2 weeks after cat scratch. Cat scratch disease is more commonly seen after kitten scratch. Rarely, cat bites can also cause tularemia.

c. Human bite: In teens, this commonly involves injury to the hand after fist-to-mouth contact. In younger children, a bite to the face or trunk is more common. Consider child abuse when human bites are involved; with self-inflicted bites, patient's psychiatric health should be assessed. Consider risk of spread of systemic infection, such as hepatitis B, herpes simplex virus, and syphilis. Organisms most commonly isolated include *Streptococcus viridans* and *Staphylococcus aureus*; in addition, *Bacteroides* and *Peptostretococcus* spp. are frequently cultured. More serious morbidity of human bites correlates with *S. aureus* and *Eikenella corrodens* infection.

d. Rodent bite: Low incidence of secondary infection; rat bite fever is rare but can present with fever, chills, headache, malaise, and rash 1–3 weeks after bite. Causative agents, *Streptobacillus moniliformis* and *Spirillum minus,* are sensitive to IV penicillin.

e. Rabbit bites: *Francisella tularensis* causing tularemia, most frequently of the ulceroglandular type, is spread to humans via rabbit bites, contact with infected animals, or ingestion of infected animals.

C. MANAGEMENT

1. **Wound hygiene:** The risk of infection can be minimized with proper irrigation (19G needle and 35mL syringe provides 8lb/in^2 water pressure, using a minimum 200mL NS) and debridement of all devitalized tissue, foreign bodies, and contaminants in the wound. Only 1% povidone–iodine should be used for cleansing, as stronger antiseptics may damage wound surface and delay healing. Peroxide should not be used because it prevents migration of white blood cells into the wound. Cultures of wounds are indicated if evidence of infection is present, which also necessitates IV antibiotics.

2. **Closure:** Wounds at high risk of infection include puncture wounds, minor hand or foot wounds, wounds with care delayed beyond 12 hours, cat or human bite wounds, and wounds in asplenic or immunosuppressed patients. In general, these wounds should not be sutured. Wounds that involve tendons, joints, deep fascial layers, or major vasculature should be evaluated by a plastic or hand surgeon and, if indicated, closed in the operating room.

a. Suturing: When indicated, closure should be done with minimal number of simple interrupted nylon sutures, and loose approximation of wound edges. Deep sutures should be avoided.

b. Head and neck: Can usually be safely sutured (with the exceptions as noted above) after copious irrigation and wound debridement if within 6–8 hours of injury and with no signs of infection. Facial wounds often require primary closure for cosmetic reasons; infection risk is lower given the good vascular supply.

TRAUMA AND BURNS

4

c. Extremities: In large hand wounds, one should close the subcutaneous dead space with minimal absorbable suture and then perform delayed cutaneous closure in 3–5 days if there is no evidence of infection.

3. **Antibiotics:** Prophylactic antibiotics are indicated for, and limited to, wounds at risk for infection, as listed under Closure. Some superficial human bites may not require prophylactic antibiotics. Antibiotics should cover for *P. multocida*, staphylococci, streptococci, and oral anaerobes. The drug of choice, considering resistant strains and spectrum of activity, would be amoxicillin/clavulanic acid. Trimethoprim–sulfamethoxazole in combination with clindamycin is an alternative for the penicillin-allergic patient. Initial doses started in emergency room; continue 3–5 days.

4. **Rabies and tetanus prophylaxis:** See pp. 353 and 369.

5. Disposition

a. Outpatient care: Careful follow-up of all bite wounds, especially those requiring surgical closure, within 24–48 hours. Extremity, especially hand wounds, should be immobilized in position of function and kept elevated. Local care is of paramount importance; wound should be kept clean and dry. Signs and symptoms of infection should be discussed.

b. Inpatient care: Consider hospitalization, for observation and/or parenteral antibiotics, for significant human bites, immunocompromised or asplenic hosts, established deep or severe infections, bites associated with systemic complaints, bites with significant functional or cosmetic morbidity, and/or unreliable follow-up or care by the parent/guardian. Hospitalization and IV antibiotics should be considered for the subsequently infected wound.

6. **The infected wound:** Drainage and debridement are required for wounds that subsequently become infected. Gram stain and aerobic/anaerobic cultures should be performed before start or change of antibiotics; in the case of cellulitis, aspirate cultures of leading edges may be useful. If deep tissue layers or structures are involved, exploration and debridement under general anesthesia may be indicated.

IV. BURNS

A. EVALUATION OF PEDIATRIC BURNS (Tables 4.3 and 4.4)

Note: The extent and severity of burn injury may change over the first few days after injury; therefore, be cautious in discussing prognosis with the victim's family.

B. BURN MAPPING (Fig. 4.3)

1. **Burn assessment chart:** Use chart to map areas of second- and third-degree burns.

TABLE 4.3

BURNS

Type of burn	Description/comment
Flame	Most common type of burn; when clothing burns, the exposure to heat is prolonged, and the severity of the burn is worse.
Scald/contact	Mortality is similar to that in flame burns when total BSA involved is equal; see p. 91 for description of patterns of scald injury and burns suspicious of intentional injury.
Chemical	Tissue damaged by protein coagulation or liquefaction rather than hyperthermic activity.
Electrical	Injury is often extensive involving skeletal muscle and other tissues in excess of the skin damage. Extent of damage may not be initially apparent. The tissues that have the least resistance are the most heat sensitive. Bone has the greatest resistance, nerve tissue the least. A cardiac arrest may occur from passage of the current through the heart.
Inhalation	Present in 30% of victims of major burns and should be considered when there is evidence of fire in enclosed space, singed nares, facial burns, charred lips, carbonaceous secretions, posterior pharynx edema, hoarseness, cough, or wheezing. Inhalation injury increases mortality.
Cold injury/frostbite	Freezing results in direct tissue injury. Toes, fingers, ears, and nose are commonly involved. Initial treatment includes rewarming in tepid (105–110°F) water for 20–40 min. Excision of tissue should not be done until complete demarcation of nonviable tissue has occurred.

4

TRAUMA AND BURNS

TABLE 4.4

BURN DEGREE

Burn depth/degree	Description/comment
First degree	Only epidermis involved; painful and erythematous
Second degree	Epidermis and dermis involved, but dermal appendages spared. Superficial second-degree burns are blistered and painful. Any blistering qualifies as second-degree burn. Deep second-degree burns may be white and painless, require grafting, and progress to full-thickness burns with wound infection.
Third degree	Full-thickness burns involving epidermis and all of the dermis, including dermal appendages; leathery and painless; require grafting.

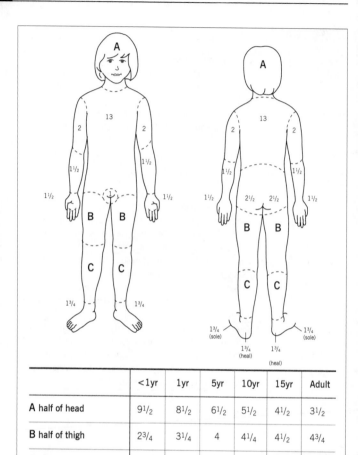

	<1yr	1yr	5yr	10yr	15yr	Adult
A half of head	9½	8½	6½	5½	4½	3½
B half of thigh	2¾	3¼	4	4¼	4½	4¾
C half of leg	2½	2½	2¾	3	3¼	3½

FIG. 4.3
Burn assessment chart. (From Barkin[5].)

2. **Calculate total BSA burned,** based only on percent of second- and third-degree burns.

C. **MANAGEMENT OF PEDIATRIC BURNS**

1. **Acute stabilization:** Special considerations of basic trauma principles.

a. Airway

1) Intubation: For pulmonary toilet or if there is evidence of inhalation. Neuromuscular blockade with succinylcholine for intubation is

appropriate for ≤48 hours postburn but is contraindicated after this time frame because of risk of worsening hyperkalemia. For alternative, see p. 3.

2) Inhalation injury: All patients with large burns and/or closed space burns should be assumed to have CO poisoning until examination and evaluation of blood carboxyhemoglobin is undertaken (see p. 27). Humidified 100% O_2 should be administered during initial assessment. Delivery of 100% O_2 counteracts the effects of CO and speeds its clearance. Carboxyhemoglobin absorbs light at the same wavelength as oxyhemoglobin, so oxygen saturation, as determined by pulse oximetry, is not altered; must obtain a Pao_2.

a) Cyanide poisoning, via inhalation of combustible materials, can produce almond-scented breath and may cause profound positive anion gap metabolic acidosis. See p. 28.

b. Breathing
1) Monitor pulmonary status with serial arterial blood gases (ABGs).
2) Increasing tachypnea may be seen in patients with pulmonary insufficiency caused by acute asphyxia and CO toxicity, upper airway obstruction secondary to edema, or overwhelming parenchymal damage.

c. Circulation: Initial fluid resuscitation: Start IV fluid resuscitation of infants with burns >10% of BSA (body surface area), children with burns >15% BSA, or children with evidence of smoke inhalation. Consider bolus of 20mL/kg LR or NS plus maintenance fluids to maintain a urine output of 0.5–2mL/kg per hour. In the hypotensive patient, manage the cardiovascular status according to basic trauma principles before initiating fluid resuscitation.

d. Secondary survey: Consider associated injuries. Electrical injury can produce deep tissue damage, intravascular thrombosis, cardiac and respiratory arrest, fractures secondary to muscle contraction, and cardiac arrhythmias. Look for exit site for electrical injury. Motor vehicle accidents, falls, or explosions may result in associated head, visceral, or bone injuries.

e. Laboratory evaluation: Consider CBC, type and crossmatch, carboxyhemoglobin, coagulation studies, chemistry panel, ABGs, and chest radiograph (may not show changes for 24–72 hours).

f. GI: Placement of nasogastric tube for decompression; make patient nothing by mouth (NPO); begin stress ulcer prophylaxis with H_2-receptor blockers and antacids.

g. Bladder decompression and urine output monitor with Foley catheter.

h. Cardiac: Consider ECG.

i. Eye: Careful examination for burns or abrasions with referral to ophthalmology if suspected.

j. Special considerations
1) Tetanus immunoprophylaxis: see p. 353.

2) Temperature management: Cooling decreases the severity of the burn if administered within 30 minutes of injury; it also helps to relieve pain. If burn <10% of BSA, apply clean towels soaked in cold water to help prevent burn progression. In patient with burns comprising >10% BSA, apply clean dry towels to burn to avoid hypothermia. Do not use grease, butter, etc.

3) Chemical burns: It is important to wash away or neutralize the chemical. Except in rare circumstances, the most efficacious first-aid treatment for chemical burns is lavaging with copious volumes of water for about 20 minutes.

4) Analgesia: IV analgesia is often necessary to treat pain. Do not attribute combativeness or anxiety to pain until adequate perfusion and oxygenation are established. Consider morphine 0.1mg/kg IV or Demerol 1mg/kg IV/PO (see pp. 586–587, for details).

2. **Triage and management of pediatric burns**
a. Outpatient management
   1) Considerations: If burn <10% of infant BSA or <15% of child's BSA, and involves no full-thickness areas, patient may be treated as an outpatient.
   2) Management
      a) Cleanse with warm saline or mild soap and water. Consider debridement with forceps or sterile gauze to pick up the edges and peel it off of the base of the burn. Leave blisters intact.
      b) Apply topical antibacterial agent (Table 4.5).
      c) Daily follow-up is recommended.
      d) Have patient cleanse burn at home twice daily with mild soap followed by application of an antibacterial agent and sterile dressing, as above. Once epithelialization has begun, may reduce to daily dressing change.
      e) Pain management: Oxycodone or ibuprofen at recommended pediatric doses.
b. Inpatient management
   1) Considerations: Inpatient management should be considered for more extensive burns; electrical or chemical burns; burns of critical areas such as face, hands, feet, perineum, or joints; burns suspicious of abuse or unsafe home environment; and burns in a child with underlying chronic illness, evidence of smoke inhalation, cyanide poisoning, or CO poisoning. Consider transfer to a burn center if any of the following conditions are satisfied: burns of at least 20–30% BSA; major burns to the hand, face, joints, perineum; electrical burns; or burns associated with potentially life-threatening injuries.
   2) Fluid therapy: Provide sufficient fluid to prevent shock and renal failure from excessive fluid losses and third spacing. Assess adequacy of perfusion using urine output, blood pressure, heart rate, peripheral circulation, and sensorium. Monitor electrolytes and ABGs for

TABLE 4.5

TOPICAL ANTIBACTERIAL AGENTS

Agent	Action	Side effects	Use
Silver sulfadiazine (Silvadene)	Broad antibacterial, painless, fair eschar penetration	Sulfonamide sensitivity, occasional leukopenia, contraindicated in pregnancy	Q12hr; cover with light dressings; leave face and chest open
Bacitracin ointment	Limited antibacterial action, poor eschar penetration, transparent, easy to apply	Rapid development of resistance; conjunctivitis if contact with eye	Q12hr, apply to small areas; acceptable with facial burns
Mafenide (Sulfamylon)	Excellent antibacterial for Gram-positive and Gram-negative and *Clostridium*, rapid eschar penetration	Painful, sulfonamide sensitivity, carbonic anhydrase inhibition may lead to acidosis	Q12hr; cover with light dressings; leave face, chest, abdomen open
Aqueous silver nitrate solution	Universal antibacterial action, poor eschar penetration	Strong tissue staining, hypochloremic alkalosis	Q12hr, light gauze dressing
Iodophores (Efodine)	Universal antibacterial action, poor eschar penetration	Strong tissue staining, iodine absorption	Q12hr, light gauze dressing

4

TRAUMA AND BURNS

acidosis. Use one of two formulas below as guidelines to estimate fluid need. Consider central venous access for burns >25% BSA.

a) Galveston formula

    i) First 24 hours: Give 5000mL/m^2 of burned surface area (burn losses) plus 2000mL/m^2 of total BSA (maintenance fluids) over the first 24 hours; infuse half of the burn losses and 1/3 of maintenance of this over the first 8 hours, calculated from time of burn injury. Deduct fluid already given en route to the referral center from burn losses calculation. For children >1 year, use LR plus 12.5g of 25% albumin/L. For infants <1 year, prepare a 1L solution of 930mL of 1/3 NS, 20mL $NaHCO_3$ (1mEq/mL), and 50mL of 25% albumin.

    ii) Second and subsequent days: Give 3750mL/m^2 of burned surface area per 24 hours (burn losses) plus 1500mL/m^2 of total BSA per 24 hours (maintenance fluids). As sodium requirements after first 24 hours are less, use D_5 1/3 NS with 20–30mEq/L potassium phosphate (because of frequent hypophosphatemia).

    iii) Reevaluate fluid requirements as wounds heal. Assess wounds weekly, and document on burn map.

b) Parkland formula: Note that this formula provides for replacement and losses, not maintenance fluids, so one must add maintenance fluid requirements.

    i) First 24 hours: Give 4mL/kg per % BSA burned over the first 24 hours; give half of total over the first 8 hours calculated from the time of injury. Give the remaining half over the next 16 hours.

    ii) Second 24 hours: Fluid requirements average 50–75% of the first day's requirements. Determine concentrations and rates by monitoring weight, serum electrolytes, urine output, nasogastric losses, etc.

    iii) Consider adding colloid after 18–24 hours (albumin 1g/kg per day) to maintain serum albumin >2g/dL.

    iv) Withhold potassium generally for the first 48 hours because of large release of potassium from damaged tissues. To manage electrolytes most effectively, monitor urine electrolytes twice weekly and replace urine losses accordingly. Urine output should be maintained at 0.5mL/kg per hour.

3. **Prevention of burns:** Measures include child-proofing the home, installing smoke detectors, and turning hot water tap temperature down to 49–52°C (it takes 2 minutes of immersion at 52°C to cause a full-thickness burn, compared with 5 seconds of immersion at 60°C).

V. ABUSE

A. **INTRODUCTION:** Involve the medical professional, social worker, and community agencies such as emergency medical service providers, police, social services, and prosecutors.

B. **MANAGEMENT:** The medical professional should suspect, diagnose, treat, report, and document all cases of child abuse, neglect, or maltreatment.

1. **Suspect:** Be suspicious whenever there is inconsistent or inadequate history of injury, inappropriate parental response to the situation, delay in seeking medical attention, discrepancy between mechanism of injury and physical examination findings, evidence of neglect or failure to thrive, evidence of disturbed emotions or expressions in a child, prior history of suspicious events, or parental substance abuse.

2. **Diagnose:** Characteristic or concerning injuries.

a. Bruises: Shape, color, and dating of bruise are important (see Table 4.1, pp. 75–76); correlate with history. Looped marks or railroad track marks may indicate injury from cords, belts, and ropes.

b. Bites: Shape, size, and location are important; correlate with history and dental anatomy of questioned perpetrator. Intercanine distances of >3cm are suggestive of human bites; they generally crush more than lacerate. Saliva samples can be taken from fresh bites.

c. Burns: Absence of splash marks and/or clearly demarcated edges are suggestive of intentional injury. Stocking glove patterns, symmetrically burned buttocks and/or lower legs, spared inguinal creases, and symmetric involvement of palms or soles all suggest intentional injury.

d. Hemorrhage: Retinal hemorrhages are suggestive of abuse and always warrant evaluation for intentional head trauma. Duodenal hematoma, causing eventual upper GI obstruction, secondary to blunt trauma is suspicious for intentional injury.

e. Skeletal injury: Correlate mechanism of injury with physical finding; rule out any underlying bony pathology.

   1) Long bones: Classic fracture of abuse is the epiphyseal/metaphyseal chip fracture, seen as the 'bucket handle' or 'corner' fracture at the end of the long bones, secondary to jerking or shaking of a child's limb. Spiral fractures may be suspicious of abuse, especially if no history of rotational force is given as mechanism of injury.

   2) Ribs: Usually nondisplaced, often posterior near attachment to spine; may not be readily visible on acute plain films. Pleural thickening, pleural fluid, and contusion may suggest an undetected rib fracture. Fractures are secondary to direct blows or severe squeezing of rib cage. Closed chest compressions from

4

TRAUMA AND BURNS

cardiopulmonary resuscitation do not appear to cause rib fractures in children.

3) Skull: Fractures suggestive of force greater than that sustained with minor household trauma are suspicious for abuse; these include fractures >3mm wide, complex fractures, bilateral fractures, and nonparietal fractures.

f. Genital injury: Vaginal bleeding in the prepubertal female or injury to external genitalia, especially posterior region, are suspicious for abuse. Hymen should be examined for irregularity outside the realm of normal variation. A normal examination does not rule out abuse. Anus should be evaluated for bruising, laceration, hemorrhoids, scars that extend beyond the anal verge, absence of anal wink, and evidence of infection such as genital warts. Circumferential hematoma of the anal sphincter is associated with forced penetration.

g. Shaken baby syndrome: Classically presents with retinal hemorrhages, long bone or rib fractures, and CNS dysfunction such as seizure, apnea, or lethargy secondary to intracranial injury; usually in children <6 months of age.

3. **Useful studies**

a. Skeletal surveys, not simply a 'babygram', are suggested to evaluate suspicious bony trauma in any child; mandatory for children <2 years of age.

b. Bone scan may be indicated to identify early or difficult-to-detect bone fractures.

c. CT scan of the head is unreliable for detection of skull fractures but useful in detecting intracranial pathology secondary to trauma.

d. MRI may identify lesions not detected by CT scan, for example, posterior fossa injury involvement and diffuse axonal injury; also provides more useful information about the dating of injuries identified.

e. Ophthalmologic evaluation for retinal hemorrhages is useful in suspected shaken baby syndrome.

4. **Treat:** Refer to basic principles of trauma management. Special attention should be paid to 'stabilizing' the existing and immediate environment of the child (utilizing available social and protective services) so as to protect the child from incurring further injury during the work-up.

5. **Report:** All health care providers are required by law to report suspected maltreatment of a child to the local police and/or welfare agency. Suspicion, supported by objective evidence, is criterion for reporting and should first be discussed with not only the rest of the involved medical team but also the family. The professional who makes such reports is immune from any civil or criminal liability.

6. **Document:** Write legibly, carefully documenting the following: reported and suspected history and mechanisms of injury; any history given by the victim in his/her own words (use quotation marks); information provided by other providers or services; and physical examination findings, including drawings of injuries and details of dimensions, color, shape, and texture. Remember, 'r/o abuse' is a plan, not a diagnosis. When in doubt, err on side of protecting the child until further evaluation or evidence can confirm or deny your suspicions.

VI. REFERENCES

1. Bracken MB, Shepard MJ, Collins WF, et al. A randomised, controlled trial of methylprednisolone or naloxone in the treatment of acute spinal-cord injury: results of the Second National Acute Spinal Cord Injury Study. *N Engl J Med* 1990; **322(20):**1405-1411.
2. May HL, ed. *Emergency medicine*, Vol. 1, 2nd edn, Boston: Little, Brown; 1992.
3. Ogden JA. *Skeletal injury in the child,* 2nd edn. Philadelphia: WB Saunders, 1990.
4. Sports Medicine Council. *Guidelines for the management of concussion in sports.* Denver: Colorado Medical Society; 1991.
5. Barkin RM, Rosen P. *Emergency pediatrics: a guide to ambulatory care,* 4th edn, St Louis: Mosby; 1994.

4

TRAUMA AND BURNS

PART II

Diagnostic and Therapeutic Information

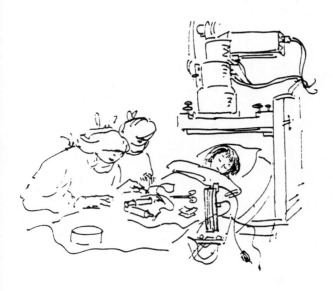

ADOLESCENT MEDICINE

Diane M. Straub, MD, MPH

I. RECOMMENDED CONTENT FOR ROUTINE ADOLESCENT HEALTH VISIT[1,2]

A. MEDICAL HISTORY: Immunizations, chronic illness, chronic medications (including hormonal contraception), recent dental care, hospitalizations, surgeries.

B. FAMILY HISTORY: Psychiatric disorders, suicide, alcoholism/substance abuse.

C. REVIEW OF SYSTEMS

1. **Dietary habits:** Typical foods consumed, types and frequency of meals skipped, vomiting, use of laxatives or other weight-loss methods, dietary sources of calcium.
2. Recent weight gain or loss

D. PSYCHOSOCIAL/MEDICOSOCIAL HISTORY (HEADSS)

1. **H(ome)**
   a. Household composition.
   b. Family dynamics and relationships with adolescent.
   c. Living/sleeping arrangements.
   d. Guns in the home.

2. **E(ducation)**
   a. School attendance/absences.
   b. Ever failed a grade(s); grades as compared to last year's?
   c. Attitude toward school.
   d. Favorite, most difficult, best subjects.
   e. Special educational needs.
   f. Goals: vocational/technical school, college, career.

3. **A(ctivities)**
   a. Physical activity, exercise, hobbies.
   b. Sports participation.
   c. Job.
   d. Weapon carrying and fighting.

4. **D(rugs)**
   a. Cigarettes/smokeless tobacco: Age at first use, packs per day.
   b. Alcohol and/or other drugs: Use at school or parties; use by friends, self; kind (i.e., beer, wine coolers), frequency, and quantity used. If yes, CAGE: Have you ever felt the need to **C**ut down; have others **A**nnoyed you by commenting on your use; have you ever felt **G**uilty about your use; have you ever needed an **E**yeopener (alcohol first thing in morning)?

5. **S(exuality)**
   a. Sexual feelings: Opposite or same sex.
   b. Sexual intercourse: Age at first intercourse, number of lifetime and current partners, recent change in partners.

   c. Contraception/sexually transmitted disease (STD) prevention.
   d. History of STDs.
   e. Prior pregnancies, abortions; ever fathered a child?
   f. History of/current nonconsensual intimate physical contact/sex.

6. S(uicide)/depression
   a. Feelings about self: Positive and negative.
   b. History of depression or other mental health problems, prior suicidal thoughts, prior suicide attempts.
   c. Sleep problems: Difficulty getting to sleep, early waking.

E. PHYSICAL EXAMINATION (MOST PERTINENT ASPECTS)
1. Skin: Acne (type and distribution of lesions).
2. Thyroid
3. Spine: Scoliosis (see pp. 116–117 for assessment and treatment).
4. Breasts: Tanner stage (Fig. 5.1 and Table 5.1), masses.
5. External genitalia
   a. Pubic hair distribution: Tanner stage (Figs 5.1 and 5.2 and Table 5.2).
   b. Testicular examination: Tanner stage (Fig. 5.2 and Table 5.3), masses.
6. Pelvic examination: Sexually active, gynecologic compliant.

F. LABORATORY TESTS
1. Purified protein derivative (PPD): If high risk.
2. Hemoglobin/hematocrit: Once during puberty for boys, once after menarche for girls.
3. Sexually active adolescents: Serologic tests for syphilis annually; offer HIV testing, especially if syphilis or other ulcerative genital disease.
   a. Males: First part voided urinalysis/leukocyte esterase screen with positive results confirmed by detection tests for gonorrhea and chlamydia (i.e., cultures, ligase/polymerase chain reaction).
   b. Females: Detection tests for gonorrhea and chlamydia (i.e., cultures, LCR/PCR), wet preparation, potassium hydroxide (KOH), cervical Gram stain, Papanicolaou smear, midvaginal pH.

G. IMMUNIZATIONS (see pp. 345–348 for specifics of dosing, route, formulation, and schedules)
1. Tetanus and diphtheria (Td): booster age 11–12 years.
2. Measles: Two doses of live attenuated vaccine are required after first birthday. Use measles, mumps, rubella (MMR) vaccine if not previously immunized for mumps or rubella. Assess pregnancy status, and do not administer rubella vaccine to woman anticipating pregnancy within 90 days.
3. Hepatitis B vaccine: Recommended for all adolescents (three doses) if not previously vaccinated.
4. Varicella vaccine: Two doses at least 1 month apart are recommended for adolescents ≥13 years old with no history of disease.

H. ANTICIPATORY GUIDANCE
1. Sexuality (e.g., abstinence, STD/pregnancy prevention)
2. Nutrition: Excessive/inadequate calories, balanced diet, calcium.
3. Coping skills/violence prevention

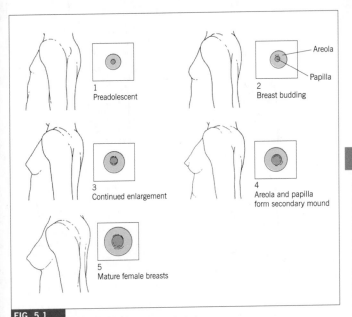

FIG. 5.1

Tanner stages of breast development in females. (Adapted from Johnson[3].)

TABLE 5.1

BREAST DEVELOPMENT

Stage	Comment (mean age +/− standard deviation)
I	Preadolescent; elevation of papilla only
II	Breast bud; elevation of breast and papilla as small mound; enlargement of areolar diameter (11.15 ± 1.10)
III	Further enlargement and elevation of breast and areola; no separation of their contours (12.15 ± 1.09)
IV	Projection of areola and papilla to form secondary mound above level of breast (13.11 ± 1.15)
V	Mature stage; projection of papilla only as a result of recession of areola to general contour of breast (15.3 ± 1.74)

From Oski[4], as adapted from Marshall[5,6].
Note: Stages IV and V may not be distinct in some patients.

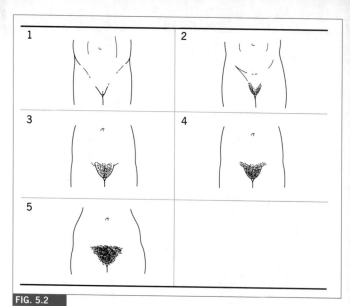

FIG. 5.2
Tanner stages of pubic hair development in females. (Adapted from Neinstein[7].)

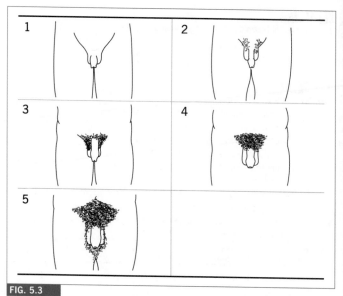

FIG. 5.3
Pubic hair and genital development in males. Tanner stages 1–5. (Adapted from Neinstein[7].)

TABLE 5.2

PUBIC HAIR (MALE AND FEMALE)

Stage	Comment (mean age +/− standard deviation)
I	Preadolescent: Vellus over pubes no further developed than that over abdominal wall (i.e., no pubic hair)
II	Sparse growth of long, slightly pigmented downy hair, straight or only slightly curled, chiefly at base of penis or along labia (male: 13.44 ± 1.09, female: 11.69 ± 1.21)
III	Considerably darker, coarser and more curled; hair spreads sparsely over junction of pubes (male: 13.9 ± 1.04, female: 12.36 ± 1.10)
IV	Hair resembles adult in type; distribution still considerably less than in adult; no spread to medial surface of thighs (male: 14.36 ± 1.08, female: 12.95 ± 1.06)
V	Adult in quantity and type with distribution of the horizontal pattern (male: 15.18 ± 1.07, female: 14.41 ± 1.12)
VI	Spread up linea alba: 'Male escutcheon'

From Oski[4], as adapted from Marshall[5,6].

TABLE 5.3

GENITAL DEVELOPMENT (MALE)

Stage	Comment (mean age +/− standard deviation)
I	Preadolescent: testes, scrotum, and penis about same size and proportion as in early childhood
II	Enlargement of scrotum and testes; skin of scrotum reddens and changes in texture; little or no enlargement of penis (11.64 ± 1.07)
III	Enlargement of penis, first mainly in length; further growth of testes and scrotum (12.85 ± 1.04)
IV	Increased size of penis with growth in breadth and development of glans; further enlargement of testes and scrotum and increased darkening of scrotal skin (13.77 ± 1.02)
V	Genitalia adult in size and shape (14.92 ± 1.10)

From Oski[4], as adapted from Marshall[5,6].

5

ADOLESCENT MEDICINE

4. **Safety:** Driving/seat belts, guns, bicycle helmets.
5. **Substance abuse prevention**

II. PUBERTAL EVENTS AND TANNER STAGE DIAGRAMS

The temporal interrelationship of the biologic and psychosocial events of adolescence are illustrated in Fig. 5.3 and Tables 5.1 –5.4. Age limits for the events and stages are approximations and may differ from those used by other authors.

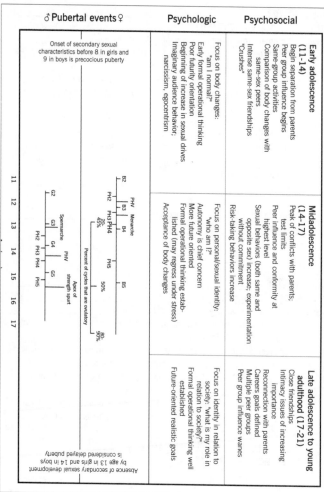

FIG. 5.4

Pubertal events and Tanner stages. B, breast (stage); G, genital (stage); PH, pubic hair (stage); PHV, peak height velocity. (Adapted from Joffe[1].)

III. CONTRACEPTIVE INFORMATION
A. METHODS OF CONTRACEPTION (Table 5.4)

TABLE 5.4

METHODS OF CONTRACEPTION

Method	Failure rate in typical user (%)	Benefits	Risk/disadvantages
Combined oral contraceptives[a]	3.0 (may be increased among adolescents)	Intercourse independent; decreased risk of dysmenorrhea, benign breast disorders, arthritis, iron deficiency anemia, ovarian and uterine cancers, ovarian cysts	Thromboembolic phenomena, cerebrovascular accident, hypertension, worsening of migraines, breakthrough bleeding, amenorrhea, nausea, weight gain, acne, depression, glucose intolerance
Injectable contraceptives (Depo-Provera)	0.3	Intercourse independent, long-acting (3 months), can be used when breast-feeding, no estrogen, decreased risk of endometrial/ovarian cancer, no drug interactions	Injection every 3 months, delayed return to fertility, menstrual irregularity/amenorrhea, weight gain
Progestin-only pill (minipill)	1.1	Fewer metabolic complications; used for patients with hypertension, diabetes, sickle cell disease	Menstrual irregularities (generally not recommended for adolescents)
Norplant	0.04	Intercourse independent, highly effective, long-lasting protection (approximately 3-5 years)	Requires minor surgical procedure for insertion, removal; menstrual irregularities, headaches, nervousness, nausea, dizziness, dermatitis, acne, change in appetite, weight gain, breast tenderness, hirsutism, hair loss

[a]See pp. 104–107 for further information on oral contraceptive pills.

5

ADOLESCENT MEDICINE

Continued

TABLE 5.4

METHODS OF CONTRACEPTION—cont'd

Method	Failure rate in typical user (%)	Benefits	Risk/disadvantages
Condom	12.0	No major risks, low cost, nonprescription, male involvement, protects against STD and cervical cancer	Decreased sensation, use with each act of coitus; polyurethane condoms are now available for those with latex allergy
Diaphragm with contraceptive cream or jelly	18.0	Some protection against many STDs	Allergy (rare), toxic shock syndrome (rare), increased incidence of urinary tract infection, vaginal ulceration, requires motivation
Spermicide	21.0	Nonprescription, no major medical risks, some STD protection	Allergy (rare), use related to coitus
Intrauterine device	3.0	Minimal demands after insertion, secrecy	Generally not recommended for adolescents, increased risk of pelvic inflammatory disease
Natural family planning	20.0	Natural, no risks, nonprescription	Not very effective with irregular menses, requires highly motivated partners

Adapted, with permission, from Wilson[8].
Hormonal methods of birth control do not afford protection against STDs.

B. ORAL CONTRACEPTIVE PILL (OCP) INFORMATION

1. **OCP contraindications** (for all OCPs containing estrogen)[9]
a. Refrain from providing (WHO category 4): History of thrombophlebitis/thromboembolic disease, stroke, ischemic structural heart disease, structural heart disease with complications, breast/liver cancer, estrogen-dependent neoplasia, acute liver disease, benign hepatic adenoma, diabetes with complications, headaches with focal neurologic symptoms, major surgery with prolonged immobilization or any surgery on the legs, hypertension with pressures 160+/100+mmHg.

b. Exercise caution (WHO category 3): Undiagnosed abnormal vaginal/uterine bleeding, use of drugs that affect liver enzymes, gallbladder disease.

c. Advantages generally outweigh disadvantages (WHO category 2): Headaches without focal neurologic symptoms, diabetes without complications, major surgery without prolonged immobilization, sickle cell disease, moderate hypertension (140–159/100–109mmHg), undiagnosed breast mass.

2. Instructions for use

a. Sunday start most common method.

b. Start with low-dose estrogen pill (≤30–35mcg).

c. 21 days hormonal pills, 7 days inactive pills.

d. Advise patient about need for back-up methods during first month of use and need for STD prevention.

e. Pelvic examination recommended at baseline or during first 3–6 months of use, then annually.

f. 2–3 visits a year to monitor for compliance, BP, side effects.

3. Side effects (ACHES)

a. *Abdominal pain* (pelvic vein/mesenteric vein thrombosis, pancreatitis).

b. *Chest pain* (pulmonary embolism).

c. *Headaches* (thrombotic/hemorrhagic stroke, retinal vein thrombosis).

d. *Eye symptoms* (thrombotic/hemorrhagic stroke, retinal vein thrombosis).

e. *Severe leg pain* (thrombophlebitis of the lower extremity).

C. **ADVICE FOR PATIENTS WHO HAVE MISSED ORAL CONTRACEPTIVE PILLS** (Fig. 5.5)

D. **EMERGENCY CONTRACEPTIVE PILL (ECP)** (Table 5.5)

1. Instructions for use[9]

a. To reduce the chance of nausea, recommend diphenhydramine dose 1 hour before the first dose of ECPs.

TABLE 5.5		
EMERGENCY CONTRACEPTIVE PILL (ECP)		
Trade name	Formulation	Pills per dose
Ovral	0.05mg ethinyl estradiol, 0.50mg norgestrel	2 white pills
Lo-Ovral	0.03mg ethinyl estradiol, 0.30mg norgestrel	4 white pills
Nordette	0.03mg ethinyl estradiol, 0.15mg levonorgestrel	4 light-orange pills
Levlen	0.03mg ethinyl estradiol, 0.15mg levonorgestrel	4 light-orange pills
Triphasil	0.03mg ethinyl estradiol, 0.125mg levonorgestrel	4 yellow pills
Trilevlen	0.03mg ethinyl estradiol, 0.125mg levonorgestrel	4 yellow pills
Alesse	0.02mg ethinyl estradiol, 0.10mg levonorgestrel	5 pink pills

Data from Program for Applied Technologies (PATH)[11].

5

ADOLESCENT MEDICINE

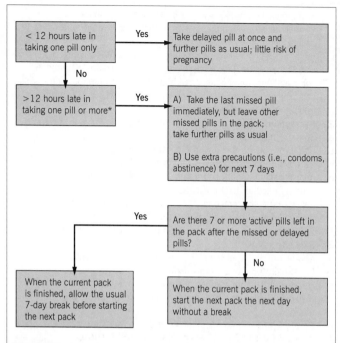

FIG. 5.5

Advice for patients who have missed oral contraceptive pills. Based on the '7-day rule' that seven consecutive pills are enough to 'put the ovaries to sleep', so a pill-free interval of >7 days risks ovulation. This algorithm is based on exogenous hormone for 21 of the 28-day cycle; in packs with 28 days of pills, the '7-day break' represents the hormone-free pills. *If two or more pills are missed, if they were all from the first 7 in the pack, and *if unprotected intercourse occurred since the end of the last pack,* emergency contraception is indicated in addition to (A) and (B) (see Table 5.4). (From Guillebaud[10].)

b. The first ECP dose should be taken as soon as possible after unprotected sex.
c. The second ECP dose should be take 12 hours after the first dose; do not take any extra pills.
d. Use only one type of pill.
e. Recommend the use of condoms, spermicides, or a diaphragm during sex after taking ECPs until the next menstrual period; ensure proper regular birth control for the future.
f. Perform pregnancy test if there is no menstrual period within 3 weeks of ECP treatment.

IV. VAGINAL INFECTIONS, GENITAL ULCERS, AND WARTS

See p. 380 for discussion of infection with *Chlamydia* sp., gonorrhea, pelvic inflammatory disease, HIV, and further discussion of syphilis. See pp. 386–399 and ch. 29 for additional information and comments regarding medications. After diagnosis of an STD, encourage patient to refrain from intercourse until full therapy is complete, partner is treated, and all visible lesions are resolved.

A. **DIAGNOSTIC FEATURES AND MANAGEMENT OF VAGINAL INFECTION** (Table 5.6)
B. **DIAGNOSTIC FEATURES AND MANAGEMENT OF GENITAL ULCERS AND WARTS** (Table 5.7)

Text continued on p. 113

5

ADOLESCENT MEDICINE

TABLE 5.6

DIAGNOSTIC FEATURES AND MANAGEMENT OF VAGINAL INFECTIONS

	Normal vaginal examination	Yeast vaginitis	Trichomoniasis	Bacterial vaginosis
Etiology	Uninfected; *Lactobacillus* predominant	*Candida albicans* and other yeasts	*Trichomonas vaginalis*	Associated with *Gardnerella vaginalis*, various anaerobic bacteria, and mycoplasma
Typical symptoms	None	Vulvar itching and/or irritation, increased discharge	Malodorous purulent discharge, vulvar itching	Malodorous, slightly increased discharge
Discharge				
Amount	Variable; usually scant	Scant to moderate	Profuse	Moderate
Color[a]	Clear or white	White	Yellow–green	Usually white or gray
Consistency	Nonhomogeneous, floccular	Clumped; adherent plaques	Homogeneous	Homogeneous, low viscosity; smoothly coating vaginal walls
Inflammation of vulvar or vaginal epithelium	No	Yes	Yes	No
pH of vaginal fluid[b]	Usually <4.5	Usually ≤4.5	Usually ≥5.0	Usually >4.5
Amine ('fishy') odor with 10% KOH	None	None	May be present	Present

Microscopy[c]	Normal epithelial cells; *Lactobacillus* predominate	Leukocytes, epithelial cells, yeast, mycelia, or pseudomycelia in 40–80%	Leukocytes; motile trichomonads seen in 50–70% of symptomatic patients, less often in the absence of symptoms	Clue cells; few leukocytes; *Lactobacillus* outnumbered by profuse mixed flora, nearly always including *G. vaginalis* plus anaerobic species, on Gram stain
Usual treatment	None	Fluconazole 150mg PO (single dose), or miconazole 200mg or clotrimazole 200mg vaginal suppository qhs for 3 days	Metronidazole 2.0g PO (single dose) or metronidazole 500mg PO BID for 7 days	Metronidazole 500mg PO BID for 7 days or metronidazole gel 0.75%, one applicator (5g) intravaginally BID for 5 days
Usual management of sex partners	None	None; topical treatment if candidal dermatitis of penis is present	Treatment recommended	Examine for STD; routine treatment not recommended

From Holmes[12] and Centers for Disease Control and Prevention[13].

[a]Color of discharge is determined by examining vaginal discharge against the white background of a swab.

[b]pH determination is not useful if blood is present.

[c]To detect fungal elements, vaginal fluid is digested with 10% KOH before microscopic examination; to examine for other features, fluid is mixed (1:1) with physiologic saline. Gram stain is also excellent for detecting yeasts and pseudomycelia and for distinguishing normal flora from the mixed flora seen in bacterial vaginosis, but it is less sensitive than the saline preparation for detection of *T. vaginalis*.

ADOLESCENT MEDICINE

5

TABLE 5.7

DIAGNOSTIC FEATURES AND MANAGEMENT OF GENITAL ULCERS AND WARTS

Infection	Clinical presentation	Presumptive diagnosis	Definitive diagnosis	Treatment/management of sex partners
Genital herpes	Grouped vesicles, painful shallow ulcers; tender inguinal adenopathy	Tzanck smear	Viral culture or antigen test	No known cure. Prompt initiation of therapy shortens duration of first episode. For severe recurrent disease, initiate therapy at start of prodrome or within 1 day of onset of lesions; see ch. 29 (formulary) for dosing of acyclovir, famciclovir, or valacylcovir. Transmission can occur during asymptomatic periods.
Primary syphilis	Indurated, well-defined, usually single painless ulcer—'chancre'; nontender inguinal adenopathy	Nontreponemal serologic test: VDRL, RPR, or STS	Treponemal serologic test: FTA-ABS or MHA-TP; Dark-field microscopy or direct fluorescent antibody tests of esion exudate or tissue	Parenteral penicillin G is preferred treatment; preparation(s), dosage, and length of treatment depend on stage and clinical manifestations (see ch. 18). Evaluation of sexual contacts is indicated for the following exposures: primary syphilis—3 months plus duration of symptoms; secondary syphilis—6 months plus duration of symptoms; latent syphilis—1 year (if <3 months since exposure, may be falsely seronegative; presumptive treatment recommended).

Chancroid	Multiple, ragged, painful, nonindurated ulcer(s); painful suppurative inguinal adenopathy	Culture of *Haemophilus ducreyi*	Azithromycin 1g PO ×1, or ceftriaxone 250mg IM ×1 or erythromycin 500mg PO QID for 7 days. Evaluation and treatment of sexual contacts within 10 days of symptoms.
	Clinical presentation and negative syphilis and herpes testing		
LGV	Transient, small ulcers, often multiple; tender inguinal adenopathy, most prominent feature, commonly unilateral	Complement fixation, Frie test, serology	Doxycycline 100mg PO BID ×21 days. Evaluation and treatment of sexual contacts within 30 days of symptoms.
		Culture of LGV-specific *Chlamydia trachomatis*	
Granuloma inguinale (donovanosis)	Granulomatous painless nodules, usually beefy red in appearance, progressing to ulceration with sharply defined border; no inguinal adenopathy, although lesions may mimic it	Biopsy of lesion; diagnostic agent is *Calymmato-bacterium granulomatis*	Doxycycline 100mg PO BID or TMP/SMX one DS tab (160mg TMP) PO BID ×21 days or until lesion completely heals. Return weekly or biweekly for evaluation until infection is healed. Evaluation and treatment of sexual contacts within 60 days of onset of symptoms and clinical signs and symptoms of disease present in contact.
		Giemsa or Wright stain demonstrating Donovan's bodies; history of travel to the Tropics substantiates clinical impression	

Continued

Adapted with permission from Centers for Disease Control and Prevention[13] and Adger[14].

FTA-ABS, fluorescent treponemal antibody absorbed; HPV, human papilloma virus; LGV, lymphogranuloma venereum; MHA-TP, microhemagglutination assay for antibody to *T. pallidum*; RPR, rapid plasma reagin; STS, serologic test for syphilis; VDRL, Venereal Disease Research Laboratory.

ADOLESCENT MEDICINE

5

TABLE 5.7

DIAGNOSTIC FEATURES AND MANAGEMENT OF GENITAL ULCERS AND WARTS—cont'd

Infection	Clinical presentation	Presumptive diagnosis	Definitive diagnosis	Treatment /management of sex partners
Genital warts (HPV infection)	Single or multiple soft, fleshy papillary or sessile, painless growth around the anus, vulvovaginal area, penis, urethra, or perineum; no inguinal adenopathy	Typical clinical presentation	Papanicolaou smear revealing typical cytologic changes	Treatment does not eradicate infection. Goal: Removal of exophytic warts. Exclude cervical dysplasia before treatment. Cryotherapy with liquid nitrogen or cryoprobe (not for vaginal warts), podophyllin 10-25% in compound tincture of benzoin (contra-indication in pregnancy), or bichloroacetic or trichloroacetic acid (no method preferred). Period of communicability is unknown.

V. RECOMMENDED COMPONENTS OF THE PREPARTICIPATION PHYSICAL EVALUATION (PPE)

A. **MEDICAL HISTORY:** Illnesses or injuries since the last check-up or PPE; chronic conditions and medications; hospitalizations or surgeries; medications used by the athletes (including those they may be taking to enhance performance); use of any special equipment or protective devices during sports participation; allergies, particularly those associated with anaphylaxis or respiratory compromise and those provoked by exercise; immunization status, including hepatitis B, MMR, tetanus, and varicella.

B. **REVIEW OF SYSTEMS/PHYSICAL EXAMINATION ITEMS[15]** (examination items in italics)

1. *Height and weight*
2. **Vision:** Visual problems, corrective lenses; *visual acuity.*
3. **Cardiac:** History of congenital heart disease; symptoms of syncope, dizziness, or chest pain during exercise; history of high blood pressure or heart murmurs; family history of heart disease; previous history of disqualification or limited participation in sports because of a cardiac problem; *blood pressure, heart rate and rhythm, pulses (including radial/femoral lag), auscultation for murmurs.*
4. **Respiratory:** Asthma, coughing, wheezing, or dyspnea during exercise.
5. **Genitourinary:** Age at menarche, last menstrual period, regularity of menstrual periods, number of periods in the last year, longest interval between periods, dysmenorrhea; *palpation of the abdomen, palpation of the testicles, examination of the inguinal canals.*
6. **Orthopedic:** Previous injuries that have limited sports participation; injuries that have been associated with pain, swelling, or the need for medical intervention; *screening orthopedic examination (Fig. 5.6); see* p. 116.
7. **Neurology:** History of a significant head injury or concussion; numbness or tingling in the extremities; severe headaches; seizure disorder.
8. **Psychosocial:** Weight control and body image; stresses at home or in school; use or abuse of drugs and alcohol; *attention to signs of eating disorders, including oral ulcerations, eroded tooth enamel, edema, lanugo hair, calluses/ulcerations on knuckles.*

5

ADOLESCENT MEDICINE

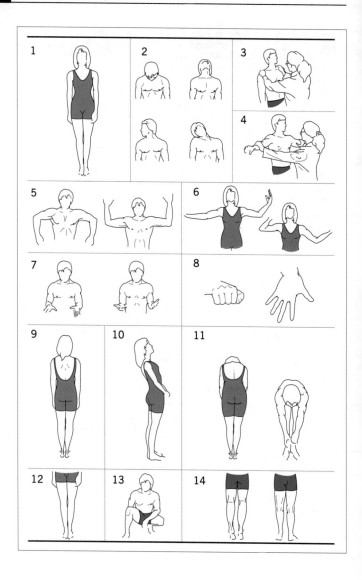

FIG. 5.6
Screening orthopedic examination. The general musculoskeletal screening examination consists of the following: (1) Inspection, athlete standing, facing examiner (symmetry of trunk, upper extremities); (2) forward flexion, extension, rotation, lateral flexion of neck (range of motion, cervical spine); (3) resisted shoulder shrug (strength, trapezius); (4) resisted shoulder abduction (strength, deltoid); (5) internal and external rotation of shoulder (range of motion, glenohumeral joint); (6) extension and flexion of elbow (range of motion, elbow); (7) pronation and supination of elbow (range of motion, elbow and wrist); (8) clenching of fist, then spreading of fingers (range of motion, hand and fingers); (9) inspection, athlete facing away from examiner (symmetry of trunk, upper extremities); (10) back extension, knees straight (spondylolysis/spondylolisthesis); (11) back flexion with knees straight, facing toward and away from examiner (range of motion, thoracic and lumbosacral spine; spine curvature; hamstring flexibility); (12) inspection of lower extremities, contraction of quadriceps muscles (alignment symmetry); (13) 'duck walk' four steps (motion of hips, knees, and ankles; strength; balance); (14) standing on toes, then on heels (symmetry, calf; strength; balance). (Adapted from American Academy of Family Physicians[16].)

VI. SCOLIOSIS[17]

Refer to Fig. 5.7 for routine screening for scoliosis. Many curves that are detected on screening are nonprogressive and/or too slight to be significant.

A. ASSESSMENT

1. **Radiographic determination of the Cobb angle** (Fig. 5.8): If clinical suspicion of significant scoliosis.
2. **Bone scan ± MRI:** If there is pain that is worse at night, progressive, well localized, or otherwise suspicious.
3. **MRI:** If presents at <10 years old or presence of 'opposite' curves (left-sided thoracic, right-sided lumbar).

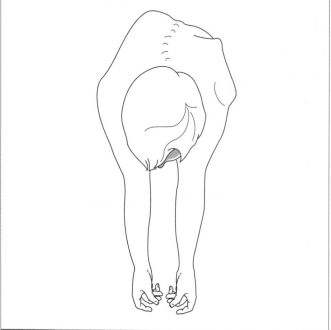

FIG. 5.7

Forward bending test. This emphasizes any asymmetry of the paraspinous muscles and rib cage.

B. TREATMENT: According to the Cobb angle and skeletal maturity, which is assessed by grading the ossification of the iliac crest.

1. **Skeletally immature**
a. <10 degrees: Single follow-up radiograph in 4–6 months to ensure no significant progression.
b. 10–20 degrees: Radiographs every 4–6 months.
c. 20–40 degrees: Bracing.
d. >40 degrees: Surgical correction.
2. **Skeletally mature**
a. <40 degrees: No further evaluation or intervention indicated.
b. >40 degrees: Surgical correction.
3. **Orthopedic referral:** This is indicated if skeletally immature with curve >20 degrees, skeletally mature with curve >40 degrees, and/or presence of suspicious pain or neurologic symptoms.

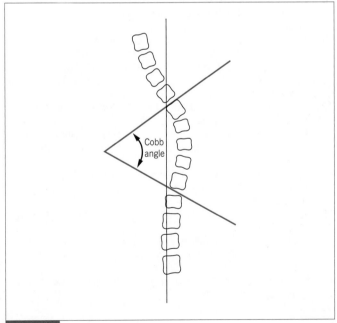

FIG. 5.8
Cobb angle. This is measured using the superior and inferior endplates of the most tilted vertebrae at the end of each curve.

ADOLESCENT MEDICINE

5

VII. REFERENCES

1. Joffe A. Adolescent medicine. In: Oski FA, DeAngelis CD, Feigin RD, et al. *Principles and practice of pediatrics.* Philadelphia: JB Lippincott; 1994.

2. Adger H, Sweet RL, Shafer MA, Schachter J. Screening for *Chlamydia trachomatis* and *Neisseria gonorrhoeae* in adolescent males: value of first-catch urine examination. *Lancet* 1984; **8409:**944.

3. Johnson TR, Moore WM, Jefferies JE. *Children are different: development psysiology,* 2nd edn., Columbus, OH: Ross Laboratories, Division of Abbott Laboratories; 1978.

4. Oski FA, DeAngelis CD, Feigin RD, et al. *Principles and practice of pediatrics.* Philadelphia: JB Lippincott; 1994.

5. Marshall WA, Tanner JM. Variations in pattern of pubertal changes in girls. *Arch Dis Child* 1969; **44:**291.

6. Marshall WA, Tanner JM. Variations in pattern of pubertal changes in boys. *Arch Dis Child* 1970; **45:**13.

7. Neinstein LS. *Adolescent health care: a practical guide,* 2nd edn. Baltimore: Urban & Schwarzenberg; 1991.

8. Wilson MD. Adolescent pregnancy and contraception. In: Oski FA, DeAngelis CD, Feigin RD, et al. *Principles and practice of pediatrics.* Philadelphia: JB Lippincott; 1994.

9. Hatcher RA, Trussell J, Steward F, et al: *Contraceptive technology,* 17th rev. edn. New York: Ardent Media, Inc.; 1998: 420–424.

10. Guillebaud J. *Fertility Control Reviews* 1995; **4(2):**18–20.

11. Program for Applied Technologies (PATH). *Emergency contraception: resource for providers.* Seattle: PATH; 1997.

12. Holmes KK, Per-Anders M, Sparling PF, et al. *Sexually transmitted diseases.* New York: McGraw-Hill; 1990.

13. Centers for Disease Control and Prevention. 1998 guidelines for treatment of sexually transmitted diseases. *MMWR* 1998; **47(RR-1):**1–118.

14. Adger H. Sexually transmitted diseases. In: Oski FA, DeAngelis CD, Feigin RD, et al. *Principles and practice of pediatrics,* Philadelphia: JB Lippincott; 1994.

15. Andrews J. Making the most of the sports physical. *Contemp Pediatr* 1997; **14:**182–205.

16. American Academy of Family Physicians. *Preparticipation physical examination,* 2nd edn. Kansas City, MO, American Academy of Family Physicians; 1997:22.

17. Kautz SM, Skaggs DL. Getting an angle on spinal deformities. *Contemp Pediatr* 1998; **15:**112–28.

BLOOD CHEMISTRIES/
BODY FLUIDS

Mary K. Choukair, MD

These values are compiled from the published literature[1-5] and from the Johns Hopkins Hospital Department of Laboratory Medicine. Normal values vary with the analytic method used. If any doubt exists, consult your laboratory for its analytic method and range of normal values. Hematologic values may be found at the end of ch. 15 and endocrine values in ch. 10.

I. REFERENCE VALUES (Table 6.1)

TABLE 6.1

REFERENCE VALUES

	Conventional units	SI units
ACID PHOSPHATASE		
(Major sources: prostate and erythrocytes[10])		
Newborn	7.4–19.4U/L	7.4–19.4U/L
2–13yr	6.4–15.2U/L	6.4–15.2U/L
Adult male	0.5–11.0U/L	0.5–11.0U/L
Adult female	0.2–9.5U/L	0.2–9.5U/L
ALANINE AMINOTRANSFERASE (ALT)		
(Major sources: liver, skeletal muscle, and myocardium[10])		
Infant	<54U/L	<54U/L
Child/adult	1–30U/L	1–30U/L
ALDOLASE		
(Major sources: skeletal muscle and myocardium[10])		
Newborn	<32U/L	<32U/L
Child	<16U/L	<8U/L
Adult	<8U/L	<8U/L
ALKALINE PHOSPHATASE		
(Major sources: liver, bone, intestinal mucosa, placenta, and kidney[10])		
Infant	150–420U/L	150–420U/L
2–10yr	100–320U/L	100–320U/L
11–18-yr-old boy	100–390U/L	100–390U/L
11–18-yr-old girl	100–320U/L	100–320U/L
Adult	30–120U/L	30–100U/L
α_1-**ANTITRYPSIN**	93–224mg/dL	0.93–2.24g/L

Continued

TABLE 6.1

REFERENCE VALUES—cont'd

	Conventional units	SI units
α-FETOPROTEIN		
>1yr–adult	<30ng/mL	<30mcg/L
Tumor marker	0–10mg/mL	

AMMONIA (heparinized venous specimen on ice analyzed within 30min)

	Conventional units	SI units
Newborn	90–150mcg/dL	64–107mcmol/L
0–2wk	79–129mcg/dL	56–92mcmol/L
>1mo	29–70mcg/dL	21–50mcmol/L
Adult	0–50mcg/dL	0–35.7mcmol/L

AMYLASE

(Major sources: pancreas, salivary glands, and ovaries[10])

	Conventional units	SI units
Newborn	0–44U/L	5–65U/L
Adult	0–88U/L	0–130U/L

ANTIHYALURONIDASE ANTIBODY

<1:256

ANTINUCLEAR ANTIBODY (ANA)

Not significant	<1:80
Likely significant	>1:320

Patterns with clinical correlation
  Centromere—CREST
  Nucleolar—Scleroderma
  Homogeneous—nDNA, antihistone Ab

ANTISTREPTOLYSIN O TITER (4× rise in paired serial specimens is significant)

Preschool	<1:85
School age	<1:170
Older adult	<1:85

Note: Alternatively, values up to 200 Todd units are normal.

ARSENIC

	Conventional units	SI units
Normal	<3mcg/dL	<0.39mcmol/L
Acute poisoning	60–930mcg/dL	7.98–124mcmol/L
Chronic poisoning	10–50mcg/dL	1.33–6.65mcmol/L

ASPARTATE AMINOTRANSFERASE (AST)

(Major sources: liver, skeletal muscle, kidney, myocardium, and erythrocytes[10])

	Conventional units	SI units
Newborn/infant	20–65U/L	20–65U/L
Child/adult	0–35U/L	0–4350U/L

TABLE 6.1

REFERENCE VALUES—cont'd		Conventional units	SI units
BICARBONATE			
Preterm		18–26mEq/L	18–26mmol/L
Full term		20–25mEq/L	20–25mmol/L
>2yr		22–26mEq/L	22–26mmol/L
BILIRUBIN (TOTAL)			
Cord	Preterm	<2mg/dL	<34mcmol/L
	Term	<2mg/dL	<34mcmol/L
0–1dy	Preterm	<8mg/dL	<137mcmol/L
	Term	<6mg/dL	<103mcmol/L
1–2dy	Preterm	<12mg/dL	<205mcmol/L
	Term	<8mg/dL	<137mcmol/L
3–5dy	Preterm	<16mg/dL	<274mcmol/L
	Term	<12mg/dL	<205mcmol/L
Thereafter	Preterm	<2mg/dL	<34mcmol/L
	Term	<1mg/dL	<17mcmol/L
Adult		0.1–1.2mg/dL	1.7–20.5mcmol/L
BILIRUBIN (CONJUGATED)		0–0.4mg/dL	0–8mcmol/L
CALCIUM (TOTAL)			
Preterm <1wk		6–10mg/dL	1.5–2.5mmol/L
Full term <1wk		7.0–12.0mg/dL	1.75–3.0mmol/L
Child		8.0–10.5mg/dL	2–2.6mmol/L
Adult		8.5–10.5mg/dL	2.1–2.6mmol/L
CALCIUM (IONIZED)			
Newborn <48hr		4.0–4.7mg/dL	1.00–1.18mmol/L
Adult		4.52–5.28mg/dL	1.13–1.32mmol/L
CARBON DIOXIDE (CO_2 CONTENT)			
Cord blood		14–22mEq/L	14–22mmol/L
Infant/child		20–24mEq/L	20–24mmol/L
Adult		24–30mEq/L	24–30mmol/L
CARBON MONOXIDE (CARBOXYHEMOGLOBIN)			
Nonsmoker		0–2% of total hemoglobin	
Smoker		2–10% of total hemoglobin	
Toxic		20–60% of total hemoglobin	
Lethal		>60% of total hemoglobin	
CAROTENOIDS (CAROTENES)			
Infant		20–70mcg/dL	0.37–1.30mcmol/L
Child		40–130mcg/dL	0.74–2.42mcmol/L
Adult		50–250mcg/dL	0.95–4.69mcmol/L

6

BLOOD CHEMISTRIES/BODY FLUIDS

Continued

TABLE 6.1
REFERENCE VALUES—cont'd

	Conventional units	SI units
CERULOPLASMIN	21–53mg/dL	210–530mg/L
CHLORIDE (SERUM)		
Pediatric	99–111mEq/L	99–111mmol/L
Adult	96–109mEq/L	96–109mmol/L
CHOLESTEROL (see Lipids)		
COPPER		
0–6mo	20–70mcg/dL	3.1–11mcmol/L
6yr	90–190mcg/dL	14–30mcmol/L
12yr	80–160mcg/dL	12.6–25mcmol/L
Adult male	70–140mcg/dL	11–22mcmol/L
Adult female	80–155mcg/dL	12.6–24.3mcmol/L
C-REACTIVE PROTEIN	0–0.5mg/dL	

(Other laboratories may have different reference values)

CREATINE KINASE (CREATINE PHOSPHOKINASE)
(Major sources: myocardium, skeletal muscle, smooth muscle, and brain[10])

Newborn	10–200U/L	10–200U/L
Man	12–80U/L	12–80U/L
Woman	10–55U/L	10–55U/L

CREATININE (SERUM)

Cord	0.6–1.2mg/dL	53–106mcmol/L
Newborn	0.3–1.0mg/dL	27–88mcmol/L
Infant	0.2–0.4mg/dL	18–35mcmol/L
Child	0.3–0.7mg/dL	27–62mcmol/L
Adolescent	0.5–1.0mg/dL	44–88mcmol/L
Man	0.6–1.3mg/dL	53–115mcmol/L
Woman	0.5–1.2mg/dL	44–106mcmol/L

ESR (refer to ch. 15)

FERRITIN

Newborn	25–200ng/mL	25–200mcg/L
1mo	200–600ng/mL	200–600mcg/L
6mo	50–200ng/mL	50–200mcg/L
6mo–15yr	7–140ng/mL	7–140mcg/L
Adult male	15–200ng/mL	15–200mcg/L
Adult female	12–150ng/mL	12–150mcg/L

TABLE 6.1		
REFERENCE VALUES—cont'd		
	Conventional units	SI units
FIBRINOGEN	200–400mg/dL	2–4g/L
FOLIC ACID (FOLATE)	3–17.5ng/mL	4.0–20.0 nmol/L
FOLIC ACID (RBCs)	153–605mcg/mL RBCs	
GALACTOSE		
Newborn	0–20mg/dL	0–1.11mmol/L
Thereafter	<5mg/dL	<0.28mmol/L
γ-GLUTAMYL TRANSFERASE (GGT)		
(Major sources: liver [biliary tree] and kidney[10])		
Cord	19–270U/L	19–270U/L
Preterm	56–233U/L	56–233U/L
0–3wk	0–130U/L	0–130U/L
3wk–3mo	4–120U/L	4–120U/L
>3mo boy	5–65U/L	5–65U/L
>3mo girl	5–35U/L	5–35U/L
1–15yr	0–23U/L	0–23U/L
Adult male	11–50U/L	11–50U/L
Adult female	7–32U/L	7–32U/L
GASTRIN	<100 pg/mL	<100ng/L
GLUCOSE (SERUM)		
Preterm	45–100mg/dL	1.1–3.6mmol/L
Full term	45–120mg/dL	1.1–6.4mmol/L
1wk–16yr	60–105mg/dL	3.3–5.8mmol/L
>16yr	70–115mg/dL	3.9–6.4mmol/L
IRON		
Newborn	100–250mcg/dL	18–45mcmol/L
Infant	40–100mcg/dL	7–18mcmol/L
Child	50–120mcg/dL	9–22mcmol/L
Adult male	65–170mcg/dL	12–30mcmol/L
Adult female	50–170mcg/dL	9–30mcmol/L
KETONES (SERUM)		
Qualitative	Negative	
Quantitative	0.5–3.0mg/dL	5–30mg/L

6

BLOOD CHEMISTRIES/BODY FLUIDS

Continued

TABLE 6.1
REFERENCE VALUES—cont'd

	Conventional units	SI units
LACTATE		
Capillary blood		
Newborn	<27mg/dL	0.0–3.0mmol/L
Child	5–20mg/dL	0.56–2.25mmol/L
Venous	5–20mg/dL	0.5–2.2mmol/L
Arterial	5–14mg/dL	0.5–1.6mmol/L

LACTATE DEHYDROGENASE (AT 37°C)
(Major sources: myocardium, liver, skeletal muscle, erythrocytes, platelets, and lymph nodes[10])

	Conventional units	SI units
Neonate	160–1500U/L	160–1500U/L
Infant	150–360U/L	150–360U/L
Child	150–300U/L	150–300U/L
Adult	0–220U/L	0–220U/L

LACTATE DEHYDROGENASE ISOENZYMES (% total)

LD_1 heart	24–34%
LD_2 heart, erythrocytes	35–45%
LD_3 muscle	15–25%
LD_4 liver, trace muscle	4–10%
LD_5 liver, muscle	1–9%

LEAD (see ch. 2)

Child	<10mcg/dL	<48mcmol/L

LIPASE   4–24U/dl

LIPIDS[6]

	Cholesterol (mg/dL)			LDL (mg/dL)		
	Desirable	Borderline	High	Desirable	Borderline	High
Child/adolescent	<170	170–199	≥200	<110	110–129	≥130
Adult	<200	200–239	≥240	<130	130–159	≥160
HDL	>45					

	Conventional units	SI units
MAGNESIUM	1.3–2.0mEq/L	0.65–1.0mmol/L
MANGANESE (BLOOD)		
Newborn	2.4–9.6mcg/dL	0.44–1.75mcmol/L
2–18yr	0.8–2.1mcg/dL	0.15–0.38mcmol/L
METHEMOGLOBIN	0–1.3% total Hgb	

TABLE 6.1

REFERENCE VALUES—cont'd

	Conventional units	SI units
OSMOLALITY	285–295mOsmol/kg	285–295mmol/kg

PHENYLALANINE

Preterm	2.0–7.5mg/dL	0.12–0.45mmol/L
Newborn	1.2–3.4mg/dL	0.07–0.21mmol/L
Adult	0.8–1.8mg/dL	0.05–0.11mmol/L

PHOSPHORUS

Newborn	4.2–9.0mg/dL	1.36–2.91mmol/L
0–15yr	3.2–6.3mg/dL	1.03–2.1mmol/L
Adult	2.7–4.5mg/dL	0.87–1.45mmol/L

PORCELAIN[12] 0.52–1.94mg/dL 0.32–9.93mmol/L

POTASSIUM

<10dy of age	4.0–6.0mEq/L	4.0–6.0mmol/L
>10dy of age	3.5–5.0mEq/L	3.5–5.0mmol/L

PREALBUMIN

Newborn–6wk	4–36mg/dL
6wk–16yr	13–27mg/dL
Adult	18–45mg/dL

PROTEINS

Protein electrophoresis (g/dL)

Age	TP	Albumin	α-1	α-2	β	γ
Cord	4.8–8.0	2.2–4.0	0.3–0.7	0.4–0.9	0.4–1.6	0.8–1.6
Newborn	4.4–7.6	3.2–4.8	0.1–0.3	0.2–0.3	0.3–0.6	0.6–1.2
1dy–1mo	4.4–7.6	2.5–5.5	0.1–0.3	0.3–1.0	0.2–1.1	0.4–1.3
1–3mo	3.6–7.4	2.1–4.8	0.1–0.4	0.3–1.1	0.3–1.1	0.2–1.1
4–6mo	4.2–7.4	2.8–5.0	0.1–0.4	0.3–0.8	0.3–0.8	0.1–0.9
7–12mo	5.1–7.3	3.2–5.7	0.1–0.6	0.3–1.5	0.4–1.0	0.2–1.2
13–24mo	3.7–7.5	1.9–5.0	0.1–0.6	0.4–1.4	0.4–1.4	0.4–1.6
25–36mo	5.3–8.1	3.3–5.8	0.1–0.3	0.4–1.1	0.3–1.2	0.4–1.5
3–5yr	4.9–8.1	2.9–5.8	0.1–0.4	0.4–1.0	0.5–1.0	0.4–1.7
6–8yr	6.0–7.9	3.3–5.0	0.1–0.5	0.5–0.8	0.5–0.9	0.7–2.0
9–11yr	6.0–7.9	3.2–5.0	0.1–0.4	0.7–0.9	0.6–1.0	0.8–2.0
12–16yr	6.0–7.9	3.2–5.1	0.1–0.4	0.5–1.1	0.5–1.1	0.6–2.0
Adult	6.0–8.0	3.1–5.4	0.1–0.4	0.4–1.1	0.5–1.2	0.7–1.7

PYRUVATE	0.3–0.9mg/dL	0.03–0.10mmol/L

Continued

TABLE 6.1

REFERENCE VALUES—cont'd

	Conventional units	SI units
RHEUMATOID FACTOR	<20	

RHEUMATON TITER (modified Waaler–Rose slide test)

	<10	

SODIUM

	Conventional units	SI units
Preterm	130–140mEq/L	130–140mmol/L
Older	135–148mEq/L	135–148mmol/L

TRANSAMINASE (SGOT) (see Aspartate aminotransferase [AST])

TRANSAMINASE (SGPT) (see Alanine aminotransferase [ALT])

TRANSFERRIN

	Conventional units	SI units
Newborn	130–275mg/dL	1.3–2.75g/L
Adult	200–400mg/dL	2.0–4.0g/L

TRIGLYCERIDES (fasting)[11]

	Male (mg/dL)	Female (mg/dL)	Male (g/L)	Female (g/L)
Cord blood	10–98	10–98	0.10–0.98	0.10–0.98
0–5yr	30–86	32–99	0.30–0.86	0.32–0.99
6–11yr	31–108	35–114	0.31–1.08	0.35–1.14
12–15yr	36–138	41–138	0.36–1.38	0.41–1.38
16–19yr	40–163	40–128	0.40–1.63	0.40–1.28
20–29yr	44–185	40–128	0.44–1.85	0.40–1.28
Adults	40–160	35–135	0.40–1.60	0.35–1.35

TROPONIN

	Conventional units	SI units
	0.03-0.15ng/mL	

UREA NITROGEN

	Conventional units	SI units
	7–22mg/dL	2.5–7.9mmol/L

URIC ACID

	Conventional units	SI units
0–2yr	2.4–6.4mg/dL	0.14–0.38mmol/L
2–12yr	2.4–5.9mg/dL	0.14–0.35mmol/L
12–14yr	2.4–6.4mg/dL	0.14–0.38mmol/L
Adult male	3.5–7.2mg/dL	0.20–0.43mmol/L
Adult female	2.4–6.4mg/dL	0.14–0.38mmol/L

VITAMIN A (retinol)

	Conventional units	SI units
Newborn	35–75mcg/dL	1.22–2.62mcmol/L
Child	30–80mcg/dL	1.05–2.79mcmol/L
Adult	30–65mcg/dL	1.05–2.27mcmol/L

TABLE 6.1

REFERENCE VALUES—cont'd

	Conventional units	SI units
VITAMIN B$_1$ (thiamine)	5.3–7.9mcg/dL	0.16–0.23mcmol/L
VITAMIN B$_2$ (riboflavin)	3.7–13.7mcg/dL	98–363mcmol/L
VITAMIN B$_{12}$ (cobalamin)	130–785pg/mL	96–579pmol/L
VITAMIN C (ascorbic acid)	0.2–2.0mg/dL	11.4–113.6mcmol/L
VITAMIN D$_3$ (1,25-dihydroxy-vitamin D)		
	25–45pg/mL	60–108pmol/L
VITAMIN E	5–20mg/dL	11.6–46.4mcmol/L
ZINC	70–150mcg/dL	10.7–22.9mcmol/L

II. EVALUATION OF PLEURAL, PERICARDIAL, AND ASCITIC FLUID

A. PROPERTIES OF TRANSUDATE VS EXUDATE (Table 6.2)

TABLE 6.2

PROPERTIES OF TRANSUDATE VS EXUDATE

Measurement[a]	Transudate	Exudate[b]
Specific gravity	<1.016	>1.016
Protein (g/dL)	<3.0	>3.0
Fluid:serum ratio	<0.5	>0.5
LDH (IU)	<200	>200
Fluid:serum ratio (isoenzymes not useful)	<0.6	>0.6
WBCs	<1000/mm^3	>1000/mm^3
RBCs	<10,000	Variable
Glucose	Same as serum	Less than serum
pH[c]	7.4–7.5	<7.4

LDH, lactate dehydrogenase; WBCs, white blood cells; RBCs, red blood cells.
[a]Always obtain serum for glucose, LDH, protein, amylase, etc.
[b]Not required to meet all the following criteria to be considered an exudate.
[c]Collect anaerobically in a heparinized syringe.

B. OTHER INFORMATION[4]

1. **Pleural fluid:** Amylase >500U/mL or pleural fluid:serum ratio >1 suggests pancreatitis.
2. **Ascitic fluid:** White blood cells (WBCs) >800 cells/mm^3 suggests peritonitis.

C. DIFFERENTIAL DIAGNOSIS OF PLEURAL EFFUSIONS (Table 6.3)

TABLE 6.3

DIFFERENTIAL DIAGNOSIS OF PLEURAL EFFUSIONS

Transudate	Exudate
Congestive heart failure	Infection
Pericardial disease	Neoplasm
Cirrhosis	Hemothorax
Nephrotic syndrome	Esophageal perforation
Peritoneal dialysis	Pancreatic disease
Chylothorax	Intraabdominal abscess
Hypothyroidism	Drugs (e.g., nitrofurantoin
Pulmonary arteriovenous malformation	and dantrolene)
Collagen vascular disease	Urinary tract obstruction
Nonimmune hydrops fetalis	
Iatrogenic hydrothorax: Catheters, VP shunts	
Pulmonary emboli	

Adapted from Loughlin[7].

III. EVALUATION OF CEREBROSPINAL FLUID (Table 6-4)

TABLE 6.4

EVALUATION OF CEREBROSPINAL FLUID

WBC COUNT

Preterm mean (range)	9 (0–25 WBCs/mm^3)	57% PMNs
Term mean (range)	8 (0–22 WBCs/mm^3)	61% PMNs
Child	0–7 WBCs/mm^3	0% PMNs

GLUCOSE

Preterm mean (range)	50 (24–63mg/dL)
Term mean (range)	52 (34–119mg/dL)
Child	40–80mg/dL

CSF GLUCOSE/BLOOD GLUCOSE

Preterm mean (range)	55–105%
Term mean (range)	44–128%
Child	50%

LACTIC ACID DEHYDROGENASE

Mean	20 (5–30U/L), or about 10% of serum value

MYELIN BASIC PROTEIN <4ng/mL

OPENING PRESSURE

Newborn	80–110 (<110mmH$_2$O)
Infant/child	<200mmH$_2$O (lateral recumbent)
Respiratory variations	5–10mmH$_2$O

PROTEIN

Preterm mean (range)	115 (65–150mg/dL)
Term mean (range)	90 (20–170mg/dL)
Child	5–40mg/dL

Adapted from Oski[8].
WBC, white blood cell; PMNs, polymorphonuclear lymphocytes; CSF, cerebrospinal fluid.

IV. EVALUATION OF SYNOVIAL FLUID (Table 6-5)

TABLE 6.5

EVALUATION OF SYNOVIAL FLUID

Group	Condition	Color/clarity	Viscosity	Mucin clot	WBC count	PMNs (%)	Miscellaneous findings
Noninflammatory	Normal	Yellow/clear	VH	G	<200	<25	—
	Traumatic arthritis	Xanthochromic/turbid	H	F-G	<2000	<25	Debris
Inflammatory	Osteoarthritis	Yellow/clear	H	F-G	1000	<25	—
	SLE	Yellow/clear	N	N	5000	10	LE cells
	Rheumatic fever	Yellow/cloudy	→	F	5000	10–50	—
	Juvenile rheumatoid arthritis	Yellow/cloudy	→	Poor	15,000–20,000	75	—
	Reiter's syndrome and Lyme disease	Yellow/opaque	→	Poor	20,000	80	Reiter's cells in Reiter's syndrome
Pyogenic	Tuberculous arthritis	Yellow–white/cloudy	→	Poor	25,000	50–60	Acid-fast bacilli
	Septic arthritis	Serosanguineous/turbid	→	Poor	50,000–300,000	>75	Low glucose, bacteria

From Cassidy[9]

↓, decreased; F, fair; G, good; H, high; N, normal; VH, very high; PMNs, polymorphonuclear neutrophils (leukocytes); SLE, systemic lupus erythematosus.

6

BLOOD CHEMISTRIES/BODY FLUIDS

V. REFERENCES

1. Meites S, ed. *Pediatric clinical chemistry*, 2nd and 3rd edns. Washington, DC: American Association for Clinical Chemistry; 1981.

2. Tietz NW. *Textbook of clinical chemistry,* Philadelphia: WB Saunders; 1986.

3. Lundberg GD. SI unit implementation: the next step. *JAMA* 1988; **260**:73.

4. Wallach J. *Interpretation of diagnostic tests*. Boston: Little, Brown & Co; 1992.

5. Berkow R. *The Merck manual of diagnosis and therapy*. Rahway, NJ: Merck Research Laboratories; 1992.

6. Summary of the NCEP Adult Treatment Panel II Report: highlights of the report of the Expert Panel on Blood and Cholesterol Levels in Children and Adolescents, 1991, U.S. Department of Health and Human Services. *JAMA* 1993; **269**.

7. Loughlin G, Eigen H. *Respiratory disease in children: diagnosis and management.* Baltimore: Williams & Wilkins; 1994.

8. Oski FA. *Principles and practice of pediatrics,* 2nd edn. Philadelphia: JB Lippincott; 1994.

9. Cassidy JT, Petty RE. *Textbook of pediatric rheumatology*, 3rd edn. Philadelphia: WB Saunders; 1995.

10. Burtis CA, Ashwood ER. *Tietz textbook of clinical chemistry,* 2nd edn. Philadelphia: WB Saunders; 1994, 787.

11. Behrman RE, Kliegman RM, Arvin AM. *Nelson textbook of pediatrics,* 15th edn. Philadelphia: WB Saunders; 1996.

12. Iannone P, Reddy U, Siberry V, Siberry V. Surviving pediatric chief residency at Hopkins. *Patience and virtue.* 1998-1999, Baltimore and Wilmington, DE.

CARDIOLOGY

Lydia Ko Chiang, MD
Alison Ensor Dunn, MD

I. THE CARDIAC CYCLE (Fig. 7.1)

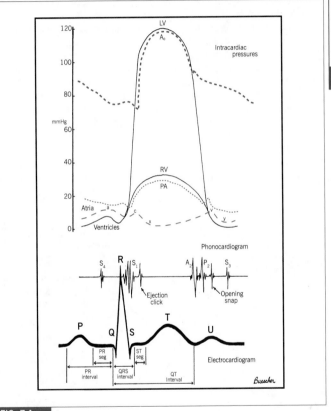

FIG. 7.1
The cardiac cycle.

II. TECHNIQUES TO ASSESS CARDIAC FUNCTION

A. PHYSICAL EXAMINATION

1. Blood pressure

a. **Pulse pressure** = Systolic pressure − Diastolic pressure.
  1) If wide (>40mmHg) consider thyrotoxicosis, arteriovenous (AV) fistula, patent ductus arteriosus, or aortic insufficiency.

2) If narrow (<25mmHg) consider pericarditis, pericardial effusion, pericardial tamponade, aortic stenosis, or significant tachycardia.

b. **Mean arterial pressure (MAP)** = Diastolic pressure + (Pulse pressure/3).

  1) In preterm infants and newborns, generally a normal MAP = gestational age in weeks + 5.

c. **Blood pressure**

  1) Four limb blood pressures can be used to assess for coarctation of the aorta; must obtain in both right and left arm because of possibility of aberrant subclavian artery (see p. 156).

  2) **Pulsus paradoxus** is an exaggeration of the normal drop in systolic blood pressure (SBP) seen with inspiration. Determine the SBP at end of exhalation and then during inhalation; if the difference in SBP is greater than 10mmHg, consider pericardial effusion, tamponade, pericarditis, asthma, or restrictive cardiomyopathies.

  3) See Figs. 7.18–7.22 and Tables 7.11 and 7.12 for blood pressure norms.

2. **Murmurs**

a. Systolic murmurs (Fig. 7.2)

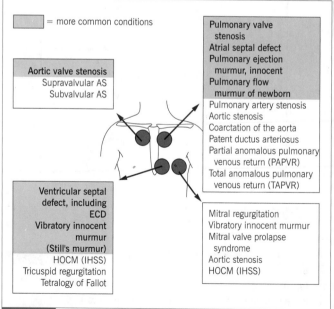

□ = more common conditions

Aortic valve stenosis
Supravalvular AS
Subvalvular AS

Pulmonary valve stenosis
Atrial septal defect
Pulmonary ejection murmur, innocent
Pulmonary flow murmur of newborn
Pulmonary artery stenosis
Aortic stenosis
Coarctation of the aorta
Patent ductus arteriosus
Partial anomalous pulmonary venous return (PAPVR)
Total anomalous pulmonary venous return (TAPVR)

Ventricular septal defect, including ECD
Vibratory innocent murmur (Still's murmur)
HOCM (IHSS)
Tricuspid regurgitation
Tetralogy of Fallot

Mitral regurgitation
Vibratory innocent murmur
Mitral valve prolapse syndrome
Aortic stenosis
HOCM (IHSS)

FIG. 7.2

The locations at which various systolic murmurs may be heard. (From Park[1].)

1) Right upper sternal border (RUSB)
   a) Aortic valve stenosis: Ejection, loudest at 3rd left intercostal space (LICS), ± thrill, ejection click, possible single S2, and transmits well to the neck; also can be heard at LUSB and apex.
   b) Subaortic stenosis: Ejection, without a click; may also have aortic regurgitation murmur during diastole.
   c) Supravalvular aortic stenosis: Ejection, ± thrill, and may transmit to the back. Evaluate for Williams syndrome.
2) Left upper sternal border (LUSB)
   a) Pulmonic stenosis (PS): Ejection, ± thrill, S2 may be widely split when mild, ± variable ejection click at 2nd LICS, and transmits to the back.
   b) Atrial septal defect (ASD): Ejection with widely split, fixed S2.
   c) Pulmonary artery stenosis: Ejection, P2 may be loud, and transmits well to back and both lung fields.
   d) Tetralogy of Fallot: Long ejection murmur, louder at middle left sternal border (MLSB) or LUSB, ± thrill, loud and single S2.
   e) Coarctation of the aorta: Ejection, loudest at the left interscapular area.
   f) Patent ductus arteriosus (PDA): Continuous murmur usually heard best at left infraclavicular area, ± thrill.
   g) Total anomalous pulmonary venous return (TAPVR): Ejection, widely split and fixed S2, quadruple or quintuple rhythm (S1, split S2, S3, S4), and diastolic rumble at left lower sternal border.
3) Left lower sternal border (LLSB)
   a) Ventricular septal defect (VSD): Regurgitant systolic, may not be holosystolic, localized to LLSB, and may have loud P2.
   b) Complete AV canal: Similar to VSD, also with diastolic rumble at LLSB, and may have a gallop rhythm in infants.
   c) Hypertrophic obstructive cardiomyopathy/idiopathic hypertrophic subaortic stenosis (HOCM/IHSS): Ejection murmur of medium pitch heard best at LLSB or apex, ± thrill. Murmur will vary with maneuvers. Venous return is decreased with Valsalva maneuver, so outflow tract obstruction will increase and the murmur becomes louder. With squatting, venous return increases, resulting in increased blood flow and dilatation of left ventricle (LV); therefore obstruction decreases and the murmur softens.
   d) Tricuspid regurgitation: Regurgitant systolic, triple or quadruple rhythm.
4) Apex
   a) Mitral regurgitation (MR): Regurgitant systolic, may not be holosystolic, which may transmit to the left axillae and may be loudest in the midprecordium.
   b) Mitral valve prolapse: Midsystolic click from valve prolapse with late systolic murmur if MR present. The click will move closer to

the first heart sound if LV volume is decreased (standing, sitting, Valsalva maneuver) and closer to the second heart sound if LV volume is increased (squatting).

b. Diastolic murmurs
   1) Early
      a) Aortic regurgitation: Decrescendo, high pitched, loudest at 3rd LICS, and radiates to apex.
      b) Pulmonary regurgitation: Medium pitched, loudest at 2nd LICS, and radiates along left sternal border (LSB).
   2) Middle and late
      a) Mitral stenosis: Best heard at the apex.
      b) Tricuspid stenosis: Best heard along LSB.

c. Continuous: Begin in systole and continue into all or part of diastole.
   1) Arteriovenous or aortopulmonary connection: PDA, AV fistula, and aorta–pulmonary window.
   2) Turbulent venous flow: Venous hum.
   3) Turbulent arterial flow: Coarctation of the aorta, peripheral pulmonary artery stenosis.

d. Benign: Heart murmurs caused by a disturbance of the laminar flow of blood, frequently produced as the diameter of the blood's pathway decreases and the velocity increases.
   1) Still's vibratory murmur (flow from the left ventricle to the aorta): Grade 2–3/6 systolic ejection murmur (SEM) heard best at the LLSB to the apex; more musical than most other murmurs; louder when supine. Usually appreciated in children 3–6 years old.
   2) Pulmonary ejection murmur (flow from right ventricle [RV] to pulmonary artery): Early–midsystolic 1–3/6 murmur heard best along LUSB with a blowing quality. Usually seen in children 8–14 years old.
   3) Peripheral PS (flow from branching of pulmonary artery to arterioles): 1–2/6 SEM heard best at the LUSB with radiations throughout the chest, axillae, and back. Found in newborns and usually disappears by 3–6 months of life.
   4) Venous hum (confluence of the jugular, subclavian, and innominate veins to the superior vena cava [SVC]): Continuous 1–3/6 murmur heard at the right or left superior infraclavicular area. Will disappear when patient is supine and will diminish with head rotation and jugular vein compression. Usually seen in children 3–6 years old.
   5) Carotid bruit (flow from aortic arch to the brachiocephalic vessels): Systolic 2–3/6 murmur heard best at the right supraclavicular area and over the carotids. Rarely there will be a carotid thrill. Can be appreciated at any age.

3. Heart sounds

a. S1 is best heard at the apex or LLSB. Wide splitting is unusual in children and may suggest Ebstein's anomaly or right bundle-branch block (RBBB).

b. S2, heard best at the LUSB, has a normal physiologic split that increases with inspiration. If the S2 split is wide and fixed, consider volume overload from an ASD or partial anomalous pulmonary venous return (PAPVR); pressure overload from PS; electrical delay from RBBB; early aortic closure from MR; or normal variation. Conditions that delay aortic valve closure or accelerate pulmonic valve closure will narrow S2. Examples are pulmonary hypertension, aortic stenosis, LBBB, and normal variant (Table 7.1).

c. S3, heard best at the apex or LLSB, can be commonly heard in healthy children and adults but may also be seen in patients with dilated ventricles (large VSD, congestive heart failure [CHF]). See Fig. 7.1.

d. S4, heard at the apex, is always considered pathologic and suggests decreased ventricular compliance.

7

CARDIOLOGY

TABLE 7.1

SUMMARY OF ABNORMAL S2

Abnormal splitting

Widely split and fixed S2

Volume overload (e.g., ASD, PAPVR)

Abnormal pulmonary valve (e.g., PS)

Electrical delay (e.g., RBBB)

Early aortic closure (e.g., MR)

Occasional normal child

Narrowly split S2

Pulmonary hypertension

AS

Occasional normal child

Single S2

Pulmonary hypertension

One semilunar valve (e.g., pulmonary atresia, aortic atresia, truncus arteriosus)

P2 not audible (e.g., TGA, TOF, severe PS)

Severe AS

Occasional normal child

Paradoxically split S2

Severe AS

LBBB, Wolff–Parkinson–White syndrome (type B)

Abnormal intensity of P2

Increased P2 (e.g., pulmonary hypertension)

Decreased P2 (e.g., severe PS, TOF, TS)

From Park[1].

PAPVR, Partial anomalous pulmonary venous return; MR, mitral regurgitation; LBBB, Left bundle-branch block; TS, tricuspid stenosis; ASD, atrial septal defect; PS, pulmonary stenosis; RBBB, right bundle-branch block; AS, aortic stenosis; TGA, transposition of the great arteries; TOF, tetralogy of Fallot.

B. CHEST RADIOGRAPH

1. **Evaluate the heart.**
a. Size: The cardiac shadow should be less than 50% of the thoracic width, which is the maximal width between inner margins of the ribs, as measured on a posteroanterior (PA) radiograph during inspiration.
b. Shape: The contour of the SVC, right atrium (RA), and inferior vena cava (IVC) (on the right) and the aorta, pulmonary artery, left atrium (LA), RV, and LV (on the left) can often be distinguished on PA and lateral chest radiographs, aiding in the diagnosis of chamber/vessel enlargement and some congenital heart disease (Fig. 7.3).
c. Situs (levocardia, mesocardia, dextrocardia).

2. **Evaluate lung fields.**
a. Decreased pulmonary blood flow: Seen in pulmonary or tricuspid stenosis/atresia, tetralogy of Fallot, pulmonary hypertension ('peripheral pruning').
b. Increased pulmonary blood flow: Increased pulmonary vascular markings with redistribution from bases to apices of lungs and extension to lateral lung fields, as with ASD, VSD, PDA, transposition of the great arteries (TGA), and TAPVR.
c. Venous congestion (CHF): Increased pulmonary vascular markings centrally, interstitial and alveolar pulmonary edema (air bronchograms), septal lines, and pleural effusions, as with TAPVR and mitral valve stenosis/regurgitation.

3. **Evaluate airway.**
a. The trachea usually bends slightly to the right above the carina in normal patients with a left-sided aortic arch. A perfectly straight or left-bending trachea suggests a right aortic arch, which may be associated

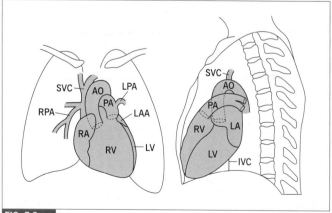

FIG. 7.3

Radiologic contours of the heart. See text for abbreviations. AO, Aorta.

with other defects (tetralogy of Fallot, truncus arteriosus, vascular rings, chromosome 22 microdeletion).

4. **Skeletal anomalies**

a. Rib notching (e.g., from collateral vessels in patients >5 years with coarctation of the aorta).

b. Sternal abnormalities (e.g., Holt–Oram syndrome; pectus excavatum in Marfan, Ehlers–Danlos, pentalogy of Cantrell and Noonan syndromes).

c. Vertebral anomalies (e.g., VATER/VACTERL syndrome: **V**ertebral anomalies, **A**nal atresia, **T**racheo**E**sophageal fistula, **R**adial and **R**enal, **C**ardiac, and **L**imb anomalies).

5. See pp. 154–158 for typical findings on chest radiograph.

C. **BASIC ELECTROCARDIOGRAPHY PRINCIPLES**

1. **Lead placement** (Fig. 7.4)

a. Unipolar limb leads

    1) aVR: Right arm is positive electrode.

    2) aVL: Left arm is positive electrode.

    3) aVF: Left foot is positive electrode.

b. Bipolar limb leads

    1) Lead I: Right arm negative to left arm positive.

    2) Lead II: Right arm negative to left leg positive.

    3) Lead III: Left arm negative to left leg positive.

c. Precordial/horizontal plane leads.

Note: For pediatric ECGs, V3R is typically recorded instead of V3 (i.e., V1, V2, V3R, V4, V5, V6).

2. **ECG complexes** (Fig. 7.1)

a. P wave: Represents atrial depolarization.

b. QRS complex: Represents ventricular depolarization.

c. T wave: Represents ventricular repolarization.

d. U wave: May follow T wave, representing late phases of ventricular repolarization.

3. **Systematic approach for evaluating ECGs**

Note: The following section provides a systematic approach to reading ECGs, with normal values given. See Figures 7.7–7.14 for interpretation of abnormal ECG findings.

a. Rate (See p. 179 for age-specific heart rate norms.)

    1) Standardization: Paper speed is 25mm/sec. One small square = 1mm = 0.04sec. One large square = 5mm = 0.2sec. Amplitude standard: 10mm = 1 millivolt.

    2) Calculation: Heart rate (beats per minute) = 60 divided by the average R–R interval in seconds or 1500 divided by R–R interval in millimeters. For a quick estimate, see Fig. 7.5.

b. Rhythm

    1) Sinus rhythm: Every QRS complex preceded by a P wave, normal PR interval (the PR interval may be prolonged, as in first-degree AV block), and normal P wave axis (upright P in lead I and aVF).

7

CARDIOLOGY

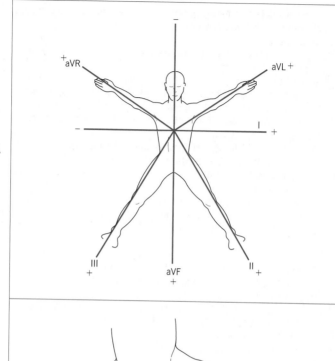

A

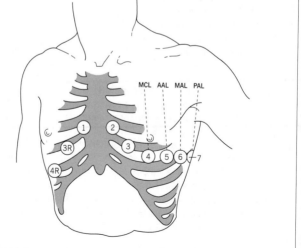

B

FIG. 7.4
A, Frontal/limb leads. **B,** Placement of precordial leads. AAL, anterior axillary line; MAL, midaxillary line; MCL, midclavicular line; PAL, posterior axillary line.

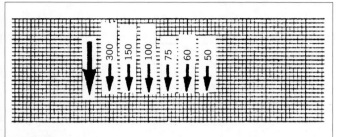

FIG. 7.5

Estimation of heart rate. (From Park[1].)

TABLE 7.2

MEAN AND RANGES OF NORMAL QRS AXES

	Age	Mean° (range)
	1 wk–1 mo	+110 (+30 to +180)
	1–3 mo	+70 (+10 to +125)
	3 mo–3 yr	+60 (+10 to +110)
	>3 yr	+60 (+20 to +120)
	Adults	+50 (−30 to +105)

From Park[1].

TABLE 7.3

T WAVE AXIS

Age	V1, V2	AVF	I, V5, V6
Birth–1 day	±	+	±
1–4 days	±	+	+
4 days to adolescent	−	+	+
Adolescent to adult	+	+	+

+, T wave positive;−, T wave negative; ±, T wave normally either positive or negative.

2) There is normal respiratory variation of the R–R interval without morphologic changes of the P wave or QRS complex.

c. Axis

1) Normal values

a) P wave axis: From 0 to +90° for sinus rhythm.

b) QRS axis: Varies with age, with right axis deviation seen in newborns secondary to RV dominance (Table 7.2).

c) T wave axis: Generally from 0 to +90° (Table 7.3).

2) Estimation of mean QRS axis

a) Use leads I and aVF to determine quadrant of mean QRS axis. For example, positive deflection in leads I and aVF yields mean axis in left lower quadrant (0 to +90°) (Fig. 7.6).

b) Next, find the lead with an isoelectric QRS complex (R = S). Mean QRS axis is perpendicular to this lead in the predetermined quadrant.

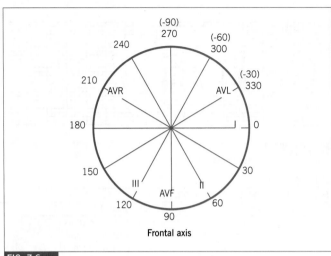

FIG. 7.6
Frontal axis.

TABLE 7.4

NORMAL PR INTERVAL RANGE FOR AGE (UPPER LIMIT OF NORMAL)

0–1 mo	1–6 mo	6–12 mo	1–3 yr
0.09–0.10 **(0.12)**	0.09–0.11 **(0.14)**	0.10–0.12 **(0.14)**	0.10–0.12 **(0.15)**

3–8 yr	8–12 yr	12–16 yr	Adult
0.12–0.15 **(0.17)**	0.14–0.16 **(0.18)**	0.15–0.16 **(0.19)**	0.15–0.17 **(0.21)**

d. Intervals: Measure the PR interval, QRS duration, and QT interval using the limb lead recordings.
  1) PR interval: Normal value varies with heart rate and age (Table 7.4).
  2) QRS duration[2]: Normal width is ≤0.1 second in all leads, but varies with age. Upper limits for children <3 years = 0.07 second, 3–8 years = 0.08 second, 8–12 years = 0.09 second, and ≥12 years = 0.10 second.
  3) QT interval: Normal value varies with heart rate and should be corrected (QTc = corrected QT interval).

  a) $QTc = \dfrac{\text{Measured QT (sec)}}{\sqrt{\text{R-R interval (sec)}}}$

The R–R interval should extend from the R wave in the QRS complex in which you are measuring QT to the preceding R wave.

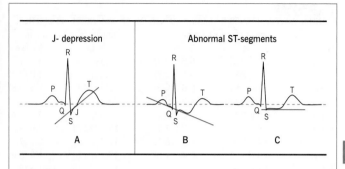

FIG. 7.7

ST segment changes. **A,** J depression. **B** and **C,** Abnormal ST segments. (From Park[1].)

    b) Normal values for QTc
       i) 0.440 second is 97th percentile for infants 3–4 days old[3].
       ii) ≤0.45 second in infants <6 months old.
       iii) ≤0.44 second in children.
       iv) ≤0.425 second in adolescents and adults.

e. P wave size and shape: Normal P wave should be <0.10 second in children, <0.08 second in infants, with amplitude <30mV (3mm in height, with normal standardization = 10mV/mm).

f. R wave progression: Generally see normal increase in R wave size and decrease in S wave size from leads V1 to V6 (with dominant S waves in right precordial leads and dominant R waves in left precordial leads), representing dominance of left ventricular forces. However, newborns and infants have a normal dominance of the right ventricle.

g. Normal Q waves: Usually <0.04 second (1mm) in duration and <25% of total QRS amplitude. Can see Q waves <5mm deep in left precordial leads and aVF; up to 8mm deep in lead III for children <3 years of age.

h. ST–T wave changes
    1) ST segment: Generally flat (isoelectric), but normal variation may include elevation or depression of up to 1mm in limb leads and 2mm in left precordial leads. J-point depression or elevation is a nonpathologic shift of the J point (the QRS and ST segment junction), with upward-sloping ST segment and no prolonged ST segment depression or elevation (Fig. 7.7).
    2) T waves: Normally inverted in aVR. In young patients, negative T waves may be normal in V1 and V2, sometimes V3 and V4 (see Table 7.3). Once T wave becomes upright in a precordial lead, all leads to left should have positive T waves.

i. Voltage: QRS amplitude varies with age (Table 7.5).

TABLE 7.5
R AND S WAVE VOLTAGES BY LEAD AND AGE (MEAN AND 98TH PERCENTILE)

	Amplitude in V1 (in mm)[a]		Amplitude in V6 (in mm)	
Age	R wave	S wave	R wave	S wave
<1 day	13.8 (26.1)	8.5 (22.7)	4.2 (11.1)	3.2 (9.6)
1–2 days	14.1 (26.9)	9.1 (20.7)	4.5 (12.2)	3.0 (9.4)
3–6 days	12.9 (24.2)	6.6 (16.8)	5.2 (12.1)	3.5 (9.8)
1–3 wk	10.6 (20.8)	4.2 (10.8)	7.6 (16.4)	34. (9.8)
1–2 mo	9.5 (18.4)	5.0 (12.4)	11.6 (21.4)	2.7 (6.4)
3–5 mo	9.8 (19.8)	5.7 (17.1)	13.1 (22.4)	2.9 (9.9)
6–11 mo	9.4 (20.3)	6.4 (18.1)	12.6 (22.7)	2.1 (7.2)
1–2 yr	8.9 (17.7)	8.4 (21.0)	13.1 (22.6)	1.9 (6.6)
3–4 yr	8.1 (18.2)	10.2 (21.4)	14.8 (24.2)	1.5 (5.2)
5–7 yr	6.7 (13.9)	12.0 (23.8)	16.3 (26.5)	1.2 (4.0)
8–11 yr	5.4 (12.1)	11.9 (25.4)	16.3 (25.4)	1.0 (3.9)
12–15 yr	4.1 (9.9)	10.8 (21.2)	14.3 (23.0)	0.8 (3.7)

Data modified from Davignon[4].

[a]In millimeters at 10mV/mm standardization.

D. SPECIFIC ECG FINDINGS
1. Arrhythmias
a. Sinus rhythms
  1) Sinus tachycardia: Normal sinus rhythm with heart rate >95th percentile for age (usually less than 230 beats/min) (see p. 179).
    a) Causes: Anxiety, fever, hypovolemia, shock, sepsis, exercise, anemia, CHF, pulmonary embolus, hyperthyroidism, myocardial disease, drugs (e.g., β-agonists, aminophylline, atropine), alcohol withdrawal.
    b) Treatment: Address underlying causes.
  2) Sinus bradycardia: Normal sinus rhythm with heart rate <5th percentile for age.
    a) Causes: Vagal stimulation, increased intracranial pressure, hypothyroidism, hypothermia, hypoxia, hyperkalemia, hypercalcemia, drugs (e.g., digoxin, β-blockers), acidosis, long QT syndrome, normal individuals and athletes.
    b) Treatment: Address underlying causes. If symptomatic, refer to inside back cover.
b. Supraventricular arrhythmia: Abnormal rhythm resulting from ectopic focus in atria or AV node, or from accessory conduction pathways. Characterized by varying P wave shape and abnormal P wave axis. QRS morphology usually normal (Fig. 7.8).
  1) Premature atrial contraction (PAC): Ectopic atrial focus causing early depolarization. Abnormal P wave and normal QRS complex appear prematurely with incomplete compensatory pause.
    a) Causes: Cardiac surgery, digitalis toxicity, otherwise healthy children with stress, caffeine, theophylline, sympathomimetic agents.

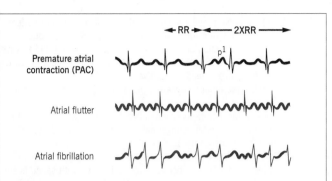

FIG. 7.8

Supraventricular arrhythmias[8]. p^1, premature atrial contraction.

b) Treatment: None necessary, except with digitalis toxicity.

2) Atrial flutter: Atrial rate between 250 and 350 beats/min, yielding characteristic flutter or sawtooth pattern (no discrete P waves), and variable ventricular response rate (with normal QRS complex).

    a) Causes: Usually associated with significant cardiac disease, such as myocardial disease, dilated atria, previous intraatrial surgery, valvular or ischemic heart disease, digitalis toxicity.

    b) Treatment: Digoxin ± propranolol, synchronized cardioversion, atrial overpacing. Consult cardiologist.

3) Atrial fibrillation: Ectopic atrial foci with atrial rate between 350 and 600 beats/min, yielding characteristic fibrillatory pattern (no discrete P waves) and irregularly irregular ventricular response rate of about 110–150 beats/min with normal QRS complex.

    a) Causes: Usually associated with significant cardiac disease, such as myocardial disease, dilated atria, previous intraatrial surgery, coronary artery disease, hypertension, valvular disease, digitalis toxicity, exacerbated by stress, alcohol.

    b) Treatment: If unstable, pharmacologic therapy with digoxin ± propranolol, synchronized cardioversion with coumadin pretreatment. Consult cardiologist.

4) Supraventricular tachycardia (SVT): Sudden run of three or more premature supraventricular beats at rate >230 beats/min, with normal (i.e., narrow) QRS complex and abnormal P wave. Either sustained (>30 seconds) or unsustained.

    a) Three types of SVT

        i) AV reentrant tachycardia: Presence of accessory 'bypass' pathway (e.g., bundle of Kent), in conjunction with AV node, establishes cyclic pattern of signal reentry, independent of sinoatrial (SA) node. Most common cause of nonsinus tachycardia in children (see 'Wolff–Parkinson–White syndrome').

      ii) AV nodal/junctional tachycardia: Cyclical reentrant pattern resulting from dual AV node pathways. Simultaneous depolarization of atria and ventricles yields invisible P wave (buried in preceding QRS or T wave) or retrograde P wave (negative in lead II, positive in aVR).

      iii) Ectopic atrial tachycardia: Rapid firing of ectopic focus in atrium.

    b) Causes: Most commonly idiopathic (over half of children with SVT); also in certain congenital heart defects (i.e., Ebstein's anomaly, transposition).

    c) Treatment: Vagal maneuvers (Valsalva, ice bag to face), adenosine (0.1mg/kg per dose, rapid IV push with saline flush; may increase by increments of 0.05mg/kg per dose every 2 minutes until maximum dose of 0.25mg/kg per dose or max. single dose of 12mg), digoxin, β-blockers, esophageal overdrive pacing. If unstable, need immediate **synchronized** cardioversion (0.5J/kg, may repeat 1J/kg). Consult cardiologist.

  5) Nodal escape beat or junctional rhythm: Abnormal rhythm driven by AV node impulse, giving normal QRS complex and invisible P wave (buried in preceding QRS or T wave) or retrograde P wave (negative in lead II, positive in aVR).

c. Ventricular arrhythmia: Abnormal rhythm resulting from ectopic focus in ventricles. Characterized by wide QRS complex, T wave pointing in opposite direction to QRS, random relation of QRS to P wave (i.e., AV dissociation) (Fig. 7.9).

  1) Premature ventricular contraction (PVC): Ectopic ventricular focus causing early depolarization. Abnormally wide QRS complex appears prematurely, usually with full compensatory pause. May be unifocal or multifocal. Bigeminy is alternating normal and abnormal QRS complexes; trigeminy is two normal QRS complexes followed by abnormal one. Couplet is two consecutive PVCs.

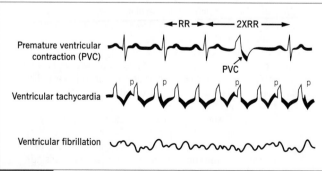

FIG. 7.9
Ventricular arrhythmias.

a) Causes: Seen in healthy children, myocarditis and myocardial injury, cardiomyopathy, long QT syndrome, congenital and acquired heart disease, toxic effect (digitalis, catecholamines, theophylline, caffeine, anesthetics), mitral valve prolapse, anxiety, hypokalemia, hypoxia, hypomagnesemia. **PVCs are more worrisome if there is underlying cardiac disease, if they are worse with activity, if patient is symptomatic, and if they are multiform (especially couplets).**

b) Treatment: None necessary, except identifying potential heart disease and addressing underlying cause.

2) Ventricular tachycardia (VT): Series of three or more PVCs at rapid rate (120–250 beats/min), with wide QRS complex and dissociated, retrograde, or no P wave. Either sustained (>30 seconds) or unsustained, monophasic, or polymorphic.

a) Causes: Same as above for PVC, but 70% have abnormal hearts.

b) Treatment: If hemodynamically stable, address underlying causes, consider lidocaine, and consult cardiologist. If hemodynamically unstable (i.e., shock), see inside back cover.

3) Ventricular fibrillation: Depolarization of ventricles in uncoordinated, asynchronous pattern, yielding abnormal QRS complexes of varying size and morphology with irregular, rapid rate. Rare in children.

a) Causes: Myocarditis, myocardial infarction (MI), postoperative state, digitalis or quinidine toxicity, drugs (e.g., catecholamines), severe hypoxia, electrolyte disturbance.

b) Treatment: Requires immediate action. See inside back cover.

2. Conduction disturbances

a. AV heart block: Disturbance in conduction of impulse from sinus node to ventricles (Fig. 7.10).

1) First-degree AV block: Abnormal but asymptomatic delay in conduction through AV node, yielding prolongation of PR interval beyond upper limits for age (see Table 7.4).

a) Causes: Seen in healthy children, acute rheumatic fever, tick-borne disease, connective tissue disease, congenital heart disease, cardiomyopathy, digitalis toxicity, after surgery.

b) Treatment: None necessary, except treating underlying disease.

2) Second-degree AV block: Impaired conduction through AV node such that there are 'dropped beats,' and some but not all P waves are followed by QRS.

a) Möbitz type I (Wenckebach): Progressive lengthening of PR interval until a QRS is not conducted and ventricular contraction does not occur. Block is at level of AV node and does not usually progress to complete heart block.

i) Causes: Seen in healthy children, myocarditis, cardiomyopathy, congenital heart disease, postsurgery, myocardial infarction, toxicity (digitalis, β-blocker).

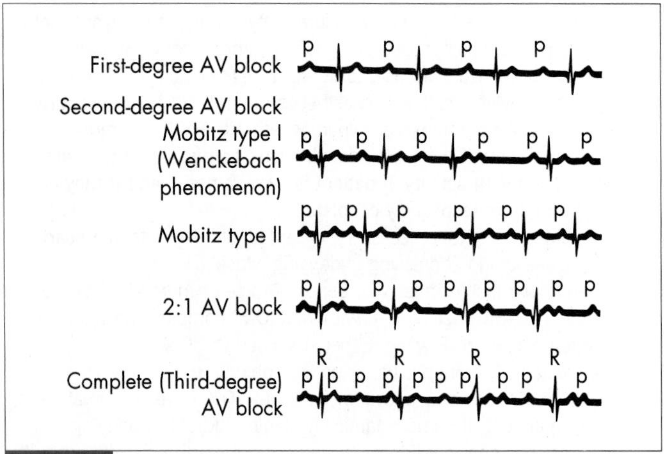

FIG. 7.10

Conduction blocks. (From Park[5].)

    ii) Treatment: Address underlying cause.

   b) Möbitz type II: Paroxysmal skipped ventricular conduction without lengthening of the PR interval. Block is at level of bundle of His and may progress to complete heart block.

    i) Causes: Same as those for type I block.

    ii) Treatment: Address underlying cause. May need pacemaker.

   c) Higher AV block: Conduction of atrial impulse at regular intervals, yielding 2:1 block (2 atrial impulses for every ventricular response), 3:1 block, etc.

  3) Third-degree (complete) AV block: Complete dissociation of atrial and ventricular conduction. P wave and PP interval regular; RR interval regular and much slower (driven by junctional or ectopic ventricular pacemaker with intrinsic rate of 30–50/minute). Width of QRS will be narrow with junctional pacemaker, wide with ventricular pacemaker.

   a) Causes: Congenital (isolated anomaly, maternal lupus or other connective tissue disease, structural heart disease such as left transposition of the great artery) or acquired (acute rheumatic fever, myocarditis, Lyme carditis, postsurgery, cardiomyopathy, myocardial infarction, drug overdose).

   b) Treatment: If bradycardic, see inside back cover and consult cardiologist.

 b. Ventricular conduction disturbance: Abnormal transmission of electrical impulse through ventricles leading to prolongation of QRS complex ($\geq$0.08 second for infants, $\geq$0.10 second for adults) (Fig. 7.11)[2].

  1) Right bundle-branch block (RBBB): Delayed right bundle conduction prolongs RV depolarization time, leading to wide QRS with terminal slurring directed right and anterior.

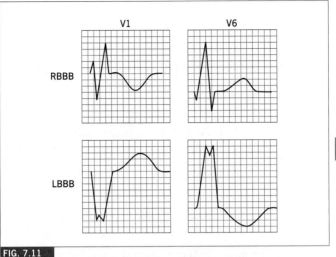

FIG. 7.11

ECG findings of right (RBBB) and left bundle-branch block (LBBB).

a) RBBB criteria: Right axis deviation, long QRS with terminal slurred R' (M-shaped RSR' or RR) in V1, V2, aVR, and wide and slurred S wave in leads I and V6.

Note: RSR' pattern in V1 can be normal in infants and young children if QRS duration and voltage are normal and R' <R.

b) Causes: ASD, surgery with right ventriculotomy, Ebstein's anomaly, coarctation in infants <6 months, endocardial cushion defect, and partial anomalous pulmonary venous return; occasionally occurs in normal children.

2) Left bundle-branch block (LBBB): Delayed left bundle conduction prolongs septal and LV depolarization time, leading to wide QRS with loss of usual septal signal; there is still a predominance of left ventricle forces. Rare in children.

a) LBBB criteria: Wide negative QS complex in lead V1 with loss of septal R wave and entirely positive, wide R or RR' complex in lead V6 with loss of septal q wave.

b) Causes: Hypertension, ischemic or valvular heart disease, cardiomyopathy.

3) Wolff–Parkinson–White syndrome (WPW): Atrial impulse transmitted via anomalous conduction pathway (i.e., bundle of Kent) to ventricles, bypassing AV node and normal ventricular conduction system. Leads to premature and prolonged depolarization of ventricles. Bypass pathway is a predisposing condition for SVT.

a) WPW criteria: Shortened PR interval (<0.08 second for <3 years old; <0.10 second for 3–16 years old; <0.12 second for

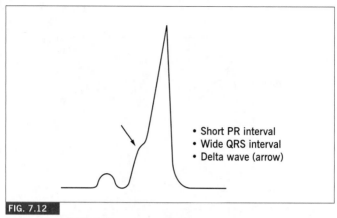

- Short PR interval
- Wide QRS interval
- Delta wave (arrow)

FIG. 7.12

ECG findings of Wolff–Parkinson–White syndrome.

>16 years old), delta wave (initial slurring of QRS upstroke), and wide QRS (Fig. 7.12)[2].

b) Treatment: Acute management of SVT if necessary as above; consider ablation of accessory pathway if recurrent SVT.

3. Atrial and ventricular enlargement

a. Atrial enlargement: Diagnosed by measuring P wave (Fig. 7.13)[1].

1) Right atrial enlargement (RAE): Initial component of P wave (representing RA depolarization) is prominent, yielding tall P waves (≥3mm) in any lead.

2) Left atrial enlargement (LAE): P wave is wide (≥0.08 second in infants; ≥0.1 second in children) and often notched in limb leads, or biphasic with deep terminal inversion in V1, representing initial RA depolarization followed by prolonged and prominent depolarization of enlarged LA.

b. Ventricular hypertrophy: Diagnosed by QRS axis, voltage, and R/S ratio (see Table 7.5, p. 142).

1) Right ventricular hypertrophy (RVH) criteria (at least one of the following):

a) Increased right and anterior QRS voltage (with normal QRS duration):

i) R in lead V1 >98th percentile for age.

ii) S in lead V6 >98th percentile for age.

b) Upright T wave in lead V1 after 3 days of age to adolescence.

c) Supplemental criteria include presence of q wave in V1 (qR or qRs pattern), right axis deviation for patient's age, and RV strain (associated with inverted T wave in V1 with tall R wave).

2) Left ventricular hypertrophy (LVH) criteria:

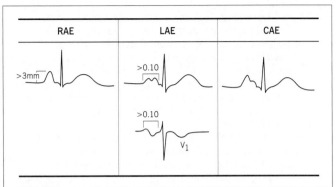

FIG. 7.13

Criteria for atrial enlargement. CAE, combined atrial enlargement; LAE, left atrial enlargement; RAE, right atrial enlargement. (From Park[1].)

a) Increased QRS voltage in leftward leads (with normal QRS duration):
i) R in lead V6 (and I, aVL, V5) >98th percentile for age.
ii) S in lead V1 >98th percentile for age.
b) Supplemental criteria include left axis deviation for patient's age, volume overload (associated with Q wave >5mm and tall T waves in V5 or V6), and LV strain (associated with inverted T wave in leads V6, I, or aVF).

4. **Myocardial infarction in children**
a. Etiology: Myocardial infarction in children is rare but could occur in children with anomalous origin of the left coronary artery, Kawasaki disease, congenital heart disease (pre- and post-surgical), and dilated cardiomyopathy. Rarely seen in children with hypertension, lupus, myocarditis, cocaine ingestion, and adrenergic drugs (e.g., β-agonists used for asthma).
b. Frequent ECG findings in children with acute MI
1) New-onset wide Q waves (>0.035 second), with or without Q wave notching, seen within first few hours (and persistent over several years)[6].
2) ST segment elevation (>2mm), seen within first few hours[6].
3) Diphasic T waves, seen within first few days (becoming sharply inverted then normalizing over time).
4) Prolonged QTc interval (>0.44 second) with accompanying abnormal Q waves[6].
5) Deep, wide Q waves in leads I, aVL, or V6, without Q waves in II, III, aVF, suggestive of anomalous origin of left coronary artery.
c. Other criteria

1) Laboratory findings such as elevated creatine phosphokinase (CPK)/MB fraction and lactate dehydrogenase (LDH) are helpful, although nonspecific for detection of acute MI in children.

2) **Cardiac troponin I** is likely to be a more sensitive indicator of early myocardial damage in children. Plasma levels become elevated within hours of cardiac injury and persist for 4–7 days. Significant elevation of cardiac troponin I (>2ng/mL) is a predictor of poor clinical outcome and is specific to cardiac injury[7].

5. **Prolonged QTc interval**

a. Causes: Hypocalcemia, hypokalemia, hypomagnesemia, myocarditis, myocardial ischemia, bradycardia, drug effect (quinidine, procainamide, phenothiazines, tricyclics, organophosphates, erythromycin, trimethoprim–sulfamethoxazole, and cisapride), and familial (specific Na+/K+ channel defects in some cases).

b. Complications: Prolonged QTc interval predisposes to ventricular arrhythmias, often initiated by a PVC occurring during the prolonged repolarization phase.

1) Symptoms of arrhythmias: Syncope, palpitations, lightheadedness, and seizure, or may degenerate into ventricular fibrillation and cardiac arrest.

2) *Torsades de pointes:* A special form of ventricular tachycardia with QRS complexes of varying amplitudes (sinusoidal), particularly seen in prolonged QTc (Fig. 7.14).

c. Treatment: Often self-limited, but need to identify underlying cause and correct it. If unstable, treat with pharmacologic agents (lidocaine, bretylium, isoproterenol, magnesium), cardiac pacing, or cardioversion. Consult with cardiologist.

6. **Potassium**: For ECG changes, see p. 240.

7. **Calcium**: Hypocalcemia presents with prolonged QTc interval. Hypercalcemia presents with shortened QTc interval.

8. **Digitalis effect**: Associated with shortened QTc interval, ST depression ('scooped' or 'sagging'), mildly prolonged PR interval, and flattened T wave.

9. **Digitalis toxicity**: Primarily arrhythmias (bradycardia, SVT, ectopic atrial tachycardia, ventricular tachycardia, AV block).

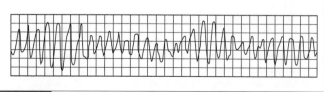

FIG. 7.14

Torsades de pointes.

10. See Table 7.6.

E. ECHOCARDIOGRAPHY

1. Specific data obtained through echocardiography

a. M-mode technique: Uses one ultrasonic beam that passes through cardiac structures in a single axis, allowing for measurement of heart wall and chamber dimensions during different phases of cardiac cycle.

   1) Important for quantifying left ventricular systolic function and contractility. Best represented by the **shortening fraction,** which measures percent change in left ventricular end-systolic dimension (LVESD) and left ventricular end-diastolic dimension (LVEDD). Very reliable index of LV function (Fig. 7.15).

   2) Shortening fraction (%) =

$$\frac{LVEDD - LVESD}{LVEDD} \times 100$$

b. Transesophageal echocardiography (TEE): Uses ultrasound transducer on end of modified endoscope to view the heart from the esophagus and stomach, allowing for better imaging of the aorta, atria, and obese or intraoperative patients. Also useful for visualizing valvular anatomy, such as valvular vegetations.

7

CARDIOLOGY

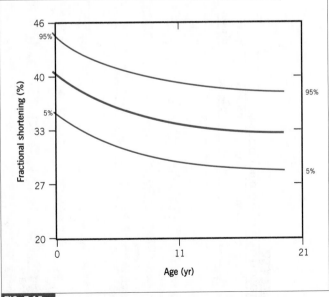

FIG. 7.15

Normal range for shortening fraction related to age. (From Colon[10].)

TABLE 7.6

SYSTEMIC EFFECTS ON ELECTROCARDIOGRAM

	Short QT	Long QT-U	Prolonged QRS	ST-T changes	Sinus tach	Sinus brady	AV block	V tach	Miscellaneous
CHEMISTRY									
Hyperkalemia			X	X			X	X	Low voltage Ps; peaked Ts
Hypokalemia		X	X	X					
Hypercalcemia	X							X	
Hypocalcemia		X			X		X		
Hypermagnesemia							X		
Hypomagnesemia		X							
DRUGS									
Digitalis	X			X			X		
Phenothiazines		T				T		T	
Phenytoin	X								
Propranolol	X					X	X		
Quinidine		X	X			T	T	T	
Tricyclics		T	T	T	T		T		
Verapamil						X	X		
Imipramine							T	T	Atrial flutter

MISCELLANEOUS

Condition						
CNS injury	X		X	X	X	Atrial flutter
Freidreich's ataxia			X	X	X	Atrial flutter
Duchenne's disease			X	X		
Myotonic dystrophy	X		X	X		
Collagen disease			X			
Hypothyroidism			X		X	Low voltage
Hyperthyroidism		Romano-Ward	X	X		
Other diseases		Lyme disease	X	X		Holt-Oram, maternal lupus

From Garson[8] and Walsh[9].

X, present; T, present only with drug toxicity.

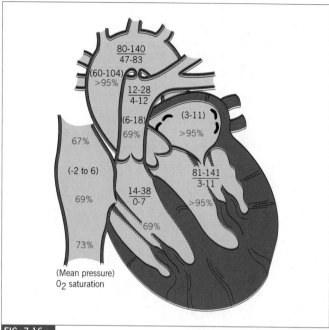

FIG. 7.16

Normal pressures and saturations obtained with cardiac catheterization.

F. INVASIVE CARDIAC MONITORING (Fig. 7.16)

III. CONGENITAL HEART DISEASE (CHD)

A. ACYANOTIC

1. **VSD:** 20–25% of CHD; this is the most common form.

a. Examination: 2–5/6 holosystolic murmur loudest at the LLSB. A systolic thrill may be felt at the LLSB. There may be an apical diastolic rumble if there is a large shunt. S2 may be narrow and the P2 component may be increased.

b. ECG: Small VSD: Normal. Medium VSD: LVH (left ventricular hypertrophy), ± LAE (left atrial enlargement). Large VSD: BVH (biventricular hypertrophy), ± LAE, pure RVH.

c. Chest radiograph: Cardiomegaly and increased PVMs (pulmonary vascular markings) dependent on the amount of L to R shunting.

2. **ASD**

a. Examination: Wide, fixed split S2 with a grade 2–3/6 SEM at the LUSB. May have middiastolic rumble at LLSB.

b. ECG: Right axis deviation (RAD) and mild RVH or RBBB with a RSR' in V1.

c. Chest radiograph: Cardiomegaly with increased PVMs.
3. **PDA:** 5–10% of CHD in term infants; 40–60% in preterm infants weighing <1500g. Embryologic connection from main pulmonary trunk to the descending aorta. The PDA usually inserts 5–10mm distal to the origin of the left subclavian artery. If it remains patent, it may produce pulmonary overload and subsequent LV failure. Prostaglandin E_2 and prostacyclin (PGI_2) maintain duct patency. Oxygen (response increases with increasing gestational age) and indomethacin close duct. PDA may be necessary in pulmonary atresia, interrupted aortic arch, coarctation, TGA, aortic atresia, and other CHDs.
a. Examination: 1–4/6 continuous 'machinery' murmur loudest at the LUSB or left infraclavicular area. May have apical diastolic rumble because of increased blood flow across the mitral valve in diastole. Bounding peripheral pulses with widened pulse pressure (>60mmHg difference between systolic and diastolic) if large shunt. Hyperactive precordium. Palmar pulses.
b. ECG: Normal or LVH in small–moderate PDA. BVH in large PDA.
c. Chest radiograph: May have cardiomegaly and increased PVMs depending on size of shunt.
d. Treatment
    1) Diuretics to decrease effects of the LV volume overload. Lasix is frequently used for short-term management.
    2) Indomethacin is a prostaglandin synthetase inhibitor that has an 80% closure rate.
        a) Contraindications to indomethacin
            i) Creatinine >1.8mg/dL, BUN (blood urea nitrogen) >25, or urine output <1ml/kg per hour.
            ii) Renal or gastrointestinal bleeding.
            iii) Necrotizing enterocolitis (NEC).
            iv) Suspected or proven sepsis.
            v) Platelet count <80,000/mm^3.
            vi) Bleeding tendency (including intracranial hemorrhage).
            vii) Hyperbilirubinemia.
        b) Complications of indomethacin use
            i) Transient decrease in GFR (glomerular filtration rate) and subsequent decreased urine output.
            ii) Transient gastrointestinal (GI) bleeding not associated with an increased incidence of NEC.
            iii) Prolonged bleeding time and disturbed platelet function for 7–9 days independent of platelet number (not associated with increased incidence of intraventricular hemorrhage).
    3) Surgical ligation of duct.
4. **AV canal:** 30–60% occur in children with Down syndrome. Complete AV canal consists of ostium primum ASD; VSD in the inlet portion of the ventricular septum; a cleft in the anterior mitral valve leaflet; a

7

CARDIOLOGY

cleft in the septal leaflet of the tricuspid valve forming common anterior and posterior cusps of the AV valve. If the ventricular septum is intact, then called 'partial AV canal'.

a. Examination: Hyperactive precordium with systolic thrill at LLSB and loud S2. There may be a grade 3–4/6 holosystolic regurgitant murmur along LLSB. May hear systolic murmur of MR at apex. May hear mid-diastolic rumble at LLSB or at apex. Gallop rhythm may be present.
b. ECG: Superior QRS axis. RVH and LVH may be present.
c. Chest radiograph: Cardiomegaly with increased PVMs.

5. **Pulmonic stenosis (PS)**
a. Examination: Ejection click at LUSB with valvular PS. Click intensity will vary with respiration, decreasing with inspiration and increasing with expiration. S2 may split widely with P2 diminished in intensity. SEM (2–5/6) ± thrill at LUSB with radiation to the back and sides.
b. ECG: Mild PS: Normal. Moderate PS: RAD and RVH. Severe PS: RAE and RVH with strain.
c. Chest radiograph: Normal heart size with normal to decreased PVMs.

6. **Aortic stenosis (AS)**
a. Examination: Systolic thrill at RUSB, suprasternal notch, or over carotids. Ejection click, which does *not* vary with respiration, if valvular AS. Harsh SEM (2–4/6) at 2nd RICS or 3rd LICS with radiation to neck and apex. May have early diastolic decrescendo murmur as a result of aortic regurgitation (AR). Narrow pulse pressure if severe stenosis.
b. ECG: Normal in mild AS. LVH ± strain in more severe disease.
c. Chest radiograph: Usually normal.

7. **Coarctation of the aorta:** 8–10% of CHD with male/female ratio of 2:1. Three presentations: (1) infant in congestive heart failure, (2) child with arterial hypertension, and (3) child with heart murmur.
a. Examination: 2–3/6 SEM at LUSB with radiation to the left interscapular area posteriorly. Bicuspid valve is often associated, therefore may also have systolic ejection click at the apex and RUSB. Blood pressure in lower extremities will be lower than in upper extremities (>10mmHg difference considered significant). Check all four limbs because anomalies or variations can occur. For example, aberrant right subclavian distal to coarctation in 3–4% will produce right arm pressures and pulses equal to lower extremity values. Pulse oximetry discrepancy of >5% between upper and lower extremities also suggestive of coarctation if ductus arteriosus is patent. May have heavy ventricular impulse (right or left depending on presence of associated pulmonary hypertension), systolic thrill in suprasternal notch, or gallop. Arterial pulses below coarctation are decreased in amplitude and delayed in timing compared with proximal pulses and may be weak and thready. May have differential cyanosis (confined to lower extremity). May have findings of Turner syndrome in females (short stature, wide-spaced nipples, webbed neck). During the first 48 hours of life there may not be a blood pressure difference if the duct is open.

b. ECG: RVH or RBBB in infancy, LVH in older children.
c. Chest radiograph: Marked cardiomegaly and pulmonary venous congestion. Rib notching from collateral circulation not seen in infants because collaterals not yet established; usually seen after 5 years of age.

B. CYANOTIC

1. **Tetralogy of Fallot:** A large VSD, overriding aorta, right ventricle outflow tract (RVOT) obstruction, right ventricular hypertrophy. The degree of RVOT obstruction will determine whether there is clinical cyanosis. If there is only mild PS, there will be an L to R shunt and the child will be acyanotic. Increasing obstruction leads to increased R to L shunting across the VSD and cyanosis.

a. Examination: Loud systolic ejection murmur at middle and upper LSB and a loud, single S2. May also have a thrill at the middle and lower LSB.
b. ECG: RAD and RVH.
c. Chest radiograph: Boot-shaped heart with normal heart size.
d. **Tet spells:** Occur in young infants, with the highest incidence at 2–4 months of age. Tet spells are the result of increased RVOT obstruction or decreased systemic resistance, which causes increased R to L shunting across the VSD. Clinically, there will be increased deep and rapid breathing, with increasing cyanosis and decreasing heart murmur. Some of the treatment options are shown in Table 7.7.

2. **Transposition of the great arteries**

a. Examination: Nonspecific findings. Extreme cyanosis. S2 will be single

7

CARDIOLOGY

TABLE 7.7

TREATMENT OPTIONS FOR 'TET SPELLS'

Treatment	Rationale
Oxygen	Reduces hypoxemia (limited value)
Knee–chest position	Decreases venous return and increases systemic resistance
Propranolol	Negative inotropic effect on infundibular myocardium; may block drop in systemic vascular resistance (0.01–0.25mg/kg slow IV push)
Morphine	Decreases venous return, depresses respiratory center, relaxes infundibulum (morphine sulfate 0.1–0.2mg/kg SC or IM). Do not try to establish IV access initially. Use the SC route.
Phenylephrine HCl	Increases systemic vascular resistance (0.02mg/kg IV)
Methoxamine	Increases systemic vascular resistance
Sodium bicarbonate	Reduces metabolic acidosis (1mEq/kg IV)
Correct anemia	Increases delivery of oxygen to tissues
Correct pathologic tachyarrhythmias	May abort hypoxic spell
Infuse glucose	Avoids hypoglycemia from increased utilization and depletion of glycogen stores

and loud. May have murmur from associated VSD or PS, but if not present, there may not be a murmur.

b. ECG: Since right ventricle acts as systemic ventricle, will have RAD and RVH. Upright T wave in V1 after 3 days old may be the only abnormality.

c. Chest radiograph: Classic finding is 'egg on a string' with cardiomegaly. Increased PVMs may also be noted.

3. **Tricuspid atresia:** Absent tricuspid valve and hypoplastic RV and PA. Must have ASD, PDA, or VSD for survival.

a. Examination: Single S2. A grade 2–3/6 systolic regurgitation murmur at the LLSB is present if there is a VSD. Occasionally, PDA murmur.

b. ECG: Superior QRS axis, RAE or CAE, and LVH.

c. Chest radiograph: Normal or slightly enlarged heart size. May have boot-shaped heart.

4. **Total anomalous pulmonary venous return:** Pulmonary veins drain into RA or other location besides LA. Must have ASD or patent foramen ovale (PFO) for survival. Four types can be distinguished:
   a) Supracardiac (most common): Common pulmonary vein drains into the SVC.
   b) Cardiac: Pulmonary vein drains into the coronary sinus or into the RA directly.
   c) Subdiaphragmatic: Common pulmonary vein drains into the IVC, portal vein, ductus venosus, or hepatic vein.
   d) Mixed type: Combination of the above.

a. Examination: Hyperactive RV impulse, quadruple rhythm, S2 fixed and widely split, 2–3/6 SEM at LUSB and middiastolic rumble at LLSB.

b. ECG: RAD, RVH (RSR' in V1). May see RAE.

c. Chest radiograph: Cardiomegaly and increased pulmonary vascular markings. Classic is the 'snowman in a snowstorm' finding, but this is rarely seen until after 4 months of age.

5. **Other:** Cyanotic CHDs that occur at a frequency of <1% each include pulmonary atresia, Ebstein's anomaly, truncus arteriosus, single ventricle, and double-outlet right ventricle.

6. **Oxygen challenge test:** Used to evaluate the etiology of cyanosis in neonates. Obtain baseline arterial blood gas (ABG) with saturation at $Fio_2 = 0.21$, then place infant in oxygen hood at $Fio_2 = 1$ for a minimum of 10 minutes, and repeat ABG. Pulse oximetry will not be useful for following the change in oxygenation once the saturations reach 100% (approximately $Pao_2 > 90$)(Table 7.8).

C. SURGICAL PROCEDURES

1. **Atrial septostomy:** Creation of intraatrial opening to allow for mixing or shunting between atria (i.e., for TGA, tricuspid atresia, mitral atresia).

a. **Park:** A knife-tipped cardiac catheter enlarges the intraatrial communication at the foramen ovale.

b. **Rashkind:** A balloon-tipped cardiac catheter is rapidly pulled across the foramen ovale to create a defect in the atrial septum.

TABLE 7.8

OXYGEN CHALLENGE TEST

INTERPRETATION

	$Fio_2 = 0.21$ Pao_2 (% saturation)	$Fio_2 = 1.00$ Pao_2 (% saturation)	$Paco_2$
Normal	70 (95)	>200 (100)	35
Pulmonary disease	50 (85)	>150 (100)	50
Neurologic disease	50 (85)	>150 (100)	50
Methemoglobinemia	70 (85)	>200 (85)	35
Cardiac disease			
Separate circulation[a]	<40 (<75)	<50 (<85)	35
Restricted PBF[b]	<40 (<75)	<50 (<85)	35
Complete mixing without restricted PBF[c]	50 (85)	<150 (<100)	35
Persistent pulmonary hypertension	Preductal	Postductal	
PFO (no R to L shunt)	70 (95)	<40 (<75)	Variable 35–50
PFO (with R to L shunt)	<40(<75)	<40 (<75)	Variable 35–50

From Lees[11]; Kitterman[12]; and Jones[13].

PBF, Pulmonary blood flow; PFO, patent foramen ovale.

[a]D-Transposition of the great arteries (D-TGA) with intact ventricular septum.

[b]Tricuspid atresia with pulmonary stenosis or atresia; pulmonary atresia or critical pulmonary stenosis with intact ventricular septum; or tetralogy of Fallot.

[c]Truncus, total anomalous pulmonary venous return, single ventricle, hypoplastic left heart, D-TGA with ventricular septal defect, tricuspid atresia without pulmonary stenosis or atresia.

7

CARDIOLOGY

2. **Palliative systemic-to-pulmonary artery shunts:** Use of systemic arterial flow to increase pulmonary blood flow in cardiac lesions with impaired pulmonary perfusion (e.g., tetralogy of Fallot, hypoplastic right heart, tricuspid atresia, pulmonary stenosis) (Fig. 7.17).
a. Blalock–Taussig shunt (classic): Direct end-to-side subclavian artery to pulmonary artery anastomosis on side opposite to arch of aorta.
b. Blalock–Taussig shunt (modified): Gore-Tex graft placed between subclavian artery and pulmonary artery.
c. Waterston–Cooley shunt: Direct ascending aorta to right pulmonary artery anastomosis (now rarely performed).
d. Potts shunt: Direct descending aorta to left pulmonary artery anastomosis (now rarely performed).
3. **Palliative cava-to-pulmonary artery shunts:** Use of systemic venous flow to increase pulmonary blood flow (usually performed in older children who have lower pulmonary vascular resistance), as intermediate step to Fontan procedure (Fig. 7.17).
a. Glenn shunt (unidirectional): SVC to right pulmonary artery (RPA) anastomosis with ligation of the proximal RPA and cardiac end of the SVC.

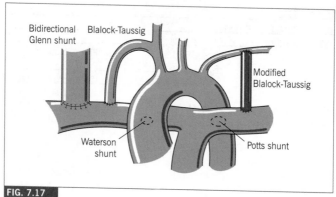

FIG. 7.17

Schematic diagram of cardiac shunts.

b. Glenn shunt (bidirectional): SVC to right pulmonary artery anastomosis with flow to both the RPA and LPA.

4. **Repair of transposition of great arteries**

a. Atrial inversion procedures: Now rarely done, these procedures connect RA to LV, which pumps out to pulmonary arteries, and connect LA to RV, which becomes systemic pump to aorta. **Mustard** procedure uses pericardial or prosthetic intraatrial baffles. **Senning** procedure uses the native atrial septum or wall as baffles.

b. Arterial switch (of Jatene): Pulmonary artery and aorta are transected above valves and switched, and coronary arteries are moved from old aortic root to new aorta (former pulmonary root).

c. Rastelli: Method of patching VSD such that LV outflow passes through VSD into aorta, and a valved conduit or graft is placed between the RV and pulmonary arteries. Used for TGAs with pulmonary stenosis.

5. **Fontan:** Anastomosis of SVC to RPA (Glenn shunt), together with anastomosis of RA and/or IVC to pulmonary arteries via conduits; separates systemic and pulmonary circulations in patients with functionally single ventricles (tricuspid atresia, hypoplastic left heart syndrome).

6. **Norwood:** Used for hypoplastic left heart syndrome.

a. Stage 1: Anastomosis of proximal main pulmonary artery (MPA) to aorta, with aortic arch reconstruction and transection and patch closure of distal MPA; modified right Blalock–Taussig shunt (subclavian artery to right PA) to provide pulmonary blood flow. ASD created to allow for adequate left to right flow.

b. Stage 2: Bidirectional Glenn shunt to reduce volume overload of single right ventricle and modified Fontan procedure to correct cyanosis.

D. **EXERCISE RECOMMENDATIONS FOR CONGENITAL HEART DISEASE** (Table 7.9)

TABLE 7.9

EXERCISE RECOMMENDATIONS FOR CONGENITAL HEART DISEASE
SPORTS ALLOWED FOR SOME SPECIFIC CARDIAC LESIONS

Diagnosis	Sports allowed
• Small ASD or VSD	All
• Mild aortic stenosis	All
• MVP (without other risk factors)	All
• Moderate aortic stenosis	IA, IB, IIA
• Mild LV dysfunction	IA, IB, IC
• Moderate LV dysfunction	IA only
• Hypertrophic cardiomyopathy	None (or IA only)
• Severe aortic stenosis	None
• Long QT syndrome	None

	Low dynamic (A)	Moderate dynamic (B)	High dynamic (C)
I. Low static	Billiards	Baseball	Badminton
	Bowling	Softball	Cross-country skiing
	Cricket	Table tennis	Field hockey[a]
	Curling	Tennis (doubles)	Orienteering
	Golf	Volleyball	Race walking
	Riflery		Racquetball
			Running (long distance)
			Soccer[a]
			Squash
			Tennis (singles)
II. Moderate static	Archery	Fencing	Basketball[a]
	Auto racing[a,b]	Field events (jumping)	Ice hockey[a]
	Diving[a,b]	Figure skating[a]	Cross-country skiing (skating technique)
	Equestrian[a,b]	Football (American)[a]	Football (Australian)[a]
	Motorcycling[a,b]	Rodeoing[a,b]	Lacrosse[a]
		Rugby[a]	Running (middle distance)
		Running (sprint)	Swimming
		Surfing[a,b]	Team handball
		Synchronized swimming[b]	
III. High static	Bobsledding[a,b]	Body building[a,b]	Boxing[a]
	Field events (throwing)	Downhill skiing[a,b]	Canoeing/kayaking
	Gymnastics[a,b]	Wrestling[a]	Cycling[a,b]
	Karate/judo[a]		Decathlon
	Luge[a,b]		Rowing
	Sailing		Speed skating
	Rock climbing[a,b]		
	Waterskiing[a,b]		
	Weight lifting[a,b]		
	Windsurfing[a,b]		

From 26th Bethesda Conference, 1994[14].
[a]Danger of bodily collision.
[b]Increased risk if syncope occurs.

7

CARDIOLOGY

IV. ACQUIRED HEART DISEASE

A. ENDOCARDITIS

1. **Common causative organisms:** About 70% are streptococcal species (*Streptococcus viridans,* enterococci); 20% are staphylococcal species (*Staphylococcus aureus, S. epidermidis*); 10% are other organisms (*Haemophilus influenzae,* Gram-negative bacteria, fungi).

2. **Clinical findings:** New heart murmur, fever, splenomegaly, petechiae, Osler's nodes (tender nodules at fingertips), Janeway's lesions (painless hemorrhagic areas on palms or soles), splinter hemorrhages, and Roth's spots (retinal hemorrhages).

3. **Bacterial endocarditis prophylaxis[15]**

a. High-risk category

   1) Prosthetic cardiac valves (bioprosthetic and homograft valves).
   2) Previous history of bacterial endocarditis.
   3) Complex cyanotic congenital heart disease (i.e., tetralogy of Fallot, transposition).
   4) Surgically constructed systemic–pulmonary shunts or conduits.

b. Moderate-risk category

   1) Most other congenital cardiac malformations (all unrepaired congenital heart disease except secundum ASD).
   2) Acquired valvular dysfunction (i.e., rheumatic heart disease).
   3) Hypertrophic cardiomyopathy.
   4) Mitral valve prolapse with valvular regurgitation and/or thickened leaflets.

c. Low-risk category: Endocarditis prophylaxis **NOT** recommended for following conditions:

   1) Isolated secundum ASD.
   2) Surgical repair of ASD, VSD, or PDA, without residua beyond 6 months.
   3) Previous coronary artery bypass graft surgery.
   4) Mitral valve prolapse without valvular regurgitation.
   5) Physiologic, functional, or innocent heart murmurs.
   6) Previous Kawasaki disease without valvular dysfunction.
   7) Previous rheumatic fever without valvular dysfunction.
   8) Cardiac pacemakers and implanted defibrillators.

d. Procedures and endocarditis: Prophylaxis is recommended for the following:

   1) All **dental procedures** likely to cause gingival bleeding, including routine professional cleaning, periodontal surgery, and dental extractions.
   2) Tonsillectomy and/or adenoidectomy.
   3) Surgical procedures that involve **respiratory or intestinal mucosa.**
   4) Bronchoscopy with a **rigid bronchoscope.**
   5) Incision and drainage or other procedures involving infected tissues.
   6) Specific **gastrointestinal (GI) procedures,** including sclerotherapy,

esophageal stricture dilatation, biliary tract surgery, and endoscopic retrograde cholangiography with biliary obstruction.

7) Specific **genitourinary (GU) tract procedures,** including cystoscopy, prostatic surgery, and urethral dilatation.

8) Any urinary tract procedure, including urethral catheterization, if there is evidence of a urinary tract infection (UTI), and any vaginal procedure, including D&C, removal of an IUD, and vaginal delivery, if there is evidence of local infection.

9) For patients in high-risk category, prophylaxis is optional for low-risk procedures involving the lower respiratory, GI, or GU tracts (flexible bronchoscopy, TEE, endoscopy, vaginal delivery, or vaginal hysterectomy).

e. Procedures for which endocarditis prophylaxis is **NOT** recommended:

1) Local intraoral anesthetic injections (nonintraligamentary).
2) Shedding of primary teeth.
3) Tympanostomy tube insertion.
4) Endotracheal intubation, flexible bronchoscopy, and endoscopy (with or without biopsy).
5) Cardiac catheterization and pacemaker placement.
6) In uninfected tissue: Urethral catheterization, D&C, therapeutic abortion, sterilization procedures, insertion and removal of IUDs, vaginal delivery, hysterectomy, cesarean section.

f. Prophylaxis for dental, oral, respiratory tract, or esophageal procedures:

1) Amoxicillin 50mg/kg (max. 2g) PO 1 hour before procedure:

Note: Postprocedure antibiotic dose no longer recommended.

2) Parenteral alternative: Ampicillin 50mg/kg (max. 2g) IM/IV within 30 minutes before procedure.
3) Penicillin-allergic patients: Clindamycin 20mg/kg (max. 600mg) or cephalexin/cefadroxil 50mg/kg (max. 2g) or azithromycin/clarithromycin 15mg/kg (max. 500mg), all PO 1 hour before procedure.

Note: Erythromycin no longer recommended because of GI upset and complicated pharmacokinetics.

4) Parenteral alternative for penicillin-allergic patients: Clindamycin 20mg/kg (max. 600mg) IV or cefazolin 25mg/kg (max. 1g) IM/IV, within 30 minutes before procedure.

g. Prophylaxis for GI and GU procedures:

1) Regimen for high-risk patients
   a) Ampicillin 50mg/kg (max. 2g) IM/IV plus gentamicin 1.5mg/kg (max. 120mg) IM/IV within 30 minutes before procedure. Then ampicillin 25mg/kg (max. 1g) IM/IV or amoxicillin 25mg/kg (max. 1g) PO 6 hours later.
   b) Penicillin-allergic patients: Vancomycin 20mg/kg (max. 1g) IV over 1–2 hours plus gentamicin 1.5mg/kg (max. 120mg) IM/IV, completed within 30 minutes before procedure.

7

CARDIOLOGY

2) Regimen for moderate-risk patients
   a) Amoxicillin 50mg/kg (max. 2g) PO 1 hour before procedure, or ampicillin 50mg/kg (max. 2g) IM/IV within 30 minutes before procedure.
   b) Penicillin-allergic patients: Vancomycin 20mg/kg (max. 1g) IV over 1–2 hours, completed within 30 minutes before procedure.

Note: Children taking penicillin/amoxicillin should be given clindamycin, azithromycin, or clarithromycin for endocarditis prophylaxis, or procedure should be delayed 9–14 days after completion of antibiotic course.

B. MYOCARDIAL DISEASE
1. **Dilated cardiomyopathy:** End result of myocardial damage, leading to atrial and ventricular dilatation with decreased contractile function of the ventricles.
   a. Etiology: Infectious, toxic (alcohol, doxorubicin), metabolic (hypothyroidism, muscular dystrophy), immunologic, collagen vascular disease.
   b. Symptoms: Fatigue, weakness, shortness of breath.
   c. Examination: Signs of congestive heart failure, including tachycardia, tachypnea, rales, cold extremities, jugular venous distention, hepatomegaly, peripheral edema, S3 gallop, and displacement of PMI to left and inferiorly.
   d. Chest radiograph: Generalized cardiomegaly, pulmonary congestion.
   e. ECG: Sinus tachycardia, LVH, possibly atrial enlargement, arrhythmias, conduction disturbances, ST segment/T wave changes.
   f. Echocardiography: Enlarged ventricles (increased end-diastolic and end-systolic dimensions) with little or no wall thickening; decreased shortening fraction.
   g. Treatment: Management of CHF (digoxin, diuretics, vasodilatation, rest). Consider anticoagulants to decrease risk of thrombi formation.
2. **Hypertrophic cardiomyopathy:** Abnormality of myocardial cells leading to significant ventricular hypertrophy, particularly LV, with small to normal ventricular dimensions. Contractile function is increased but filling is impaired secondary to stiff ventricles. Most common is asymmetric septal hypertrophy (IHSS) with variable degrees of obstruction. There is a 4–6% incidence of sudden death in children and adolescents.
   a. Etiology: Genetic (autosomal dominant, 60% of cases) or sporadic (40% of cases).
   b. Symptoms: Easy fatiguability, anginal pain, shortness of breath, occasional palpitations.
   c. Examination: Usually adolescents or young adults; left ventricular heave, sharp upstroke of arterial pulse, murmur of mitral regurgitation.
   d. Chest radiograph: Globular-shaped heart with LV enlargement.
   e. ECG: LVH, prominent Q waves (septal hypertrophy), ST segment/T wave changes, arrhythmias.

f.   Echocardiography: Diagnostic study, showing extent and location of hypertrophy, obstruction, increased contractility.

g.   Treatment: Moderate restriction of physical activity, negative inotropes (β-blocker, calcium channel blocker) to help improve filling, systemic bacterial endocarditis (SBE) prophylaxis.

3. **Restrictive cardiomyopathy:** Myocardial/endocardial disease (usually infiltrative or fibrotic) resulting in stiff ventricular walls with restriction of diastolic filling but normal contractile function. Results in atrial enlargement. Very rare in children.

a.   Etiology: Amyloidosis, sarcoidosis, hemochromatosis, glycogen storage diseases, neoplastic infiltration.

b.   Symptoms: Exercise intolerance, weakness, chest pain, shortness of breath.

c.   Examination: Jugular venous distention, hepatomegaly, signs of pulmonary congestion (rales, tachypnea), S3 gallop, systolic murmur of mitral/tricuspid regurgitation.

d.   Chest radiograph: Cardiomegaly, pulmonary congestion, pleural effusion.

e.   ECG: Occasionally, atrial fibrillation, SVT.

f.   Echocardiography: Normal LV and RV dimensions, but enlarged atria. Normal LV systolic function until later stages.

g.   Treatment: Diuretics; consider anticoagulants or antiplatelet agents to decrease risk of thrombi formation.

4. **Myocarditis:** Inflammation of myocardial tissue.

a.   Etiology: Viral (coxsackievirus, echovirus, poliomyelitis, mumps, rubella, cytomegalovirus, HIV, arbovirus, adenovirus, influenza), bacterial, rickettsial, fungal, or parasitic infection; immune-mediated disease (Kawasaki disease, acute rheumatic fever); collagen vascular disease; toxin-induced condition.

b.   Symptoms: Nonspecific and inconsistent, depending on severity of disease. Variably see anorexia, lethargy, emesis, lightheadedness, cold extremities, shortness of breath.

c.   Examination: Signs of CHF (tachycardia, tachypnea, jugular venous distention, rales, gallop, hepatomegaly); occasionally, soft systolic murmur, arrhythmias.

d.   Chest radiograph: Variable cardiomegaly and pulmonary edema.

e.   ECG: Low QRS voltages throughout (<5mm), ST segment/T wave changes (e.g., decreased T wave amplitude), prolongation of QT interval, arrhythmias (especially premature contractions, first- or second-degree AV block).

f.   Echocardiography: Enlargement of heart chambers, impaired LV function.

g.   Treatment: Bedrest, diuretics, inotropes (dopamine, dobutamine, isoproterenol), digoxin, gamma globulin (2g/kg over 24 hours), afterload reducer (e.g., ACE inhibitor), possibly steroids. May require heart transplantation.

7

CARDIOLOGY

C. PERICARDIAL DISEASE

1. **Pericarditis:** Inflammation of visceral and parietal layers of pericardium.
   a. Etiology: Viral/idiopathic (especially echovirus, coxsackievirus B), tuberculous, bacterial, uremia, neoplastic disease, collagen vascular disease, post-MI or postpericardiotomy, radiation-induced, drug-induced (e.g., procainamide, hydralazine).
   b. Symptoms: Chest pain (retrosternal or precordial, radiating to back or shoulder, pleuritic in nature, alleviated by leaning forward, aggravated by supine position), dyspnea.
   c. Examination: Pericardial friction rub, fever, tachypnea.
   d. ECG: Diffuse ST segment elevation in almost all leads (representing inflammation of adjacent myocardium); PR segment depression.
   e. Treatment: Often self-limited. Treat underlying condition and provide symptomatic treatment with rest, analgesia, and antiinflammatory drugs.

2. **Pericardial effusion:** Accumulation of excess fluid in pericardial sac.
   a. Etiology: Associated with acute pericarditis (exudative fluid) or serous effusion resulting from increased capillary hydrostatic pressure (e.g., CHF), decreased plasma oncotic pressure (e.g., hypoproteinemia), and increased capillary permeability (transudative fluid).
   b. Symptoms: Can present with no symptoms, dull ache in left chest, or symptoms of cardiac tamponade, discussed below.
   c. Examination: Muffled distant heart sounds, dullness to percussion of posterior left chest (secondary to atelectasis from large pericardial sac), hemodynamic signs of cardiac compression (see next section).
   d. Chest radiograph: Globular, symmetric cardiomegaly.
   e. ECG: Decreased voltage of QRS complexes, **electrical alternans** (variation of QRS axis with each beat secondary to swinging of heart within pericardial fluid).
   f. Echocardiography: Fluid within pericardial cavity visualized by M-mode and two-dimensional (2-D) echocardiography.
   g. Treatment: Address underlying condition. Observe if asymptomatic; use pericardiocentesis if there is sudden increase in volume or hemodynamic compromise.

3. **Cardiac tamponade:** Accumulation of pericardial fluid under high pressure, causing compression of cardiac chambers, limiting filling, and decreasing stroke volume and cardiac output.
   a. Etiology: As above for pericardial effusion. Most commonly associated with neoplasm, uremia, viral infection, and acute hemorrhage.
   b. Symptoms: Dyspnea, fatigue, cold extremities.
   c. Examination: Jugular venous distention, hepatomegaly, peripheral edema, tachypnea, and rales (from increased systemic and pulmonary venous pressure); hypotension, tachycardia, **pulsus paradoxus** (decrease in systolic BP by >10mmHg with each inspiration), and decreased capillary refill (from decreased stroke volume and cardiac output); quiet precordium and muffled heart sounds.
   d. ECG: Sinus tachycardia, decreased voltage, **electrical alternans.**

e. Echocardiography: RV collapse in early diastole, RA/LA collapse in end-diastole and early systole.

f. Treatment: Pericardiocentesis (with temporary catheter left in place if necessary), pericardial window or stripping if recurrent condition (see p. 60).

D. KAWASAKI DISEASE

Leading cause of acquired heart disease in children in developed countries. Seen almost exclusively in children under 8 years of age. Patients present with acute febrile vasculitis, which may lead to long-term cardiac complications from vasculitis of coronary arteries. Peaks in winter and spring.

1. **Etiology:** Unknown. Thought to be immune regulated, in response to infectious agents and/or environmental toxins.

2. **Diagnosis:** Based on clinical criteria. These include high fever lasting >5 days plus at least four of the following five criteria:

a. Bilateral bulbar conjunctival injection without exudate.

b. Erythematous mouth and pharynx, strawberry tongue, and/or red, cracked lips.

c. Polymorphous exanthem (may be morbilliform, maculopapular, or scarlatiniform).

d. Swelling of hands and feet with erythema of palms and soles.

e. Cervical lymphadenopathy (>1.5cm in diameter), usually single and unilateral.

Note: Atypical Kawasaki disease, more often seen in infants, consists of fever with fewer than four of the above criteria, but findings of coronary artery abnormalities.

3. **Other clinical findings:** Often see extreme irritability, abdominal pain, diarrhea, vomiting. Also see anterior uveitis (80%), arthritis/arthralgias (35%), aseptic meningitis (25%), pericardial effusion or arrhythmias (20%), gallbladder hydrops (<10%), carditis (<5%), and perineal rash with desquamation.

4. **Laboratory findings:** Leukocytosis with shift to left, neutrophils with vacuoles or toxic granules, elevated CRP (C-reactive protein) or ESR (seen acutely), thrombocytosis (after first week, peaking at 2 weeks), normocytic/normochromic anemia, sterile pyuria (70%), increased LFTs (40%).

5. **Subacute phase (11–25 days after onset of illness):** Resolution of fever, rash, and lymphadenopathy. Often, desquamation of fingertips/toes and thrombocytosis occur.

6. **Cardiovascular complications:** If untreated, 15–25% develop coronary artery aneurysms and dilatation in this phase (peak prevalence about 2–4 weeks after onset of disease; rarely appears after 6 weeks) and are at risk for coronary thrombosis acutely and coronary stenosis chronically. Carditis; aortic, mitral, and tricuspid regurgitation; pericardial effusion; CHF; MI; LV dysfunction; and ECG changes may also occur.

7

CARDIOLOGY

7. **Convalescent phase:** ESR, CRP, and platelet count return to normal. Those with coronary artery abnormalities are at increased risk for MI, arrhythmias, and sudden death.

8. **Management**[16]

a. **Intravenous gamma globulin (IVGG)** has been shown to reduce incidence of coronary artery dilatation to <3% and decrease duration of fever if given in first 10 days of illness. Current recommended regimen: Single dose of **IVGG 2g/kg over 10–12 hours.**

b. **Aspirin** is recommended for both its antiinflammatory and its antiplatelet effects. Some recommend **initial high-dose aspirin (80–100mg/kg per day divided in four doses)** until fever resolves. Then continue with **3–5mg/kg per day** Q24hr for 6–8 weeks or until platelet count and ESR are normal (if there are no coronary artery abnormalities), *or indefinitely* if coronary artery abnormalities persist. Others recommend starting with low-dose aspirin (3–5mg/kg per day) and continuing as above.

c. Dipyridamole 4mg/kg divided in three doses sometimes used as alternative to aspirin.

d. Follow-up: Serial echocardiography recommended to assess coronary arteries and LV function (at time of diagnosis, at 6–8 weeks, and at 6–12 months). More frequent intervals and longer term follow-up recommended if abnormalities seen on echocardiography (Table 7.10).

TABLE 7.10
GUIDELINES FOR TREATMENT AND FOLLOW-UP OF CHILDREN WITH KAWASAKI DISEASE

Risk level	Pharmacologic therapy	Physical activity	Follow-up and diagnostic testing	Invasive testing
I (no coronary artery changes at any stage of illness)	None beyond initial 6–8 weeks	No restrictions beyond initial 6–8 weeks.	None beyond first year unless cardiac disease suspected.	None recommended.
II (transient coronary artery ectasia that disappears during acute illness)	None beyond initial 6–8 weeks	No restrictions beyond initial 6–8 weeks.	None beyond first year unless cardiac disease suspected. Physician may see patient at 3- to 5-year intervals.	None recommended.
III (small to medium solitary coronary artery aneurysm)	3–5mg/kg aspirin per day, at least until abnormalities resolve	For patients in first decade of life, no restriction beyond initial 6–8 weeks. For patients in second decade, physical activity guided by stress testing every other year. Competitive contact athletics with endurance training discouraged.	Annual follow-up with echocardiogram ± electro-cardiogram in first decade of life.	Angiography, if stress testing or echocardiography suggests stenosis.

Continued

7

CARDIOLOGY

TABLE 7.10

GUIDELINES FOR TREATMENT AND FOLLOW-UP OF CHILDREN WITH KAWASAKI DISEASE—cont'd

Risk level	Pharmacologic therapy	Physical activity	Follow-up and diagnostic testing	Invasive testing
IV (one or more giant coronary artery aneurysms or multiple small to medium aneurysms, without obstruction)	Long-term aspirin (3–5 mg/kg per day) ± warfarin	For patients in first decade of life, no restriction beyond initial 6–8 weeks. For patients in second decade, annual stress testing guides recommendations. Strenuous athletics are strongly discouraged. If stress test rules out ischemia, non-contact recreational sports allowed.	Annual follow-up with echocardiogram ± electro-cardiogram ± chest x-ray ± additional electrocardiogram at 6-month intervals. For patients in first decade of life, pharmacologic stress testing should be considered.	Angiography, if stress testing or echocardiography suggests stenosis. Elective catheterization may be done in certain circumstances.
V (coronary artery obstruction)	Long-term aspirin (3–5 mg/kg per day) ± warfarin. Use of calcium channel blockers should be considered to reduce myocardial oxygen consumption.	Contact sports, isometrics, and weight training should be avoided. Other physical activity recommendations guided by outcome of stress testing or myocardial perfusion scan.	Echocardiogram and electro-cardiogram at 6-month intervals and annual Holter and stress testing.	Angiography recommended for some patients to aid in selecting therapeutic options. Repeat angiography with new-onset or worsening ischemia.

V. NORMAL VALUES
A. BLOOD PRESSURE (Figs 7.18–7.22; Tables 7.11 and 7.12)

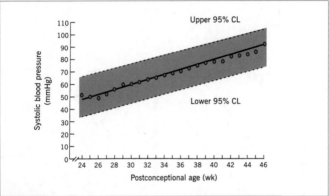

FIG. 7.18
Linear regression of mean systolic blood pressure on postconceptional age (gestational age in weeks + weeks after delivery). (From Zubrow[17].)

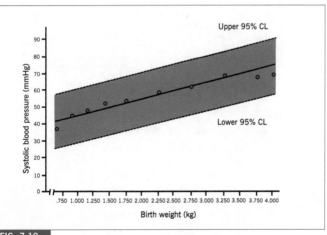

FIG. 7.19
Linear regression of mean systolic blood pressure on birth weight on day 1 of life. (From Zubrow[17].)

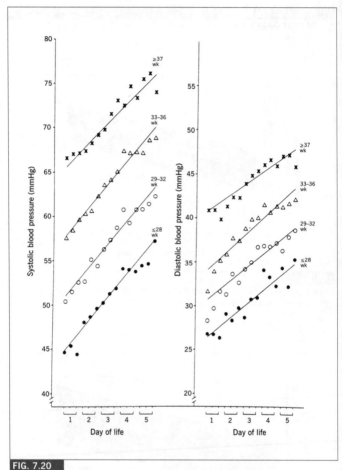

FIG. 7.20
Systolic and diastolic blood pressure in the first 5 days of life. (From Zubrow[17].)

7

CARDIOLOGY

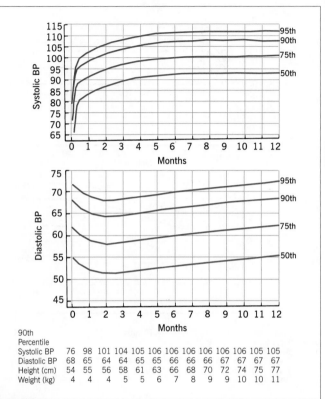

90th Percentile												
Systolic BP	76	98	101	104	105	106	106	106	106	106	106	105	105
Diastolic BP	68	65	64	64	65	65	66	66	66	67	67	67	67
Height (cm)	54	55	56	58	61	63	66	68	70	72	74	75	77
Weight (kg)	4	4	4	5	5	6	7	8	9	9	10	10	11

FIG. 7.21

Age-specific percentiles of BP measurements in **girls** from birth to 12 months of age; Korotkoff phase IV (K4) used for diastolic BP. (From Horan[18].)

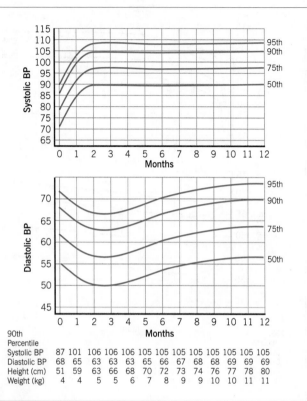

FIG. 7.22

Age-specific percentiles of BP measurements in **boys** from birth to 12 months of age; Korotkoff phase IV (K4) used for diastolic BP. (From Horan[18].)

TABLE 7.11

BLOOD PRESSURE LEVELS FOR THE 90TH AND 95TH PERCENTILES OF BLOOD PRESSURE FOR *GIRLS* AGED 1–17 YEARS BY PERCENTILES OF HEIGHT

Percentiles Age (yr)	Height[a] → BP[b] ↓	Systolic BP (mmHg) by percentile of height							Diastolic BP (DBP) (mmHg) by percentile of height						
		5%	10%	25%	50%	75%	90%	95%	5%	10%	25%	50%	75%	90%	95%
1	90th	97	98	99	100	102	103	104	53	53	53	54	55	56	56
	95th	101	102	103	104	105	107	107	57	57	57	58	59	60	60
2	90th	99	99	100	102	103	104	105	57	57	58	58	59	60	61
	95th	102	103	104	105	107	108	109	61	61	62	62	63	64	65
3	90th	100	100	102	103	104	105	106	61	61	61	62	63	63	64
	95th	104	104	105	107	108	109	110	65	65	65	66	67	67	68
4	90th	101	102	103	104	106	107	108	63	63	64	65	65	66	67
	95th	105	106	107	108	109	111	111	67	67	68	69	70	71	71
5	90th	103	103	104	106	107	108	109	65	66	66	67	68	69	69
	95th	107	107	108	110	111	112	113	69	70	70	71	72	73	73
6	90th	104	105	106	107	109	110	111	67	67	68	69	69	70	71
	95th	108	109	110	111	112	114	114	71	71	72	73	73	74	75
7	90th	106	107	108	109	110	112	112	69	69	69	70	71	72	72
	95th	110	110	112	113	114	115	116	73	73	73	74	75	76	76
8	90th	108	109	110	111	112	113	114	70	70	71	71	72	73	74
	95th	112	112	113	115	116	117	118	74	74	75	75	76	77	78
9	90th	110	110	112	113	114	115	116	71	72	72	73	74	74	75
	95th	114	114	115	117	118	119	120	75	76	76	77	78	78	79

Continued

7

CARDIOLOGY

TABLE 7.11

BLOOD PRESSURE LEVELS FOR THE 90TH AND 95TH PERCENTILES OF BLOOD PRESSURE FOR *GIRLS* AGED 1–17 YEARS BY PERCENTILES OF HEIGHT—cont'd

Percentiles Age (yr)	Height[a] → BP[b] →	Systolic BP (mmHg) by percentile of height							Diastolic BP (DBP) (mmHg) by percentile of height						
		5%	10%	25%	50%	75%	90%	95%	5%	10%	25%	50%	75%	90%	95%
10	90th	112	112	114	115	116	117	118	73	73	73	74	75	76	76
	95th	116	116	117	119	120	121	122	77	77	77	78	79	80	80
11	90th	114	114	116	117	118	119	120	74	74	75	75	76	77	77
	95th	118	118	119	121	122	123	124	78	78	79	79	80	81	81
12	90th	116	116	118	119	120	121	122	75	75	76	76	77	78	78
	95th	120	120	121	123	124	125	126	79	79	80	80	81	82	82
13	90th	118	118	119	121	122	123	124	76	76	77	78	78	79	80
	95th	121	122	123	125	126	127	128	80	80	81	82	82	83	84
14	90th	119	120	121	122	124	125	126	77	77	78	79	79	80	81
	95th	123	124	125	126	128	129	130	81	81	82	83	83	84	85
15	90th	121	121	122	124	125	126	127	78	78	79	79	80	81	82
	95th	124	125	126	128	129	130	131	82	82	83	83	84	85	86
16	90th	122	122	123	125	126	127	128	79	79	79	80	81	82	82
	95th	125	126	127	128	130	131	132	83	83	83	84	85	86	86
17	90th	122	123	124	125	126	128	128	79	79	79	80	81	82	82
	95th	126	126	127	129	130	131	132	83	83	83	84	85	86	86

[a]Height percentile determined by standard growth curves.

TABLE 7.12

BLOOD PRESSURE LEVELS FOR THE 90TH AND 95TH PERCENTILES OF BLOOD PRESSURE FOR *BOYS* AGED 1–17 YEARS BY PERCENTILES OF HEIGHT

Age (yr)	Height[a] → BP[b] ↓	Systolic BP (mmHg) by percentile of height							Diastolic BP (DBP) (mmHg) by percentile of height						
		5%	10%	25%	50%	75%	90%	95%	5%	10%	25%	50%	75%	90%	95%
1	90th	94	95	97	98	100	102	102	50	51	52	53	54	54	55
	95th	98	99	101	102	104	106	106	55	55	56	57	58	59	59
2	90th	98	99	100	102	104	105	106	55	55	56	57	58	59	59
	95th	101	102	104	106	108	109	110	59	59	60	61	62	63	63
3	90th	100	101	103	105	107	108	109	59	59	60	61	62	63	63
	95th	104	105	107	109	111	112	113	63	63	64	65	66	67	67
4	90th	102	103	105	107	109	110	111	62	62	63	64	65	66	66
	95th	106	107	109	111	113	114	115	66	67	67	68	69	70	71
5	90th	104	105	106	108	110	112	112	65	65	66	67	68	69	69
	95th	108	109	110	112	114	115	116	69	70	70	71	72	73	74
6	90th	105	106	108	110	111	113	114	67	68	69	70	70	71	72
	95th	109	110	112	114	115	117	117	72	72	73	74	75	76	76
7	90th	106	107	109	111	113	114	115	69	70	71	72	72	73	74
	95th	110	111	113	115	116	118	119	74	74	75	76	77	78	78
8	90th	107	108	110	112	114	115	116	71	71	72	73	74	75	75
	95th	111	112	114	116	118	119	120	75	76	76	77	78	79	80
9	90th	109	110	112	113	115	117	117	72	73	73	74	75	76	77
	95th	113	114	116	117	119	121	121	76	77	78	79	80	80	81

Continued

7

CARDIOLOGY

TABLE 7.12
BLOOD PRESSURE LEVELS FOR THE 90TH AND 95TH PERCENTILES OF BLOOD PRESSURE FOR *BOYS* AGED 1–17 YEARS BY PERCENTILES OF HEIGHT—cont'd

Age (yr)	Height[a] → BP[b] →	Systolic BP (mmHg) by percentile of height							Diastolic BP (DBP) (mmHg) by percentile of height						
		5%	10%	25%	50%	75%	90%	95%	5%	10%	25%	50%	75%	90%	95%
10	90th	110	112	113	115	117	118	119	73	74	74	75	76	77	78
	95th	114	115	117	119	121	122	123	77	78	79	80	80	81	82
11	90th	112	113	115	117	119	120	121	74	74	75	76	77	78	78
	95th	116	117	119	121	123	124	125	78	79	79	80	81	82	83
12	90th	115	116	117	119	121	123	123	75	75	76	77	78	78	79
	95th	119	120	121	123	125	126	127	79	79	80	81	82	83	83
13	90th	117	118	120	122	124	125	126	75	76	76	77	78	79	80
	95th	121	122	124	126	128	129	130	79	80	81	82	83	83	84
14	90th	120	121	123	125	126	128	128	76	76	77	78	79	80	80
	95th	124	125	127	128	130	132	132	80	81	81	82	83	84	85
15	90th	123	124	125	127	129	131	131	77	77	78	79	80	81	81
	95th	127	128	129	131	133	134	135	81	82	83	83	84	85	86
16	90th	125	126	128	130	132	133	134	79	79	80	81	82	82	83
	95th	129	130	132	134	136	137	138	83	83	84	85	86	87	87
17	90th	128	129	131	133	134	136	136	81	81	82	83	84	85	85
	95th	132	133	135	136	138	140	140	85	85	86	87	88	89	89

[a]Height percentile determined by standard growth curves.
[b]Blood pressure percentile determined by a single measurement.

B. HEART RATE (Table 7.13)

TABLE 7.13

AGE-SPECIFIC HEART RATES (BEATS/MIN)

Age	2%	Mean	98%
<1 day	93	123	154
1–2 days	91	123	159
3–6 days	91	129	166
1–3 wk	107	148	182
1–2 mo	121	149	179
3–5 mo	106	141	186
6–11 mo	109	134	169
1–2 yr	89	119	151
3–4 yr	73	108	137
5–7 yr	65	100	133
8–11 yr	62	91	130
12–15 yr	60	85	119

7

CARDIOLOGY

VI. REFERENCES

1. Park MK. *Pediatric cardiology for practitioners,* 3rd edn. St Louis: Mosby; 1996.
2. Goldberger AL. *Clinical electrocardiography.* St Louis: Mosby; 1994.
3. Schwartz PJ, Stramba-Badiale M, Segantini A, Austoni P, Bosi G, Giorgetti R, Grancini F, Marni ED, Perticone F, Rosti D, Salice P. Prolongation of the QT interval and the sudden infant death syndrome. *N Engl J Med* 1998; **338:**1709–1714.
4. Davignon A et al. Normal ECG standards for infants and children. *Pediatr Cardiol* 1979; **1:**123–131.
5. Park MK, Guntheroth WG. *How to read pediatric ECGs,* 3rd edn. St Louis: Mosby; 1992.
6. Towbin JA, Bricker JT, Garson A Jr. Electrocardiographic criteria for diagnosis of acute myocardial infarction in childhood. *Am J Cardiol* 1992; **69:**1545.
7. Hirsch R, Landt Y, Porter S, Canter CE, Jaffe AS, Ladenson JH, Grant JW, Landt M. Cardiac troponin I in pediatrics: normal values and potential use in assessment of cardiac injury. *J Pediatr* 1997; **130:**872–877.
8. Garson A Jr. *The electrocardiogram in infants and children: a systematic approach.* Philadelphia: Lea & Febiger; 1983.
9. Walsh EP. In: Fyler DC, Nadas A, eds. *Pediatric cardiology.* Philadelphia: Hanley & Belfus; 1992.
10. Colon SD, Parness IA, Spevak PJ, Sanders SP. Developmental modulation of myocardial mechanics: age- and growth-related alterations in afterload and contractility. *J Am Coll Cardiol* 1992; **19:**619.

11. Lees MH. Cyanosis of the newborn infant: recognition and clinical evaluation. *J Pediatr* 1970; **77**:484.

12. Kitterman JA. *Pediatr Rev* 1982; **4**:13.

13. Jones RW, Baumer JH, Joseph MC, Shinebourne EA. Arterial oxygen tension and response to oxygen breathing in differential diagnosis of heart disease in infancy. *Arch Dis Child* 1976; **51**:667.

14. 26th Bethesda Conference, 1994.

15. Dajani AS, Taubert KA, Wilson W, Bolger AF, Bayer A, Ferrieri P, Gewitz MH, Shulman ST, Nouri S, Newburger JW, Hutto C, Pallasch TJ, Gage TW, Levison ME, Peter G, Zuccaro G Jr. Prevention of bacterial endocarditis: recommendations by the American Heart Association. *JAMA* 1997; **277**:1794.

16. Dajani AS, Taubert KA, Takahashi M, Bierman FZ, Freed MD, Ferrieri P, Gerber M, Shulman ST, Karchmer AW, Wilson W et al. Guidelines for the long-term management of patients with Kawaski disease: report from the Committee on Rheumatic Fever, Endocarditis, and Kawasaki Disease, Council on Cardiovascular Disease in the Young, American Heart Association. *Circulation* 1994; **89**:916.

17. Zubrow AB, Hulman S, Kushner H, Falkner B. Determinants of blood pressure in infants admitted to neonatal intensive care units: a prospective multicenter study—Philadelphia Neonatal Blood Pressure Study Group. *J Perinatol* 1995; **15**:470.

18. Horan MJ. *Pediatrics* 1987; **79**:1.

CONVERSION FORMULAS AND BIOSTATISTICS

George K. Siberry, MD, MPH

I. CONVERSION FORMULAS

A. TEMPERATURE

1. Calculation

a. To convert degrees Celsius to degrees Fahrenheit:
   ([9/5] × Temperature) + 32.
b. To convert degrees Fahrenheit to degrees Celsius:
   (Temperature − 32) × (5/9).

2. Temperature equivalents (Table 8.1)

8

TABLE 8.1			
TEMPERATURE EQUIVALENTS			
Celsius	Fahrenheit	Celsius	Fahrenheit
34.0	93.2	38.6	101.4
34.2	93.6	38.8	101.8
34.4	93.9	39.0	102.2
34.6	94.3	39.2	102.5
34.8	94.6	39.4	102.9
35.0	95.0	39.6	103.2
35.2	95.4	39.8	103.6
35.4	95.7	40.0	104.0
35.6	96.1	40.2	104.3
35.8	96.4	40.4	104.7
36.0	96.8	40.6	105.1
36.2	97.1	40.8	105.4
36.4	97.5	41.0	105.8
36.6	97.8	41.2	106.1
36.8	98.2	41.4	106.5
37.0	98.6	41.6	106.8
37.2	98.9	41.8	107.2
37.4	99.3	42.0	107.6
37.6	99.6	42.2	108.0
37.8	100.0	42.4	108.3
38.0	100.4	42.6	108.7
38.2	100.7	42.8	109.0
38.4	101.1	43.0	109.4

TABLE 8.2

WEIGHT CONVERSION TABLE

Ounces	1lb	2lb	3lb	4lb	5lb	6lb	7lb	8lb
0	454g	907	1361	1814	2268	2722	3175	3629
1	482	936	1389	1843	2296	2750	3204	3657
2	510	964	1418	1871	2325	2778	3232	3686
3	539	992	1446	1899	2353	2807	3260	3714
4	567	1021	1474	1928	2381	2835	3289	3742
5	595	1049	1503	1956	2410	2863	3317	3771
6	624	1077	1531	1985	2438	2892	3345	3799
7	652	1106	1559	2013	2466	2920	3374	3827
8	680	1134	1588	2041	2495	2948	3402	3856
9	709	1162	1616	2070	2523	2977	3430	3884
10	737	1191	1644	2098	2552	3005	3459	3912
11	765	1219	1673	2126	2580	3033	3487	3941
12	794	1247	1701	2155	2608	3062	3515	3969
13	822	1276	1729	2183	2637	3090	3544	3997
14	851	1304	1758	2211	2665	3119	3572	4026
15	879	1332	1786	2240	2693	3147	3600	4054

1 lb = 16 oz = 454g; 1 kg = 2.2 lb. To convert pounds to grams, multiply by 454. To convert kilograms to pounds, multiply by 2.2.

B. LENGTH AND WEIGHT
1. **Length:** To convert inches to centimeters, multiply by 2.54.
2. **Weight** (Table 8.2): To convert pounds to kilograms, divide by 2.2.

II. BIOSTATISTICS FOR MEDICAL LITERATURE

A. STUDY DESIGN COMPARISON (Table 8.3)

B. MEASUREMENTS IN CLINICAL STUDIES (Table 8.4)

1. **Prevalence**
a. Proportion of study population who have a disease (at one point or period in time).
b. Number of old cases and new cases divided by total population.
c. In cross-sectional studies (use Table 8.4): $(A + B)/(A + B + C + D)$.

2. **Incidence**
a. Number of people in study population who newly develop an outcome (disease) per total study population per given time period.
b. Number of new cases divided by the total population over a given time period (use Table 8.4).
c. For cohort studies and clinical trials: $(A + B)/(A + B + C + D)$.

3. **Relative risk (RR)**
a. Ratio of incidence of disease among people with risk factor to incidence of disease among people without risk factor.

TABLE 8.3

STUDY DESIGN COMPARISON

Design type	Definition	Advantages	Disadvantages
Case–control (often called retrospective)	Define diseased subjects (cases) and nondiseased subjects (controls); compare proportion of cases with exposure (risk factor) with proportion of controls with exposure (risk factor).	Good for rare diseases Smaller sample size Faster (not followed over time) Less expensive	Highest potential for biases (recall, selection and others) Weak evidence for causality No prevalence, PPV, NPV
Cohort (usually prospective; occasionally retrospective)	In study population, define exposed group (with risk factor) and nonexposed group (without risk factor). Over time, compare proportion of exposed group with outcome (disease), with proportion of nonexposed group with outcome (disease).	Defines incidence Stronger evidence for causality Decreases biases (sampling, measurement, reporting)	Expensive Long study times May not be feasible for rare diseases/outcomes Factors related to exposure and outcome may falsely alter effect of exposure on outcome (confounding)
Cross-sectional	In study population, concurrently measure outcome (disease) and risk factor. Compare proportion of diseased group with risk factor, with proportion of nondiseased group with risk factor.	Defines prevalence Short time to complete	Selection bias Weak evidence for causality
Clinical trial (experiment)	In study population, assign (randomly) subjects to receive treatment or receive no treatment. Compare rate of outcome (e.g., disease cure) between treatment and nontreatment groups.	Randomized blinded trial is gold standard Randomization reduces confounding. Best evidence for causality	Expensive Risks of experimental treatments in humans Longer time Bad for rare outcomes/diseases

NPV, negative predictive value; PPV, positive predictive value.

CONVERSION FORMULAS AND BIOSTATISTICS

8

TABLE 8.4

GRID FOR CALCULATIONS IN CLINICAL STUDIES

		Exposure or risk factor or treatment	
		Positive	Negative
Disease or outcome	Positive	A	B
	Negative	C	D

b. For cohort studies or clinical trials (use Table 8.4):
   $[A/(A + C)]/[B/(B + D)]$.
c. RR = 1 means no effect of exposure (or treatment) on outcome (or disease). RR <1 indicates exposure or treatment protective against disease. RR >1 indicates exposure/treatment increases probability of outcome/disease.

4. **Odds ratio (OR)**
a. For case–control studies, ratio of odds of having risk factor in people with disease (A/B) to odds of having risk factor in people without disease (C/D), or $(A/B)/(C/D) = (A \times D)/(B \times C)$. (Use Table 8.4.)
b. Good estimate of RR if disease is rare. OR = 1 means no risk factor–disease association. OR >1 suggests risk factor associated with increased disease, and OR <1 suggests risk factor protective against disease.

5. **α (significance level of statistical test)**
a. Probability of finding a statistical association by chance alone when there truly is no association (type I error).
b. Often set at 0.05; low α especially important when interpreting a finding of an association.

6. **Power (of a statistical test)**
a. β = Probability of finding no statistical association when there truly is one (type II error).
b. Power = $1 - \beta$ = Probability of finding a statistical association when there truly is one.
c. Power often set at 0.80; high power especially important when interpreting a finding of no association.

7. **Sample size**
a. Number of subjects required in a clinical study to achieve a sufficiently high power and sufficiently low α to obtain a clinically relevant result.

8. **p value**
a. Probability of a finding by chance alone.
b. If p value < preset α level (often 0.05), then finding is interpreted as sufficiently unlikely to be due to chance as to be accepted as real.

9. **Confidence interval (95%)**
a. 95% probability that the reported interval contains the true value.

TABLE 8.5

GRID FOR EVALUATING A CLINICAL TEST

		Disease status	
		Positive	Negative
Test result	Positive	A (true positive)	B (false positive)
	Negative	C (false negative)	D (true negative)

C. MEASUREMENTS FOR EVALUATING A CLINICAL TEST (Table 8.5)

1. Sensitivity (Sens)

a. Proportion of all diseased who have positive test (use Table 8.5): $A/(A + C)$.

b. Use highly sensitive test to help exclude a disease. (Low false-negative rate. High likelihood ratio [LR] negative. This is good for screening.)

2. Specificity (Spec)

a. Proportion of all nondiseased who have a negative test (use Table 8.5): $D/(B + D)$.

b. Use highly specific test to help confirm a disease. (Low false-positive rate. High LR positive.)

3. Positive predictive value (PPV)

a. Proportion of all those with positive tests who truly have disease (use Table 8.5): $A/(A + B)$.

b. Increased PPV with higher disease prevalence and higher specificity (and, to a lesser degree, higher sensitivity).

4. Negative predictive value (NPV)

a. Proportion of all those with negative tests who truly do not have disease (use Table 8.5): $D/(C + D)$.

b. Increased NPV with lower prevalence (rarer disease) and higher sensitivity.

5. Likelihood ratio (LR)

a. LR positive: Ability of positive test result to confirm diseased status: LR positive = $(Sens)/(1 - Spec)$.

b. LR negative: Ability of negative test result to confirm nondiseased status: LR negative = $(Spec)/(1 - Sens)$. [Alternative LR negative = $(1 - Sens)/Spec$.]

c. Good tests have LR ≥ 10. (Good tests ≤ 0.1 if using alternative LR negative formula.) Physical examination findings often have LR of about 2.

d. LR is not affected by disease prevalence. LR can be used to calculate increase in probability of disease from baseline prevalence with positive test (LR positive) and decrease in probability of disease from baseline prevalence with negative test (using alternative LR negative) for any level of disease prevalence (Fig. 8.1).

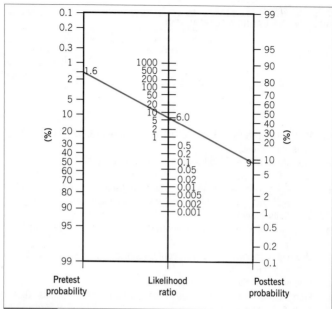

FIG. 8.1

Nomogram for calculating the change in probability by applying tests with known LRs. For example, the prevalence (i.e., pretest probability) of occult bacteremia in a well-appearing 3–36-month-old with temp $\geq 39°$ C without source is 1.6%[2]. LR positive for WBC $>20 \times 10^9$/L is 6.0. For such infants, then, with a WBC $>20 \times 10^9$/L, you can use the nomogram to determine the increased probability from the positive test. Anchor a straight edge at 1.6% on the left pretest probability column and direct the straight edge through the central column at the LR of 6.0. The straight edge will intersect the right column with your answer to give a posttest probability of approximately 9%. It is then up to you to decide the clinical importance of a 9% probability of bacteremia. (From Fagan[1].)

III. REFERENCES

1. Fagan TJ. Nomogram for Bayes' theorem. *N Engl J Med* 1975; **293:** 257.
2. Lee GM, Harper MB. Risk of bacteremia for febrile young children in the post–*Haemophilus influenzae* type b era. *Arch Pediatr Adolesc Med* 1998; **152:**624–628.

DEVELOPMENT

Adrianna Maria Bravo, MD

I. INTRODUCTION

Developmental disabilities are a group of interrelated, chronic, non-progressive, neurologic disorders occurring in childhood. This chapter focuses on screening and assessment of neurodevelopment to identify possible developmental disability.

A. DEVELOPMENT: This can be divided into three major streams or skill areas: Motor, cognitive, and behavior. Each stream has a spectrum of normal and abnormal presentation. Abnormal assessment in one stream increases the risk of deficit in another stream and should therefore alert the examiner to consider a careful assessment of all three streams. A developmental diagnosis is a functional description and classification that does not specify an etiology or medical diagnosis. One useful way to think about the development of a child is to format each stream along the side of a triangle as depicted in Fig. 9.1.

9

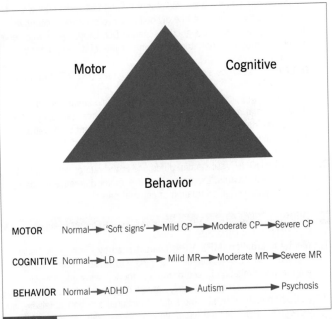

FIG. 9.1
Streams of development.

1. The motor stream includes assessment of both fine motor and gross motor skills. In addition, a full CNS examination should be performed on any child when a motor assessment is being made; this includes examination of tone, strength, coordination, deep tendon reflexes (DTRs), primitive reflexes, and postural reactions.
2. The cognitive stream includes assessment of language skills (expressive and receptive) and of problem-solving/visual-motor skills.
3. The behavior stream, commonly referred to as the psychosocial stream, includes assessment of social skills, activities of daily living, affect, temperament, and interpersonal communication/interaction.

II. DEFINITIONS

A. DEVELOPMENTAL QUOTIENT (DQ)
1. The DQ can be calculated for any given stream:
$$DQ = (Developmental\ age/Chronological\ age) \times 100$$
2. The DQ reflects the child's rate of development over time and holds considerable predictive value in children with delay whose deficits are static. Two separate developmental assessments over time are more predictive than a single assessment. Testing should be performed in several areas of skill.
3. Language remains the best predictor of future intellectual endowment. Language development can be divided into two streams – receptive and expressive – each assigned a separate DQ. Language should serve as the common denominator comparing its rate of development with other skill areas.

B. DELAY: Performance significantly below average (DQ <70) in a given area of skill.

C. DEVIANCY: Atypical development within a single stream, such as developmental milestones occurring out of sequence. Deviancy does not necessarily imply abnormality. Example: An infant who walks before crawling, or an infant with early development of hand preference.

D. DISSOCIATION: A substantial difference in the rate of development between two streams. Example: Cognitive–motor difference in some children with mental retardation or cerebral palsy.

III. DISORDERS

A. COGNITIVE DISORDERS
1. **Mental retardation (MR):** MR is characterized by significantly below-average intellectual functioning (IQ <70–75), existing concurrently with related limitation in two or more of the following adaptive skill areas: communication, self-care, home living, social skills, community use, self-direction, health and safety, functional academics, leisure, and work (Table 9.1). Mental retardation manifests itself before age 18. Formal psychometric testing is needed to make the diagnosis of MR.

TABLE 9.1

MENTAL RETARDATION

Level	IQ	Academic potential	Daily living	Work
Borderline	70–80	Educable to about the 6th grade	Fully independent	Employable; may need training to be competitive
Mild	50–69	Reading and writing to 4th–5th grade or less	Relatively independent with some training	Employable, often need training
Moderate	35–49	Limited reading to 1st or 2nd grade	Dress without help, use toilet, prepare food	Likely to need sheltered employment
Severe	20–34	Very unlikely to read or write	Can be toilet trained, dress with help	Sheltered employment
Profound	<20	None	Occasionally can be toilet trained, dress with help	Very limited

9

DEVELOPMENT

Patients should be referred to a developmental pediatrician for such testing if the DQ for any given stream is <70 or if there is significant learning difficulty.

2. **Communication disorders:** A group of disorders that can be subdivided into expressive language disorders, mixed receptive–expressive language disorders, and phonologic disorders. Developmental language disorders can be characterized by deficits of comprehension, production, or use of language. These deficits can be seen in children with more global disorders such as MR, autism, and pervasive developmental disorder; in addition, they can be seen as a specific language disability. All children suspected of having a communication disorder should undergo a hearing assessment.

3. **Learning disabilities (LD):** A heterogeneous group of disorders that manifest as significant difficulties in one or more of seven areas (as defined by the Federal Government): Basic reading skills, reading comprehension, oral expression, listening comprehension, written expression, mathematical calculation, and mathematical reasoning. Specific learning disabilities are diagnosed when the individual's achievement on standardized tests in a given area is substantially (i.e., 2 standard deviations) below that expected for age, schooling, and level of intelligence.

B. MOTOR DISORDERS

1. **Cerebral palsy (CP):** Cerebral palsy is a disorder of movement and posture resulting from a permanent, nonprogressive lesion of the immature brain. Manifestations, however, may change with brain growth and development. A child with significant motor impairment can be identified at any age. The diagnosis of CP should be made before age 12 months; however, the mean age of diagnosis is 13 months. CP is best classified in terms of clinical and topographic characteristics (Table 9.2). For further information, see Capute[1].

C. BEHAVIOR DISORDERS

1. **Attention deficit/hyperactivity disorder (ADHD):** This is a neurobehavioral disorder characterized by inattention, impulsivity, and hyperactivity which are more frequent and severe than typically observed in individuals of the same developmental age. (See pp. 552–553 for further details.)

D. COMBINED DISORDERS

1. **Pervasive developmental disorders (PDD):** PDD is characterized by severe and pervasive impairment in the following areas of development: Reciprocal social interaction skills; communication skills; or presence of

TABLE 9.2

CLINICAL CLASSIFICATION OF CEREBRAL PALSY

	Type	Pattern of involvement
I. SPASTIC		
	Hemiplegia	Homolateral arm and leg; arm worse than leg
	Diplegia	All four extremities; legs much worse than arms
	Quadriplegia	All four extremities impaired; legs worse than arms
	Double hemiplegia	All four extremities; arms notably worse than legs
	Monoplegia	One extremity, usually upper; probably reflects a mild hemiplegia
	Triplegia	One upper extremity and both lower; probably represents a hemiplegia plus a diplegia or incomplete quadriplegia
	Paraplegia	Involves legs only with normal upper extremities; almost always spinal cord injury, not CP
II. EXTRAPYRAMIDAL		
	Choreoathetosis	Complex movement/tone disorders reflecting basal ganglia pathology
	Rigidity	
	Dystonia	
	Ataxia	Movement and tone disorders reflecting cerebellar origin
	Tremor	
	Hypotonia	Usually related to diffuse, often severe, cerebral and/or cerebellar cortical damage

stereotyped behavior, interests, and activities. Disorders include the following:

a. Autism: Infantile autism is at the severe end of the PDD spectrum. To make the diagnosis of autism, one must meet a set of criteria as outlined in the DSM-IV[2]. Criteria include: Impaired social interactions; impaired communication; restricted, repetitive, and stereotyped patterns of behavior, interests or activities; onset before age 3.

b. PDD not otherwise specified (PDD NOS) is along the spectrum of autism, but not severe enough to meet the criteria for making the diagnosis of autism.

c. Others: These include Rett syndrome, Asperger syndrome, and childhood disintegrative disorder.

2. **Minimal brain dysfunction (MBD):** This is an old but useful diagnostic term applied to children who exhibit some degree, often subtle, of abnormality across all three domains of developmental function: Neuromotor (subtle neurologic abnormalities referred to as 'soft signs'; these may include, but are not limited to, mild generalized hypotonia, presence of facial expressions while performing rapid alternating movements, or posturing of hands and arms when asked to walk with inverted or everted feet); cognitive (learning disability or perceptual deficits); and behavior (ADHD symptoms). For more detailed information, see Capute[3].

IV. DEVELOPMENTAL SCREENING

A. DENVER DEVELOPMENT ASSESSMENT (DENVER II) (see foldout)

1. **Use:** The Denver II is meant to be used as a tool for screening of the apparently normal child between the ages of 0 and 6 years; its use is suggested at every well-child visit. This screen will allow the practitioner to identify those children who *may* have developmental delay and should therefore be further evaluated for the purpose of definitive diagnosis. The test evaluates the child in four areas: personal–social, fine motor, gross motor, language.

2. **Supplies:** The Denver II screening manual supplies detailed information about the standardization, administration, and interpretation of the assessment. In brief, supplies provided in the Denver II kit include red yarn, raisins, rattle, 10 wooden blocks, glass bottle with $\frac{5}{8}$-inch opening, small bell, tennis ball, red pencil, small plastic doll with feeding bottle, plastic cup with handle, blank paper.

3. **Explanation of form:** Test items are arranged in one of four sectors corresponding to the streams of development. Age scales appear across the top and bottom of the form. Each item is represented by a bar that spans the ages at which 25%, 50%, 75%, and 90% of the standardized sample passed that item. Some items contain a small footnote referring to instructions on the back of the form. Items that can be passed by report of the caregiver are denoted with the letter 'R.'

9

DEVELOPMENT

4. **Calculation of age:** The child's age needs to be calculated accurately. For children born more than 2 weeks before the expected date of delivery and who are <2 years of age, the calculated age must be adjusted by subtracting the number of days of prematurity (based on a 30-day or 4-week month, and a 7-day week) from the chronologic age. Once the preterm child reaches 2 years of age, this correction is no longer necessary. An 'age line' should be drawn from the top to the bottom of the form connecting the appropriate age markers of the child.

5. **Evaluation**

a. Item score: Items intersected by and just adjacent to the age line should be tested. Items should be marked as 'P' for pass, 'F' for failed, 'NO' for no opportunity, or 'R' for refused to cooperate or attempt.

b. Item assessment: Each item should be assessed as one of the following:

   1) Advanced: Child passes item that falls completely to the right of age line.
   2) Normal: Child passes, fails, or refuses item on which the age line falls between the 25th and 75th percentile.
   3) Caution: Child fails or refuses item on which the age line falls between 75th and 90th percentile.
   4) Delayed: Child fails or refuses item that falls completely to the left of age line.

c. Global assessment: When two or more 'delays' are noted, the child is considered to have failed the screening and thereby warrants referral. A child warrants reevaluation in 3 months if there is one 'delay' and/or two or more 'cautions.' A child is normal with no 'delays' and a maximum of one 'caution'. In addition, some children may be termed 'untestable' if there is a significant number of 'refusal' or 'no opportunity' items; these children should be retested in 2–3 weeks; if the same result occurs at this time then referral is warranted.

V. DEVELOPMENTAL EVALUATIONS

Use of the following test is meant to define delays suggested by prior screening tools such as the Denver Developmental Assessment.

A. **DEVELOPMENTAL MILESTONES** (Table 9.3): In assessing for delay, an individual DQ can be calculated for any given milestone; if the quotient is <70%, a diagnosis of delay can be made and warrants further evaluation and/or referral. For example, a 13-month-old child who does not yet walk alone but is able to walk when led with two hands held, i.e., a 10-month level of motor development, has a DQ of $10/13 = 77\%$ and is not considered delayed.

B. **POSTURAL REACTIONS AND PRIMITIVE REFLEXES** (Tables 9.4 and 9.5): Intrauterine/birth reflexes, or primitive reflexes, are present at birth and disappear by 6–9 months. Postural reactions appear after suppression of the birth reflexes and precede voluntary motor function. A reflex/reaction profile can be helpful in identifying infants at risk for cerebral palsy or other developmental disability. An infant with an abnormally absent, asymmetric, or obligatory reflex/reaction is at high risk for developmental disability.

C. **CLAMS/CAT** (Capute Scales) (Table 9.6): The Capute Scales are an assessment tool that gives quantitative developmental quotients for visual-motor/problem-solving and language abilities. The CLAMS (Clinical Linguistic and Auditory Milestone Scale) was developed, standardized, and validated for assessment of language development from birth to 36 months of age. The CAT (Clinical Adaptive Test) consists of problem-solving items, for ages from birth to 36 months, adapted from standardized infant psychological tests.

1. **Supplies:** The kit includes the following items: red ring, cup, ten cubes, pegboard with six holes and two pegs, metal bell, crayon and paper, tissues, card with four pictures, card with six pictures, bottle and pellets, round stick, glass/Plexiglas, formboard with three shapes.

2. **Responses:** Responses to the test item are recorded as 'yes' for pass and 'no' for fail. A basal age is determined when all items for two consecutive months are scored as 'yes.' Items for tests at the next higher age group are administered until two consecutive levels of all 'no' responses are obtained. Items marked with an asterisk must be answered or demonstrated by the child and not per report of the parent/caregiver.

3. **Scoring:** Scoring is done by calculating the basal age as the highest age group where a child accomplishes all of the test tasks correctly. The age equivalent is then determined by adding the decimal number (recorded in parentheses) next to each correctly scored item passed at age groups beyond the basal age to the basal age itself. This is done to calculate the language age equivalent and the problem-solving age equivalent. Each of these age equivalents is then divided by the child's chronologic age and multiplied by 100 to determine a developmental quotient. Again, a DQ <70% constitutes delay and warrants referral for evaluation to rule out MR or auditory/visual impairment. For example, a 6-month-old child who *can* orient to voice, laugh out loud, and orient toward bell laterally, but who *cannot* ah-goo or razz has a basal age (age where child accomplishes all tasks correctly) of 4 months. An additional 0.3 is added for the ability to orient toward bell laterally, as per the decimal number recorded in parentheses. Together, this gives an age-equivalent of 4.3. The DQ of this patient's linguistic and auditory skills is 4.3 (age equivalent) ÷ 6.0 (chronologic age) × 100 = 71.7.

D. **EVALUATION OF VISUAL-MOTOR SKILLS AND PROBLEM-SOLVING SKILLS:** For these tests, it is important to observe *how* they are done as well as the final product.

Text continued on p. 202

DEVELOPMENTAL MILESTONES

Age	Gross motor	Visual-motor/problem-solving
1mo	Raises head slightly from prone, makes crawling movements	Birth: visually fixes 1mo: has tight grasp, follows to midline
2mo	Holds head in midline, lifts chest off table	No longer clenches fist tightly, follows object past midline
3mo	Supports on forearms in prone, holds head up steadily	Holds hands open at rest, follows in circular fashion, responds to visual threat
4mo	Rolls front to back, supports on wrists and shifts weight	Reaches with arms in unison, brings hands to midline
5mo	Rolls back to front, sits supported	Transfers objects
6mo	Sits unsupported, puts feet in mouth in supine position	Unilateral reach, uses raking grasp
7mo	Creeps	
8mo	Comes to sit, crawls	Inspects objects
9mo	Pivots when sitting, pulls to stand, cruises	Uses pincer grasp, probes with forefinger, holds bottle, throws objects
10mo	Walks when led with both hands held	—
11mo	Walks when led with one hand held	—
12mo	Walks alone	Uses mature pincer grasp, releases voluntarily, marks paper with pencil
13mo	—	—
14mo	—	—
15mo	Creeps up stairs, walks backwards	Scribbles in imitation, builds tower of 2 blocks in imitation
17mo	—	—
18mo	Runs, throws objects from standing without falling	Scribbles spontaneously, builds tower of 3 blocks, turns 2–3 pages at a time

Language	Social/adaptive	Age
Alerts to sound	Regards face	1mo
Smiles socially (after being stroked or talked to)	Recognizes parent	2mo
Coos (produces long vowel sounds in musical fashion)	Reaches for familiar people or objects, anticipates feeding	3mo
Laughs, orients to voice	Enjoys looking around environment	4mo
Says 'ah-goo,' razzes, orients to bell (localizes laterally)		5mo
Babbles	Recognizes strangers	6mo
Orients to bell (localized indirectly)		7mo
'Dada' indiscriminately	Fingerfeeds	8mo
'Mama' indiscriminately, gestures, waves bye-bye, understands 'no'	Starts to explore environment; plays gesture games (e.g., pat–a–cake)	9mo
'Dada/mama' discriminately; orients to bell (directly)	—	10mo
One word other than 'dada/mama,' follows 1-step command with gesture	—	11mo
Uses two words other than 'dada/mama,' immature jargoning (runs several unintelligible words together)	Imitates actions, comes when called, cooperates with dressing	12mo
Uses three words	—	13mo
Follows 1-step command without gesture	—	14mo
Uses 4–6 words	15–18mo: uses spoon, uses cup independently	15mo
Uses 7–20 words, points to 5 body parts, uses mature jargoning (includes intelligible words in jargoning)	—	17mo
Uses 2-word combinations	Copies parent in tasks (sweeping, dusting), plays in company of other children	18mo

9

DEVELOPMENT

Continued

TABLE 9.3

DEVELOPMENTAL MILESTONES—cont'd

Age	Gross motor	Visual-motor/ problem-solving
19mo	—	—
21mo	Squats in play, goes up steps	Builds tower of 5 blocks
24mo	Walks up and down steps without help	Imitates stroke with pencil, builds tower of 7 blocks, turns pages one at a time, removes shoes, pants, etc.
30mo	Jumps with both feet off floor, throws ball overhand	Holds pencil in adult fashion, performs horizontal and vertical strokes, unbuttons
3yr	Can alternate feet when going up steps, pedals tricycle	Copies a circle, undresses completely, dresses partially, dries hands if reminded
4yr	Hops, skips, alternates feet going down steps	Copies a square, buttons clothing, dresses self completely, catches ball
5yr	Skips alternating feet, jumps over low obstacles	Copies triangle, ties shoes, spreads with knife

From Caputo[5–7]. Rounded norms form Caputo[8].

TABLE 9.4

POSTURAL REACTIONS

Postural reaction	Age of appearance
Head righting	6wk–3mo
Landau response	2–3mo
Derotational righting	4–5mo
Anterior propping	4–5mo
Parachute	5–6mo
Lateral propping	6–7mo
Posterior propping	8–10mo

Adapted from Milani-Comparetti[9]; Caputo[10,11]; and Palmer[12].

Language	Social/adaptive	Age
Knows 8 body parts	—	19mo
Uses 50 words, 2-word sentences	Asks to have food and to go to toilet	21mo
Uses pronouns (I, you, me) inappropriately, follows 2-step commands	Parallel play	24mo
Uses pronouns appropriately, understands concept of '1,' repeats 2 digits forward	Tells first and last names when asked; gets self drink without help	30mo
Uses minimum 250 words, 3-word sentences; uses plurals, past tense; knows all pronouns; understands concept of '2'	Group play, shares toys, takes turns, plays well with others, knows full name, age, sex	3yr
Knows colors, says song or poem from memory, asks questions	Tells 'tall tales,' plays cooperatively with a group of children	4yr
Prints first name, asks what a word means	Plays competitive games, abides by rules, likes to help in household tasks	5yr

9

DEVELOPMENT

Description	Importance
Lifts chin from tabletop in prone position	Necessary for adequate head control and sitting
Extension of head, then trunk and legs when held prone	Early measure of developing trunk control
Following passive or active head turning, the body rotates to follow the direction of the head	Prerequisite to independent rolling
Arm extension anteriorly in supported sitting	Necessary for tripod sitting
Arm extension when falling	Facial protection when falling
Arm extension laterally in protective response	Allows independent sitting
Arm extension posteriorly	Allows pivoting in sitting

TABLE 9.5

PRIMITIVE REFLEXES

Primitive reflexes	Elicitation
Moro reflex (MR, 'embrace' response) of fingers, wrists, and elbows	Supine: sudden neck extension; allow head to fall back about 3cm
Galant reflex (GR)	Prone suspension: stroking paravertebral area from thoracic to sacral region
Asymmetric tonic neck reflex (ATNR, 'fencer' response)	Supine: rotate head laterally about 45–90°
Symmetric tonic neck reflex (STNR, 'cat' reflex)	Sitting: head extension/flexion
Tonic labyrinthine supine (TLS)	Supine: extension of the neck (alters relation of labyrinths)
Tonic labyrinthine prone (TLP)	Prone: flexion of the neck
Positive support reflex (PSR)	Vertical suspension; bouncing hallucal areas on firm surface
Stepping reflex (SR, walking reflex)	Vertical suspension; hallucal stimulation
Crossed extension reflex (CER)	Prone; hallucal stimulation of a LE in full extension
Plantar grasp (PG)	Stimulation of hallucal area
Palmar grasp	Stimulation of palm
Lower extremity placing (LEP)	Vertical suspension; rubbing tibia or dorsum of foot against edge of tabletop
Upper extremity placing (UEP)	Rubbing lateral surface of forearm along edge of tabletop from elbow to wrist to dorsum
Downward thrust (DT)	Vertical suspension; thrust LEs downward

UE, upper extremity; LE, lower extremity.

Response	Timing
Extension, adduction, and then abduction of UEs, with semiflexion	Present at birth, disappears by 3–6mo
Produces truncal incurvature with concavity towards stimulated side	Present at birth, disappears by 2–6mo
Relative extension of limbs on chin side and flexion on occiput side	Present at birth, disappears by 4–9mo
Extension of UEs and flexion of LEs/flexion of UEs and LE extension	Appears at 5mo; not present in most normal children; disappears by 8–9mo
Tonic extension of trunk and LEs, shoulder retraction and adduction, usually with elbow flexion	Present at birth, disappears by 6–9mo
Active flexion of trunk with protraction of shoulders	Present at birth, disappears by 6–9mo
Neonatal: momentary LE extension followed by flexion; **mature:** extension of LEs and support of body weight	Present at birth; disappears by 2–4mo; appears by 6mo
Stepping gait	Disappears by 2–3mo
Initial flexion, adduction, then extension of contralateral limb	Present at birth; disappears by 2–3mo
Plantar flexion grasp	Present at birth; disappears by 9mo
Palmar grasp	Present at birth; disappears by 4mo
Initial flexion, then extension, the placing of LE on tabletop	Appears at 1dy
Flexion, extension, then placing of hand on tabletop	Appears at 3mo
Full extension of LEs	Appears at 3mo

9

DEVELOPMENT

TABLE 9.6

CLAMS/CAT[a]

Age (mo)	CLAMS	Yes	No	CAT	Yes	No
1	1. Alerts to sound (0.5)*	—	—	1. Visually fixates momentarily upon red ring (0.5)	—	—
	2. Soothes when picked up (0.5)	—	—	2. Chin off table in prone (0.5)	—	—
2	1. Social smile (1.0)*	—	—	1. Visually follows ring horizontally and vertically (0.5)	—	—
		—	—	2. Chest off table prone (0.5)	—	—
3	1. Cooing (1.0)	—	—	1. Visually follows ring in circle (0.3)	—	—
				2. Supports on forearms in prone (0.3)	—	—
				3. Visual threat (0.3)	—	—
4	1. Orients to voice (0.5)*	—	—	1. Unfisted (0.3)	—	—
	2. Laughs aloud (0.5)	—	—	2. Manipulates fingers (0.3)	—	—
		—	—	3. Supports on wrists in prone (0.3)	—	—
5	1. Orients toward bell laterally (0.3)*	—	—	1. Pulls down rings (0.3)	—	—
	2. Ah-goo (0.3)	—	—	2. Transfers (0.3)	—	—
	3. Razzing (0.3)	—	—	3. Regards pellet (0.3)	—	—
6	1. Babbling (1.0)	—	—	1. Obtains cube (0.3)	—	—
				2. Lifts cup (0.3)	—	—
				3. Radial rake (0.3)	—	—
7	1. Orients toward bell (1.0)* (upwardly/indirectly 90°)	—	—	1. Attempts pellet (0.3)	—	—
				2. Pulls out peg (0.3)	—	—
				3. Inspects ring (0.3)	—	—
8	1. 'Dada' inappropriately (0.5)	—	—	1. Pulls out ring by string (0.3)	—	—
	2. 'Mama' inappropriately (0.5)	—	—	2. Secures pellet (0.3)	—	—
				3. Inspects bell (0.3)	—	—
9	1. Orients toward bell (upward directly 180°) (0.5)*	—	—	1. Three finger scissor grasp (0.3)	—	—
	2. Gesture language (0.5)	—	—	2. Rings bell (0.3)	—	—
				3. Over the edge for toy (0.3)	—	—

[a]See p. 193 for instructions.

TABLE 9.6

CLAMS/CAT—cont'd

Age (mo)	CLAMS	Yes	No	CAT	Yes	No
10	1. Understands 'no' (0.3)	—	—	1. Combine cube–cup (0.3)	—	—
	2. Uses 'dada' appropriately (0.3)	—	—	2. Uncovers bell (0.3)	—	—
	3. Uses 'mama' appropriately (0.3)			3. Fingers pegboard (0.3)	—	—
11	1. One word (other than 'mama' and 'dada') (1.0)	—	—	1. Mature overhand pincer movement (0.5)	—	—
				2. Solves cube under cup (0.5)	—	—
12	1. One-step command with gesture (0.5)	—	—	1. Release one cube in cup (0.5)	—	—
	2. Two-word vocabulary (0.5)	—	—	2. Crayon mark (0.5)	—	—
14	1. Three-word vocabulary (1.0)	—	—	1. Solves glass frustration (0.6)	—	—
	2. Immature jargoning (1.0)	—	—	2. Out–in with peg (0.6)	—	—
				3. Solves pellet–bottle with demonstration (0.6)	—	—
16	1. Four- to six-word vocabulary (1.0)	—	—	1. Solves pellet-bottle spontaneously (0.6)	—	—
	2. One-step command without gesture (1.0)	—	—	2. Round block on form board (0.6)	—	—
				3. Scribbles in imitation (0.6)	—	—
18	1. Mature jargoning (0.5)	—	—	1. Ten cubes in cup (0.5)	—	—
	2. 7–10 word vocabulary (0.5)	—	—	2. Solves round hole in form board reversed (0.5)	—	—
	3. Points to one picture (0.5)*	—	—	3. Spontaneous scribbling with crayon (0.5)	—	—
	4. Body parts (0.5)	—	—	4. Pegboard completed spontaneously (0.5)	—	—

Continued

9

DEVELOPMENT

TABLE 9.6

CLAMS/CAT—cont'd

Age (mo)	CLAMS	Yes	No	CAT	Yes	No
21	1. 20-word vocabulary (1.0)	—	—	1. Obtains object with stick (1.0)	—	—
	2. Two-word phrases (1.0)	—	—	2. Solves square in form board (1.0)	—	—
	3. Points to two pictures (1.0)*	—	—	3. Tower of three cubes (1.0)	—	—
24	1. 50-word vocabulary (1.0)	—	—	1. Attempts to fold paper (0.7)	—	—
	2. Two-step command (1.0)	—	—	2. Horizontal four cube train (0.7)	—	—
	3. Two word sentences (1.0)	—	—	3. Imitates stroke with pencil (0.7)	—	—
				4. Completes form board (0.7)	—	—
30	1. Uses pronouns appropriately (1.5)	—	—	1. Horizontal-vertical stroke with pencil (1.5)	—	—
	2. Concept of one (1.5)*	—	—	2. Form board reversed (1.5)	—	—
	3. Points to seven pictures (1.5)*	—	—	3. Folds paper with definite crease (1.5)	—	—
	4. Two digits forward (1.5)*	—	—	4. Train with chimney (1.5)	—	—
36	1. 250-word vocabulary (1.5)	—	—	1. Three cube bridge (1.5)	—	—
	2. Three-word sentence (1.5)	—	—	2. Draws circle (1.5)	—	—
	3. Three digits forward (1.5)*	—	—	3. Names one color (1.5)	—	—
	4. Follows two prepositional commands (1.5)*	—	—	4. Draw-a-person with head plus one other part of body (1.5)	—	—

1. **Goodenough–Harris Draw-a-Person Test**
a. Procedure: Give the child a pencil (preferably a no. 2 with eraser) and a sheet of blank paper. Instruct child to 'Draw a person; draw the best person you can.' Supply encouragement if needed (i.e., 'Draw a whole person'); however, do not suggest specific supplementation or changes.
b. Scoring: Ask the child to describe or explain the drawing to you. Give the child one point for each detail present using the guide in Table 9.7. (Maximum score = 51.)
c. Age norms (Table 9.8).

TABLE 9.7

GOODENOUGH–HARRIS SCORING

General:	☐ Head present		Proportion:	☐	Head: 10% to 50% of trunk area
	☐ Legs present			☐	Arms: Approx. same length as
	☐ Arms present				trunk
Trunk:	☐ Present			☐	Legs: 1–2 times trunk length;
	☐ Length greater than breadth				width less than
	☐ Shoulders				trunk width
Arms/legs:	☐ Attached to trunk			☐	Feet: to leg length
	☐ At correct point			☐	Arms and legs in two dimensions
Neck:	☐ Present			☐	Heel
	☐ Outline of neck continuous with head, trunk, or both.		Motor coordination:	☐	Lines firm and well connected
Face:	☐ Eyes			☐	Firmly drawn with correct joining
	☐ Nose			☐	Head outline
	☐ Mouth			☐	Trunk outline
	☐ Nose and mouth in two dimensions			☐	Outline of arms and legs
	☐ Nostrils			☐	Features
Hair:	☐ Present		Ears:	☐	Present
	☐ On more than circumference; nontransparent			☐	Correct position and proportion
Clothing:	☐ Present		Eye detail:	☐	Brow or lashes
	☐ Two articles; nontransparent			☐	Pupil
	☐ Entire drawing and trousers) nontransparent (sleeves			☐	Proportion
	☐ Four articles			☐	Glance directed front in profile drawing
	☐ Costume complete		Chin:	☐	Present; forehead
Fingers:	☐ Present			☐	Projection
	☐ Correct number		Profile:	☐	Not more than one error
	☐ Two dimension; length, breadth			☐	Correct
	☐ Thumb opposition				
	☐ Hand distinct from fingers and arm				
Joints:	☐ Elbow, shoulder or both				
	☐ Knee, hip, or both				

TABLE 9.8

GOODENOUGH AGE NORMS

Age (yr)	3	4	5	6	7	8	9	10	11	12	13
Points	2	6	10	14	18	22	26	30	34	38	42

From Taylor[13].

2. **Gesell figures** (Fig. 9.2): One should note that the examiner is not supposed to demonstrate the drawing of the figures for the patient; however, most developmentalists do demonstrate and do not feel that it makes a difference.

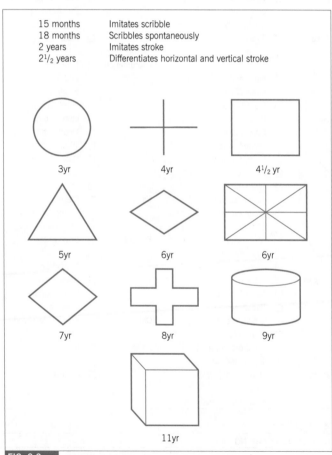

15 months	Imitates scribble
18 months	Scribbles spontaneously
2 years	Imitates stroke
2½ years	Differentiates horizontal and vertical stroke

3yr 4yr 4½ yr

5yr 6yr 6yr

7yr 8yr 9yr

11yr

FIG. 9.2
Gesell figures. (From Illingsworth[14] and Cattel[15].)

3. **Block skills:** The structures in Fig. 9.3 should be demonstrated for the child. Figure 9.4 includes the developmental age at which each structure can usually be accomplished.

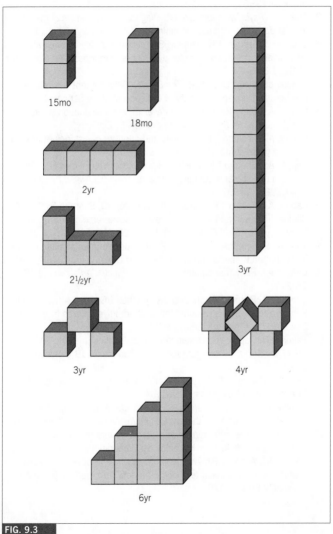

FIG. 9.3
Block skills. (From Capute[16].)

VI. REFERENCES

1. Capute AJ, Accardo PJ, eds. Cerebral palsy. *Developmental disabilities in infancy and childhood*, 2nd edn, vol 2, *The spectrum of developmental disabilities,* part II, Cerebral palsy. Baltimore: Paul H Brookes; 1996.

2. American Psychiatric Association. *Diagnostic and statistical manual of mental disorders*, 4th edn. Washington, DC: The Association; 1994.

3. Capute AJ, Shapiro BK, Palmer FB. Spectrum of developmental disabilities: continuum of motor dysfunction. *Orthoped Clin North Am* 1981; **12**:15–21.

4. Frankenburg WE, Dodds JB. *The Denver Development Assessment (Denver II).* Denver: University of Colorado Medical School; 1990.

5. Capute AJ, Biehl RF. Functional developmental evaluation: prerequisite to habilitation. *Pediatr Clin North Am* 1973; **20**:3.

6. Capute AJ, Accardo PJ. Linguistic and auditory milestones during the first two years of life. *Clin Pediatr* 1978; **17**:847.

7. Capute AJ, Shapiro BK, Wachtel RC, Gunther VA, Palmer FB. The clinical linguistic and auditory milestone scale (CLAMS). *Am J Dis Child* 1986; **140**:694.

8. Capute AJ, Palmer FB, Shapiro BK, Wachtel RC, Schmidt S, Ross A. Clinical linguistic and auditory milestone scale: prediction of cognition in infancy. *Dev Med Child Neurol* 1986; **28**:762.

9. Milani-Comparetti A, Gidoni EA. Routine developmental examination in normal and retarded children. *Dev Med Child Neurol* 1967; **9**:631.

10. Capute AJ. Early neuromotor reflexes in infancy. *Pediatr Ann* 1986; **15**:217.

11. Capute AJ, Palmer FB, Shapiro BK, Wachtel RC, Ross A, Accardo PJ. Primitive reflex profile: a quantitation of primitive reflexes in infancy. *Dev Med Child Neurol* 1984; **26**:375.

12. Palmer FB, Capute AJ. Developmental disabilities. In: Oski FA, ed. *Principles and practice of pediatrics*. Philadelphia: JB Lippincott; 1994.

13. Taylor E. *Psychological appraisal of children with cerebral defects*. Boston: Harvard University; 1961.

14. Illingsworth RS. *The development of the infant and young child, normal and abnormal*, 5th edn. Baltimore: Williams & Wilkins; 1972.

15. Cattel P. *The measurement of intelligence of infants and young children*. New York: The Psychological Corporation; 1960.

16. Capute AJ, Accardo PJ. *The pediatrician and the developmentally disabled child: a clinical textbook on mental retardation*. Baltimore: University Press; 1979.

ENDOCRINOLOGY

Jeffrey Renn Keefer, MD, PhD

I. COMMON MANAGEMENT ISSUES

A. DIABETIC KETOACIDOSIS (DKA): Defined by hyperglycemia, ketonemia, ketonuria, and metabolic acidosis (pH <7.30, bicarbonate <15mEq/L).

1. Assessment

a. History: In known diabetic child, determine usual insulin regimen, last dose, history of infection, or inciting event. In suspected diabetic child, determine history of polydypsia, polyuria, polyphagia, weight loss, vomiting, or abdominal pain.

b. Examination: Assess for dehydration, Kussmaul's breathing, fruity breath, change in mental status, and current weight.

c. Laboratory tests: Check blood glucose, blood gas, electrolytes, and urinalysis (for glucose and ketones). Consider sending $HgbA_{1c}$ as an index of chronic hyperglycemia and if needed for diagnostic workup consider sending Islet cell antibodies, thyroid antibodies, and thyroid function tests.

2. Initial management

a. Overview: The most critical concept for successful management of DKA is to frequently reevaluate the clinical status and laboratory data of the patient and make changes in the treatment strategy based on these findings. Fluid and electrolyte requirements of patients in DKA may vary greatly, and therefore the following guidelines should be taken as a starting point for therapy that must be individualized based on the dynamics of the patient. Cerebral edema is the most important complication of DKA management. Overaggressive hydration and overly rapid correction of hyperglycemia may play a role in the development of cerebral edema and should be avoided.

b. Fluids: Assume 5–10% dehydration (dictated by clinical examination). Give 10–20ml/kg bolus of NS or LR over 1 hour then run 0.45 NS (with other appropriate electrolytes – see below) at a rate calculated to replace the remaining fluid deficit equally over 36–48 hours *plus* provide maintenance requirements. For the maintenance requirements some clinicians simply calculate the fluid rate based on weight in the usual manner, regardless of urine output. However, if urine output is very high other clinicians would include these ongoing losses in the maintenance calculation for the first few hours until the osmotic diuresis slows. In this case the maintenance portion of your rate should equal urine output plus insensible losses (approximated as 40% of standard maintenance calculation). Finally, some DKA protocols recommend using NS rather than 0.45 NS during part of the replacement period in an effort to further decrease risk of cerebral edema.

c. Insulin: Begin insulin drip after first NS/LR bolus is completed if hemodynamically stable.

      1) IV insulin infusion is preferred over IM or SC injections.

      2) Give 0.1U/kg per hour regular insulin as continuous drip. Some protocols include an initial 0.1U/kg regular insulin IV bolus.

  d. Glucose

      1) Measure hourly. Rate of glucose fall should not exceed 80–100mg/dL per hour.

      2) If glucose falls faster than 100mg/dL per hour, continue insulin infusion (0.1U/kg per hour) and add D_5 to intravenous fluid (IVF). As glucose approaches 250–300mg/dL, add D_5 to IVF regardless of rate of fall.

  e. Electrolytes

      1) Sodium (Na^+): Use 0.45 NS or NS for rehydration. Serum Na^+ should rise as blood glucose falls.

      2) Potassium (K^+): Patients with DKA are total body K^+ depleted and are at risk for severe hypokalemia during DKA therapy. However, serum K^+ levels may be normal or elevated as a result of the shift of K^+ to the extracellular compartment in the setting of acidosis. Usually begin with 20–40mEq/L of K^+ in fluids and follow electrolytes closely (Q2hr). Give no K^+ initially if K^+ level is elevated or patient is not urinating.

      3) Phosphate (PO_4^{3-}): Depleted in DKA and will drop further with insulin therapy. PO_4^{3-} improves release of oxygen to tissues. Consider replacing K^+ as half KCl and half K_3PO_4 for the first 8 hours, then all as KCl. Excessive PO_4^{3-} may induce hypocalcemic tetany.

      4) Bicarbonate (HCO_3^-): Rarely used in routine DKA management. Consider only in cases of extreme acidosis (pH <7.10). Use with caution.

  f. Laboratory test schedule: Follow blood glucose hourly; blood gas and electrolytes (including PO_4^{3-}) Q2hr. Monitor urine for ketones and glucose with each void.

Note: Remember that pH is a good indicator of insulin deficiency, and if acidosis is not resolving, the patient may need more insulin, whereas the degree of hyperglycemia is often a reflection of hydration status.

3. Further management

  a. When acidosis and ketosis are resolved, start SC insulin and discontinue insulin drip 1 hour after SC dose. At this time the patient should begin tolerating solids and liquids PO.

  b. For previously diagnosed diabetics, begin their usual insulin regimen.

  c. For newly diagnosed diabetics:

      1) For the first 24 hours after insulin drip is discontinued, give 0.1–0.25U regular insulin/kg SC Q6–8hr to determine a daily insulin requirement.

      2) The next 24 hours, give two thirds of the previous day's total insulin dose as a morning (am) dose and one third as an evening (pm) dose. For the am dose, two thirds should be NPH (neutral protamine Hagedorn) and one third should be regular insulin. For the pm dose,

one half should be NPH and one half should be regular. If needed, give additional regular insulin 0.1U/kg before each meal (Fig. 10.1).

d. Usual daily maintenance dose in children: 0.5–1.0U/kg per 24 hour; in adolescents during growth spurt: 0.8–1.2U/kg per 24 hour.

B. ADRENAL INSUFFICIENCY

1. Acute adrenal crisis

a. Assessment: Characterized by hypoglycemia, hyponatremia, hyperkalemia, metabolic acidosis, and shock. If the diagnosis is suspected, obtain blood for electrolytes and glucose. Serum cortisol, 17-hydroxyprogesterone, and adrenocorticotropic hormone (ACTH) should be obtained in infants with possible congenital adrenal hyperplasia before steroid administration, but treatment should not be delayed. The older patient should have measurement of serum cortisol, ACTH, renin, and aldosterone obtained before treatment.

b. Management: Requires rapid volume expansion, glucose infusion, and corticosteroid administration. Specifically, give NS (20ml/kg) to support blood pressure and sufficient dextrose to maintain blood glucose. For corticosteroids, give approximately 50mg/m^2 of hydrocortisone IV bolus (rapid estimate: infants = 25mg; children = 50–100mg). Follow bolus with 50–100mg/m^2 per 24 hours as continuous drip (most desirable) or divided Q3–4hr. Only hydrocortisone and cortisone provide the necessary mineralocorticoid effects.

2. Daily management of adrenal insufficiency

a. Glucocorticoid maintenance: Physiologic glucocorticoid production is approximately 9–12mg/m^2 per day; therefore 12.5mg/m^2 per day of hydrocortisone IV/IM or 25mg/m^2 per day PO (given 50% bioavailability) is considered a maintenance dose. For congenital adrenal hyperplasia, this dose is recommended for daily maintenance to allow for suppression of the ACTH axis. For pure adrenal insufficiency, daily dosing of 9–12mg/m^2 of hydrocortisone PO is often sufficient and helps decrease the toxic effects seen at higher doses.

b. Mineralocorticoid maintenance for salt-losing forms of adrenal insufficiency is 0.05–0.2mg/day of fludrocortisone acetate PO once daily. Note that IV hydrocortisone at 50mg/m^2 per day (four times production) will also supply a maintenance amount of

10

ENDOCRINOLOGY

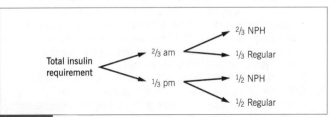

FIG. 10.1

Conversion to daily insulin dosing. NPH, neutral protamine Hagedorn.

mineralocorticoid activity for patients who cannot take PO. Always monitor BP and electrolytes when supplementing mineralocorticoids.

c. Stress dose glucocorticoids: Indication is for severe illness or surgery. The stress dose is $37.5mg/m^2$ per day hydrocortisone IV/IM or $75mg/m^2$ per day PO.

Note: See pp. 908–909 for relative potencies and dosing of other steroids.

3. Specifics about congenital adrenal hyperplasia

a. Definition: Group of autosomal recessive disorders characterized by a defect in one of the enzymes required in the synthesis of cortisol from cholesterol. Cortisol deficiency results in oversecretion of ACTH and hyperplasia of the adrenal cortex. Enzymatic defect results in impaired synthesis of the glucocorticoids, mineralocorticoids, and sex steroids beyond the enzymatic block, and overproduction of the precursors before the block. These precursers are diverted to alternative metabolic pathways.

b. Etiology: 21-Hydroxylase deficiency is the most common form (also the most common cause of ambiguous genitalia), accounting for 90% of cases. The incidence of 21-hydroxylase deficiency in Caucasians is 1/15,000. There are two types:

1) Simple virilizing form (partial enzyme deficiency): Adrenal insufficiency tends to occur only under stress.
2) Na^+-losing form (more complete enzyme deficiency): Adrenal insufficiency occurs under basal conditions and manifests as adrenal crisis in the neonatal period or soon after.

c. Diagnostic features: Signs and symptoms of adrenal insufficiency are not present at birth and rarely occur before 3–4 days of life. Adrenal crisis in untreated patients occurs at 1–2 weeks of life. Diagnosis should be considered in neonates when any of the following are present:

1) Females with virilization of the genitalia.
2) Males with nonpalpable gonads $\pm$ hyperpigmentation of the areolae or genitalia.
3) Any infant exhibiting signs or symptoms of adrenal insufficiency/crisis.
4) Adrenal crisis is marked by lethargy, emesis, poor appetite, dehydration, hypotension, shock, hyperkalemia, hyponatremia, hypoglycemia, seizures resulting from hyponatremia or hypoglycemia, and metabolic acidosis. In classic 21-hydroxylase deficiency, serum levels of 17-hydroxyprogesterone, as well as levels of serum testosterone and urinary 17-ketosteroids, are elevated (most reliable at >3 days of life in term babies).

C. SYNDROME OF INAPPROPRIATE ADH SECRETION (SIADH)

1. Definition: The hallmark of SIADH is hyponatremia with inappropriately concentrated urine in the setting of euvolemia or hypervolemia. It is associated with many conditions, including CNS trauma and CNS infection. Definitive therapy is to identify and to treat the underlying cause.

2. **Management:** Hyponatremia should be corrected slowly with fluid restriction. A reasonable goal is a 10% increase in Na^+ per 24 hours.

3. **Emergency management of complicated hyponatremia:** In the setting of coma or seizures, more rapid Na^+ correction should be undertaken by treating with hypertonic saline. See p. 233 for details.

D. CENTRAL DIABETES INSIPIDUS (VASOPRESSIN DEFICIENCY)

1. **Definition:** The hallmark of diabetes insipidus is an impaired ability to concentrate urine (specific gravity is usually <1.005). Central diabetes insipidus is associated with many CNS insults, including trauma and tumors, and as with SIADH, definitive therapy is to identify and to treat the underlying cause. For further diagnostic information, see water-deprivation test, p. 224, and vasopressin test, p. 225.

2. **Management:** DDAVP (desmopressin acetate) in either nasal spray or oral preparation is used for management of central diabetes insipidus. See p. 686 for dosing of DDAVP. Titrate all DDAVP dosing to urine output, aiming for at least one period of diuresis per day that is sufficient to stimulate thirst. Monitor electrolytes closely.

E. THYROID STORM

1. **Definition:** Defined as a form of hyperthyroidism manifested by acute onset, hyperthermia, tachycardia, and restlessness. Untreated, this may progress to delirium, coma, and death.

2. **Management:** Treat with propylthiouracil (PTU) 5–7mg/kg per day divided Q8hr (adult dose = 100mg Q8hr) or with methimazole 0.4–0.7mg/kg per day divided Q8–Q24hr) (adult dose = 10mg Q8hr). These are agents that inhibit formation of thyroid hormone. Propranolol at 0.5–2mg/kg per day divided Q6–Q8hr (adult dose = 20–40mg Q6hr) is used to suppress signs and symptoms of thyrotoxicosis. Iodide, in a variety of preparations, may also be used for acute hyperthyroid management. Adult doses are 50–500mg daily.

F. HYPOPARATHYROIDISM

1. **Definition:** True hypoparathyroidism results from a decrease in PTH. Patients may also have a PTH resistance (pseudohypoparathyroidism) in which PTH is normal or elevated. Clinical manifestations of hypoparathyroidism range from asymptomatic or mild muscle cramps to hypocalcemic tetany and convulsion.

2. **Laboratory abnormalities:** These include low calcium, elevated phosphorus, normal to low alkaline phosphatase, and low 1,25-hydroxy-vitamin D_3.

3. **Management:** Therapy is calcium supplementation for documented hypocalcemia (see pp. 651–654 for dosing information) and vitamin D supplementation with calcitriol (active vitamin D) at 0.01–0.05mcg/kg per 24 hours PO divided Q12hr. Monitor serum calcium and phosphorus carefully during therapy and never exceed 50mg/min with calcium gluconate infusions.

10

ENDOCRINOLOGY

G. LABORATORY ABNORMALITIES IN COMMON ENDOCRINE DISORDERS (Table 10.1)

TABLE 10.1
LABORATORY ABNORMALITIES IN ENDOCRINE DISEASE

Disorder	Laboratory findings
Diabetes insipidus	Low urine specific gravity (<1.005)
	Low urine osmolarity (50–200)
	Low vasopressin (<0.5pg/mL)
SIADH	Low serum Na^+ and chloride with normal HCO_3^-
	Hypouricemia
	Inappropriately concentrated urine
Hypoparathyroidism	Low serum calcium
	High serum phosphorus
	Normal or low alkaline phosphatase
	Low 1,25-hydroxy-vitamin D_3
	Low PTH (may be normal or elevated in pseudohypoparathyroidism)
Hyperparathyroidism	High serum calcium
	Low serum phosphorus
	Normal or high alkaline phosphatase
	High PTH
Congenital adrenal hyperplasia (classic 21-hydroxylase deficiency [Na^+ losing])	Low serum Na^+ and chloride
	High serum potassium
	High renin
	Low cortisol
	Elevated androgens and cortisol precursors
	Hypoglycemia

II. NORMAL VALUES (Tables 10.2–10.24)

Normal values may differ among laboratories because of variation in technique and in type of radioimmunoassay used. Unless otherwise noted, the values below are reference ranges from the Johns Hopkins Hospital Laboratories or from SmithKline Beecham clinical laboratories in Baltimore, Maryland. *Text continued on p. 219*

TABLE 10.2
GONADOTROPINS

Age	FSH (mIU/mL)	LH (mIU/mL)
Prepubertal children	0.0–2.8	0.0–1.6
Men	1.4–14.4	1–10.2
Women, follicular phase	3.7–12.9	0.9–14

Normal infants have a transient rise in FSH (follicle-stimulating hormone) and LH (luteinizing hormone) to pubertal levels or higher within the first 3 mo, which then declines to prepubertal values by the end of the first year. There is no rise with central gonadotropin deficiency. FSH and LH levels may be elevated in primary hypogonadism and low with pituitary adenomas or McCune–Albright syndrome.

TABLE 10.3

TESTOSTERONE

Age	Testosterone, serum total (ng/dL)	Testosterone, unbound (pg/mL)
Prepubertal children	10–20	0.15–0.6
Men	275–875	52–280
Women	23–75	1.1–6.3
Pregnancy	35–195	

Testosterone may be elevated in male precocious puberty, gonadal and adrenocortical tumors, or congenital adrenal hyperplasia. Low testosterone is associated with primary or secondary hypogonadism syndromes (e.g., Klinefelter syndrome).

TABLE 10.4

DIHYDROTESTOSTERONE (DHT)

Age	Males (ng/dL)	Females (ng/dL)
Prepubertal children	<3–13	<3–10
Tanner 2	5–17	4–12
Tanner 3	7–35	9–21
Tanner 4	12–52	9–23
Tanner 5	13–17	<3–36
Adults	30–100	6–33

TABLE 10.5

ESTRADIOL

Age	pg/ml
Prepubertal children	<25
Men	6–44
Women	
Luteal phase	15–260
Follicular phase	10–200
Midcycle	120–375

Normal infants have an elevated estradiol at birth, which decreases to prepubertal values during the first week of life. Estradiol levels increase again between 1 and 2 mo of age and return to prepubertal values by 6–12 mo of age. Estradiol may be elevated in McCune–Albright syndrome, granulosa cell tumors, or follicular cysts, and may be low in primary or secondary hypogonadism syndromes (e.g., Turner syndrome).

TABLE 10.6
ANDROSTENEDIONE, SERUM

Age	Male (ng/dL)	Female (ng/dL)
Preterm infants		
26–28wk to dy4 of life	92–892	92–892
31–35wk to dy4 of life	80–446	80–446
Full-term infants		
1–7dy	20–290	20–290
1–12mo	6–68	6–68
Prepubertal children	8–50	8–50
Tanner 2	31–65	42–100
Tanner 3	50–100	80–190
Tanner 4	48–140	77–225
Tanner 5	65–210	80–240
Adults	78–205	85–275

Androstenedione is increased in most forms of congenital adrenal hyperplasia.

TABLE 10.7
DEHYDROEPIANDROSTERONE (DHEA)

Age	HEA (ng/D/mL)	DHEA sulfate (mcg/dL)
Newborn infants	—	1.7–3.6
Prepubertal children	0–100	0.1–0.6
Men	195–915	1.4–7.9 (to age 30)
Women	215–855	0.7–4.5 (to age 30)

These compounds may be increased in congenital adrenal hyperplasia, adrenocortical tumors, and premature adrenarche.

TABLE 10.8
17-HYDROXYPROGESTERONE, SERUM

Age	Males (ng/dL)	Females (ng/dL)
Prepubertal	0–81	0–92
Adult	36–154	15–102 (follicular)
		150–386 (luteal)

17-Hydroxyprogesterone may be increased in most forms of congenital adrenal hyperplasia. Levels are also normally increased in newborns for the first few days of life. Finally, be aware that infant serum contains substances that may cross-react in the assay for 17-hydroxyprogesterone and artificially elevate the level, unless they are separated by chromatography. Before interpreting results on infants, be sure that your laboratory has prepared their samples appropriately.

TABLE 10.9

CORTISOL, SERUM WITH ACTH STIMULATION TEST

Condition	mcg/dL
Any sex/any age/pre-ACTH, 8am	5.7–16.6
1 hour post-ACTH	16–36

See p. 223, for interpretation of this test.

TABLE 10.10

CORTISOL, URINE

Age	mcg/g creatinine	mcg/24hr
Prepubertal children	7–25	3–9
Men	7–45	11–84
Women	9–32	10–34

TABLE 10.11

17-KETOSTEROIDS, URINE

Age	mg/24hr
<1 month	<2.0
1 month–5yr	<0.5
6–8yr	1.0–2.0
Men	9–22
Women	5–15

17-Ketosteroids are increased in congenital adrenal hyperplasia, adrenocortical tumors, and Cushing syndrome. Levels may be decreased in Addison's disease and hypopituitary states. Fractionated 17-ketosteroids are also now available in some laboratories.

TABLE 10.12

17-HYDROXYCORTICOSTEROIDS, URINE

Children (body weight variable)	$3 \pm 1 mg/m^2$ per 24hr
Men	3–9mg/24hr
Women	2–8mg/24hr

17-Hydroxycorticosteroids are decreased in hypopituitary states, Addison's disease, hypothyroidism and 21-hydroxylase–deficient congenital adrenal hyperplasia. Levels are elevated in Cushing syndrome, hyperthyroidism, 11-hydroxylase–deficient congenital adrenal hyperplasia, and stress.

10

ENDOCRINOLOGY

TABLE 10.13

CATECHOLAMINES, URINE

Compound	Amount/24hr urine collection
Dopamine	100–440mcg
Epinephrine	<15mcg
Norepinephrine	15–86mcg
Metanephrines	<0.4mg
Normetanephrines	<0.9mg
Homovanillic acid (HVA)	0–10mg
Vanillyl mandelic acid (VMA)	2–10mg

Catecholamines are elevated in a variety of tumors including neuroblastoma, ganglioneuroma, ganglioblastoma, and pheochromocytoma.

TABLE 10.14

CATECHOLAMINES, SERUM

Compound	Supine (mcg)	Sitting (mcg)
Dopamine	<87	<87
Epinephrine	<50	<60
Norepinephrine	110–410	120–680

TABLE 10.15

DIABETES-RELATED VALUES (INSULIN, C-PEPTIDE, AND HEMOGLOBIN A_{1c})

Compound	Value
Insulin (fasting)	1.8–24.6mcU/mL
C-peptide (fasting)	0.8–4.0ng/mL
Hemoglobin A_{1c}	4.5–6.1%

TABLE 10.16

INSULIN-LIKE GROWTH FACTOR 1 (IGF-1)

Age	Males (units)	Females (units)
2mo–6yr	17–248	17–248
6–9yr	88–474	88–474
9–12yr	110–565	117–771
12–16yr	202–957	261–1096
16–26yr	182–780	182–780
>26yr	123–463	123–463

Values may be decreased in growth hormone deficiency.

TABLE 10.17

INSULIN–LIKE GROWTH FACTOR–BINDING PROTEIN (IGF-BP3)

Age (years)	Males (mg/L)	Females (mg/L)
0–2	0.94–1.76	0.66–2.51
2–4	1.12–2.33	0.84–3.77
4–6	1.16–3.13	1.32–3.60
6–8	1.32–3.38	1.21–4.66
8–10	1.35–3.94	1.58–3.99
10–12	1.53–5.02	1.93–6.46
12–14	1.73–5.11	1.78–6.08
14–16	1.90–6.40	2.02–5.44
16–18	1.70–6.04	1.88–5.29
18–20	1.52–6.01	1.63–6.02
20–22	1.79–5.41	1.82–5.35
Adult (continues to vary with age)	1.15–5.18	1.19–5.69

Values may be decreased in growth hormone deficiency.

TABLE 10.18

PTH

Protein	pg/mL
Intact PTH	<10–65 (with normal calcium)
C-terminal	50–340
N-terminal	4–19

TABLE 10.19

CALCITONIN

Age	Males (pg/mL)	Females (pg/mL)
Newborns	70–348	70–348
Children	<13.8	<6.4
Adults	<40	<20

From Endocrine Sciences Laboratory, Calabasas Hills, CA.

TABLE 10.20

VITAMIN D

Compound	Value
25-Hydroxy-vitamin D	ng/mL
Newborns	8–21
Children	17–54
Adults	10–55
1,25-Dihydroxy-vitamin D	pg/ml
Newborns	8–72
Children	15–90
Adults	24–64

Note that 1,25-dihydroxy-vitamin D is the physiologically active form; however, 25-hydroxyvitamin D is the value to monitor for vitamin D deficiency, since this approximates body stores of vitamin D.

TABLE 10.21

ROUTINE STUDIES (THYROID)

Test	Age	Normal	Comments
T_4 RIA	Cord	6.6–17.5	Measures total T_4 by
(mcg/dl)	1–3dy	11.0–21.5	radioimmunoassay.
	1–4wk	8.2–16.6	
	1–12mo	7.2–15.6	
	1–5yr	7.3–15.0	
	6–10yr	6.4–13.3	
	11–15yr	5.6–11.7	
	16–20yr	4.2–11.8	
	21–50yr	4.3–12.5	
T_3 RU (%)	—	25–35	Measures thyroid hormone binding, not T_3.
T index	—	1.25–4.20	T_4 RIA $\times$ T_3 RU.
Free T_4	1–10dy	0.6–2.0	Metabolically active form. The normal
(ng/dL)	>10dy	0.7–1.7	range for free T_4 is very assay dependent.
T_3 RIA	Cord	14–86	Measures T_3 by RIA.
(ng/dL)	1–3dy	100–380	
	1–4wk	99–310	
	1–12mo	102–264	
	1–5yr	105–269	
	6–10yr	94–241	
	11–15yr	83–213	
	16–20yr	80–210	
	21–50yr	70–204	
TSH	Cord	<2.5–17.4	TSH surge peaks from 80–90mIU/mL
(mIU/ml)	1–3dy	<2.5–13.3	in term newborn by 30min after
	1–4wk	0.6–10.0	birth. Values after 1wk
	1–12mo	0.6–6.3	are within adult normal range.
	1–15yr	0.6–6.3	Elevated values suggest primary
			hypothyroidism, whereas suppressed
	16–50yr	0.2–7.6	values are the best indicator of hyperthyroidism.
TBG	Cord	0.7–4.7	
(mg/dL)	1–3dy	–	
	1–4wk	0.5–4.5	
	1–12mo	1.6–3.6	
	1–5yr	1.3–2.8	
	6–20yr	1.4–2.6	
	21–50yr	1.2–2.4	
Reverse T_3	Newborns	90–250	Reach adult range by 1 wk.
(ng/dL)	Children	10–50	
	Adults	10–50	

From Fisher[1]; and LaFranchi[2].

RIA, radioimmunoassay; RU, resin uptake; T_3, triiodothyronine; T_4, thyroxine; TBG, thyroxine-binding globulin; TSH, thyroid-stimulating hormone.

TABLE 10.22

THYROID ANTIBODIES

Interpretation	Antithyroglobulin	Antimicrosomal
Insignificant	≤1:40	<1:400
Borderline	1:80	1:400
Significant	1:160–1:640	1:1600–1:6400
Very significant	>1:640	>1:6400

TABLE 10.23

SERUM T₄ (mcg/dL) IN PRETERM AND TERM INFANTS

	Estimated gestational age (wk)				
Age	30–31	32–33	34–35	36–37	Term
Cord	4.5–8.5	3.3–11.7	4.3–9.1	1.9–13.1	4.6–11.8
12–72hr	7.3–15.7	5.9–18.7	6.2–18.6	10.3–20.7	14.8–23.2
3–10dy	4.1–11.3	4.7–12.3	5.2–14.8	7.7–17.7	9.9–21.9
11–20dy	3.9–11.1	5.1–11.5	6.9–14.1	5.4–17.0	8.2–16.2
21–45dy	4.8–10.8	4.6–11.4	6.7–11.9	3.0–19.8	9.1–15.1
46–90dy	6.2–13.0	6.2–13.0	6.2–13.0	6.2–13.0	6.4–14.0

From Cuestas[3].

TABLE 10.24

FREE T₄ (ng/dL) IN PRETERM AND TERM INFANTS

GA (wk)	29–30	31–32	33–34	35–36	37–38
Free T₄ (ng/dL)	0.3–1.2	0.2–1.6	0.5–1.4	0.5–1.7	0.6–1.9

From Travert[4].
GA, estimated gestational age (wk). Normal range for free thyroxine (T_4) is very assay dependent.

10

ENDOCRINOLOGY

III. TESTS AND PROCEDURES

A. SEXUAL DEVELOPMENT

1. **Karyotype:** The purpose is to determine the chromosomal sex in patients with ambiguous genitalia. Y-chromosome–specific markers are available.

2. **Vaginal smear[5]**

a. Purpose: To test for estrogenization of vaginal mucosa; useful in evaluating precocious puberty.

b. Method: Make a wet mount of internal vaginal secretions with NS. Methylene blue may be used to stain nuclei, but an unstained preparation can also be read. To make a permanent slide for cytopathology, place in 95% ethanol fixative.

c. Interpretation:

1) Low-estrogen states: Predominance of round or oval parabasal cells with thick cytoplasm and vesicular nuclei displaying chromatin detail.

2) High-estrogen states: Predominance of polygonal squamous (superficial) cells with small pyknotic nuclei and thin cytoplasm.

3) Intermediate cells with squame-like cytoplasm and nuclei with a reticular chromatin pattern may be variably present, but will predominate in high-cortisol or high-progestin states (e.g., the second half of the menstrual cycle).

3. **Dexamethasone suppression test (DST)[6]** (see p. 224 for further methodologic details)

a. Purpose: To evaluate premature adrenarche or precocious puberty.

b. Interpretation: Incomplete suppression of 17-ketosteroids suggests that the patient has entered puberty. Markedly increased, nonsuppressible 17-ketosteroids suggest the presence of an androgen-producing tumor, most likely adrenal in origin. Congenital adrenal hyperplasia is characterized by extremely high levels of 17-ketosteroid that are suppressible. (For normal 17-ketosteroid values see Table 10.11.)

4. **Gonadotropin-releasing hormone (GnRH or LHRH) stimulation test[7]**

a. Purpose: Measures pituitary luteinizing hormone (LH) and follicle-stimulating hormone (FSH) reserve. Helpful in the differential diagnosis of precocious or delayed sexual development.

b. Interpretation: Normal prepubertal children should show no or minimal increase in LH and FSH to an GnRH injection. An exaggerated response of a rise of LH into the adult range is obtained in central precocious puberty and in primary gonadal failure (e.g., Turner syndrome). (For normal gonadotropin values see Table 10.2.)

5. **Human chorionic gonadotropin (HCG) stimulation test:** Used to differentiate cryptorchidism (undescended testes) from anorchia (absent testes). In cryptorchidism after IM HCG, testosterone rises to adult levels; in anorchia there is no rise.

B. **GROWTH**

1. **Height prediction**

a. Genetic potential formula, using mean parental stature:

1) Boys: (Paternal height + Maternal height + 5 inches)/2.

2) Girls: (Paternal height + Maternal height − 5 inches)/2.

Target height is midparental height ± 2SD, with 1SD being about 2 inches.

b. Growth curves: Available for those who mature early, normal, and late. Predict height percentile by plotting patient's height and extrapolating to adult height at the same percentile.

2. **Growth hormone (GH) detection:** Tests for GH deficiency include several screening tests as well as a more definitive pharmacologic stimulation test. Patients failing screening tests should proceed to stimulation test (a patient must have two abnormal stimulation tests to make the diagnosis of classic GH deficiency). Measurement of insulin-like growth factor I (IGF-I) and IGF-binding protein 3 (IGFBP-3)

(proteins involved in GH action) may also be helpful in diagnosing GH deficiency, especially in partial deficiency states.

a. Screening tests for GH[8]

1) Sleep specimen: Draw GH samples 30 and 60 minutes after onset of sleep. Most subjects will have a rise in GH 45–60 minutes after the onset of nocturnal sleep.

2) Exercise test: After fasting the patient for at least 4 hours, get baseline GH level. Obtain a GH sample immediately after exercising (e.g., steady jogging for 20 minutes); most people will release significant amounts of GH after vigorous exercise.

b. Stimulation tests[8]: GH secretion may be stimulated by arginine, insulin-induced hypoglycemia, L-dopa, glucagon, and clonidine. A GH level >10ng/mL effectively rules out GH deficiency. (Note that some laboratories use 7ng/mL as the cut-off for normal vs abnormal.) Values between 7 and 10ng/mL are equivocal. This may indicate partial deficiency and requires further evaluation. Results <7ng/mL are definitely abnormal.

c. Ancillary tests:

1) IGF-I (somatomedin-C): May be drawn at any time during the day. May be useful in detecting patients with quantitative or qualitative deficiencies in GH not picked up by standard stimulation tests. A clearly normal IGF-I level argues against GH deficiency, although in young children there is considerable overlap between normals and those with GH deficiency. (For normal values see Table 10.16.)

2) IGFBP-3: May be drawn at any time during the day. Levels below the 5th percentile suggest a GH deficiency. This test may have greater discrimination than the IGF-I test in younger patients. (For normal values see Table 10.17.)

C. **ADRENAL AND PITUITARY FUNCTION** (see Fig. 10.2 **for steroid hormone pathway**)

1. **Urinary 17-hydroxycorticosteroids (17-OHCSs)** (for normal values see Table 10.12)

a. Measures approximately a third of the endproducts of cortisol metabolism.

b. Method: Collect a 24-hour urine specimen. Refrigerate during collection and process immediately (17-OHCSs are destroyed at room temperature).

c. Interpretation

1) Decreased in inanition states (anorexia nervosa); pituitary disorders involving ACTH; Addison's disease; administration of synthetic, potent corticosteroids (prednisone, dexamethasone, triamcinolone); 21-hydroxylase deficiency; liver disease; hypothyroidism; and newborn period (as a result of decreased glucuronidation).

10

ENDOCRINOLOGY

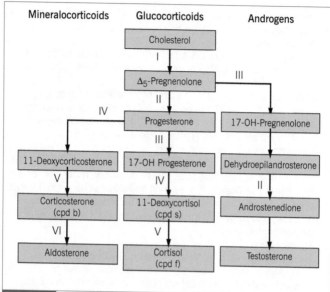

FIG. 10.2

Steroid hormone pathway and the enzymatic deficiencies in congenital adrenal hyperplasia. Enzyme deficiency: I, cholesterol (20, 22) desmolase; II, 3-B-hydroxysteroid dehydrogenase; III, 17-hydroxylase; IV, 21-hydroxylase; V, 11-hydroxylase; VI, 18- 'oxidation' defect; Cpd, compound. (From Bacon[9].)

2) Increased in Cushing syndrome; ACTH, cortisone, or cortisol therapy; medical or surgical stress; obesity (occasionally); hyperthyroidism; and 11-hydroxylase deficiency.

3) Urinary free cortisol (see Table 10.10) can also be measured, eliminating some of the nonspecificity of 17-OHCS measurement. Interpretation is similar to that for 17-OHCSs.

2. **Urinary 17-ketosteroids** (for normal values see Table 10.11)

a. Measures some endproducts of androgen metabolism.

b. Method: Collect and refrigerate 24-hour urine specimen.

c. Interpretation

1) Increased in adrenal hyperplasia (in congenital adrenal hyperplasia it may take 1–2 weeks for 17-ketosteroids to rise above the normally high newborn levels). Also increased in virilizing adrenal tumors; Cushing syndrome; exogenous ACTH, cortisone, or androgen administration (except methyltestosterone); stressful illness (burns, radiation illness, etc.); and androgen-producing gonadal tumors.

2) Decreased in Addison's disease, anorexia nervosa, and panhypopituitarism.

3. **Plasma corticosteroids** (for normal values, see Table 10.9)

a. Method: Collect heparinized blood and separate plasma immediately. Measure cortisol (corticosterone and 11-deoxycortisol may sometimes be needed). Because of the diurnal variation in cortisol concentration, 8am (the time of peak cortisol level) is the best time to draw plasma cortisol level.

b. Interpretation: Same as for 17-OHCS (see p. 221), except usually normal in anorexia nervosa, liver disease, hypothyroidism, hyperthyroidism, and obesity. Elevated levels by protein binding assay occur during pregnancy and estrogen administration.

4. **Plasma 17-hydroxyprogesterone** (for normal values see Table 10.8)

a. Method: Collect heparinized blood and separate plasma immediately.

b. Interpretation: Measures cortisol precursor, which is elevated with 21- and 11-hydroxylase deficiency forms of CAH.

5. **Adrenal capacity test (ACTH stimulation test)[10]**

a. Purpose: Used to evaluate adrenal insufficiency: Primary (Addison's disease), secondary (ACTH deficiency), or from adrenal suppression after long-term steroid treatment.

b. Interpretation: With a normal pituitary–adrenal axis, there is a rise in serum cortisol after IV ACTH (Table 10.9). With ACTH deficiency or prolonged adrenal suppression, there is no rise in cortisol after a single IV dose because this does not produce adrenal reactivation. After 3 days of IM ACTH, however, there will be adrenal reactivation with a rise in urinary 17-OHCSs. A lack of response to the IM ACTH stimulation is pathognomonic of Addison's disease. A subnormal response may be seen with adrenal hyperplasia.

6. **Pituitary ACTH capacity (metyrapone) test[10]:** Metyrapone inhibits 11-hydroxylase in the adrenal and blocks cortisol production. This causes a rise in ACTH, which increases production of cortisol precursors; these accumulate (the measured precursor is 17-deoxycortisol) and are excreted as 17-OHCSs. A failure of 17-deoxycortisol and 17-OHCSs to rise occurs with pituitary ACTH deficiency, hypothalamic tumors, and pharmacologic doses of steroids. An exaggerated response after metyrapone occurs in pituitary-dependent Cushing syndrome, hypothyroidism, and diabetes mellitus.

Warning: Test can precipitate adrenal crisis.

7. **Insulin-induced hypoglycemia:** With insulin-induced (or spontaneous) hypoglycemia, plasma cortisol normally rises by >10mcg/dL or to a level of >20mcg/dL.

8. **Dexamethasone suppression test (DST)[10]**

a. Dexamethasone suppresses secretion of ACTH by the normal pituitary, decreasing endogenous production of cortisol and, hence, the excretion of 17-OHCSs. Dexamethasone is not excreted as 17-OHCSs.

10

ENDOCRINOLOGY

b. Indication: Useful in determining the etiology of glucocorticoid or adrenal androgen overproduction.

c. Standard low-dose and high-dose DST

1) Method: Give dexamethasone PO for 3 days (low dose: $1.25mg/m^2$ per day; high dose: $3.75mg/m^2$ per day divided Q6hr) and collect 24-hour urine for 17-OHCSs. (If using DST to evaluate premature adrenarche, also measure urinary 17-ketosteroids and pregnanetriol.)

2) Interpretation: Normally, and in obesity, low-dose DST causes 17-OHCSs to fall to $<1mg/m^2$ per day. In Cushing syndrome secondary to adrenal hyperplasia, 17-OHCS levels are not suppressed by the low-dose DST, but fall with the high-dose DST, unless the hyperplasia is the result of ectopic ACTH production (lung, mediastinal tumor, etc.). With Cushing syndrome caused by adrenocortical carcinoma, and with some hypothalamic tumors, 17-OHCS levels are not suppressed even with the high-dose DST.

d. Overnight screening DST: Give 1mg dexamethasone at 11pm. At 8 or 9am the following day, draw a fasting serum cortisol level. In normal or obese patients, the serum cortisol should fall below 5mcg/dL.

9. **Water deprivation test[9]**

a. Used to diagnose diabetes insipidus. Requires careful supervision because dehydration and hypernatremia may occur.

b. Method: Begin the test in the morning after a 24-hour period of adequate hydration and stable weight. Have the patient empty his or her bladder and obtain a baseline weight. Restrict fluids for 7 hours. Measure body weight and urinary specific gravity and volume hourly. Check serum Na^+ and urine and serum osmolality every 2 hours. Hematocrit and blood urea nitrogen (BUN) may also be obtained at these times but are not critical. Monitor carefully to ensure that fluids are not ingested during the test. Terminate the test if weight loss approaches 5%.

c. Interpretation

1) Normal individuals who are water deprived will concentrate their urine between 500 and 1400mOsmol/L and plasma osmolality will range between 288 and 291mOsmol/L. In normal children and those with psychogenic diabetes insipidus, urinary specific gravity rises to at least 1.010 and usually more. The urinary:plasma osmolality ratio is >2. Urine volume decreases significantly, and there should be no appreciable weight loss.

2) In patients with ADH-deficient or nephrogenic diabetes insipidus, specific gravity remains <1.005. Urine osmolality remains <150mOsmol/L with no significant reduction of urine volume. A weight loss of up to 5% usually occurs. At the end of the test, a serum osmolality >290mOsmol/L, Na^+ >150mEq/L, and a rise of BUN and hematocrit provide evidence that the patient did not receive water.

10. Vasopressin test[9]

a. To test for nephrogenic vs ADH-deficient (central) diabetes insipidus, vasopressin is given SC, preferably at the end of the water deprivation test. Urine output, urine concentration, and water intake are monitored. Intranasal vasopressin is not recommended for this test.

b. Interpretation: Patients with ADH-deficient diabetes insipidus concentrate their urine (≥ 1.010) and demonstrate a reduction of urine volume and decreased fluid intake. Patients with nephrogenic diabetes insipidus have no significant change in intake, urine volume, or specific gravity. Constant intake associated with decreased output and increased specific gravity suggests psychogenic diabetes insipidus.

D. THYROID FUNCTION[11]

1. **Thyroid function tests:** TSH is most diagnostic for hyperthyroidism. T_4 and TSH are most informative for hypothyroidism depending on the etiology. For interpretation see Table 10.25 (see also Table 10.21 for information about specific tests and test definitions).

2. **Thyroid scan:** Used to assess thyroid clearance, to localize ectopic thyroid tissue, and to study structure and function of the thyroid. Localizes hyperfunctioning and nonfunctioning thyroid nodules. Uptake is increased in most types of dyshormonogeneses.

3. **Technetium uptake:** Measures uptake of technetium by thyroid gland during the first 20 minutes after administration. Normal: 0.24–3.4%. Increased in hyperthyroidism. Decreased in TBG (thyroxine-binding globulin) deficiency and in hypothyroidism (except dyshormonogenesis, when it may be increased).

4. **Pituitary thyroid-stimulating hormone (TSH) reserve test:** Synthetic thyroid-releasing hormone (TRH) can be given IV, which will normally cause a rise in TSH. No rise in TSH and a high T_4 (thyroxine) confirm hyperthyroidism. A low TSH that does not increase after TRH and a low T_4 suggest pituitary dysfunction. An exaggerated delayed peak in TSH response is suggestive of hypothalamic hypothyroidism, but the distinction from normal is not always clear.

10 ENDOCRINOLOGY

TABLE 10.25
THYROID FUNCTION TESTS: INTERPRETATION

	T_4 RIA	T_3 RU	T index	Free T_4	TSH
Primary hypothyroidism	L	L	L	L	H
Secondary hypothyroidism	L	L	L	L	N, L, or H
TBG deficiency	L	H	N	N	N
Hyperthyroidism	H	H	H	H	L

H, high; L, low; N, normal; RIA, radioimmunoassay; RU, resin uptake; T_3, triiodothyronine; T_4, thyroxine; TBG, thyroxine-binding globulin; TSH, thyroid-stimulating hormone.

E. PANCREATIC ENDOCRINE FUNCTION

1. **Diabetes diagnostic criteria:** Under the American Diabetes Association's new guidelines, there are three separate criteria on which the diagnosis of diabetes mellitus can be made:
   a. Symptoms of diabetes (polyuria, polydipsia, and weight loss) and a random blood glucose of >200mg/dL.
   b. Fasting blood glucose (no caloric intake for at least 8 hours) of >126mg/dL.
   c. Oral glucose tolerance test with a 2-hour post-load blood glucose of >200mg/dL.

   One of these criteria must be met on 2 separate days for definitive diagnosis.

2. **Oral glucose tolerance test (OGTT)**
   a. Pretest preparation: Calorically adequate diet required for 3 days before the test, with 50% of total calories as carbohydrate.
   b. Delay test 2 weeks after period of illness. Discontinue all hyperglycemic and hypoglycemic agents (salicylates, diuretics, oral contraceptives, phenytoin, etc.).
   c. Method: Give 1.75g/kg (max. 100g) of glucose orally after a 12-hour fast, allowing up to 5 minutes for ingestion. Mix glucose with water and lemon juice as a 20% dilution. Quiet activity is permissible during the OGTT. Draw blood samples at 0, 30, 60, 120, 180, and 240 minutes.
   d. Interpretation: 2-hour post-oral load blood glucose value of <140mg/dL is normal. A value of 140–199mg/dL suggests impaired glucose tolerance; ≥200mg/dL is diagnostic of diabetes mellitus.

IV. SEXUAL DEVELOPMENT

A. **PENILE LENGTH:** Measured from pubic ramus to tip of glans while traction is applied along length of phallus to point of increased resistance. Penile length >2.5SD below mean is considered abnormal (Table 10.26)[12-14].

B. **TESTICULAR SIZE:** Testicular growth is the earliest sign of puberty. Testicular volume of >4mL or a long axis >2.5cm is evidence that pubertal testicular growth has begun (Table 10.27)[14].

C. **CLITORIS**
1. **Anogenital ratio:** Distance between anus and posterior fourchette divided by distance between anus and base of clitoris. It is independent of body size and gestational age. Ratio >0.5 suggests virilization with labioscrotal fusion[15].
2. **Length:** Newborn (mean ± SD) = 4.3 ± 1.1mm.
3. **Preterm infants:** Clitoris is normally more prominent because clitoral size is fully developed by 27 weeks' gestation and there is less fat in labia majora.

D. **SECONDARY SEX CHARACTERISTICS:** See p. 98–102, for discussion and diagnosis of Tanner stages.

TABLE 10.26

MEAN STRETCHED PENILE LENGTH (cm)

Age	Mean ± SD	−2.5SD
Birth		
30wk gestation	2.7±0.5	1.5
34wk gestation	3.0±0.4	2.0
Full term	3.5±0.4	2.5
0–5mo	3.8±0.8	1.8
6–12mo	4.1±0.8	2.1
1–2yr	4.6±0.8	2.6
2–3yr	5.0±0.8	3.0
3–4yr	5.4±1.0	2.9
4–5yr	5.6±0.7	3.4
5–7yr	6.0±0.9	3.8
7–9yr	6.3±1.0	3.8
9–11yr	6.3±1.0	3.8
11–14yr	6.3±2.0	5.0
14–16yr	8.6±2.4	6.0
16–18yr	9.9±1.7	4.3
18–20yr	11.0±1.1	2.8
Adult	12.4±1.6	4.0

SD, standard deviation.

10

ENDOCRINOLOGY

TABLE 10.27

TESTICULAR SIZE

Age (yr)	Length (cm) (mean±SD)	Corresponding volume (mL) (approximate)	Tanner stage (genital)
<2	1.4±0.4		
2–4	1.2±0.4		
4–6	1.5±0.6	1	
6–8	1.8±0.3		
8–10	2.0±0.5	2	1
10–12	2.7±0.7	5	2
12–14	3.4±0.8	10	3
14–16	4.1±1.0	20	4
16–18	5.0±0.5	29	5
18–20	5.0±0.3	29	

SD, standard deviation.

V. REFERENCES

1. Fisher DA. The thyroid. In: Rudolf AM, ed. *Pediatrics*. Norwalk, CT: Appleton & Lange; 1991.

2. LaFranchi SH. Hyperthyroidism. *Pediatr Clin North Am* 1979; **26(1)**:33–51.

3. Cuestas RA. Thyroid function in healthy premature infants. *J Pediatr* 1978; **92(6)**:963–967.

4. Travert G, Lemonnier F, Fernandez Y. Free thyroxin measured in dried blood spots: results for 10,000 euthyroid and 29 hypothyroid newborns. *Clin Chem* 1985; **31**:1830–1833.

5. Gold JJ, Josimovich JB. *Gynecological endocrinology*, 4th edn. New York: Plenum Medical Book Co.; 1987.

6. Rosenfield R, Watson A. Adrenocortical disorders in infancy and childhood. In: Becker G, ed. *Principles and practice of endocrinology and metabolism*. Philadelphia: JB Lippincott; 1995.

7. Rosen D, Kelch RP. Precocious and delayed puberty. In: Becker G, ed. *Principles and practice of endocrinology and metabolism*. Philadelphia: JB Lippincott; 1995.

8. Plotnik L. Growth, growth hormone, and pituitary disorders. In: Oski F, ed. *Principles and practice of endocrinology and metabolism*. Philadelphia: JB Lippincott; 1994.

9. Bacon GE et al. *A practical approach to pediatric endocrinology*, 3rd edn. Chicago: Year Book Medical Publishers; 1990.

10. Migeon CJ. Adrenal cortex. In: Rudolf AM, ed. *Pediatrics*. Norwalk, CT: Appleton & Lange; 1987.

11. Lee WP. Disorders of the thyroid – Part 1: Thyroid physiology and thyroid function tests. In: Kaplan SA, ed. *Clinical pediatric and adolescent endocrinology*. Philadelphia: WB Saunders; 1982.

12. Winter J, Faiman C. Pituitary–gonadal relations in male children and adolescents. *Pediatr Res* 1972; **6**:126–135.

13. Feldman KW, Smith DW. Fetal phallic growth and penile standards for newborn male infants. *J Pediatr* 1975; **86**:395.

14. Lee PA, O'Dea L. Testes and variants of male sexual development. In: Hung W, ed. *Clinical pediatric endocrinology*. St Louis, Mosby; 1992.

15. Callegari C. Anogenital ratio: measure of fetal virilization in premature and full-term newborns. *J Pediatr* 1987; **111**:240.

FLUIDS AND ELECTROLYTES

Mary K. Choukair, MD

I. MAINTENANCE REQUIREMENTS

A. **CALORIC EXPENDITURE METHOD:** This method is based on the understanding that water and electrolyte requirements parallel caloric expenditure but not body weight. It is effective for all ages, shapes, and clinical states.

1. Determine the child's standard basal caloric (SBC) expenditure as approximated by resting energy expenditure (REE) (see Table 23.4 on p. 484).

2. Adjust caloric expenditure needs by various factors (e.g., fever, activity) as described on, p. 483.

3. For each 100 calories metabolized in 24 hours, the average patient will need 100–120mL H_2O, 2–4mEq Na^+, and 2–3mEq K^+, as derived from Table 11.1.

B. **HOLLIDAY–SEGAR METHOD:** This is a quick, simple formula that estimates caloric expenditure from weight alone; it assumes that for each 100 calories metabolized, 100mL H_2O will be required. This method is not suitable for neonates <14 days old; generally, it overestimates fluid needs in neonates compared with the caloric expenditure method (Table 11.2).

C. **BODY SURFACE AREA METHOD** (Table 11.3)**:** This method is based on the assumption that caloric expenditure is proportional to surface

11

TABLE 11.1

AVERAGE WATER AND ELECTROLYTE REQUIREMENTS PER 100 CALORIES PER 24 HOURS

Clinical state	H_2O (cc)	Na^+ (mEq)	K^+ (mEq)
Average patient receiving parenteral fluids[a]	100–120	2–4	2–3
Anuria	45	0	0
Acute CNS infections and inflammation	80–90	2–4	2–3
Diabetes insipidus	Up to 400	Var	Var
Hyperventilation	120–210	2–4	2–3
Heat stress	120–240	Var	Var
High-humidity environment	80–100	2–4	2–3

Var, Variable requirement.
[a]Adequate maintenance solution: Dextrose 5–10% (as needed) in 0.2% NaCl + 20mEq/L KCl.

TABLE 11.2

HOLLIDAY–SEGAR METHOD

Body weight	Water		Electrolytes (mEq/100mL H₂O)
	mL/kg per day	mL/kg per hr	
First 10kg	100	÷ 24 hr/day ≈4	Na⁺ 3
Second 10kg	50	÷ 24 hr/day ≈2	Cl⁻ 2
Each additional kg	20	÷ 24 hr/day ≈1	K⁺ 2

EXAMPLE: 8-YEAR-OLD WEIGHING 25kg

mL/kg per day	mL/kg per hr
100 (for 1st 10kg) × 10kg = 1000mL/day	4 (for 1st 10kg) × 10kg = 40mL/hr
50 (for 2nd 10kg) × 10kg = 500mL/day	2 (for 2nd 10kg) × 10kg = 20mL/hr
20 (per add'l kg) × 5kg = 100mL/day	1 (per add'l kg) × 5kg = 5mL/hr
25kg 1600mL/day	25kg 65mL/hr

TABLE 11.3

STANDARD VALUES FOR USE IN BODY SURFACE AREA METHOD

H₂O	1500mL/m² per 24hr
Na⁺	30–50mEq/m² per 24hr
K⁺	20–40mEq/m² per 24hr

From Finberg[1], Behrman[2], and Hellerstein[3].

area. It should not be used for children <10 kg. It provides no convenient method of taking into account changes in metabolic rate. See p. 295 for body surface area nomogram and conversion formula.

II. DEFICIT THERAPY

The most precise method of assessing fluid deficit is based on preillness weight, calculated as follows:

Fluid deficit (L) = Preillness weight (kg) − Illness weight (kg)

$$\% \text{ Dehydration} = \frac{\text{Preillness weight} - \text{Illness weight}}{\text{Preillness weight}} \times 100\%$$

If this is not available, then clinical observation may be used, as described below.

A. CLINICAL ASSESSMENT

1. **Clinical observations** (Table 11.4)
a. Hypotonic (hyponatremic) dehydration
   1) Serum Na⁺ <130mEq/L.
   2) Implies excess Na⁺ loss
b. Isotonic (isonatremic) dehydration: Serum Na⁺ 130–150mEq/L.
c. Hypertonic (hypernatremic) dehydration
   1) Serum Na⁺ >150mEq/L.
   2) Implies free water (FW) loss.

TABLE 11.4

CLINICAL OBSERVATIONS IN DEHYDRATION[a]

Examination	Older child: 3% (30mL/kg) Infant: 5% (50mL/kg)	6% (60mL/kg) 10% (100mL/kg)	9% (90mL/kg) 15% (150mL/kg)
Dehydration	Mild	Moderate	Severe
Skin turgor	Normal	Tenting	None
Skin—touch	Normal	Dry	Clammy
Buccal mucosa/lips	Moist	Dry	Parched/cracked
Eyes	Normal	Deep set	Sunken
Crying/tears	Present	Reduced	None
Fontanelle	Flat	Soft	Sunken
CNS	Consolable	Irritable	Lethargic/obtunded
Pulse	Regular	Slightly increased	Increased
Urine output	Normal	Decreased	Anuric

From Oski[4].

[a]For the same clinical observations, fluid deficit is greater in hypernatremic dehydration and smaller in hyponatremic dehydration.

3) The skin may appear thick and doughy with normal turgor, and children with such skin may be excessively irritable on examination.

B. GENERAL GUIDELINES FOR DEFICIT CALCULATION

1. Intracellular fluid (ICF) and extracellular fluid (ECF) compartments

a. Estimate of percent dehydration from extracellular and intracellular compartments related to duration of illness (Table 11.5).

b. Normal ICF and ECF composition (Table 11.6).

TABLE 11.5

PERCENT DEHYDRATION FROM EXTRACELLULAR AND INTRACELLULAR COMPARTMENTS

Duration of illness	% fluid of fluid deficit from ECF	% fluid of fluid deficit from ICF
<3 days	80	20
>3 days	60	40

TABLE 11.6

INTRACELLULAR AND EXTRACELLULAR FLUID COMPOSITION

	Intracellular (mEq/L)	Extracellular (mEq/L)
Na^+	20	135–145
K^+	150	3–5
Cl^-	—	98–110
HCO_3^-	10	20–25
PO_4^{3-}	110–115	5
Protein	75	10

11

FLUIDS AND ELECTROLYTES

c. Electrolyte deficit (from ECF and ICF losses)
   1) Na^+ deficit is the amount of Na^+ that was lost from the Na^+-containing extracellular fluid (ECF) compartment during the dehydration period, such that:
   Na^+ deficit (mEq) =

Fluid deficit (L) × Percent from ECF × Na^+ concentration (mEq/L) in ECF
   Intracellular Na^+ is negligible as a proportion of total; therefore it can be disregarded.
   2) K^+ deficit is the amount of K^+ that was lost from the K^+-containing intracellular fluid (ICF) compartment during the dehydration period, such that:
   K^+ deficit (mEq) =

Fluid deficit (L) × Percent from ICF × K^+ concentration (mEq/L) in ICF

2. **Electrolyte deficits** (in excess of ECF/ICF electrolyte losses)
a. Formula

$$mEq \ required = (CD - CA) \times fD \times wt$$

   where:
   CD = concentration desired (mEq/L)
   CA = concentration present (mEq/L)
   fD = distribution factor as fraction of body weight (L/kg)
   wt = baseline weight before illness (kg)

b. Apparent distribution factor (fD)
   1) HCO_3^-: 0.4–0.5
   2) Cl^-: 0.2–0.3
   3) Na^+: 0.6–0.7

3. **FW deficit in hypernatremic dehydration:** Calculation is based on the amount of FW required to decrease the serum Na^+ by 1mEq/L and is based on the patient's actual serum Na^+. The general calculation is as follows[5]:

$$\frac{[Na]_{actual} - [Na]_{desired}}{[Na]_{actual}} \times 1000mL/L \times 0.6L/kg \ of \ body \ weight* = mL/kg$$

   Example: If serum Na^+ = 145mEq/L (normal), then:

$$\frac{145mEq/L - 144mEq/L}{145mEq/L} \times 1000mL/L \times 0.6L/kg \ of \ body \ weight \ in \ kg =$$

$$\frac{600}{145} = 4mL/kg \ FW \ to \ reduce \ serum \ sodium \ from \ 145 \ to \ 144$$

   An estimate of FW needed to decrease the serum Na^+ by 1mEq/L is **4mL/kg (or 3 mL/kg if Na >170 because less FW is required to change the serum Na^+ by 1 mEqL at higher concentrations).**

---

*This assumes that the FW deficit is distributed throughout the total body water, which is approximately 0.6L/kg of body weight.

C. OVERVIEW OF PARENTERAL REHYDRATION

1. **Phase I (emergency) management:** If the patient is hemodynamically **unstable,** this should be carried out regardless of the type of dehydration (isotonic, hypotonic, or hypertonic) suspected.

a. Symptomatic dehydration or shock requires one or more boluses of 20mL/kg isotonic fluid (i.e., LR or 0.9% NS) in the first 30 minutes.

b. Consider blood or plasma (10mL/kg) if there is no response after two boluses of isotonic fluid or if there is acute blood loss.

c. For seizures caused by hyponatremic dehydration secondary to Na^+ loss, as an initial estimate give 10–12mL/kg of 3% saline over 60 minutes. Alternatively, to calculate the volume of 3% NaCl needed to raise the serum Na^+ by X mEq/L[6]:

$$\text{Amount of 3\% NaCl (mL)} = \frac{[X\,\text{mEq/L} \times \text{Body weight (kg)}] \times 0.6\text{L/kg}}{0.513\text{mEq Na/mL 3\% NaCl}}$$

where $X = (125\text{mEq/L} - \text{actual serum [Na]})$ to initially raise the serum Na^+ rapidly to 125 mEq/L.

2. **Phase II deficit (replacement, maintenance, and ongoing losses)**

a. Calculate deficit volume using percent dehydration (including free water deficit in hypernatremic dehydration).

b. Calculate electrolyte deficit (including excess deficit in hyponatremic dehydration).

c. Calculate maintenance fluids.

d. Calculate maintenance electrolytes.

e. Give half of the replacement therapy in addition to maintenance needs over the first 8 hours and the second half over the next 16 hours.

Note: This may be different in case of hypernatremic dehydration (see p. 232).

f. Take into consideration ongoing losses, such as continued diarrhea, excessive urinary losses, and surgical or enteral drains[7].

11

FLUIDS AND ELECTROLYTES

3. **Sample calculations**

a. Isonatremic (isotonic) dehydration: Na^+ = 130–150mEq/L.
   Example: 5-month-old with 10% dehydration over 4 days. Present
   weight = 6.3kg. Serum Na = 137mEq/L (Table 11.7).
   1) Deficit calculations
      a) Fluid deficit: Preillness weight (kg) − Present weight (kg).

   $$\text{Preillness weight} = \frac{\text{Present weight} \times 100}{100 - \% \text{ Dehydration}} = \frac{6.3\text{kg} \times 100}{100 - 10} = 7\text{kg}$$

      In this case therefore the fluid deficit is 7.0kg − 6.3kg = 0.7kg
      = 0.7L.
      b) Na^+ deficit in an illness lasting >3 days: Na^+ deficit = [ECF
         Na^+] × 60% of total fluid deficit.
         145mEq/L × (0.6 × 0.7L) = 61mEq Na^+ (refer to p. 232)
      c) K^+ deficit = [ICF K^+] × 40% of total fluid deficit.
         150mEq/L × (0.4 × 0.7L) = 42mEq K^+ (refer to p. 232)
   2) Maintenance calculations
      a) Maintenance fluid based on a preillness weight of 7kg: 7kg ×
         100mL/kg per day = 0.7L/day.
      b) Na^+ requirements: 3mEq/100mL × 700mL = 21mEq.
      c) K^+ requirements: 2mEq/100mL × 700mL = 14mEq.
   3) 24-hour requirements
      a) Total fluid requirement: 0.7L + 0.7L = 1.4L (remember to
         subtract boluses).
      b) Total Na^+ requirement: 61mEq + 21mEq = 82mEq (remember
         to subtract Na^+ given in boluses).
      c) Total K^+ requirement: 42mEq + 14mEq = 56mEq.
   4) Fluid schedule: Half of the fluid and electrolyte deficit should be
      replaced over the first 8 hours with the second half to be replaced
      over the next 16 hours, as outlined in Table 11.7. **A convenient
      fluid for this patient would be D_5 ½NS + 40mEq/L KCl or
      potassium acetate to run at 75mL/hr for the first 8 hours and the
      same fluid at 50mL/hr over the next 16 hours.**
b. Hyponatremic (hypotonic) dehydration:
   Example: 5-month-old with 10% dehydration over 4 days. Present
   weight = 6.3kg. Serum Na = 115mEq/L (Table 11.8).
   1) Calculate fluid deficit, electrolyte deficit, and maintenance fluid and
      electrolytes as in isonatremic dehydration (section 3a above).
   2) Calculate excess Na^+ deficit, seen in hypotonic dehydration:
   Excess Na^+ deficit (mEq required) = (CD − CA) × fD × Weight =
                 (135mEq/L − 115mEq/L) × 0.6L/kg × 7kg = 84mEq Na^+
   3) Total Na^+ deficit = Na^+ deficit (as in the isonatremic case) +
      excess Na^+ deficit = 61 mEq Na^+ + 84 mEq Na^+ = 145 mEq
      Na^+. Therefore Na^+ requirement over first 24 hours = total Na^+
      deficit + maintenance Na^+ = 145mEq + 21mEq = 166mEq Na^+
      required over 24 hours.

TABLE 11.7				
ISONATREMIC DEHYDRATION CALCULATIONS[a]				
Example: 7kg infant with 10% dehydration (>3 days).				
Serum Na = 137. Illness weight = 6.3kg.				
		H₂O (mL)	Na (mEq)	K (mEq)
Maintenance		700	21	14
Deficit		700		
	60% ECF × 700 = 420		61	—
	40% ICF × 700 = 280		—	42
24 HOUR TOTAL		1400	82	56
Fluid schedule:				
1st 8hr	⅓ maintenance	233	7	5
	+½ deficit	350	31	21
	1ST 8HR TOTAL	583	38	26
Exact calculations: 583mL/8hr=73mL/hr; 38mEq Na/0.583L=65mEq/L=0.42 NS; 24mEq K/0.583L=45mEq/L)				
Next 16hr	⅔ maintenance	467	14	9
	+½ deficit	350	30	21
	NEXT 16HR TOTAL	817	44	30
Exact calculations: 817mL/16hr=51mL/hr; 44mEq Na/0.817L=54mEq/L=0.35 NS; 30mEq K/0.817L=37mEq/L)				
[a]See p. 234 for complete explanation.				

11

4) Half of the fluid and electrolyte deficit should be given over the first 8 hours with the second half to be given over the second 16 hours (Table 11.8). **A convenient fluid for this patient would be D₅ NS + 40mEq/L of KCl or potassium acetate to run at 75mL/hr for the first 8 hours and D₅ ½NS + 40mEq/L of KCl or potassium acetate to run at 50mL/hr for the next 16 hours.**

5) In adults, rapid correction of hyponatremia may be associated with central pontine myelinolysis. Rapid increases in serum Na⁺ level should therefore be reserved for symptomatic patients only. In asymptomatic patients, the target rate of rise should not exceed 2–4mEq/L every 4 hours or about 20mEq/L in 24 hours.

c. Hypernatremic (hypertonic) dehydration
   Example: 5-month-old with 10% dehydration over 4 days. Present weight = 6.3kg. Serum Na = 155mEq/L (Table 11.9).
   1) Fluid deficit, maintenance fluid, and maintenance electrolytes as in isonatremic dehydration (section 3a, p. 234).
   2) FW deficit (as per p. 232) = [Observed Na⁺ − Ideal Na⁺] × 4mL/kg × Weight (kg) = (155mEq/L − 145mEq/L) × 4mL/kg × 7kg = 280mL (for Na >170, use 3mL/kg FW per 1mEq Na drop).
   3) Solute fluid deficit = Total fluid deficit − FW deficit = 700mL − 280mL = 420mL.

FLUIDS AND ELECTROLYTES

TABLE 11.8

HYPONATREMIC DEHYDRATION CALCULATIONS[a]

Example: 7kg infant with 10% dehydration (>3 days).
Serum Na = 115. Illness weight = 6.3kg.

		H_2O (mL)	Na (mEq)	K (mEq)
Maintenance		700	21	14
Deficit		700		
	60% ECF × 700 = 420		61	—
	40% ICF × 700 = 280		—	42
Excess Na deficit			84	—
24HR TOTAL		1400	166	56
Fluid schedule:				
1st 8hr	⅓ maintenance	233	7	5
	+½ deficit	350	73	21
	1ST 8HR TOTAL	583	80	26

Exact calculations: 583mL/8hr=73mL/hr; 80mEq Na/0.583L=137mEq/L=0.89 NS; 26mEq K/0.583L=45mEq/L)

Next 16hr	⅔ maintenance	467	14	9
	+½ deficit	350	72	21
	NEXT 16HR TOTAL	817	86	30

Exact calculations: 817mL/16hr=51mL/hr; 86mEq Na/0.816L=105mEq/L=0.68 NS; 30mEq K/0.817L=37mEq/L)

[a]See p. 234 for complete explanation.

4) Electrolyte deficits
   a) Na^+ deficit = [ECF Na^+] × 60% × Solute fluid deficit = 145mEq/L × 0.6 × 0.42L = 36.5mEq Na^+.
   b) K^+ deficit = [ICF K^+] × 40% × Solute fluid deficit = 150mEq/L × 0.4 × 0.42L = 25mEq K^+.
5) In hypernatremic dehydration, half of the FW deficit and all of the solute deficit can be replaced over 24 hours (Table 11.9). **An appropriate fluid for this patient would be D_5 ¼NS + 30mEq/L KCl or potassium acetate to run at 40mL/hr for 48 hours.** Reevaluate after the first day of fluids to determine the appropriate fluids for the second day.
6) Avoid dropping the serum Na^+ >15mEq/L per 24 hours to minimize cerebral edema. Thus for total Na^+ corrections of >30 (i.e., serum Na^+ >175), FW deficit replacement will need to be spread over >48 hours.
7) Follow serum Na^+ level every 4 hours initially until stable[7].
4. Probable deficits of water and electrolytes in severe dehydration (Table 11.10)
5. Ongoing losses

TABLE 11.9

HYPERNATREMIC DEHYDRATION CALCULATIONS[a]

Example: 7kg infant with 10% dehydration (>3 days).
Serum Na = 155. Illness weight = 6.3kg.

		H_2O (mL)	Na (mEq)	K (mEq)
24hr maintenance		700	21	14
Deficit		700		
Free water	280			
Solute fluid	420			
60% ECF × 420 = 252			37	—
40% ICF × 420 = 168			—	25
24 HOUR TOTAL		1400	58	39
Fluid schedule:				
1st 24hr	24hr maintenance	700	21	14
	½ **FW deficit**	140	—	—
	Solute fluid deficit	420	—	—
	Na/K deficits	—	37	25
	1st DAY TOTAL	1260	58	39

Calculations: 1260mL/24hr=53mL/hr; 58mEq Na/1.26L=46mEq/L=0.30 NS; 39mEq K/1.26L=31mEq/L)

[a]See p. 235 for complete explanation.

11

FLUIDS AND ELECTROLYTES

TABLE 11.10

DEFICITS OF WATER AND ELECTROLYTES IN SEVERE DEHYDRATION

Condition	H_2O (mL/kg)	Na^+ (mEq/kg)	K^+ (mEq/kg)	Cl^- (mEq/kg)
DIARRHEAL DEHYDRATION				
Hypotonic				
$[Na^+]$[a] <130mEq/L	20–100	10–15	8–15	10–12
Isotonic				
$[Na^+]$ = 130–150mEq/L	100–120	8–10	8–10	8–10
Hypertonic				
$[Na^+]$ >150mEq/L	100–120	2–4	0–6	0–3
PYLORIC STENOSIS	100–120	8–10	10–12	10–12
DIABETIC KETOACIDOSIS	100	8	6–10	6

From Hellerstein[3].
[a][Na] refers to the serum or plasma sodium concentration.

a. Use Table 11.11 to estimate ongoing electrolyte losses for various body fluids.
b. Losses should be determined and may require replacement Q6–8hr. Because of the wide range of normal values, specific analyses are suggested in individual cases.

TABLE 11.11

ELECTROLYTE COMPOSITION OF VARIOUS BODY FLUIDS

Fluid	Na$^+$ (mEq/L)	K$^+$ (mEq/L)	Cl$^-$(mEq/L)	Protein (g/dL)
Gastric	20–80	5–20	100–150	—
Pancreatic	120–140	5–15	40–80	—
Small bowel	100–140	5–15	90–130	—
Bile	120–140	5–15	80–120	—
Ileostomy	45–135	3–15	20–115	—
Diarrhea	10–90	10–80	10–110	—
Burns	140	5	110	3–5

D. ORAL REHYDRATION THERAPY

1. Applications of oral rehydration therapy

a. Indications: Mild to moderate dehydration.

b. Contraindications: Shock, severe dehydration, intractable vomiting, >10mL/kg per hour stool losses, coma, or severe gastric distention.

c. In patients with severe dehydration, IV therapy (20mL/kg boluses) should be used initially until pulse, blood pressure, and level of consciousness return to normal. At that time, oral hydration can be safely instituted.

2. Technique

a. If the patient is vomiting, give 5–10mL of oral rehydration fluid (using a syringe, teaspoon, or cup) every 5–10 minutes, and gradually increase amount as tolerated. Monitor this phase of rehydration.

b. Occasionally (<5% of cases), severe vomiting may necessitate IV fluids. Small amounts of vomiting should not warrant abandoning this mode of rehydration.

3. Deficit replacement

a. Mild dehydration: 50mL/kg ORS over 4 hours.

b. Moderate dehydration: 100mL/kg ORS over 4 hours[9].

4. Oral rehydration solutions (ORS) (Table 11.12)

5. Commonly consumed fluids: Approximate electrolyte composition (Table 11.13). These fluids are not recommended for rehydration.

6. Maintenance phase

a. Goal: Provide usual diet in addition to replacing ongoing losses.

b. Breast-fed infants should resume breastfeeding ad lib, and formula-fed infants should resume their regular formula.

TABLE 11.12

ORAL REHYDRATION SOLUTIONS

	CHO (g/dL)	Na⁺ (mEq/L)	K⁺ (mEq/L)	Cl⁻ (mEq/L)	Base (mEq/L)	mOsm/kg H₂O
Cerealyte	4.0	70	20	60	30	220
Infalyte (formerly Ricelyte)	3.0	50	25	45	30	200
Naturalyte	2.5	45	20	35	48	265
Pedialyte	2.5	45	20	35	30	250
Rehydralyte	2.5	75	20	65	30	310
WHO/UNICEF ORS[a]	2.0	90	20	80	30	310

From Snyder[8]

CHO, Carbohydrate.

[a]Available from Jianas Bros. Packaging Co., 2533 SW Boulevard, Kansas City, MO 64108.

TABLE 11.13

APPROXIMATE ELECTROLYTE COMPOSITION OF COMMONLY CONSUMED FLUIDS[a]

	CHO (g/dL)	Na⁺ (mEq/L)	K⁺ (mEq/L)	Cl⁻ (mEq/L)	HCO₃⁻ (mEq/L)	mOsm/kg H₂O
Apple juice	11.9	0.4	26	—	—	700
Coca-Cola	10.9	4.3	0.1	—	13.4	656
Gatorade	5.9	21	2.5	17	—	377
Ginger ale	9.0	3.5	0.1	—	3.6	565
Milk	4.9	22	36	28	30	260
Orange juice	10.4	0.2	49	—	50	654

From Behrman[2].

CHO, carbohydrate.

[a]Values vary slightly depending on source.

11

FLUIDS AND ELECTROLYTES

c. Children should continue with their regular diet (there is no role for bowel rest).
   1) Foods to encourage
      a) Starchy foods (rice, baked potatoes, noodles, crackers, toast, cereals that are not sugar coated).
      b) Soups (clear broths with rice, noodles, or vegetables).
      c) Yogurt, vegetables (without butter), fresh fruits (not canned in syrup).
   2) Foods to minimize
      a) Foods that are high in fat or simple sugars (fried foods, juices, sodas, or jello-water).
      b) Plain water should not be the only source of oral fluid.
d. Replacement of ongoing losses: Regardless of the degree of dehydration, give approximately 10mL/kg or 4 ounces of rehydration solution for each diarrheal stool.

III. SERUM ELECTROLYTE DISTURBANCES

A. POTASSIUM

1. Hypokalemia

a. Etiologies and laboratory data (Table 11.14).
b. Clinical manifestations[7,10]: Skeletal muscle weakness or paralysis, ileus, and cardiac dysrhythmias. ECG changes include delayed depolarization with flat or absent T waves and in extreme cases, U waves.
c. Laboratory data
   1) Blood: Electrolytes with BUN/Cr, CPK, glucose, renin, ABG, cortisol.
   2) Urine: Urinalysis, K^+, Na^+, Cl^-, osmolality, 17-ketosteroids.
   3) Other: ECG.
d. Management: Rapidity of treatment should be proportional to severity of symptoms.
   1) Acute: Calculate electrolyte deficit and replace with potassium acetate or potassium chloride. (Consult ch. 29 [formulary] for dosing.)
   2) Chronic: Calculate daily requirements and replace with potassium chloride or potassium gluconate.

2. Hyperkalemia

a. Etiologies (Table 11.15).
b. Clinical manifestations[7,10] (Table 11.16).
c. Management
   1) Mild to moderate (K^+ = 6.0–7.0): Goal is to enhance excretion of K^+.
      a) Place patient on monitor.

TABLE 11.14

CAUSES OF HYPOKALEMIA

Decreased stores			
	Normal BP		
Hypertension	Renal	Extrarenal	Normal stores
Renovascular disease	RTA	Skin losses	Alkalosis
Excess renin	Fanconi syndrome	GI losses	↑Insulin
Congenital adrenal hyperplasia[a]	Bartter syndrome	High CHO diet	Leukemia
	DKA	Enema abuse	B$_2$ catecholamines
Excess mineralocorticoid	Antibiotics	Laxative abuse	Familial hypokalemic
Cushing syndrome	Diuretics	Anorexia nervosa	periodic paralysis
LABORATORY DATA			
↑Urine K$^+$	↑Urine K$^+$	↓Urine K$^+$	↑Urine K$^+$

RTA, renal tubular acidosis; CHO, carbohydrate; DKA, diabetic ketoacidosis.
[a]May also be normotensive.

TABLE 11.15

CAUSES OF HYPERKALEMIA

Increased stores		Normal stores
Increased urine K$^+$	Decreased urine K$^+$	
Transfusion with aged blood	Renal failure	Cell breakdown
NaCl substitutes	Hypoaldosteronism	Leukocytosis
Spitzer syndrome	Aldosterone insensitivity	Thrombocytosis >750×10^3/mm^3
	↓Insulin	Metabolic acidosis[a]
	K$^+$-spuring diuretics	Blood drawing (hemolyzed sample)

[a]For every 0.1-unit reduction in arterial pH, there is an approximately 0.2–0.4mEq/L increase in plasma K$^+$.

11

FLUIDS AND ELECTROLYTES

b) Na$^+$ polystyrene resin (Kayexalate) 1–2g/kg with 3mL of sorbitol per gram of resin given PO Q6hr or with 5mL of sorbitol per gram of resin as retention enema over 4–6 hours.

2) Severe (K$^+$>7.0): Goal is to move K$^+$ into cells acutely.

   a) Insulin, regular, 0.1U/kg IV with 25% glucose as 0.5g/kg (2mL/kg) over 30 minutes. May repeat this dose in 30–60 minutes or begin infusion of D$_{25}$W 1–2mL/kg per hour with regular insulin 0.1U/kg per hour. Monitor glucose hourly.

   b) NaHCO$_3$ 1–2mEq/kg IV given over 5–10 minutes. (May be used even in the absence of acidosis.)

TABLE 11.16

CLINICAL MANIFESTATIONS OF K^+ DISTURBANCES

Serum K^+	ECG changes	Other symptoms
~2.5	AV conduction defect, prominent U wave, ventricular dysrhythmia, ST segment depression	Apathy, weakness, paresthesias,
~7.5	Peaked T waves	Weakness, paresthesias
~8.0	Loss of P wave, widening of QRS	—
~9.0	ST segment depression, further widening of QRS	Tetany
~10	Bradycardia, sine wave QRS-T, first-degree AV block, ventricular dysrhythmias, cardiac arrest	—

From Feld[10].
ECG, electrocardiogram; AV, atrioventricular.

    c) With onset of ECG changes, urgent reversal of membrane effects is required. Calcium gluconate (10%) 100mg/kg per dose (1mL/kg per dose) over 3–5 minutes. May repeat in 10 minutes (does not lower serum K^+ concentration).

Note: Calcium gluconate solution is not compatible with $NaHCO_3$. Flush lines between infusions.

    d) Dialysis if these measures are unsuccessful.

B. SODIUM

1. Hyponatremia

a. Etiologies (Table 11.17).

b. Factitious etiologies

    1) Hyperlipidemia: Na^+ ↓ by 0.002 × lipid (mg/dL).

    2) Hyperproteinemia: Na^+ ↓ by 0.25 × [protein (g/dL) − 8].

    3) Hyperglycemia: Na^+ ↓ 1.6mEq/L for each 100mg/dL rise in glucose.

c. Clinical manifestations[7,10]: Na^+ ≤120mEq/L often symptomatic (convulsion, shock, lethargy). If the change was less acute or chronic over several months, the patient may be relatively asymptomatic.

d. For hyponatremia not caused by dehydration (SIADH, water intoxication), the principal treatment is fluid restriction until Na levels normalize.

2. Hypernatremia

a. Etiologies (Table 11.18).

b. Clinical manifestations[7,10]: Predominantly neurologic symptoms: lethargy, weakness, altered mental status, irritability, and seizures. Additional symptoms may include muscle cramps, depressed deep tendon reflexes, and respiratory failure.

TABLE 11.17

HYPONATREMIA

Decreased weight		Increased or normal weight
Renal losses	Extrarenal losses	
CAUSE		
Na⁺-losing nephropathy	GI losses	Nephrotic syndrome
Diuretics	Skin losses	Congestive heart failure
Adrenal insufficiency	Third space	SIADH
Hyperglycemia		Acute renal failure
		Water intoxication
		Cirrhosis
LABORATORY DATA		
↑Urine Na⁺	↓Urine Na⁺	↓Urine Na⁺ᵃ
↑Urine volume	↓Urine volume	↓Urine volume
↓Specific gravity	↑Specific gravity	↑Specific gravity
↓Urine osmolality	↑Urine osmolality	↑Urine osmolality
MANAGEMENT		
Replace losses	Replace losses	Restrict fluids
Treat cause	Treat cause	Treat cause

GI, gastrointestinal; SIADH, syndrome of inappropriate antidiuretic hormone secretion.
ᵃUrine Na⁺ may be appropriate for level of Na⁺ intake in patients with SIADH and water intoxication.

TABLE 11.18

HYPERNATREMIA

Decreased weight		Increased weight
Renal losses	Extrarenal losses	
CAUSE		
Nephropathy	GI losses	Exogenous Na⁺
Diuretic use	Respiratoryᵃ	Mineralocorticoid excess
Diabetes insipidus	Skin/other sites	Hyperaldosteronism
LABORATORY DATA		
↑ Urine volume	↓ Urine volume	Relative ↓ urine volume
↑ Urine Na⁺	↓ Urine Na⁺	Relative ↓ urine Na⁺
↓ Specific gravity	↑ Specific gravity	Relative ↑ specific gravity
MANAGEMENT		

Replace FW losses based on calculations on p. 232 and treat cause. Consider a natriuretic agent if there is increased weight.

ᵃThis cause of hypernatremia is usually secondary to free water loss so that the fractional excretion of sodium may be decreased or normal.

C. CALCIUM

1. Hypocalcemia

a. Etiologies: Hypoparathyroidism (decreased PTH levels or ineffective PTH response), vitamin D deficiency, hyperphosphatemia, pancreatitis, malabsorption states (malnutrition), drug therapy (anticonvulsants), hypomagnesemia, and maternal hyperparathyroidism if patient is a neonate.

b. Clinical manifestations[7,10]: Neuromuscular irritability with weakness, paresthesia, fatigue, cramping, altered mental status, seizures, laryngospasm, and cardiac dysrhythmias. ECG changes include prolonged QT interval. Clinically, it may be detected by carpal pedal spasm after arterial occlusion of an extremity for 3 minutes (Trousseau sign) or percussion of the facial nerve with muscle twitching (Chvostek sign).

c. Laboratory data
   1) Blood: Ca^{2+} (total and ionized), phosphate, alkaline phosphatase, Mg^{2+}, total protein, albumin (a change in serum albumin of 1g/dL changes serum Ca^{2+} in the same direction by 0.8mg/dL), BUN, Cr, PTH, pH (acidosis increases ionized calcium, whereas alkalosis decreases it), 25(OH)vit D.
   2) Urine: Ca^{2+}, phosphate, Cr.
   3) Other: ECG, chest film (to visualize thymus), ankle and wrist films for rickets[6].

d. Management
   1) Treat the underlying disease.
   2) Chronic: Consider use of oral supplements of calcium carbonate, calcium gluconate, calcium glubionate, or calcium lactate.
   3) Acute symptomatic: Consider use of IV forms, such as calcium gluconate, calcium gluceptate, or calcium chloride (cardiac arrest dose).
      a) Significant hyperphosphatemia should be corrected before correction of hypocalcemia because soft tissue calcification may occur if total $[Ca^{2+}] \times [PO_4] > 80$ (see p. 246).
      b) Symptoms of hypocalcemia that are refractory to Ca^{2+} supplementation may be caused by hypomagnesemia.

2. **Hypercalcemia**

a. Etiologies: Hyperparathyroidism, vitamin D intoxication, malignancy, prolonged immobilization, and diuretics (thiazides), granulomatous disease.

b. Clinical manifestations[7,10]: Weakness, irritability, lethargy, seizures, and coma in addition to abdominal cramping, anorexia, nausea, vomiting, polyuria, polydipsia, renal calculi, and pancreatitis. ECG changes include shortened QT interval.

c. Laboratory data
   1) Blood: Ca^{2+} (total and ionized), phosphate, alkaline phosphatase, total protein, albumin, BUN, Cr, PTH, and vitamin D.
   2) Urine: Ca^{2+}, phosphate, Cr.
   3) Other: ECG; KUB; and renal ultrasound (for renal stones)[6].

    d. Management
      1) Treat the underlying disease.
      2) Hydrate to increase urine output and Ca^{2+} excretion. If GFR and BP are stable, may give NS + K^+ supplement at two to three times maintenance rate until $[Ca^{2+}]_i$ is in normal range.
      3) Diuresis with furosemide.
      4) Consider hemodialysis.
      5) Steroids (for malignancy, granulomatous disease, and vitamin D toxicity) to decrease vitamin D and Ca^{2+} absorption. Hydrocortisone or prednisone may be given.
      6) Severe or persistently elevated Ca^{2+}.
        a) Give calcitonin or bisphosphonate (in consultation with an endocrinologist).

D. MAGNESIUM

1. Hypomagnesemia

a. Etiologies: Increased urinary loss (diuretic use, renal tubular acidosis, hypercalcemia, chronic adrenergic stimulants), gastrointestinal (malabsorption syndromes, severe malnutrition, diarrhea/vomiting, short bowel syndromes, enteric fistulas), and endocrine (diabetes mellitus, PTH disorders, hyperaldosterone states).

b. Clinical manifestations[7,10]: Anorexia, nausea, weakness, malaise, depression, nonspecific psychiatric symptoms, hyperreflexia, carpopedal spasm, clonus, and tetany. ECG changes include both atrial and ventricular ectopy and torsades de pointes.

c. Laboratory data: Mg^{2+} and Ca^{2+} (total and ionized).

d. Management
    1) Acute: Give magnesium sulfate.
    2) Chronic: Magnesium oxide, magnesium gluconate, magnesium sulfate[6].

2. Hypermagnesemia

a. Etiologies: Renal failure, and excessive administration (eclampsia/preeclampsia states, cathartics, enemas).

b. Clinical manifestations[7,10]: Depressed deep tendon reflexes, lethargy, confusion, and, in extreme cases, respiratory failure.

c. Laboratory data: Mg^{2+}, BUN, Cr, and Ca^{2+}.

d. Management
    1) Stop supplemental Mg^{2+}.
    2) Diurese.
    3) Give Ca^{2+} supplements[11]
      a) Calcium chloride (use cardiac arrest doses).
      b) Calcium gluceptate.
      c) Calcium gluconate.
    4) Dialysis if life-threatening levels are present[12].

11

FLUIDS AND ELECTROLYTES

E. PHOSPHATE

1. Hypophosphatemia

a. Etiologies: Starvation, protein–energy malnutrition, malabsorption syndromes, intracellular shifts associated with respiratory or metabolic alkalosis, during the treatment of diabetic ketoacidosis, and after the administration of corticosteroids, increased renal loss, vitamin D–deficient and vitamin D–resistant rickets, and very-low-birthweight (VLBW) infants when intake does not meet demand.

b. Clinical manifestations[7,10]: Becomes symptomatic only at very low levels <1.0mg/dL) with irritability, paresthesias, confusion, seizures, and coma.

c. Laboratory data

   1) Blood: Phosphate, Ca^{2+} (total and ionized), electrolytes including BUN/Cr (follow for low K^+, Mg^{2+}, Na^+), vitamin D, PTH.

   2) Urine: Ca^{2+}, phosphate, Cr, pH.

d. Management

   1) Insidious onset of symptoms: Give oral potassium phosphate or sodium phosphate.

   2) Acute onset of symptoms: Give IV potassium phosphate or sodium phosphate.

2. Hyperphosphatemia

a. Etiologies: Hypoparathyroidism (but rarely occurs in the absence of renal insufficiency), reduction of GFR <25%, excessive administration of phosphate (PO, IV, or enemas), and use of cytotoxic drugs to treat malignancies.

b. Clinical manifestations[7,10]: Symptoms of the resulting hypocalcemia.

c. Laboratory data

   1) Blood: Phosphate, Ca^{2+} (ionized and total), electrolytes including BUN/Cr, CBC, vitamin D, PTH, ABG.

   2) Urine: $Ca2^+$, phosphate, Cr, urinalysis.

d. Management

   1) Restrict dietary phosphate.

   2) Give phosphate binders (calcium carbonate, aluminum hydroxide; use with caution in renal failure).

   3) For cell lysis (with normal renal function), NS bolus and IV mannitol.

   4) If poor renal function, may consider dialysis[12].

IV. ANION GAP

A. DEFINITION: The anion gap (AG) represents anions other than bicarbonate and chloride required to balance the positive charge of Na^+. Clinically it is measured by:

$$AG = Na^+ - (Cl^- + CO_2)$$

(Normal: 12mEq/L ± 2mEq/L)

B. METABOLIC ACIDOSIS WITH NORMAL ANION GAP (HYPERCHLOREMIC ACIDOSIS)

1. **Gastrointestinal loss of bicarbonate**
a. Diarrhea (secretory).
b. Fistula or drainage of the small bowel or pancreas.
c. Surgery for necrotizing enterocolitis.
d. Ureteral sigmoidoscopy or ileal loop conduit.
e. Ileoileal pouch.
f. Use of anion exchange resins in presence of renal impairment.
2. **Renal loss of bicarbonate** (see Table 21-8. p. 452).
3. **Other causes**
a. Addition of HCl, NH_4Cl, arginine, or lysine hydrochloride.
b. Hyperalimentation.
c. Dilutional acidosis.

C. METABOLIC ACIDOSIS WITH INCREASED ANION GAP

1. **Increased acid production (noncarbonic acid)**
a. Increased β-hydroxybutyric acid and acetoacetic acid production
   1) Insulin deficiency (diabetic ketoacidosis).
   2) Starvation or fasting.
   3) Ethanol intoxication.
b. Increased lactic acid production
   1) Tissue hypoxia.
   2) Muscular exercise.
   3) Ethanol ingestion.
   4) Systemic diseases (leukemia, diabetes mellitus, cirrhosis, pancreatitis).
   5) Inborn errors of metabolism (carbohydrates, urea cycles, amino acids, organic acids).
c. Increased short fatty acids (acetate, propionate, butyrate, D-lactate) from colonic fermentation
   1) Viral gastroenteritis.
   2) Other causes of carbohydrate malabsorption.
d. Conditions in which the nature of the organic acid responsible for the acidosis has not been clearly established
   1) Methanol intoxication.
   2) Ethylene glycol intoxication.
   3) Paraldehyde intoxication.
   4) Salicylate intoxication.
   5) NSAID intoxication.
   6) Methylmalonic aciduria.
   7) Propionyl-CoA carboxylase deficiency.
e. Increased sulfuric acid
   1) Methionine administration.
2. **Decreased acid excretion:** Acute and chronic renal failure[13].

V. MISCELLANEOUS

A. CONVERSION FORMULA OF MG TO MEq/L (Table 11.19)[2]

$$mEq/L = mg/L \text{ per equivalent weight}$$
$$\text{Equivalent weight} = \text{Atomic weight/Valence of element}$$

TABLE 11.19
FACTORS FOR CONVERSION[a]

Element or radical	mEq/L to mg/dL		mg/dL to mEq/L	
Na^+	1	2.30	1	0.4348
K^+	1	3.91	1	0.2558
Ca^{++}	1	2.005	1	0.4988
Mg^{++}	1	1.215	1	0.8230
Cl^-	1	3.55	1	0.2817
Bicarbonate (HCO_3^-)	1	6.1	1	0.1639
Phosphorus valence 1	1	3.10	1	0.3226
Phosphorus valence 1.8	1	1.72	1	0.5814

From Behrman[2].
[a]From milliequivalents per liter to milligrams per deciliter and vice versa.

B. SERUM OSMOLALITY

1. Defined as the number of particles per liter. May be approximated by:

$$2[Na^+] + \frac{\text{Glucose (mg/dL)}}{18} + \frac{\text{BUN (mg/dL)}}{2.8}$$

2. Normal range: 285–295mOsm/L.

VI. PARENTERAL FLUID COMPOSITION (Table 11.20)

TABLE 11.20
COMPOSITION OF FREQUENTLY USED PARENTERAL FLUIDS

Liquid	CHO (g/100mL)	Protein[a] (g/100mL)	cal/L	Na$^+$ (mEq/L)	K$^+$ (mEq/L)	Cl$^-$ (mEq/L)	HCO$_3$$^{-b}$ (mEq/L)	Ca^{2+} (mEq/L)
D$_5$W	5	—	170	—	—	—	—	—
D$_{10}$W	10	—	340	—	—	—	—	—
NS (0.9% NaCl)	—	—	—	154	—	154	—	—
½NS (0.45% NaCl)	—	—	—	77	—	77	—	—
D$_5$ (0.2% NaCl)	5	—	170	34	—	34	—	—
3% saline	—	—	—	513	—	513	—	—
8.4% sodium bicarbonate (1mEq/mL)	—	—	—	1000	—	—	1000	—
Ringer's	0–10	—	0–340	147	4	155.5	—	≈4
Lactated Ringer's	0–10	—	0–340	130	4	109	28	3
Amino acid 8.5% (Travasol)	—	8.5	340	3	—	34	52	—
Plasmanate	—	5	200	110	2	50	29	—
Albumin 25% (salt poor)	—	25	1000	100–160	—	<120	—	—
Intralipid[d]	2.25	—	1100	2.5	0.5	4.0	—	—

CHO, carbohydrate; HCO$_3$$^-$, bicarbonate.

[a]Protein or amino acid equivalent.

[b]Bicarbonate or equivalent (citrate, acetate, lactate).

[c]Approximate values: actual values may vary somewhat in various localities depending on electrolyte composition of water supply used to reconstitute solution.

[d]Values are approximate; may vary from lot to lot. Also contains ≈ 1.2% egg-phosphatides.

FLUIDS AND ELECTROLYTES 11

VII. REFERENCES

1. Finberg L, Kravath RE, Fleishman AR. *Water and electrolytes in pediatrics.* Philadelphia: WB Saunders; 1982.
2. Behrman RE, Kliegman RM, Arvin AM. *Nelson textbook of pediatrics,* 15th edn. Philadelphia: WB Saunders; 1996.
3. Hellerstein S. Fluids and electrolytes: clinical aspects. *Pediatr Rev* 1993; **14(3):**103–115.
4. Oski FA. *Principles and practice of pediatrics.* Philadelphia: JB Lippincott; 1994.
5. Segar WE: Parenteral fluid therapy. *Curr Probl Pediatr* 1972; **3(2):**3–40.
6. Fleisher G, Ludwig S. *Textbook of pediatric emergency medicine.* Baltimore: Williams & Wilkins; 1993.
7. Barkin R. *Pediatric emergency medicine,* 2nd edn. St Louis: Mosby; 1997.
8. Snyder J. *Semin Pediatr Infect Dis* 1994; **5:**231.
9. Duggan C, Santosham M, Glass RI. The management of acute diarrhea in children: oral rehydration, maintenance, and nutritional therapy: Centers for Disease Control and Prevention. *MMWR* 1992; **41(RR-16):**1–20.
10. Feld LG, Kaskel FJ, Schoeneman MJ. The approach to fluid and electrolyte therapy in pediatrics. *Adv Pediatr* 1988; **35:**497–535.
11. *American hospital formulary service drug information,* 1995, p. 2195.
12. Fonser L. *Pediatr Ann* 1995; **24:**44.
13. Hanna J, Scheinman J, Chan J. The kidney in acid–base balance. *Pediatr Clin North Am* 1995; **42(6):**1365.

GASTROENTEROLOGY

B. Kelly Gleason, MD

I. GASTROINTESTINAL BLEEDING

A. INITIAL EVALUATION AND TREATMENT (Fig. 12.1)

1. ABCs and hemodynamic stabilization.
2. Physical examination looking for evidence of bleeding.
3. Verify blood and obtain baseline laboratory tests. Consider CBC with platelets, PT/aPTT, type and crossmatch, reticulocyte count, blood smear, BUN/Cr, electrolytes, DIC panel.
4. Assess for ongoing losses.
5. Specific therapy based on assessment and site of bleeding.
6. **Consider transfusion:** If there is continued bleeding, symptomatic anemia and/or hematocrit <20%.

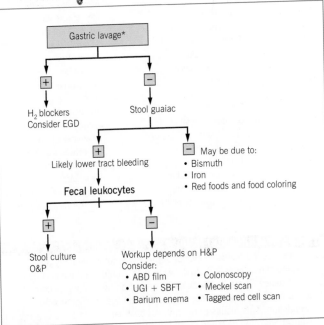

FIG 12.1

Evaluation of GI bleeding.*May use G tube if present; use with caution if esophageal varices suspected.

B. DIFFERENTIAL DIAGNOSIS OF GI BLEEDING (Table 12.1)

TABLE 12.1

DIFFERENTIAL DIAGNOSIS OF GI BLEEDING, IN ORDER OF FREQUENCY

	Upper GI bleed	Lower GI bleed
Newborns	Swallowed maternal blood	Anal fissure
	Hemorrhagic gastritis	Allergic proctocolitis
	Stress ulcer	Infectious diarrhea
	Idiopathic	Hirschsprung disease
	Coagulopathy	Necrotizing colitis
	Gastric outlet obstruction	Volvulus
	Gastric volvulus	Stress ulcer
	Pyloric stenosis	Vascular malformation
	Antral/pyloric webs	GI duplication
Infants	Epistaxis	Anal fissure
	Gastritis	Infectious diarrhea
	Esophagitis	Allergic proctocolitis
	Stress ulcer	Meckel diverticulum
	Gastric/duodenal ulcer	Intussusception
	Foreign bodies	GI duplication
	Gastric volvulus	Peptic ulcer
	Esophageal varices	Foreign body
Children	Epistaxis	Anal fissure
	Tonsillitis/sinusitis	Polyp
	Gastritis	Infectious diarrhea
	Gastric/duodenal ulcer	Lymphonodular hyperplasia
	Medications	Inflammatory bowel disease
	Mallory–Weiss tear	Henoch–Schönlein purpura
	Tumors	Meckel's diverticulum
	Hematologic disorders	Peptic ulcer
	Esophageal varices	Hemolytic uremic syndrome
	Munchausen by proxy	Vascular malformations

II. CONSTIPATION AND ENCOPRESIS

Constipation is the failure to evacuate the lower colon regularly and is defined clinically as <3 stools/week with painful passage and hard consistency. There is a wide variation in normal stooling patterns from once daily to weekly. Encopresis is the leakage of stool around impaction. This results from chronic constipation and there is a loss of sensation in the distended rectal vault. Encopresis is a common disorder, occurring in 1–4% of 4- to 10-year-old children. Most cases of encopresis and constipation occur in the setting of functional fecal retention. Other underlying disorders need to be considered and excluded.

A. DIFFERENTIAL DIAGNOSIS OF NONFUNCTIONAL CONSTIPATION

1. **Neurologic** (e.g., Hirschsprung's, spinal pathology, botulism).
2. **Obstructive** (e.g., anal ring, small left colon, meconium ileus, mass).
3. **Endocrine/metabolic** (e.g., collagen vascular disease, hypothyroidism).
4. **Medicinal** (e.g., opiates, iron, tricyclic antidepressants, chemotherapy agents such as vincristine).

B. COMPLICATIONS

1. Abdominal pain.
2. Rectal fissures, ulcers, and prolapse.
3. Urinary tract infection (UTI) and urinary incontinence, ureteral obstruction.
4. Stasis syndrome with bacterial overgrowth.
5. Social isolation.

C. TREATMENT OF FUNCTIONAL CONSTIPATION: The treatment of chronic constipation requires long-term behavioral modification along with medication. The goal is eventual weaning of medication once normal colorectal sensation and stooling patterns have been established. The three stages of treatment include:

1. **Disimpaction (2–5 days):** Enemas may be attempted at home once daily for 3–5 days. Prolonged use may result in hypophosphatemia and hypocalcemia. Refractory constipation may require colonic lavage with isotonic polyethylene glycol solution (GoLYTELY). This usually requires hospitalization and nasogastric tube placement.
   a. Enema (see ch. 29 (formulary) for dosing)
      - Mineral oil: See p. 776.
      - Hypertonic phosphate (Fleets): See p. 849.
      - Milk and molasses 50:50 mix up to 6oz max.
   b. Oral/nasogastric
      - Mineral oil: Use with caution <1 yr age due to risk of aspiration.
      - Polyethylene glycol (GoLYTELY): See p. 819 for oral/nasogastric doses.

2. **Sustained evacuation (usually ≥3–12 months):** This stage restores normal colorectal tone and requires habitual toilet use with positive rewards and behavioral therapy. Initial diet should be low in fiber with a transition to a high-fiber diet once disimpaction has occurred. Medications include lubricants, hyperosmolar sugars, and stimulants. See ch. 29 for specific dosages. Generic and brand names of medications follow:
   a. Fiber supplements: Barley malt (barley cereal, Maltsupex); cellulose (Citrucel); psyllium (Metamucil, Fiberall); polycarbophil (Fibercon, Konsyl).

12

GASTROENTEROLOGY

b. Lubricants: Mineral oil (Kondremul, Agarol); surfactant (Docusate).
c. Hyperosmolar sugars: Fructose/sorbitol (prune juice); lactulose (do not use <6 months).
d. Stimulants: Salts (Milk of Magnesia, magnesium citrate); senna (Senekot); diphenylmethane (Bisacodyl); prokinetics (cisapride, metoclopramide). Phenolphthalein and castor oil should not be used in children.
3. **Gradually wean from medications.**

III. DIARRHEA

Usual stool output is <10g/kg per day in children and <200g/day in adults. Diarrhea is increased water in stool, resulting in increased stool frequency or loose consistency. Chronic diarrhea is diarrhea lasting more than 14 days. Acute diarrhea is most commonly of an infectious, usually viral, etiology. Oral rehydration is almost always successful and should be attempted with an appropriate oral rehydration solution. See ch. 11 for calculation of deficit and maintenance fluid requirements and oral rehydration composition. Breast-feeding should continue, and a regular diet should be restarted as soon as patient is rehydrated. The etiology of diarrhea may be infectious or malabsorptive, and the mechanism is osmotic or secretory.

A. **CHARACTERISTICS OF OSMOTIC DIARRHEA**
1. **Stool volume:** Depends on diet and decreases with fasting.
2. **Fecal Na^+:** <60mosmol/L.
3. **Fecal osmolarity** <plasma osmolarity.
B. **CHARACTERISTICS OF SECRETORY DIARRHEA**
1. **Stool volume:** Increased and does not vary with diet.
2. **Fecal Na^+:** >60mosmol/L.
3. **Fecal osmolarity:** <plasma osmolarity.
a. Calculation of stool osmotic gap

Osmotic gap (mOsm/L) = $290 - 2$ (Stool Na^+ + Stool K^+)

b. Interpretation
   1) Stool Na^+ >70mEq/L and osmotic gap <100mOsm/L suggest a secretory diarrhea.
   2) Stool Na^+ <70mEq/L and osmotic gap >100 mOsm/L suggest malabsorption due to an excessive osmotic load.
C. **INFECTIOUS DIARRHEA**
1. **Viral:** The most common cause of acute gastroenteritis is viral infection causing malabsorption. Common etiologic agents include rotavirus, enteric adenovirus, Norwalk virus, astrovirus, and calicivirus.
2. **Bacterial:** A bacterial etiology is more common in bloody diarrhea; it is usually secretory or dysenteric. Dysentery is defined as diarrhea with blood and mucus resulting from invasion of bowel mucosa. Specific antibiotic therapy depends on the organism, the site of infection, host factors, and culture sensitivities. See Table 12.2 for general treatment information.

TABLE 12.2
TREATMENT RECOMMENDATIONS FOR BACTERIAL ENTERIC INFECTIONS

Organism	Clinical syndrome	Treatment recommendations	Therapy*
Salmonella	Diarrhea	No treatment, can prolong carriage	
	Invasive disease or:	Treatment recommended: length of treatment depends on site of infection; relapses are common, and re-treatment recommended	Amoxicillin
	<3 months of age		TMP/SZX
	Malignancy		Cefotaxime
	Hemoglobinopathy		
	Immunosuppressed		
	Chronic GI disease		
	Severe colitis		
Shigella	Diarrhea or dysentery	Treatment shortens duration of signs and symptoms, eliminates organism from feces, prevents spread of organism	TMP/SZX
Yersinia	Noninvasive diarrhea	Treatment in normal host does not have established benefit	
	Septicemia and infection other than GI tract	Treatment recommended	TMP/SZX
			Ceftriaxone
Campylobacter	Diarrhea or dysentery	Treatment shortens duration of illness; prevents relapse	Erythromycin

*Definitive therapy should be based on culture sensitivities.
HUS, hemolytic uremic syndrome.

Continued

12

GASTROENTEROLOGY

TABLE 12.2

TREATMENT RECOMMENDATIONS FOR BACTERIAL ENTERIC INFECTIONS—cont'd

Organism	Clinical syndrome	Treatment recommendations	Therapy*
E. coli			
EHEC (O157) (enterohemorrhagic)	HUS	Antimicrobial therapy does not appear to prevent progression to HUS and role of antimicrobials uncertain	
EPEC (enteropathogenic)	Diarrhea	Nonabsorbable oral antibiotics	Neomycin/Gentamycin
	Chronic carriage	Absorbable oral antibiotics	TMP/SZX
ETEC (enterotoxigenic)	Diarrhea	Disease usually self-limited and no treatment recommended	TMP/SZX
EIEC (enteroinvasive)	Diarrhea	Treatment recommended	

*Definitive therapy should be based on culture sensitivities.
HUS, hemolytic uremic syndrome.

3. **Parasitic:** The most common cause of parasitic diarrhea is *Giardia lamblia* (giardiasis); the most common cause of parasitic dysentery is amebae (amebiasis). Treatment recommendations are listed in Table 12.3. (Testing is listed on p. 259.)

TABLE 12.3

TREATMENT OF PARASITIC ENTERIC INFECTIONS

Organism	Clinical syndrome	Treatment recommendations	Antiparasitic
Giardia lamblia	Asymptomatic carriage	No treatment unless household member with: Pregnancy Cystic fibrosis Hypogammaglobulinemia	Metronidazole
	Diarrhea	Symptomatic disease should be treated	Metronidazole Furazolidone
Amebae	Asymptomatic	Treatment recommended for all infection	Paromomycin
	Diarrhea/dysentery Extraintestinal	Treatment recommended for all infection	Metronidazole followed by iodoquinol

D. **MALABSORPTIVE DIARRHEA:** Malabsorption may be generalized or specific for a carbohydrate, fat, or protein. The most commonly malabsorbed carbohydrate is lactose. Lactose malabsorption may be primary or secondary. Primary lactose malabsorption occurs from lack of lactase and is found in 80% of adults worldwide, presenting no earlier than 9–10 years of age. Secondary lactase deficiency results from temporary mucosal injury, commonly from infection. Fat malabsorption, steatorrhea, is defined as absorption of <90% of ingested fat. The mechanism includes inadequate lipase activity or biliary digestion and mucosal disease. (Testing is listed on pp. 262–264.)

IV. HYPERBILIRUBINEMIA

Bilirubin is the product of hemoglobin metabolism. There are two forms: direct (conjugated) and indirect (unconjugated). Hyperbilirubinemia is usually the result of increased hemoglobin load, reduced hepatic uptake, reduced hepatic conjugation, or decreased excretion. Direct hyperbilirubinemia is defined as direct bilirubin >15% of total bilirubin >2mg/dL.

A. **INDIRECT HYPERBILIRUBINEMIA**

1. **Transient neonatal jaundice:** Physiologic jaundice; breast-feeding jaundice; breast milk jaundice; Lucey–Driscoll syndrome; reabsorption of extravascular blood; polycythemia. (See p. 431 for treatment guidelines.)

2. **Hemolytic disorders**
a. Blood group incompatibility including ABO/Rh/minor Ag.
b. Hemoglobinopathies: Sickle-cell anemia; thalassemia major.
c. Red cell membrane disorders: Spherocytosis; elliptocytosis.
d. Microangiopathies: Hemolytic uremic syndrome; hemangioma.
e. Red cell enzyme deficiencies: Glucose-6-phosphate dehydrogenase; fructokinase; pyruvate kinase; glutathione peroxidase, '5 pyrimidine nucleosidase deficiencies.
f. Autoimmune disease: Viral infection; systemic lupus erythematosus (SLE).
3. **Enterohepatic recirculation:** Hirschsprung disease; cystic fibrosis; ileal atresia; pyloric stenosis.
4. **Disorders of bilirubin metabolism:** Crigler–Najjar syndrome; Gilbert syndrome; hypothyroidism; hypoxia; acidosis.
5. **Miscellaneous:** Sepsis; dehydration; hypoalbuminemia; drugs.
B. **DIRECT HYPERBILIRUBINEMIA**
1. **Biliary obstruction:** Biliary atresia; paucity of intrahepatic bile ducts (Alagille syndrome); choledochal cyst; inspissated bile syndrome; fibrosing pancreatitis; primary sclerosing cholangitis; gallstones; neoplasm; Caroli's disease.
2. **Infection:** Sepsis; UTI; cholangitis; liver abscess; viral hepatitis (hepatitis A, B, C; CMV; EBV); other viral infections (coxsackievirus, herpes simplex, varicella, echovirus, reovirus, parvovirus); syphilis; toxoplasmosis; tuberculosis; leptospirosis; histoplasmosis; visceral larva migrans (toxocariasis).
3. **Metabolic disorders:** α_1-Antitrypsin deficiency; cystic fibrosis; galactosemia; galactokinase deficiency; Wilson's disease; hereditary fructose intolerance; Niemann–Pick disease; Wolman's disease; glycogen storage disease; Zellweger syndrome; Gaucher's disease; Dubin–Johnson syndrome; Rotor syndrome; other disorders of bilirubin metabolism.
4. **Chromosomal abnormalities:** Turner syndrome; trisomy 18; trisomy 21.
5. **Drugs:** Aspirin; acetaminophen; iron; isoniazid; vitamin A; erythromycin; sulfonamides; oxacillin; rifampin; ethanol; steroids; tetracycline; methotrexate.
6. **Miscellaneous:** Neonatal hepatitis syndrome; hyperalimentation; Reye syndrome; histiocytosis; neonatal SLE.

V. EVALUATION OF LIVER FUNCTION TESTS (LFTS)
A. **SUGGESTIVE OF LIVER CELL INJURY:** AST, ALT, LDH, NH_3.
B. **SUGGESTIVE OF CHOLESTASIS:** Increased bilirubin, urine bilinogen, GGT, alkaline phosphatase, 5'-nucleotidase, serum bile acids.

C. **TESTS OF SYNTHETIC FUNCTION:** Albumin, prealbumin, prothrombin time (PT), activated partial prothrombin time (aPTT), cholesterol. Elevated NH_3 is evidence of decreased ability to detoxify ammonia. See Table 12.4 for evaluation and interpretation of LFTs (see pp. 260–261).

Note: See pp. 410–411 for serology of hepatitides and pp. 356–358 for immunization recommendations.

VI. MISCELLANEOUS TESTS

A. **FETAL HEMOGLOBIN (APT TEST)**
1. **Purpose:** To differentiate fetal blood from swallowed maternal blood.
2. **Method:** Mix specimen with an equal quantity of tap water and centrifuge or filter. Add 1 part of 0.25mMol/L (1%) NaOH to 5 parts of supernatant.

Note: Specimen must be bloody, and supernatant must be pink for proper interpretation.

3. **Interpretation:** A pink color persisting over 2 minutes indicates fetal hemoglobin. Transition from pink to yellow within 2 minutes indicates adult hemoglobin.

B. **FECAL LEUKOCYTES**
1. **Purpose:** To aid in the diagnosis of diarrhea by noting the presence or absence of leukocytes in the stool.
2. **Method:** Place a small amount of stool or mucus (ideally from a rectal swab) on a glass slide. Mix thoroughly with two drops of 0.5% methylene blue (Wright or Gram stain can also be used). Wait 2–3 minutes, cover with a coverslip, and examine under low power.
3. **Interpretation:** Sheets of polymorphonuclear cells suggest an inflammatory enterocolitis, such as that seen with *Shigella, Salmonella, Yersinia, Campylobacter,* invasive *Escherichia coli, Clostridium difficile,* ulcerative colitis, and Crohn's disease. Eosinophilia may indicate allergic colitis.

C. **PARASITES** (See Table 12.3)
1. **Direct smear:** Place a small amount of stool in a drop of saline on a glass slide, mix, remove particulate matter, and cover with a coverslip. Add iodine stain for identification of protozoan cysts.
2. **Laboratory identification:** Specimen must be fresh. If delay is expected, preserve with a commercially available kit.
3. *Giardia lamblia:* In addition to stool examination for cysts, a string test collection system (e.g., Entero/Test) can assist in identification. An antigen detection test is also now widely available and commonly used.
4. **Pinworms.** Obtain specimen in the morning before the child has had a bath. Apply sticky side of cellophane tape to the perianal area, transfer tape to a glass slide sticky side down, and examine for ova.
a. Treatment: Mebendazole, pyrantel pamoate, albendazole.

D. *HELICOBACTER PYLORI:* A variety of different tests is available for diagnosing *H. pylori* infection, including the following:

TABLE 12.4

EVALUATION OF LIVER FUNCTION TESTS

Enzyme	Source	Increased	Decreased	Comments
AST/ALT	Liver	Hepatocellular injury	Vitamin B$_6$ deficiency	ALT more specific than AST for liver
	Heart	Rhabdomyolosis	Uremia	AST >ALT in hemolysis
	Skeletal muscle	Muscular dystrophy		AST/ALT >2 in 90% of alcohol disorders in adults
	Pancreas	Hemolysis		
	RBCs	Liver cancer		
	Kidney			
Alkaline phosphatase	Liver	Hepatocellular injury	Low phosphate	Highest in cholestatic conditions
	Osteoblasts	Bone growth, disease, trauma	Wilson's disease	Must be differentiated from bone source
	Small intestine	Pregnancy	Zinc deficiency	
	Kidney	Familial	Hypothyroidism	
	Placenta		Pernicious anemia	

GGT	Bile ducts Renal tubules Pancreas Small intestine Brain	Cholestasis Newborn period Induced by drugs	Estrogen therapy Artificially low in hyperbilirubinemia	Not found in bone Increased in 90% primary liver disease Biliary obstruction Intrahepatic cholestasis Induced by alcohol Specific for hepatobiliary disease in nonpregnant patient
5'-NT	Liver cell membrane Intestine Brain Heart Pancreas	Cholestasis		Specific for hepatobiliary disease in nonpregnant patient
NH$_3$	Bowel Bacteria Protein metabolism	Hepatic disease secondary to urea cycle dysfunction Hemodialysis Valproic acid rx Urea cycle enzyme deficiency Organic acidemia and carnitine deficiency		Converted to urea in liver

Alk phos, alkaline phosphatase; AST/ALT, aspartate aminotransferase/alanine aminotransferase; GGT, γ-glutamyl transpeptidase; 5'-NT, 5'-nucleotidase.

GASTROENTEROLOGY

12

1. **Endoscopy tests:** Histologic examination of biopsy specimens obtained by endoscopy.
2. **Test for urease:** pH-sensitive dye tests for urease (e.g., CLO test) performed on biopsy specimens (*H. pylori* produces urease, which hydrolyzes urea to ammonia [a base] and CO_2).
3. **Breath urea tests:** These measure labeled CO_2 in expired air after oral administration of radiolabeled urea (after being formed, CO_2 diffuses into the bloodstream and is expired).
4. **Serologic tests:** These are for IgG antibody against *H. pylori*. Antibody may be positive after effective treatment.
5. **Treatment:** Antibiotics (e.g., clarithromycin) and proton pump inhibitors (e.g., omeprazole).

E. **TESTS FOR CARBOHYDRATE MALABSORPTION**
1. **Fecal pH**
a. Purpose: To screen for carbohydrate malabsorption.
b. Method: Dip a portion of nitrazine pH paper into the liquid portion of a fresh stool specimen and compare with the color chart provided.
c. Interpretation: pH <5.5 suggests carbohydrate malabsorption.
2. **Stool reducing substances**
a. Purpose: To screen for carbohydrate malabsorption by measuring reducing substances (lactose, maltose, fructose, galactose) in stool.
b. Method: Place a small amount of fresh liquid stool in a test tube and dilute with twice its volume of water. Centrifuge and place 15 drops of the supernatant in a second test tube containing a Clinitest tablet. Compare the resulting color with the chart provided for urine testing. To screen for malabsorption of sucrose (not a reducing substance) use 1mol/L HCl instead of water and boil for 30 seconds before centrifuging.
c. Interpretation
   1) >0.5% reducing substance suggests carbohydrate malabsorption.
   2) 0.25–0.5% is indeterminate.
   3) <0.25% is normal.
3. **Breath hydrogen test**
a. Purpose: To diagnose malabsorption of a specific carbohydrate by measuring hydrogen gas in expired air after an oral load of the carbohydrate in question.
b. Method: Have infants fast for 4–6 hours, older children for 12 hours. Give a 2g/kg (max. 50g) oral load of the desired carbohydrate as a 20% solution (10% in infants <6 months of age). Place nasal prongs or an air-tight face mask attached to a 20mL syringe with stopcock (other collection systems available) on the child, and aspirate 5mL of end-expiratory air for four consecutive breaths before the carbohydrate load and every 30 minutes for 3 hours thereafter. Inject samples into red-topped glass tubes and send for measurement of H_2 by gas chromatography.

Note: Do not give antibiotics for 1 week before test.

c. Interpretation: H_2 is produced by bacterial fermentation of undigested carbohydrate in the bowel, diffuses into the blood, and is expelled in expired air. A rise in H_2 >20 ppm above the lowest test value obtained suggests malabsorption of the test carbohydrate. An elevated baseline and/or a rise in H_2 >20 ppm above baseline within 30 minutes suggests small bowel bacterial overgrowth.

4. **Monosaccharide and disaccharide absorption**
a. Purpose: To diagnose malabsorption of a specific carbohydrate (glucose [a monosaccharide] or lactose, maltose, fructose, galactose, or sucrose [disaccharides]) by measuring the change in blood glucose after an oral load of the carbohydrate in question. Most useful when breath test is not available.
b. Method: Have patient fast for 4–6 hours before test. Give a 2g/kg (max. 50g) oral load of the desired carbohydrate as a 10% solution. For maltose give 1g/kg. Measure serum glucose before carbohydrate dose and 30, 60, 90, and 120 minutes after the dose. Test all stools passed during and for 8 hours after the test for pH and reducing substances.
c. Interpretation
   1) Rise in blood glucose <20mg/dL over the baseline suggests malabsorption of the test carbohydrate.
   2) Malabsorption is also suggested if, during or within 8 hours of the test, the patient develops diarrhea, stool pH of <5.5, or >0.5% of stool-reducing substances.

5. **D-Xylose test**
a. Purpose: To screen for small bowel malabsorption by measuring the amount of D-xylose absorbed after an oral load. Unreliable in patients with edema, renal disease, delayed gastric emptying, severe diarrhea, rapid transit time, or small bowel bacterial overgrowth.
b. Method: Have infants fast for 4–6 hours, older children for 8 hours. Give a 14.5g/m^2 (max. 25g) oral load of D-xylose as a 10% water solution. Ensure adequate urine output using supplementary oral or IV fluid, collect all urine for 5 hours, and send for quantitation. Alternatively, send serum specimens for D-xylose concentration before the load and 30, 60, 90, and 120 minutes after the load.
c. Interpretation (urine)
   1) Children >6 months old
      a) 5 hours urinary excretion of <15% of the oral load suggests malabsorption.
      b) 15–24% is indeterminate.
      c) ≥25% is normal.
   2) Infants <6 months old: 5 hours urinary excretion <10% suggests malabsorption.
d. Interpretation (serum): Failure of the serum level to exceed 25mg/dL in any of the postabsorptive specimens suggests malabsorption.

F. TESTS FOR FAT MALABSORPTION: QUANTITATIVE FECAL FAT

1. **Purpose:** To screen for fat malabsorption by quantitating fecal fat excretion.

2. **Method:** Patient should be on a normal diet (<35% fat) with the amount of calories and fat ingested recorded for 2 days before the test and during the test itself. Collect and freeze all stools passed within 72 hours, and send to the laboratory for determination of total fecal fatty acid content.

3. **Interpretation**

a. Total fecal fatty acid excretion of >5g fat/24 hours may suggest malabsorption.

Note: Results will vary with amount of fat ingested and normal values have not been established for children <2 years old.

b. The coefficient of absorption (CA) is a more accurate indicator of malabsorption and does not vary with fat intake:

$$CA = (\text{g fat ingested} - \text{g fat excreted})/(\text{g fat ingested}) \times 100$$

c. Malabsorption is suggested by the following:

1) Preterm infants: CA <60–75%.

2) Full-term infants: CA <80–85%.

3) 10 months to 3 years old: CA <85–95%.

4) >3 years old: CA <95%.

Note: Quantitative fecal fat is recommended over qualitative methods (e.g., staining with Sudan III), which depend on spot checks and are thus unreliable for diagnosing fat malabsorption.

G. OCCULT BLOOD

1. **Purpose:** To screen for the presence of blood through detection of heme in stool.

2. **Method:** Smear a small amount of stool on the test areas of an occult blood test card (such as Hemoccult) and allow to air dry. Apply developer as directed.

3. **Interpretation:** A blue color resembling that of the control indicates the presence of heme. Brisk transit of ingested red meat and inorganic iron may yield a false-positive result.

Note: Low pH diminishes the sensitivity of a Hemoccult card. Use a Gastroccult or similar card when testing gastric contents for the presence of heme.

REFERENCE

1. Mezo H et al. *Contemp Pediatr* 1994; **2**:60–92.

GENETICS

Amy B. Hirshfeld, MD

When evaluating any child for a genetic disorder, one of the most valuable tools is the **three-generation pedigree.** For each family member, note age, sex, and medical status or cause of death. Specifically ask about family history of neonatal or childhood deaths, mental retardation, developmental delay, birth defects, seizure disorders, known genetic disorders, ethnicity, consanguinity, infertility, miscarriages, and stillbirths.

13

I. INBORN ERRORS OF METABOLISM: ABNORMALITIES OF BIOCHEMICAL PATHWAYS

Inborn errors of metabolism (IEMs) may present any time from the neonatal period to adulthood. Although these disorders are often thought of as rare, when considered collectively, they represent significant treatable causes of morbidity and mortality. For further details on IEMs see references[1-4].

A. PRESENTATIONS

1. **Neonatal onset:** Commonly presents as a previously healthy full-term neonate, who at 24–72 hours of age develops anorexia, lethargy, vomiting, and/or seizures. One in five sick **full-term** neonates with no risk factors for infection will have metabolic disease.

2. **Late onset (>28 days old):** Many IEMs can present beyond the newborn period if the defect is partial. In addition, some disorders characteristically present late.

a. Typical symptoms: Vomiting, respiratory distress, and changes in mental status, including confusion, lethargy, irritability, aggressive behavior, hallucinations, seizures, and coma. A history of unusual dietary preferences (e.g., protein avoidance) may be elicited.

b. Symptoms are usually brought on by intercurrent illness, prolonged fast, dietary indiscretion, or any process causing increased catabolism.

c. Examples of late-onset disorders

  1) Medium-chain acyl-CoA dehydrogenase deficiency (MCAD): Most common age of onset 3–18 months; may present earlier or later. (See p. 271 for further details.)

  2) Symptomatic ornithine transcarbamylase (OTC) heterozygote

   a) Presentation: Girls with vomiting and change in mental status.

   b) The only urea cycle defect that is X-linked recessive.

   c) Laboratory findings: Elevated ammonium, respiratory alkalosis; plasma amino acids and urine orotic acid are diagnostic.

d) Therapy
  i) Acute management (see p. 268).
  ii) Long-term therapy of protein restriction, citrulline supplementation, and oral sodium phenylbutyrate (Buphenyl).

B. **FAMILY HISTORY:** Initially inquire about sibling deaths, male deaths on the mother's side, and consanguinity. When the patient is stable, obtain a full three-generation pedigree (see p. 265).

C. **LABORATORY EVALUATION OF SUSPECTED METABOLIC DISEASE**

1. **Initial laboratory tests:** For sample collection requirements, see Table 13.1.

TABLE 13.1

SAMPLE COLLECTION

Specimen	Volume (mL)	Tube[a]	Handling
Plasma ammonium	1–3	Green top	On ice; immediate transport to laboratory; levels rise rapidly on standing.
Plasma amino acids[b]	1–3	Green top	On ice; if must store, spin down, separate plasma and freeze.
Plasma carnitine	1–3	Green top	On ice.
Acylcarnitine profile	Saturate newborn screen filter paper with blood		Dry and mail to reference laboratory.
Lactate	3	Gray top	On ice.
Karyotype	3	Green top	Room temperature.
Very-long-chain fatty acids	3	Purple top	Room temperature.
White blood cells for enzymes/DNA	3	Purple top	Room temperature.
Urine organic acids	5–10	—	Deliver immediately or freeze.
Urine amino acids	5–10	—	Deliver immediately or freeze.
Skin biopsy		Tissue culture medium or patient's plasma	Refrigerate; do not freeze.

[a]Additives in tubes: purple, K_3EDTA; green, lithium heparin; gray, potassium oxalate and sodium fluoride.
[b]Obtain after a 3-hour fast.

a. Blood
   1) Complete blood count.
   2) Electrolytes (calculate anion gap), aspartate aminotransferase (AST), alanine aminotransferase (ALT), total and direct bilirubin.
   3) Glucose.

Note: Infants and children with profound hypoglycemia should have laboratory tests listed on p. 268 before treatment with glucose.
   4) Blood gas.
   5) Plasma ammonium.
   6) Plasma lactate.

b. Urine
   1) Dipstick: pH, ketones, glucose, protein, bilirubin.
   2) Odor (Table 13.2).
   3) Urine-reducing substances: For method, see p. 443. Disorders associated with a positive test include[5]:
      a) Galactose: Galactosemia, galactokinase deficiency, severe liver disease.
      b) Fructose: Hereditary fructose intolerance, essential fructosuria.
      c) Glucose: Diabetes mellitus, renal tubular defects.
      d) *p*-Hydroxyphenylpyruvic acid: Tyrosinemia.
      e) Xylose: Pentosuria.

Note: The evaluation of jaundice in a neonate should include urine-reducing substances to rule out galactosemia.
2. **Further laboratory tests:** If the initial evaluation is suspicious for metabolic disease, obtain the following tests and consult a geneticist. **Early diagnosis and appropriate therapy are essential for preventing irreversible brain damage and death.**
a. Plasma amino acids.
b. Quantitative plasma carnitine.
c. Urine organic acids.

13

GENETICS

TABLE 13.2

UNUSUAL URINE ODORS

Disease	Odor
ACUTE DISEASE	
Maple syrup urine disease	Maple syrup, burned sugar
Isovaleric acidemia	Cheesy or sweaty feet
Multiple carboxylase deficiency	Cat's urine
3-OH,3-methyl glutaryl-CoA lyase deficiency	Cat's urine
NONACUTE DISEASE	
Phenylketonuria	Musty
Hypermethioninemia	Rancid butter, rotten cabbage
Trimethylaminuria	Fishy

d. If lactate elevated, obtain serum pyruvate and repeat lactate.
e. If lumbar puncture performed, freeze 1–2mL of cerebrospinal fluid for later analysis.

D. DIFFERENTIAL DIAGNOSIS

1. **Abnormal urine odors** (Table 13.2 on p. 267)
2. **Interpretation of initial laboratory findings** (Table 13.3)
3. **Differential diagnosis of hyperammonemia** (Fig. 13.1 on p. 270)

E. GENERAL ACUTE MANAGEMENT OF IEMS

1. Stop dietary sources of protein.
2. D_{10} at 1.5–2 times maintenance delivers 10–15mg/kg per minute of glucose to stop catabolism. (A catabolic state results in an endogenous protein load.)
3. Add Na^+/K^+ based on degree of dehydration and electrolyte results.
4. In severe dehydration give bolus of NS. D_{10} should still be piggybacked in at 1.5–2 times maintenance to stop catabolism.
5. HCO_3^- replacement for severe acidosis (pH <7.1) only.
6. In cases of hyperammonemia give sodium benzoate 250mg/kg (5.5g/m^2) IV and sodium phenylacetate 250mg/kg (5.5g/m^2) IV, and arginine-HCl (10% solution) 6mL/kg (12g/m^2) IV. (Benzoate and phenylacetate are substrates for alternate pathways of nitrogen excretion; arginine supplementation allows continued operation of the urea cycle in defects in which the block is proximal to arginine.)

Note: These are experimental drugs and should be used only in consultation with a geneticist. Overdose may cause death.

a. Give these doses as a bolus over 90 minutes.
b. Repeat the same doses over 24 hours as a maintenance dose.
c. Ondansetron may be used to decrease nausea and vomiting associated with these drugs.

7. If unresponsive to this medical management, institute hemodialysis promptly.

a. Hemodialysis will probably be required in neonates because of the inherently catabolic state.
b. Hemodialysis is 10 times more efficient than peritoneal dialysis.
c. Exchange transfusion should *not* be used.

II. RECURRENT HYPOGLYCEMIA

This may result from endocrine disorders or IEMs, including defects in gluconeogenesis, glycogen breakdown (glycogen storage diseases), and fatty acid oxidation, as well as toxic impairment of gluconeogenesis (organic acidemias).

A. LABORATORY EVALUATION: The following tests should be drawn before giving glucose:

1. Blood gas.
2. Electrolytes.
3. Chemistry panel.

TABLE 13.3

DIFFERENTIAL DIAGNOSIS OF SUSPECTED METABOLIC DISEASE

Deficient pathway	Amino acid metabolism	Urea cycle	Carbohydrate metabolism	Fatty acid oxidation	Organic acid metabolism	Energy metabolism
Example	Maple syrup urine disease	OTC deficiency	Glycogen storage disease type I	Medium-chain acyl-coA dehydrogenase deficiency	Methylmalonic acidemia	Pyruvate dehydrogenase complex deficiency
Test						
Blood pH	Acidic	Alkaline	Acidic	Variable	Acidic	Acidic
Anion gap	↑	Normal	↑	±	↑	↑
Ketones	↑	Negative	↑	Inappropriately low	↑	– or ↑
Lactate	Normal	Normal	↑	Slight ↑	Normal or ↑	Markedly ↑
Glucose	Variable	Normal	↓	→	Normal or ↑	± →
NH_4^+	Normal or slight ↑	Markedly ↑	Normal	Moderate ↑	Normal or ↑	± ↑
FTT	Yes	Yes	Yes	No	Yes	Yes
Developmental delay	Yes	Yes	No	No	Yes	Yes
Neurologic signs	Lethargy to coma, hypertonia	Irritable, combative, coma, hypotonia	Hypoglycemic seizures	Lethargy to coma	Lethargy to coma, hypotonia	Lethargy to coma, hypotonia

13

GENETICS

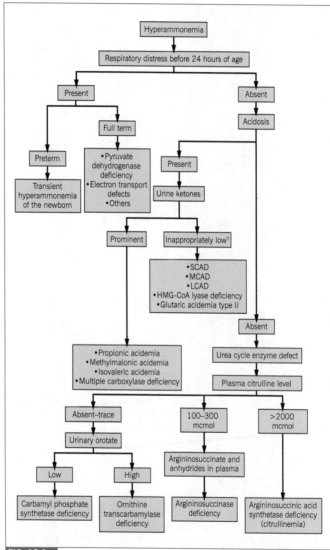

FIG. 13.1

Differential diagnosis of hyperammonemia. Dagger indicates hypoglycemia present when symptomatic. HMG-CoA, hydroxymethylglutaryl-CoA; LCAD, long-chain acyl-CoA dehydrogenase; MCAD, medium-chain acyl-CoA dehydrogenase; SCAD, short-chain acyl-CoA dehydrogenase.

4. Gray-top glucose.
5. Plasma lactate.
6. Insulin, growth hormone, and cortisol.
7. Plasma amino acids, acylcarnitine profile, quantitative carnitine levels, and urine for ketones should also be sent but may be obtained after giving glucose.

B. **GLYCOGEN STORAGE DISEASE TYPES I AND III**
1. **Presentation:** Hepatomegaly, symptomatic hypoglycemia.
a. Type I (glucose-6-phosphatase deficiency) typically presents at 1–2 months of age; prominent hepatomegaly; symptomatic with fasting >3 hours.
b. Type III (glycogen debrancher deficiency) often presents at >6 months of age; when trying to get a child to sleep through the night; symptomatic with fasting for about 8–12 hours.
2. **Laboratory findings:** Hypoglycemia and lactic acidemia after short fast; elevated AST, ALT, cholesterol, uric acid (type I only), and lactate at baseline.
3. **Definitive diagnosis:** Liver biopsy for enzyme assay.
4. **Therapy:** Frequent feedings, nocturnal nasogastric feedings; uncooked cornstarch.

C. **FATTY ACID OXIDATION DEFECTS:** Defects of the carnitine cycle or of β-oxidation: short-, medium-, long-, and very-long-chain acyl-CoA dehydrogenase deficiency, abbreviated as SCAD, MCAD, LCAD, and VLCAD, respectively. For each chain length there is a corresponding hydroxyacyl-CoA dehydrogenase deficiency: SCHAD, MCHAD, LCHAD, and VLCHAD.
1. **Presentation:** Change in mental status, emesis, or seizures after a prolonged fast or at time of increased caloric need; hepatomegaly; in some defects cardiomyopathy, dysrhythmias, or skeletal muscle weakness.
2. **Laboratory findings:** Hypoglycemia with **inappropriately low ketones** is the hallmark; moderately elevated LFTs and ammonia, low total carnitine, mild metabolic acidosis; different defects have characteristic patterns on organic acid, acylcarnitine, and acylglycine analyses.
3. **Therapy**
a. Acute: See p. 268; carnitine supplementation.
b. Chronic: Carnitine supplementation, avoidance of fasting, IV fluid with D_{10} if unable to maintain PO intake as a result of illness.

III. NEURODEGENERATIVE DISORDERS: ABNORMALITIES OF ORGANELLE FUNCTION

Note: Many other neurodegenerative disorders exist; an exhaustive list is beyond the scope of this chapter.

A. **LYSOSOMAL DISORDERS (e.g., THE MUCOPOLYSACCHARIDOSES):** Neurodegeneration with systemic storage resulting from lysosomal enzyme defects (Hurler, Hunter, Scheie, Sanfillipo, and Sly syndromes).

1. **Presentation:** Hepatosplenomegaly, corneal clouding (except Hunter), dysostosis multiplex, coarse features, neurologic deterioration.
2. **Laboratory findings:** Inclusion bodies on peripheral blood smear, positive urine mucopolysaccharide (MPS) spot; characteristic findings on eye examination and skeletal survey.
3. **Definitive diagnosis:** Assay of skin fibroblasts for specific lysosomal hydrolases.
4. **Therapy:** Experimental therapy with exogenous enzyme; bone marrow transplantation may provide some enzyme activity but cannot reverse brain damage.
B. **PEROXISOMAL DISORDERS:** Refsum syndrome, X-linked adrenoleukodystrophy (ALD), Zellweger syndrome, and others.
1. **Presentation:** Seizures, loss of milestones, loss of white matter on MRI. Progressive neurodegeneration, eventually death.
2. **Laboratory findings:** elevated very-long-chain fatty acids, pipecolic acid, phytanic acid, and plasmalogens.
3. **Definitive diagnosis:** Enzyme assays in cultured skin fibroblasts and microscopy of peroxisomes.
4. **Therapy:** Treat adrenal insufficiency if present; vitamin K. Research protocols: dietary lipid therapy, bone marrow transplant, and immunosuppression.

IV. NEWBORN METABOLIC SCREEN

All states screen for phenylketonuria and hypothyroidism; 15 of 50 states screen for various additional disorders.

A. **TIMING**
a. Screen after at least 24 hours of normal protein and lactose feeding.
b. Formula-fed infants may not have a diagnostic abnormality before 36 hours of age.
c. Breast-fed infants may not have a diagnostic abnormality before 48–72 hours of age.
d. Recommendations from American Academy of Pediatrics[6]:
   1) Screen all infants before hospital discharge. For normal term infants, screen as close as possible to hospital discharge.
   2) All infants should be screened by 7 days of age.
   3) If first screen is before 24 hours of age, rescreen by 14 days of age.

Note: Many geneticists recommend rescreening at 3 days of age if the first screen is before 24 hours of age.

B. **MANAGEMENT OF POSITIVE SCREENING RESULTS**
1. Sickle cell screen: See p. 310.
2. IEMs and hypothyroidism (Table 13.4 on pp. 274–275): State health departments have protocols for ongoing follow-up.

V. DYSMORPHOLOGY

The suspicion for many syndromes and chromosomal anomalies is often raised by major or minor anomalies noted on physical examination. The most common anomalies and commonly used diagnostic tests are listed. For more complete information see references[8,9].

A. PHYSICAL EXAMINATION

1. **Eyes**
   a. Hypotelorism and hypertelorism (outer and inner canthal distance [Figs. 13.2 and 13.3]). There are racial differences in interpupillary distance. See reference[13].
   b. Palpebral fissure length (Fig. 13.4) and angle.
   c. Epicanthal folds.
2. **Philtrum:** Long, short, or flat.
3. **Ears:** Ear pits or tags; low-set or posteriorly rotated ears.
4. **Jaw:** Micrognathia, retrognathia.
5. **Hands and feet:** Abnormal hand creases, fifth finger clinodactyly, syndactyly, polydactyly.
6. **Bone lengths**
   a. Rhizomelic shortening (shortening of proximal long bones) is typical of conditions such as achondroplasia.
   b. Proportionate dwarfism is characteristic of growth hormone deficiency.
   c. Upper:lower segment ratio (Fig. 13.5) is low in Marfan syndrome. Also measure arm span, equal to height in normal individuals. Other features of Marfan syndrome include arachnodactyly, scoliosis, and loose jointedness.

B. STRUCTURAL DIAGNOSTIC TESTS

1. **Brain MRI:** For structural defects in children with developmental delay.
2. **Ophthalmologic examination:** For optic atrophy, coloboma, cataracts, retinal abnormalities, lens subluxation, or corneal abnormalities.
3. **Echocardiography:** For structural defects.
4. **Abdominal ultrasonography:** For polysplenia or asplenia (liver–spleen scan is more accurate), absent or horseshoe kidney, ureteral or bladder defects, and abdominal situs.
5. **Skeletal survey:** For abnormalities of bone length or structure.

C. GENETIC DIAGNOSTIC TESTS

1. **Karyotype:** Detects abnormal numbers of chromosomes and deletions, duplications, translocations, and inversions large enough to be seen by light microscopy. For indications, see section VII.
2. **Fluorescence in situ hybridization (FISH):** Hybridization of a fluorescently tagged DNA probe to chromosomes allows detection of submicroscopic deletions and duplications. FISH assays are commonly available for the following syndromes: Williams (7q11), Prader–Willi and Angelman (15q11), Miller–Dieker (17p13.3), Smith–Magenis (17p11.2), velocardiofacial and DiGeorge (22q11).

Text continued on p. 278

13

GENETICS

TABLE 13.4

INITIAL MANAGEMENT OF ABNORMAL NEWBORN METABOLIC SCREEN RESULTS (MARYLAND)

Disease	Normal value	Abnormal value and response[a]		Definitive tests
		• Clinical evaluation[b] • Repeat screen within 48 hours	• Clinical evaluation[b] • Send definitive test • Telephone contact with referral center	• Clinical evaluation • Send definitive test • Immediate transfer to referral center	
Phenylketonuria (Phe in mg/dL)	Phe <2	Phe 2–6	Phe 6–12	Phe >12	Plasma amino acids (Phe, Tyr), biopterins
Maple syrup urine disease[c] (Leu in mg/dL)	Leu <2	Leu 2–4 *Check urine ketones; if positive, transfer to referral center*	Leu 4–8 *Restrict protein to 1.5g/kg per day; check urine ketones; if positive, transfer to referral center*	Leu > 8	Plasma amino acids (Val, Leu, Ile)
Homocystinuria (Met in mg/dL)	Met <1	Met 1–6	Met >6	—	Plasma amino acids (Met), plasma homocysteine
Tyrosinemia (Tyr in mg/dL)	Tyr <12	Tyr = 12	Tyr >12, ≤20 *Limit diet to 2g protein/kg per day, 120 kcal/kg per day*	Tyr > 20	Plasma amino acids (Tyr, Phe); urine for succinylacetone

Galactosemia[c] (sugar in mg/dL) Note: sugar = galactose + galactose-1-P	Beutler FST nl sugar <10	Beutler FST and sugar 10–40 or Beutler FST abnl and sugar <10 *Check urine reducing subs; if positive, remove lactose from diet, contact referral center*	Beutler FST abnl and sugar ≥10 or Beutler FST nl and sugar >40 *Check urine reducing subs; remove lactose from diet*	Galactose-1-P uridyltransferase; UDP galactokinase; gal-4-epimerase; galactose; galactose-1-phosphate
Biotinidase deficiency	Colorimetric biotinidase assay nl	Colorimetric biotinidase assay abnl	—	Plasma biotinidase RIA, urine organic acids
Hypothyroidism Term infant ≤1 week old	T_4 within 2SD of mean; TSH <30mcIU/mL	T_4 >2SD below mean; TSH <100mcIU/mL	T_4 >2SD below mean; TSH >100mcIU/mL *Start levothyroxine after drawing tests*	T_4, free T_4, TSH; thyroid-binding globulin or T_3 resin uptake
Hypothyroidism Term infant >1 week old	T_4 within 2SD of mean; TSH <30mcIU/mL	T_4 >2SD below mean; TSH <50mcIU/mL	T_4 >2 SD below mean; TSH >50mcIU/mL *Start levothyroxine after drawing tests*	—

Adapted from Maryland Department of Health and Human Hygiene Newborn Screening Follow-up Protocol and Elsas[7].

nl, normal; abnl, abnormal.

[a] Disease-specific responses in italics.

[b] More aggressive interventions should be undertaken if clinical evaluation is worrisome.

[c] Maple syrup urine disease and galactosemia can be rapidly fatal if untreated; err on the side of aggressive evaluation and treatment.

13

GENETICS

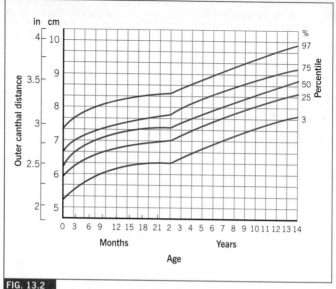

FIG. 13.2

Outer canthal distance. (Redrawn from Feingold[10].)

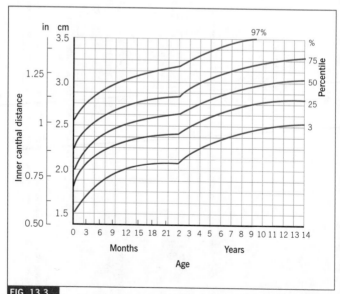

FIG. 13.3

Inner canthal distance.

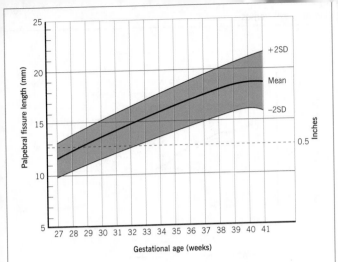

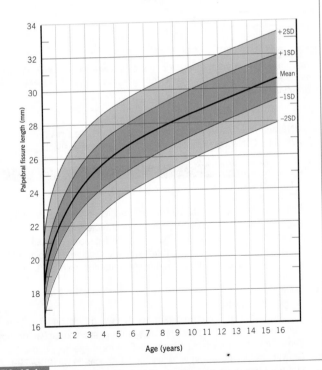

FIG. 13.4
Palpebral fissure length. **A,** Preterm infants. **B,** Children up to 16 years old. (Redrawn from Hall[8].)

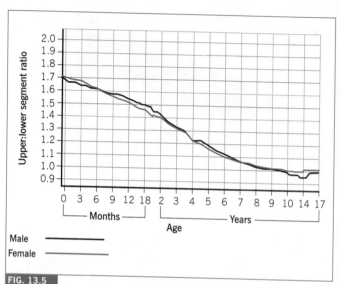

FIG. 13.5
Normal upper:lower segment ratio by age. The lower segment = distance from pubic symphysis to floor. Ratio = Upper segment/Lower segment = [Height − Lower segment]/Lower segment.

3. **DNA analysis:** Many monogenic disorders now have DNA tests available. Contact your laboratory for a list of those available.

VI. COMMON SYNDROMES

A. TRISOMY 21

1. **Incidence:** 1:660.
2. **Features:** Presence of 6 of 10 cardinal features in the neonate is highly suggestive of the diagnosis: Hypotonia, poor Moro reflex, hyperflexibility, excess skin on back of neck, flat facies, slanted palpebral fissures, anomalous auricles, pelvic dysplasia, dysplasia of the midphalanx of fifth finger, and single transverse palmar (Simian) crease.
3. **Testing**
   a. Diagnosis: Karyotype.
   b. Follow-up testing: Echocardiogram, yearly thyroid function tests, LFTs, CBC, and audiologic evaluation; radiographs of atlantooccipital junction and ophthalmologic examination by 3–5 years of age[11].
   c. Growth charts for children with trisomy 21 appear on pp. 296–299.
4. **Natural history:** Cardiac defects (50%), GI atresias (12%), mental retardation (100%), leukemia (1%), thyroid disease (15%), hearing loss (75%), serous otitis media (50–70%), and eye disease (60%).

Fifty percent of those with congenital heart defects survive to age 30; eighty percent of those without congenital heart defects survive to age 30.

B. **TRISOMY 18**
1. **Incidence:** 1:3000 with 3:1 female predominance.
2. **Features:** Clenched hand with index finger overlapping third and fifth finger overlapping fourth, intrauterine growth retardation, decreased fetal activity, low-arch dermal ridge pattern, inguinal or umbilical hernia, cardiac defects, prominent occiput, low-set ears, micrognathia, rocker bottom feet.
3. **Testing:** Karyotype with FISH analysis allows results within 24–48 hours.
4. **Natural history:** Apnea, severe failure to thrive; 50% die by 1 week, 90% by 1 year; profound mental retardation in survivors.

C. **TRISOMY 13**
1. **Incidence:** 1:5000.
2. **Features:** Holoprosencephaly, polydactyly, scalp skin defects, seizures, deafness, microcephaly, sloping forehead, cleft lip, cleft palate, retinal anomalies, microphthalmia, abnormal ears, single umbilical artery, inguinal hernia, omphalocele, cardiac defects, urinary tract malformations.
3. **Testing:** Karyotype with FISH analysis allows results within 24–48 hours.
4. **Natural history:** 44% die within 1 month; >70% die by 1 year; profound mental retardation in survivors.

D. **45,X (TURNER SYNDROME)**
1. **Incidence:** 1:5000.
2. **Features:** Short female with broad chest, wide-spaced nipples, webbed neck, congenital lymphedema. Gonadal dysgenesis (90%), renal anomalies (60%), cardiac defects (20%), most commonly coarctation of the aorta, hearing loss (50%).
3. **Testing**
a. Diagnosis: Karyotype.
b. Follow-up testing: Baseline echocardiogram, renal ultrasound; BP, hearing, and scoliosis screen with each examination; thyroid function tests and echocardiogram every 1–2 years[12].
c. Growth charts for girls with Turner syndrome appear on p. 300.
4. **Natural history:** Infertility, normal lifespan, mean IQ 90, short stature.

E. **FRAGILE X**
1. **Incidence:** 1:1500 males; 6% of boys with mental retardation; 0.3% of girls with mental retardation.
2. **Features:** Boys: Mild to profound mental retardation, cluttered speech, autism (60%), macrocephaly, large ears, prognathism, **postpubertal** macroorchidism, tall stature. Phenotype most prominent in boys; girls may have only learning disabilities.

13

GENETICS

3. Testing
a. Karyotype of lymphocytes cultured in folate-deficient medium reveals nonstaining gap present at Xq27.3, site of a CGG expansion. The number of CGG repeats correlates with disease severity.
b. DNA analysis.
4. **Natural History:** Normal lifespan.

VII. GENETIC CONSULTATION

A. INDICATIONS FOR REFERRAL
1. Known or suspected hereditary disorder.
2. Major physical anomalies, unusual body proportions, short stature, dysmorphic features.
3. Major organ malformation.
4. Developmental delay or mental retardation; learning disabilities in females who have brothers with mental retardation.
5. Complete or partial blindness or hearing loss.
6. Deterioration of motor or speech abilities in a previously thriving child.
7. Maternal exposure to drugs, alcohol, or radiation during pregnancy.
8. Strong family history of cancer.
9. Failure to thrive if routine evaluation unrevealing.

B. INDICATIONS FOR PRENATAL COUNSELING
1. Genetic disorder or birth defect in one partner.
2. Known carrier of a genetic disorder.
3. Previous child with known or suspected genetic disorder.
4. Maternal age >35 years.
5. Family history of known or suspected chromosomal anomaly.
6. Multiple early miscarriages or stillbirths.
7. Member of an ethnic group known to have a high incidence of a specific genetic disorder.

C. INDICATIONS FOR KARYOTYPE
1. Two major OR one major and two minor malformations (include small for gestational age and mental retardation as major).
2. Features of a specific chromosomal syndrome.
3. At risk for familial chromosomal aberration.
4. Ambiguous genitalia.
5. More than two spontaneous abortions or infertility (karyotype both partners).
6. Girls with short stature.

VIII. REFERENCES

1. Scriver CR, Beaudet AL, Sly WS, Valle D. *The molecular and metabolic bases of inherited disease,* 7th edn. New York: McGraw-Hill; 1995.
2. Epstein CJ, assoc. ed. Genetic disorders and birth defects. In: Rudolph AM, Hoffman JIE, Rudolph CD, eds. *Rudolph's pediatrics,* 20th edn. Norwalk, CT: Appleton & Lange; 1996.

3. Seidel HM, Rosenstein BJ, Pathak A. *Primary care of the newborn,* 2nd edn. St Louis: Mosby; 1997.

4. Seashore M, Wappner R. *Genetics in primary care and clinical medicine.* Norwalk, CT: Appleton & Lange; 1996.

5. Burton BK, Nadler HL. Clinical diagnosis of the inborn errors of metabolism in the neonatal period. *Pediatrics* 1978; **61:**398–405.

6. American Academy of Pediatrics, Committee on Genetics. Issues in newborn screening. *Pediatrics* 1992; **89:**345–349.

7. Elsas LJ. Newborn screening. In: Rudolph AM, Hoffman JIE, Rudolph C. *Rudolph's pediatrics,* 20th edn. Norwalk, CT: Appleton & Lange; 1996, 282–288.

8. Hall JG, Froster-Iskenius UG, Allanson JE. *Handbook of normal physical measurements.* Oxford, England: Oxford Medical Publications, 1989.

9. Jones K. *Smith's recognizable patterns of human malformation,* 5th edn. Philadelphia: WB Saunders; 1997.

10. Feingold M, Bossert WH. Normal values for selected physical parameters: an aid to syndrome delineation. *Birth Defects Orig Artic Ser* 1974; **10**(13):1–16.

11. American Academy of Pediatrics, Committee on Genetics. Health supervision for children with Down syndrome. *Pediatrics* 1994; **93:**855–859.

12. American Academy of Pediatrics, Committee on Genetics. Health supervision for children with Turner syndrome. *Pediatrics* 1995; **96:**1166–1173.

13. Pirnick EK, Rivas ML, Tolley EA, Smith SD, Presbury GJ. Interpupillary distance in a normal black population. *Clin Genet* 1999; **55:**182–191.

13

GENETICS

GROWTH CHARTS

George K. Siberry, MD, MPH

14

I. PRETERM INFANTS (Fig. 14.1)

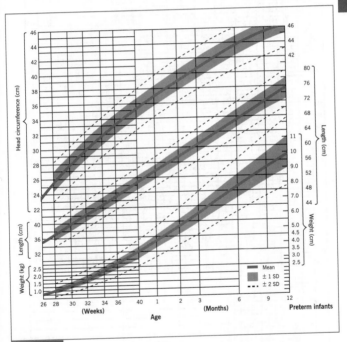

FIG. 14.1
Length, weight, and head circumference for preterm infants. (Adapted from Babson[1].)

II. GIRLS: BIRTH TO 36 MONTHS
A. LENGTH AND WEIGHT (Fig. 14.2)

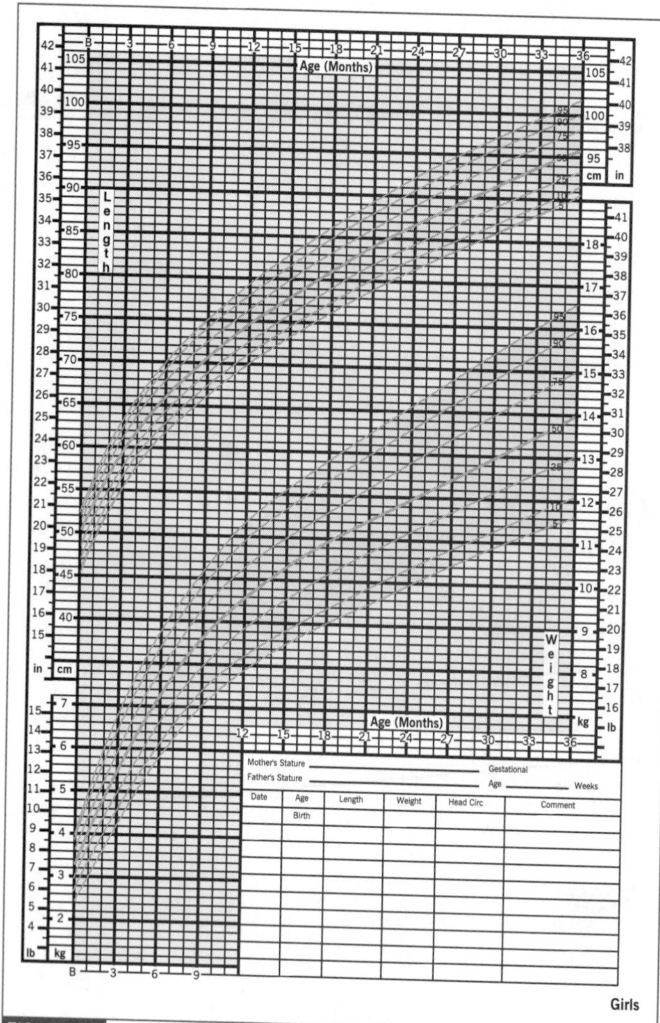

FIG. 14.2

Length and weight for girls from birth to 36 months. (Adapted from Hamill[2]. Data from the Fels Longitudinal Study, Wright State University School of Medicine, Yellow Springs, Ohio. Courtesy Ross Laboratories 1982.)

B. HEAD CIRCUMFERENCE AND LENGTH–WEIGHT RATIO (Fig. 14.3)

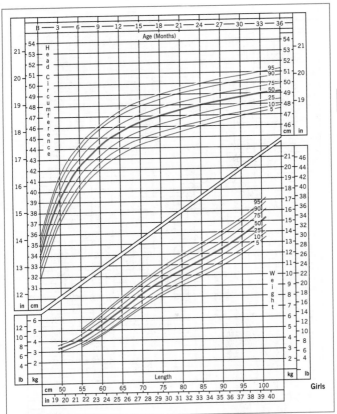

FIG. 14.3

Head circumference and length–weight ratio for girls, from birth to 36 months. (Adapted from Hamill[2]. Data from the Fels Longitudinal Study, Wright State University School of Medicine, Yellow Springs, Ohio. Courtesy Ross Laboratories 1982.)

Note: Revised CDC/NCHS growth charts are expected in 1999. They include length, weight, head circumference, and weight-for length for birth to 36 months of age and stature, weight, and BMI for 2–19 years of age.

III. BOYS: BIRTH TO 36 MONTHS
A. LENGTH AND WEIGHT (Fig. 14.4)

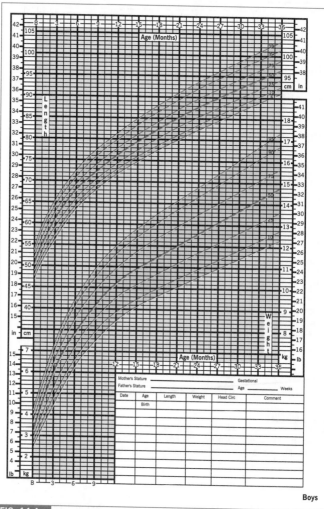

FIG. 14.4

Length and weight for boys from birth to 36 months. (Adapted from Hamill[2]. Data from the Fels Longitudinal Study, Wright State University School of Medicine, Yellow Springs, Ohio. Courtesy Ross Laboratories 1982.)

B. HEAD CIRCUMFERENCE AND LENGTH–WEIGHT RATIO (Fig. 14.5)

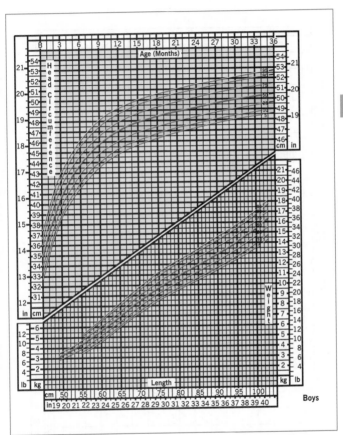

FIG. 14.5

Head circumference and length–weight ratio for boys from birth to 36 months.
(Adapted from Hamill[2]. Data from the Fels Longitudinal Study, Wright State University
School of Medicine, Yellow Springs, Ohio. Courtesy Ross Laboratories 1982.)

IV. GIRLS: 2–18 YEARS
A. STATURE AND WEIGHT (Fig. 14.6)

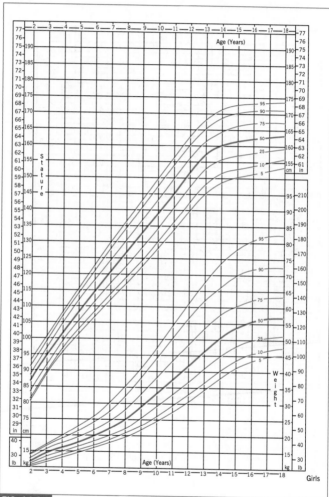

FIG. 14.6

Stature and weight for girls 2–18 years. (Adapted from Hamill[2].)

B. STATURE–WEIGHT RATIO (Fig. 14.7)

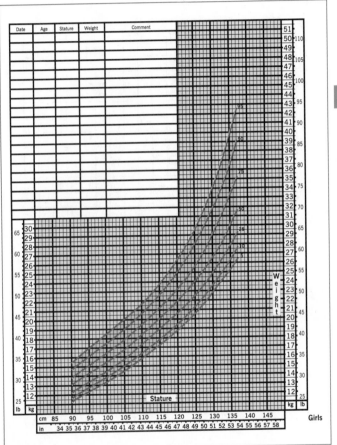

14

GROWTH CHARTS

FIG. 14.7

Stature–weight ratio for girls 2–18 years. (Adapted from Hamill[2].)

C. HEIGHT VELOCITY (Fig. 14.8)

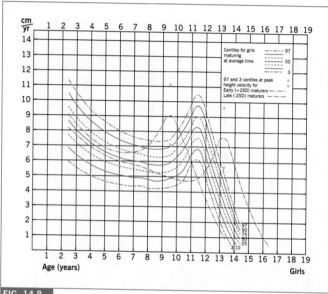

FIG. 14.8
Height velocity for girls 2–18 years. (Adapted from Tanner[3]. Courtesy Castlemead Publications, 1985. Distributed by Sereno Laboratories.)

V. BOYS: 2–18 YEARS
A. STATURE AND WEIGHT (Fig. 14.9)

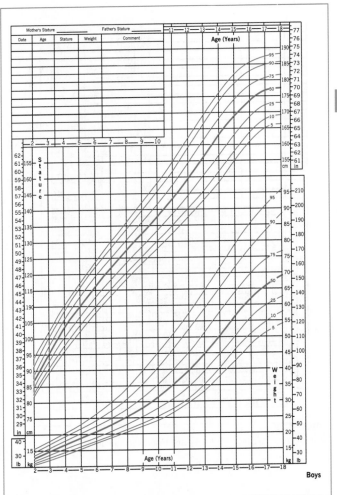

14

GROWTH CHARTS

FIG. 14.9
Stature and weight for boys 2–18 years. (Adapted from Hamill[2].)

B. STATURE–WEIGHT RATIO (Fig. 14.10)

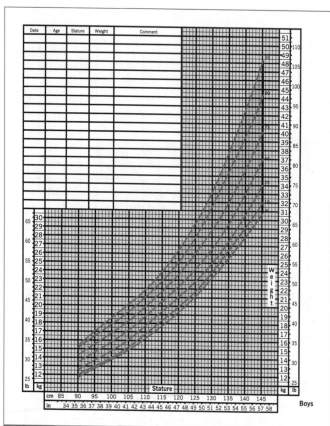

FIG. 14.10

Stature–weight ratio for boys 2–18 years. (Adapted from Hamill[2].)

C. HEIGHT VELOCITY (Fig. 14.11)

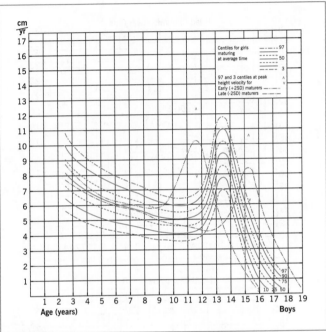

FIG. 14.11
Height velocity for boys 2–18 years. (Adapted from Tanner[3]. Courtesy Castlemead Publications, 1985. Distributed by Sereno Laboratories.)

VI. HEAD CIRCUMFERENCE: GIRLS AND BOYS 2–18 YEARS
(Fig. 14-12)

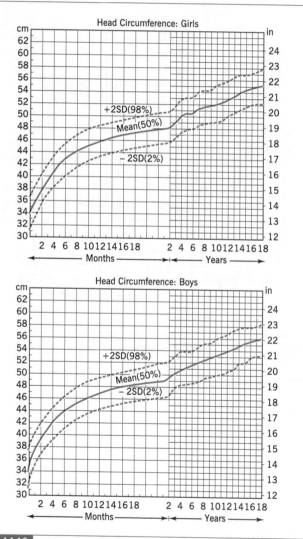

FIG. 14.12
Head circumference for boys and girls 2–18 years. (Adapted from Nelhaus[4].)

VII. BODY SURFACE AREA NOMOGRAM AND EQUATION
(Fig. 14.13)

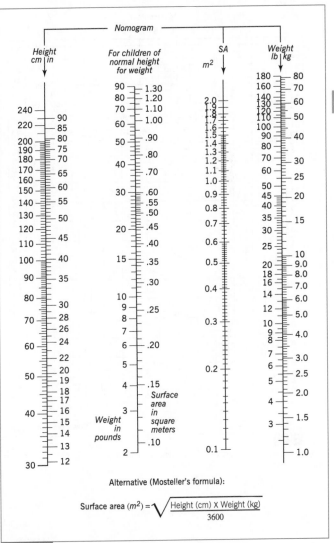

Alternative (Mosteller's formula):

$$\text{Surface area } (m^2) = \sqrt{\frac{\text{Height (cm) X Weight (kg)}}{3600}}$$

FIG. 14.13
Body surface area nomogram and equation. (Data from Briars[5].)

VIII. DOWN SYNDROME

A. LENGTH AND WEIGHT FOR BOYS WITH DOWN SYNDROME FROM BIRTH TO 36 MONTHS (Fig. 14.14)

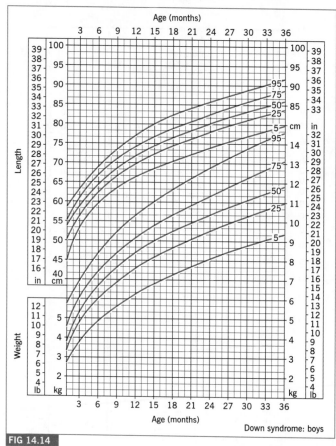

FIG 14.14

Length and weight for boys with Down syndrome, from birth to 36 months. (Adapted from Cronk[6].)

B. LENGTH AND WEIGHT FOR GIRLS WITH DOWN SYNDROME FROM BIRTH TO 36 MONTHS (Fig. 14.15)

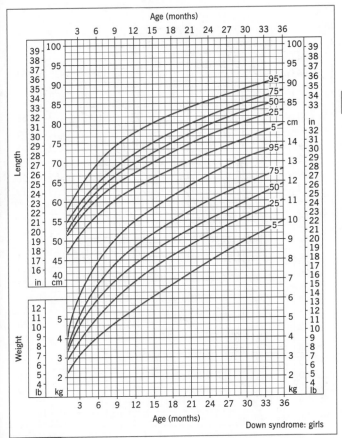

FIG 14.15

Length and weight for girls with Down syndrome, from birth to 36 months. (Adapted from Cronk[6].)

C. **STATURE AND WEIGHT FOR BOYS WITH DOWN SYNDROME FROM 2–18 YEARS** (Fig. 14.16)

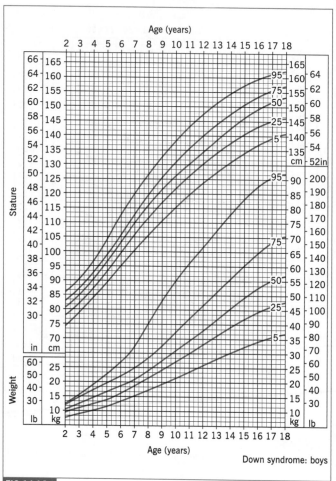

FIG 14.16

Stature and weight for boys with Down syndrome 2–18 years. (Adapted from Cronk[6].)

D. STATURE AND WEIGHT FOR GIRLS WITH DOWN SYNDROME FROM 2–18 YEARS (Fig. 14.17)

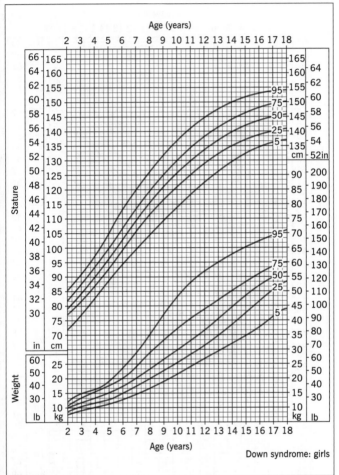

FIG 14.17

Stature and weight for girls with Down syndrome 2–18 years. (Adapted from Cronk[6].)

IX. TURNER SYNDROME: PHYSICAL GROWTH FOR GIRLS 2–18 YEARS (Fig. 14.18)

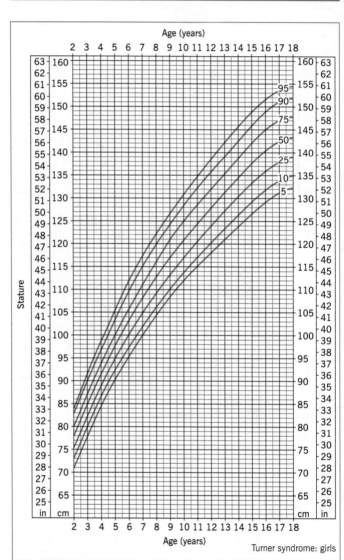

FIG 14.18

Stature for girls with Turner's syndrome 2–18 years. (From Lyon[7]. Courtesy Genentech, Inc, 1987.)

X. ACHONDROPLASIA

A. HEIGHT FOR BOYS WITH ACHONDROPLASIA FROM BIRTH TO 18 YEARS (Fig. 14.19)

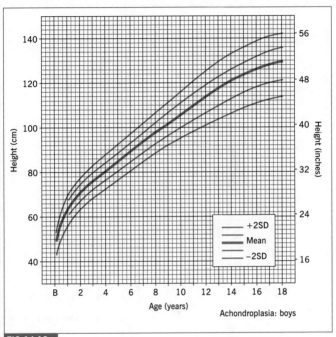

FIG 14.19

Height for boys with achondroplasia, from birth to 18 years. (From Horton[8].)

B. **HEIGHT FOR GIRLS WITH ACHONDROPLASIA FROM BIRTH TO 18 YEARS** (Fig. 14.20)

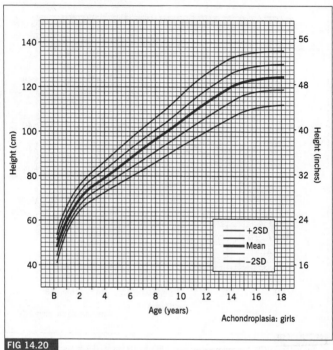

FIG 14.20
Height for girls with achondroplasia, from birth to 18 years. (From Horton[8].)

C. HEAD CIRCUMFERENCE FOR BOYS WITH ACHONDROPLASIA FROM BIRTH TO 18 YEARS (Fig. 14.21)

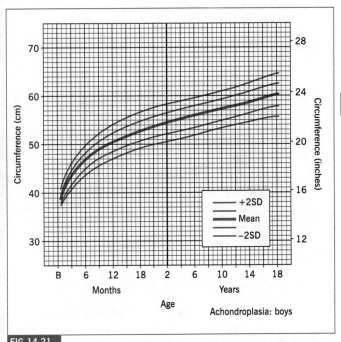

14

GROWTH CHARTS

FIG 14.21
Head circumference for boys with achondroplasia, from birth to 18 years. (From Horton[8].)

D. **HEAD CIRCUMFERENCE FOR GIRLS WITH ACHONDROPLASIA FROM BIRTH TO 18 YEARS** (Fig. 14.22)

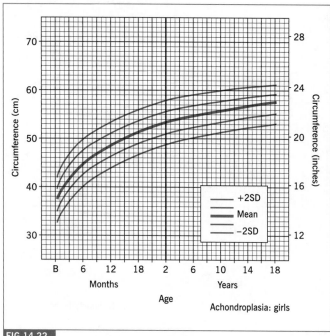

FIG 14.22
Head circumference for girls with achondroplasia, from birth to 18 years. (From Horton[8].)

XI. REFERENCES FOR GROWTH CHARTS IN OTHER CONDITIONS
A. **SICKLE CELL ANEMIA**[9]
B. **CYSTIC FIBROSIS**[10]

XII. DENTAL DEVELOPMENT (Table 14.1)

TABLE 14.1

CHRONOLOGY OF HUMAN DENTITION OF PRIMARY OR DECIDUOUS
AND SECONDARY OR PERMANENT TEETH

	Age at eruption		Age at shedding	
	Maxillary	Mandibular	Maxillary	Mandibular
PRIMARY TEETH				
Central incisors	6–8mo	5–7mo	7–8yr	6–7yr
Lateral incisors	8–11mo	7–10mo	8–9yr	7–8yr
Cuspids (canines)	16–20mo	16–20mo	11–12yr	9–11yr
First molars	10–16mo	10–16mo	10–11yr	10–12yr
Second molars	20–30mo	20–30mo	10–12yr	11–13yr
SECONDARY TEETH				
Central incisors	7–8yr	6–7yr		
Lateral incisors	8–9yr	7–8yr		
Cuspids (canines)	11–12yr	9–11yr		
First premolars (bicuspids)	10–11yr	10–12yr		
Second premolars (bicuspids)	10–12yr	11–13yr		
First molars	6–7yr	6–7yr		
Second molars	12–13yr	12–13yr		
Third molars	17–22yr	17–22yr		

From Behrman[11].

XIII. REFERENCES

1. Babson SG, Benda GI. Growth graphs for the clinical assessment of infants of varying gestational age. *J Pediatr* 1976; **89**:815.
2. Hamill PV, Drizd TA, Johnson CL, Reed RB, Roche AF, Moore WM. Physical growth: National Center for Health Statistics percentiles. 1979; **32**:607–629.
3. Tanner JM, Davis PS. Clinical longitudinal standards for height and height velocity for North American children. *J Pediatr* 1985; **107**:317–329.
4. Nelhaus G. *J Pediatr* 1968; **41**:106.
5. Briars GL, Bailey BJ. Surface area estimation: pocket calculator v nomogram. *Arch Dis Child* 1994; **70**:246–247.
6. Cronk C, Crocker AC, Pueschel SM, Shea AM, Zackai E, Pickens G, Reed RB. Growth charts for children with Down syndrome: 1 month to 18 years of age. *Pediatrics* 1988; **81**:102–110.
7. Lyon AJ, Preece MA, Grant DB. Growth curve for girls with Turner syndrome. *Arch Dis Child* 1985; **60**:932–935.

8. Horton WA, Rotter, JI, Rimoin DL, Scott CI, Hall JG. Standard growth curves for achondroplasia. *J Pediatr* 1978; **93**:435–438.

9. Platt OS, Rosenstock W, Espeland MA. Influence of sickle hemoglobinopathies on growth and development. *N Engl J Med* 1984; **311**:7–12.

10. Cystic Fibrosis Foundation, 1985.

11. Behrman RE, Kliegman RM, Arvin AM. *Nelson textbook of pediatrics,* 15th edn. Philadelphia: WB Saunders; 1996.

HEMATOLOGY

Beth E. Ebel, MD, MSc
Leslie Raffini, MD

I. HEMATOLOGIC INDICES

See Fig. 15.3 and Table 15.8 for age-specific red cell indices.

A. HEMATOCRIT (HCT): Packed cell volume. Volume percentage of red blood cells (RBCs) in plasma.

a. Falsely high HCTs caused by increased plasma trapping occur with short centrifugation time and in disorders with decreased RBC deformability (e.g., iron deficiency). Most HCTs are now done by automated methods and are not affected by centrifugation.

B. MEAN CORPUSCULAR VOLUME (MCV): Average RBC volume, directly measured by automatic cell counters, in femtoliters (10^{-15}L).

C. MEAN CORPUSCULAR HEMOGLOBIN (MCH): Average quantity of hemoglobin per RBC, in picograms (10^{-12}g).

D. MEAN CORPUSCULAR HEMOGLOBIN CONCENTRATION (MCHC): Grams of hemoglobin per 100mL packed RBCs—high in congenital spherocytosis and normal newborns; may be high in hemoglobin SC or SS disease; low in microcytic anemia, including iron deficiency.

E. RED CELL DISTRIBUTION WIDTH (RDW): Coefficient of variation in RBC size. Increased in anisocytosis, reticulocytosis, iron deficiency, and hemolysis, and in newborns.

F. RETICULOCYTE COUNT: Reticulocytes are young RBCs with remnants of cytoplasmic RNA. A special stain such as brilliant cresyl blue is used to count reticulocytes.

1. **Corrected reticulocyte count (CRC):** Corrected for differences in HCT, CRC is an indicator of erythropoietic activity. CRC >1.5 suggests increased RBC production as a result of hemolysis or blood loss.

$$CRC = \% \text{ Reticulocytes} \times \text{Patient HCT/Normal HCT}$$

II. ANEMIA

A. GENERAL EVALUATION: Anemia is defined by age-specific norms. See Table 15.8. Evaluation includes the following:

1. **Complete history:** Includes symptoms of anemia, blood loss, fatigue, pica, medication exposure, growth and development, nutritional history, ethnic background, and family history of anemia, splenectomy, or cholecystectomy.

2. **Physical examination:** Includes tachypnea, tachycardia, cardiac murmur, pallor, scleral icterus, jaundice, hepatosplenomegaly, glossitis, and signs of systemic illness.

3. **Initial laboratory tests:** These may include a complete blood count (CBC) with RBC indices, reticulocyte count, blood smear, stool for occult blood, urinalysis, and serum bilirubin.

B. **DIAGNOSIS:** Anemias may be categorized as macrocytic, microcytic, or normocytic. Table 15.1 gives a differential diagnosis of anemia based on RBC production and cell size. Note that normal hemoglobin and MCV are age dependent. Table 15.2 outlines the common causes of microcytic anemia.

C. **EVALUATION OF SPECIFIC CAUSES OF ANEMIA**

1. **Iron deficiency anemia:** Hypochromic/microcytic anemia with a low reticulocyte count and an elevated RDW.

a. Serum ferritin reflects total body iron stores after 6 months of age and is the first value to fall in iron deficiency. Ferritin is an acute phase reactant, and may be falsely elevated with inflammation or infection.

TABLE 15.1

CLASSIFICATION OF ANEMIA

Reticulocyte count	Microcytic anemia	Normocytic anemia	Macrocytic anemia

Low	Iron deficiency
	Lead poisoning
	Chronic disease
	Aluminum toxicity
	Copper deficiency
	Protein malnutrition
		Chronic disease
		RBC aplasia
		  (TEC, infection,
		  drug induced)
		Malignancy
		Juvenile rheumatoid
		  arthritis
		Endocrinopathies
		Renal failure
			Folate deficiency
			Vitamin B_{12} deficiency
			Aplastic anemia
			Congenital bone
			  marrow dysfunction
			  (Diamond–Blackfan or
			  Fanconi syndromes)
			Drug induced
			Trisomy 21
			Hypothyroidism

Normal	Thalassemia trait Sideroblastic anemia	Acute bleeding Hypersplenism Dyserythropoietic anemia II	—

High	Thalassemia
	  syndromes
	Hemoglobin C
	  disorders
		Antibody-mediated
		  hemolysis
		Hypersplenism
		Microangiopathy
		  (HUS, TTP, DIC,
		  Kasabach–Merritt)
		Membranopathies
		  (spherocytosis,
		  elliptocytosis)
		Enzyme disorders
		  (G6PD, pyruvate
		  kinase)
		Hemoglobinopathies
			Dyserythropoietic
			  anemia I, III
			Active hemolysis

From Oski[13].

TEC, transient erythroblastopenia of childhood; HUS, hemolytic uremic syndrome; TTP, thrombotic thrombocytopenic purpura; DIC, disseminated intravascular coagulation; G6PD, glucose-6-phosphate

b. Other indicators include a low serum iron or transferrin, and an elevated total iron-binding capacity (TIBC).

c. Free erythrocyte protoporphyrin (FEP) accumulates when the conversion of protoporphyrin to heme is blocked. Elevated in iron deficiency, plumbism, and erythrocyte protoporphyria. Levels >300mcg/dL generally found only with lead intoxication.

d. Iron therapy (see p. 744) should result in an increased reticulocyte count in 2-3 days and an increase in HCT after 1–4 weeks of therapy.

2. **Hemolytic anemia:** Rapid RBC turnover. Etiologies includes congenital membranopathies, hemoglobinopathies, enzymopathies, metabolic defects, and immune-mediated destruction. Useful studies include:

a. Reticulocyte count: Usually elevated and indicates increased production of RBCs to compensate for increased destruction.

b. Increased plasma aspartate transaminase (AST) and lactate dehydrogenase (LDH) from release of intracellular enzymes.

c. Haptoglobin: Binds free hemoglobin; decreased with intravascular and extravascular hemolysis.

d. Hemopexin: Binds free heme groups; decreased primarily with intravascular hemolysis.

e. Direct Coombs' test (DCT): Tests for the presence of antibody on patient RBCs. Can be falsely negative if affected cells have already been destroyed or antibody titer is low.

f. Glucose-6-phosphate dehydrogenase (G6PD) assay: Used to diagnose G6PD deficiency, an X-linked disorder. May be normal immediately after a hemolytic episode as older, more enzyme-deficient cells have been lysed. See Table 31.4, p. 913, for a list of oxidizing drugs.

15

HEMATOLOGY

TABLE 15.2

COMMON CAUSES OF MICROCYTIC ANEMIA

	Iron deficiency	β-Thalassemia trait	Chronic inflammation
Reticulocyte count	Low	Normal to ↑	Normal
RDW	↑	↓	Normal
Ferritin	↓	Normal to ↑	Normal to ↑
FEP	↑	Normal	↑
Iron	↓	Normal	↓
TIBC	↑	Normal	↓
Electrophoresis	Normal	↑ HbA₂	Normal
ESR	Normal	Normal	↑
Smear	Hypochromic, target cells, microcytic, fine basophilic stippling	Normochromic, microcytic, coarse basophilic stippling	Variable

ESR, erythrocyte sedimentation rate; FEP, free erythrocyte protoporphyrin; Hb, hemoglobin; RDW, red cell distribution width; TIBC, total iron-binding capacity.

g. Osmotic fragility test: Useful in diagnosis of hereditary spherocytosis.

h. Heinz body preparation: Precipitated hemoglobin within RBCs; present in unstable hemoglobinopathies and during oxidative stress (e.g., G6PD deficiency).

3. **Red cell aplasia:** Normocytic or macrocytic, low reticulocyte count, variable platelet and white blood cell count.

a. Congenital aplasias (macrocytic), including the following:

1) Diamond–Blackfan–Oski syndrome: Autosomal recessive pure RBC aplasia; presents in the first year of life. Associated with congenital anomalies in one third, including triphalangeal thumb, short stature, and cleft lip.

2) Fanconi's anemia: Autosomal recessive; usually presents before 10 years of age; and may present with pancytopenia. May have absent thumbs, renal anomalies, microcephaly, or short stature. Chromosomal fragility studies (e.g., diepoxybutane) may be diagnostic.

b. Transient erythroblastopenia of childhood (TEC): Occurs from age 6 months to 4 years; >80% after 1 year of age. Normal or slightly low MCV, low reticulocyte count; usual spontaneous recovery within 4–8 weeks.

c. Infectious causes, including parvovirus in children with rapid RBC turnover (infects RBC precursors), Epstein–Barr virus (EBV), cytomegalovirus (CMV), human herpes virus 6 (HHV-6).

d. Aplastic anemia.

e. Bone marrow aspiration: Evaluates RBC precursors in the marrow to look for bone marrow dysfunction, neoplasm, or specific signs of infection. May not be necessary for the diagnosis of TEC or aplastic crisis.

III. HEMOGLOBINOPATHIES

A. **HEMOGLOBIN ELECTROPHORESIS:** Separation of hemoglobin variants based on molecular charge and size. All positive sickle preparations and solubility tests for sickle hemoglobin (e.g., Sickledex) should be confirmed with electrophoresis or isoelectric focusing (a component of the mandatory newborn screen in many states) (Table 15.3).

B. **SICKLE CELL ANEMIA:** Genetic defect in β-globin present in 1:500 African–Americans; 8% of African-Americans are carriers.

1. **Diagnosis:** Often made on newborn screen with hemoglobin electrophoresis. The sickle preparation and Sickledex are both rapid tests that are positive in all sickle hemoglobinopathies (sickle trait [AS], sickle cell anemia [SS], sickle-C [SC], sickle β–thalassemia [Sβ-thal], and others). May get false negatives in neonates and other patients with a high percentage of fetal hemoglobin.

C. **THALASSEMIAS:** Defects in α- or β-globin production. α-Thalassemia minor (two-gene deletion) occurs in 1.5% of African–Americans and is common in Southeast Asians. β-Thalassemia is found throughout the Mediterranean, Middle East, India, and Southeast Asia. It can be difficult to distinguish between α- and β-thalassemia and iron deficiency. The Mentzer index is useful: MCV/RBC >13.5 suggests iron deficiency; <11.5 is suggestive of thalassemia minor. Electrophoresis in β-thalassemia minor will show 3–8% HbA_2 and may show 2–4% fetal hemoglobin(Table 15.3). Hemoglobin electrophoresis in α-thalassemia minor will be normal (except in a neonate in whom there will be some HbA_2 and 1–2% HbBarts (γ_4)). There are many other abnormal hemoglobins, including unstable forms and those with variations in oxygen affinity.

TABLE 15.3
NEONATAL HEMOGLOBIN (Hb) ELECTROPHORESIS PATTERNS[a]

FA	Fetal Hb and adult normal Hb; the normal newborn pattern.
FAV	Indicates the presence of both HbF and HbA. However, an anomalous band (V) is present, which does not appear to be any of the common Hb variants.
FAS	Indicates fetal Hb, adult normal HbA and HbS, consistent with benign sickle cell trait.
FS	Fetal and sickle HbS without detectable adult normal HbA. Consistent with homozygous sickle Hb genotype (S/S) or sickle β–thalassemia, with manifestations of sickle cell anemia during childhood.
FC[b]	Designates the presence of HbC without adult normal HbA. Consistent with clinically significant homozygous HbC genotype (C/C), resulting in a mild hematologic disorder presenting during childhood.
FSC	HbS and HbC present. This heterozygous condition could lead to the manifestations of sickle cell disease during childhood.
FAC	HbC and adult normal HbA present, consistent with benign HbC trait.
$FSAA_2$	Heterozygous HbS/β-thalassemia, a clinically significant sickling disorder.
FAA_2	Heterozygous HbA/β-thalassemia, a clinically benign hematologic condition.
F[b]	Fetal HbF is present without adult normal HbA. Although this may indicate a delayed appearance of HbA, it is also consistent with homozygous β-thalassemia major, or homozygous hereditary persistence of fetal HbF.
FV[b]	Fetal HbF and an anomalous Hb variant (V) are present.
AF	May indicate prior blood transfusion. Submit another filter paper blood specimen when the infant is 4mo of age, at which time the transfused blood cells should have been cleared.

[a]Hemoglobin variants are reported in order of decreasing abundance; for example, 'FA' indicates more fetal than adult hemoglobin.
[b]Repeat blood specimen should be submitted to confirm the original interpretation.

IV. NEUTROPENIA

A. DEFINITION: Neutropenia is defined as an absolute neutrophil count less than 1500/mm^3, though neutrophil counts vary with age (see Table 15.9). See Table 15.4 for a differential diagnosis of neutropenia. Children with significant neutropenia are at risk of bacterial and fungal infections. Granulocyte colony stimulating factor (GCSF) may be indicated. See p. 716. For management of fever and neutropenia, see p. 519.

TABLE 15.4

DIFFERENTIAL DIAGNOSIS OF CHILDHOOD NEUTROPENIA

Acquired	Congenital
Infection	Cyclic neutropenia
Immune	Severe congenital neutropenia (Kostmann syndrome)
Hypersplenism	
Vitamin B$_{12}$, folate, copper deficiency	Chronic benign neutropenia of childhood
Drugs or toxic substances	Schwachman syndrome
Aplastic anemia	Fanconi syndrome
Malignancies or preleukemic disorders	Metabolic disorders (amino acidopathies, glycogenosis)
Ionizing radiation	
	Osteopetrosis

V. THROMBOCYTOPENIA

A. DEFINITION: Platelet count less than 150,000/mm^3 (see Table 15.8).

B. DIFFERENTIAL DIAGNOSIS

1. **Idiopathic thrombocytopenic purpura (ITP):** Diagnosis of exclusion; can be acute or chronic. White cell count and hemoglobin are normal. Hemorrhagic complications are rare with platelet counts >20,000/mm^3. Many patients require no therapy. Treatment options include Rh (D) immune globulin (useful only in Rh-positive patients), intravenous immune globulin (IVIG), or corticosteroids, (see pp. 907–913). Splenectomy or chemotherapy may be considered in chronic cases. Platelet transfusions are not generally helpful, but may be necessary in life-threatening bleeding.

2. **Platelet alloimmunization:** A common cause of thrombocytopenia in newborns: Transplacental maternal antibodies (usually against PLA-1 antigen) cause fetal platelet destruction and in utero bleeding. If severe, a transfusion of maternal platelets will be more effective in raising the platelet count than random donor platelets. Diagnosis may be confirmed as follows:

   1) Mixing study of maternal plasma and paternal platelets.
   2) Absence of maternal PLA-1 antigen.
   3) Mixing study with patient plasma and a panel of known minor platelet antigens.

3. Other causes of thrombocytopenia include microangiopathic hemolytic anemias such as disseminated intravascular coagulation (DIC) and

hemolytic uremic syndrome (HUS), infection causing marrow suppression, drug-induced thrombocytopenia, marrow infiltration, cavernous hemangiomas (Kasabach–Merritt syndrome), thrombocytopenia with absent radii syndrome (TAR), thrombosis, hypersplenism, and other rare inherited disorders (e.g., Wiscott–Aldrich syndrome).

VI. COAGULATION (Figs 15.1 and 15.2)

A. **TESTS OF COAGULATION:** Note: An incorrect anticoagulant:blood ratio will give inaccurate results. See Table 15.10 for normal hematologic values.

1. **Activated partial thromboplastin time (aPTT):** Measures intrinsic system; requires factors V, VIII, IX, X, XI, XII, fibrinogen, and prothrombin. May be prolonged in heparin administration, hemophilia, von Willebrand's disease (VWD), DIC, and the presence of circulating inhibitors (e.g., lupus anticoagulants or other antiphospholipid antibodies).

2. **Prothrombin time (PT):** Measures extrinsic pathway; requires fibrinogen, prothrombin, and factors V, VII, and X. May be prolonged in deficiencies of vitamin K–associated factors, malabsorption, liver disease, DIC, coumadin administration, and circulating inhibitors.

15

HEMATOLOGY

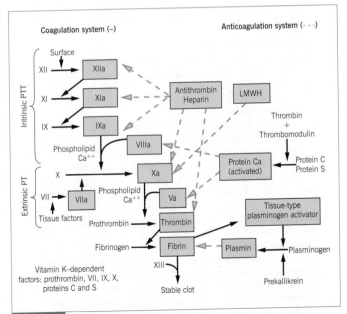

FIG. 15.1
Coagulation cascade. (Modified from Rosenberg[8].)

3. **Bleeding time (BT):** Evaluates clot formation, including platelet number and function, and von Willebrand's factor. (vWF). Performed at patient bedside.

Note: Always assess platelet number, and history of ingestion of platelet inhibitors such as NSAIDs, before bleeding time test.

B. **HYPERCOAGULABLE STATES:** Presents clinically as venous or arterial thrombosis.

1. **Congenital or genetic thrombotic risks:** Carefully assess family history of stroke, thrombosis, spontaneous abortion, etc.

a. Natural anticoagulants: Decreased levels of protein C, protein S, antithrombin III, or activated protein C resistance (factor V Leiden).

1) Protein C or protein S deficiency: Hereditary, autosomal dominant. In its homozygous form, it presents as neonatal purpura fulminans. Heterozygotes have a 3–6fold increased risk of venous thrombosis.

2) Antithrombin III deficiency: Hereditary, autosomal dominant. Homozygotes die in infancy; heterozygotes have increased risk of thrombus.

3) Activated protein C resistance (factor V Leiden): 2–5% of Caucasians are heterozygotes (5–10fold venous thrombosis risk); 1:1000 are homozygotes (80–100fold venous thrombosis risk).

b. Hyperhomocysteinemia: Increased levels of homocysteine associated with venous and arterial thromboses.

c. Others include prothrombin mutations, plasminogen abnormalities, and dysfibrinogenemia.

2. **Acquired thrombotic risks**

a. Endothelial damage: Indwelling vascular catheter, hypertension, surgery, smoking, diabetes, hyperlipidemia, and birth control pills.

b. Hyperviscosity: Macroglobulinemia, sickle-cell disease, and polycythemia.

c. Platelet activation: Essential thrombocytosis, oral contraceptives, and heparin-associated thrombocytopenia.

d. Antiphospholipid syndromes: Venous or arterial thrombosis and spontaneous abortions. Occurs commonly in patients with systemic lupus erythematosus or malignancies, and may occur transiently after a viral infection or during pregnancy. Characterized by prolonged aPTT, antibody detection, and prolonged dilute Russell's viper venom time (dRVVT).

e. Other: Includes procoagulant factors such as drugs (e.g., L-asparaginase), malignancies, liver disease, renal disease, nephrotic syndrome, infection, inflammatory disease, diabetes, and paroxysmal nocturnal hemoglobinuria.

3. **Laboratory evaluation**

a. Exclude common acquired causes as discussed previously. Initial laboratory screening includes coagulation studies; dRVVT; factor V Leiden PCR or activated protein C resistance assay; PCR for prothrombin 20210 mutation; activity assays for antithrombin III, protein C, and protein S; and total plasma homocysteine levels.

Note: The identification of one risk factor such as an in dwelling vascular
   catheter does not preclude the search for others, especially when
   accompanied by a family history of thrombus.

4. Treatment of thromboses

a. Heparin therapy: For deep venous thrombus or pulmonary embolus.
   1) Loading dose: 50–75units/kg IV over 30 minutes to 1 hour, followed
      by maintenance continuous infusion of heparin at 28 units/kg per
      hour if patient is <1 year old, or 20 units/kg per hour if ≥1 year
      old.
   2) Obtain aPTT level 6 hours after loading dose and adjust per Table
      15.5. Goal is aPTT at 1.5–2.5 times baseline aPTT.
   3) Heparin may be reversed with protamine (see p. 831).

b. Low-molecular-weight heparin (LMWH): This may be useful in
   children, although it is less studied and more costly than heparin.
   LMWH has more specific anti-Xa activity, a longer half-life, and a more
   predictable dose:efficacy ratio.
   1) Doses depend on preparation. Enoxaparin is given at a dose of
      1mg/kg SC or IV every 12 hours (see p. 704). Infants require higher
      doses (1.6mg/kg average); IV administration has not been studied in
      infants. One half of the treatment dose may be given for prophylaxis.

15

HEMATOLOGY

TABLE 15.5

ADJUSTMENT AND MONITORING OF HEPARIN THERAPY

aPTT control ratio	Rebolus/dose interruption	Heparin infusion adjustment
<1.2 ×	Repeat original load.	Increase by 5u/kg/hr.
1.2–1.4 ×	Repeat half original load.	Increase by 3u/kg/hr.
1.5–2.5 ×	None.	No change.
2.6–3.2 ×	None.	Decrease by 3u/kg/hr.
3.3–4.0 ×*	Stop infusion, recheck aPTT in 1hr. Restart infusion when aPTT is in or is projected to be in therapeutic range.	Decrease by 5u/kg/hr.
4.0–5.0 ×*	Stop infusion, recheck aPTT in 2hr. Restart infusion when aPTT is in or is projected to be in therapeutic range.	Decrease by 7u/kg/hr.
>5.0 ×*	Stop infusion; call hematologist on call immediately.	

From Johns Hopkins Hospital laboratory guidelines, 10/98.
Note: Draw aPTT 6hr after bolus dose, and repeat 6–8hr after every dose adjustment. Repeat daily
during stable dosing period. Check platelet count every third day until heparin is discontinued.
*Make sure sample not drawn from heparinized line.

2) Monitor LMWH therapy by following anti-Xa activity/mL. Therapeutic range is 0.6-1.0 unit/mL for full anticoagulation and 0.2-0.4 unit/mL for prophylactic dosing. The utility of monitoring levels is under investigation.

c. Coumadin: This may be used for long-term anticoagulation, although it carries significant risk for morbidity and mortality.

Note: Patient must be heparinized while initiating coumadin therapy secondary to hypercoagulability from decreased protein C and S levels.

1) Coumadin is usually administered orally at a loading dose of 0.1–0.2mg/kg per day for 2–3 days, followed by a daily dose sufficient to maintain the PT INR (international normalized ratio) in the desired range, usually 2–3 times baseline. Infants often require higher daily doses of coumadin. In all patients, levels should be followed every 1–2 weeks.

Note: Coumadin efficacy is greatly affected by dietary intake of vitamin K.

Note: as coumadin is protein bound, many drugs alter the therapeutic level, so concomitant medicines should be carefully reviewed.

2) Coumadin effect can be reversed with IV fresh frozen plasma (FPP) or the administration of vitamin K (see p. 885).

d. Thrombolytic therapy: consider urokinase or streptokinase.

Cautionary note: Children receiving anticoagulation therapy should be protected from trauma. Intramuscular injections are contraindicated. The use of antiplatelet agents and arterial punctures should be avoided.

C. **BLEEDING DISORDERS** (Fig. 15.2)
1. Disorders of platelet number or function
2. Inherited abnormalities of coagulation factors

a. Factor VIII deficiency (hemophilia A; X-linked disorder): Prolonged aPTT, reduced factor VIII activity. PT (prothrombin time) and BT are normal. Treat with factor VIII concentrate. Recombinant factor VIII is preferred to reduce risk of infection. The factor level is usually raised by 2% per 1 unit of factor VIII/kg (see Table 15.6 for desired level). Factor may need to be redosed based on the clinical scenario. The first dose has a shorter half-life, and a second dose, if needed, is given after 4–8 hours. Thereafter, the half-life is approximately 8–12 hours, and subsequent doses are usually Q12hr. Continuous infusion is often required for surgical patients—usually with a 50 unit/kg loading dose, followed by 3–4 units/kg per hour.

Units of factor VIII = Weight (kg) × Desired % replacement × 0.5

b. Factor IX deficiency (hemophilia B, Christmas disease; X-linked): Laboratory studies include a prolonged aPTT and low factor IX activity. Treat with factor IX concentrate. The factor level is usually raised by 1% for each unit of factor IX concentrate/kg; it has a half-life of 18–24

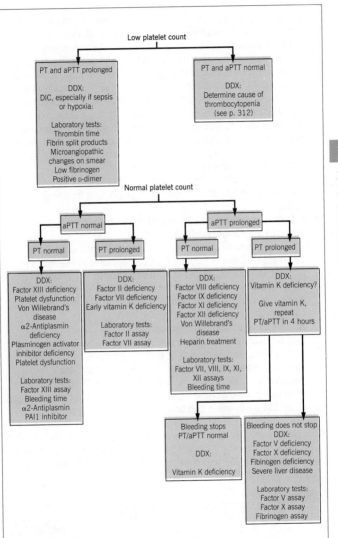

FIG. 15.2

Differential diagnosis of (DDX) bleeding disorders.

hours. As with factor VIII, a second dose, if needed, should be given at a shorter interval. Recombinant factor IX has a shorter half-life; consider evaluation of in vivo factor survival in each patient.

c. Von Willebrand's disease: The vWF binds platelets to subendothelial surfaces and carries factor VIII. Typical vWF type I is characterized by a prolonged BT and normal platelet count. The aPTT is usually mildly or moderately prolonged, and there is decreased ristocetin cofactor activity. Factor VIII and vWF levels are decreased in type 1 disease, but may be normal in variants with dysfunctional vWF. In patients with a proven response to desmopressin acetate (DDAVP), bleeding or minor surgical procedures may be treated with DDAVP, intravenously or intranasally (see p. 686), given over 20–30 minutes.

d. Aminocaproic acid, 100mg/kg IV or PO Q6hr (up to 24g/dy); may be useful for treatment of oral bleeds and prophylaxis for dental extractions.

Note: DDAVP is contraindicated in vWF type IIb because it may exacerbate thrombocytopenia.

For more severe disease or patients with dysfunctional vWF, the treatment of choice is Humate P (heat-inactivated vWF-enriched concentrate: 40mcg/kg), a similar product containing active vWF, or cryoprecipitate; note the associated infectious risks of these pooled blood products. Concentrates are preferred because they are virally inactivated.

3. Acquired coagulation factor abnormalities

a. DIC: Characterized by a prolonged PT and aPTT, decreased fibrinogen and platelets, increased fibrin degradation products and D-dimer. Treatment includes identifying and treating the underlying disorder. Replacement of depleted coagulation factors with FFP may be necessary in severe cases; 10–15mL/kg will raise the clotting factors by about 20%. Fibrinogen can be given as cryoprecipitate. Platelet transfusions may also be necessary.

b. Liver disease: The liver is the major site of synthesis for the following clotting factors: V, VII, IX, X, XI, XII, XIII, prothrombin, and fibrinogen. Treatment with FFP and platelets is as needed, but be aware that this

TABLE 15.6

DESIRED FACTOR REPLACEMENT IN HEMOPHILIA

Bleeding site	Desired level (%)
Joint or simple hematoma	20–40
Simple dental extraction	50
Major soft tissue bleed	80–100
Serious oral bleeding	80–100
Head injury	100+
Major surgery (dental, orthopedic, other)	100+

will increase the protein load. Vitamin K should be given to patients with liver disease and clotting abnormalities (see p. 885).

c. Vitamin K deficiency: Factors II, VII, IX, X and protein C and protein S are vitamin K dependent. Early vitamin K deficiency may present with isolated prolonged PT because factor VII has the shortest half-life.

d. Hemolytic uremic syndrome (HUS/TTP): Characterized by a microangiopathic hemolytic anemia, uremia, and thrombocytopenia. HUS does not typically include severe coagulation abnormalities, such as those seen in DIC.

VII. BLOOD COMPONENT REPLACEMENT

A. BLOOD VOLUME: Age specific (Table 15.7)

B. BLOOD PRODUCT COMPONENTS

1. **RBCs:** RBCs are given to improve tissue oxygenation and expand intravascular volume. The decision to transfuse RBCs should be made with consideration of clinical symptoms and signs, the degree of cardiorespiratory or CNS disease, the cause and course of anemia, and options for alternative therapy, noting the risks of transfusion-associated infections.

a. Packed RBC (PRBC) transfusion: Concentrated RBCs, with HCT of 55–70%. Typed, crossmatched product preferred where possible; O-negative or O-positive blood may be used if transfusion cannot be delayed. O-negative is preferred for females of or below child-bearing age to reduce risks of Rh sensitization.

b. Unless rapid replacement is required for acute blood loss or shock, infuse no faster than 2–3mL/kg per hour (generally 10mL/kg aliquots over 4 hours) to avoid congestive heart failure. A rule of thumb in severe compensated anemia is to give an 'x'mL/kg aliquot, where $x =$ hemoglobin (mg/dL); that is, if Hb = 5, transfuse 5mL/kg over 4 hours.

$$\text{Volume of PRBCs (mL)} = \text{EBV (mL)} \times \frac{\text{Desired HCT} - \text{Actual HCT}}{\text{HCT of PRBCs}}$$

where *EBV* is the estimated blood volume and *HCT of PRBC* is usually 55–70%.

15

HEMATOLOGY

TABLE 15.7

APPROXIMATE BLOOD VOLUME

Age	Total blood volume (mL/kg)	Age	Total blood volume (mL/kg)
Preterm infants	90–105	4–6yr	80–86
Term newborns	78–86	7–18yr	83–90
1–12mo	73–78	Adults	68–88
1–3yr	74–82		

From Nathan[3].

c. Leukocyte-poor PRBCs
   1) Leukocyte-poor filtered RBCs: 99.9% of white cells removed from product; used for cytomegalovirus-negative (CMV-negative) patients to reduce risk of CMV transmission. Also reduces likelihood of a nonhemolytic febrile transfusion reaction.
   2) Washed: 92–95% of white cells removed from product. Similar advantages to leukocyte-poor filtered RBCs. Although filtered leukocyte-poor blood is now more commonly used, washing may be helpful if a patient has preexisting antibodies to blood products such as patients who have complete IgA deficiency or who have a history of urticarial transfusion reactions.
   3) Use of leukocyte-poor PRBCS reduces the risk of subsequent acute febrile transfusion reactions from donor leukocytes.
d. Irradiated blood products
   1) Many blood products (PRBCs, platelet preparations, leukocytes, FFP, and others) contain viable lymphocytes capable of proliferation and engraftment in the recipient, causing graft-versus-host disease (GVHD). Irradiation with 1500cGy before transfusion may prevent GVHD, but does not prevent antibody formation against donor white cells. Engraftment is most likely in young infants, immuno-compromised patients, or patients receiving blood from first-degree relatives.
   2) Indications: Intensive chemotherapy, leukemia, lymphoma, bone marrow transplantation, solid organ transplantation, known or suspected immune deficiencies, intrauterine transfusions, and transfusions in neonates.
e. CMV-negative blood: Obtained from donors who test negative for CMV. May be given to neonates or other immunocompromised patients, including those awaiting organ or marrow transplant who are CMV negative.

2. **Platelets:** Treat severe or symptomatic thrombocytopenia.
a. Pooled concentrates: Pooled from multiple donors.
b. Single donor product: Hemopheresis product; preferred for patients with antiplatelet antibodies because of multiple transfusions.
c. Leukocyte-poor: Use if history of significant acute, febrile platelet transfusion reactions.
d. Usually give 4 units/m^2, or approximately 10mL/kg of normally concentrated platelet product. The platelet count is raised by 10,000–15,000/mm^3 by giving 1 unit/m^2. For infants and children, 10mL/kg will increase the platelet count by approximately 50,000/mm^3. Hemorrhagic complications are rare with platelet counts >10,000/mm^3. Platelet count >50,000/mm^3 is advisable for minor procedures such as lumbar puncture; >100,000/mm^3 is advisable for major surgery or intracranial operation. Peak posttransfusion concentration is reached 45–60 minutes after transfusion.

Note: Platelet products should not be refrigerated because this promotes premature platelet activation and clumping.

3. **FFP:** Contains all clotting factors except platelets. Used in severe clotting factor deficiencies with active bleeding or to reverse the effects of coumadin. Also may replace anticoagulant factors (antithrombin III, protein C, protein S). Used in treatment of DIC, vitamin K deficiency with active bleeding, or thrombotic thrombocytopenic purpura (TTP). Usual amount is 10–15mL/kg; repeat doses as needed. In TTP plasma exchange is often preferred.

4. **Cryoprecipitate:** Enriched for factor VIII (5–10 units/mL), vWF, and fibrinogen. Useful for children with factor VIII, fibrinogen, or vWF deficiency in the context of active bleeding.

5. **Monoclonal factor VIII:** Highly purified factor, derived from pooled human blood.

6. **Recombinant factor VIII or IX:** Highly purified, with less infectious risk than pooled human products. Risk of inhibitor formation, as with other products.

C. **PARTIAL PRBC EXCHANGE TRANSFUSION:** May be indicated for sickle cell patients with acute chest syndrome, stroke, intractable pain crisis, or refractory priapism. Replace with Sickledex-negative cells. Goal is to reduce percent HbSS to <40%. Follow HCT carefully during transfusion to avoid hyperviscosity, maintaining HCT <35%. To calculate the volume of PRBC needed for a double PRBC volume exchange:

$$\frac{EBV\ (mL) \times Patient\ HCT \times 2}{HCT\ of\ PRBC\ (55–70\%)}$$

where *EBV* is the estimated blood volume in milliliters and is age dependent (see Table 15.7).

D. **COMPLICATIONS OF TRANSFUSIONS**

1. **Acute transfusion reactions.**

a. Acute hemolytic reaction: Most often the result of blood group incompatibility. Signs and symptoms include fever, chills, tachycardia, hypotension, and shock. Treatment includes immediate cessation of blood infusion and institution of supportive measures. Laboratory findings include DIC, hemoglobinuria, and positive Coombs' test.

b. Febrile nonhemolytic reaction: Usually the result of host antibody response to donor leukocyte antigens, common in previously transfused patients. Symptoms include fever, chills, and diaphoresis. Stop transfusion and evaluate as previously described. Prevention includes premedication with antipyretics, antihistamines, and corticosteroids (see pp. 907–912).

c. Urticarial reaction: Reaction to donor plasma proteins. Stop transfusion immediately; treat with antihistamines and epinephrine if respiratory compromise. Use washed or filtered RBCs with next transfusion.

15

HEMATOLOGY

d. Evaluation of acute transfusion reaction.
   1) Patient's urine: Test for hemoglobin.
   2) Patient's blood: Confirm blood type, screen for antibodies, and repeat DCT on pretransfusion and posttransfusion sera.
   3) Donor blood: Culture for bacteria.

2. **Delayed transfusion reaction:** Minor blood group antigen incompatibility. Occurs 3–10 days after transfusion. Symptoms include fatigue, jaundice, and dark urine. Laboratory findings include anemia, a positive Coombs' test, new RBC antibodies, and hemoglobinuria.

3. **Transmission of infectious diseases:** Low incidence at present with increased vigilance in blood product screening. Data from 1991 to 1993 estimate the risk of transmitting infection as follows: human immunodeficiency virus, 1 in 493,000; human T-cell leukemia/lymphoma virus, 1 in 641,000; hepatitis B, 1 in 63,000; hepatitis C, 1 in 103,000. The aggregate risk was 1 in 34,000 (88% resulted from hepatitis viruses)[12]. Another transmitted infection included CMV.

4. **Sepsis:** This occurs secondary to a bacterial infection, which may occur in contaminated products, particularly platelets, as they are stored at room temperature.

VIII. TECHNIQUES

A. HCT TECHNIQUE

1. **Microhematocrit:** Fill standard microhematocrit tube with blood; seal one end with clay. Centrifuge (12,000 g) for 5 min. Now rarely performed because of the high risk of infection.

2. **Automatic cell counter:** Most laboratories generate a calculated HCT. Differences from manual counts include an inability to identify band neutrophils and confusion of reticulocytes with white blood cells.

B. WRIGHT'S STAINING TECHNIQUE

1. **Methodology:** Place air-dried blood smears, film side up, on staining rack. Cover smear with undiluted Wright's stain and leave for 2–3 minutes. Add equal volume of distilled water, and blow gently on the surface until a greenish metallic sheen appears. Leave diluted stain on smear for 2–6 minutes. Without disturbing the slide, flood with water and wash until stained smear is light red. Blot dry.

2. **Interpretation of blood smear** (see Plates 1–12): Examine the smear in an area where the RBCs are nearly touching but do not overlap.

a. RBCs: Look at RBC size, shape, and color.

b. White blood cells: A rough estimation of the count can be made by looking at the smear under high power ($100\times$ magnification with a $10\times$ objective and $10\times$ lens). Every 1 white cell per high-powered field correlates with approximately $500/mm^3$.

c. Platelets: Rough approximation: 1 platelet/oil immersion field corresponds to $10,000–15,000/mm^3$. Platelet clumps usually indicate $>100,000$ platelets/mm^3.

IX. REFERENCE TABLES

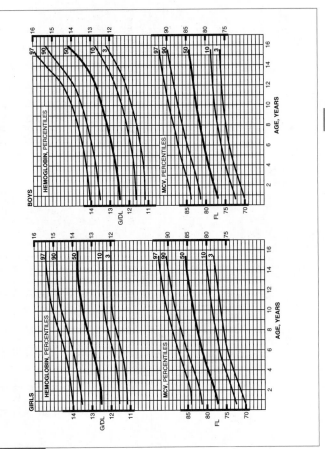

FIG. 15.3

Hemoglobin and mean corpuscular volume by age. (From Dallman[7].)

TABLE 15.8

AGE-SPECIFIC BLOOD CELL INDICES

Age	Hb (g%)[a]	HCT (%)[a]	MCV (fL)[a]	MCHC (g/% RBC)[a]	Reticulocytes	WBCs (×10³/mm³)[b]	Platelets (10³/mm³)[b]
26–30wk gestation[c]	13.4	41.5	118.2	37.9	—	4.4	254
	(11)	(34.9)	(106.7)	(30.6)		(2.7)	(180–327)
28wk	14.5	45	120	31.0	(5–10)	—	275
32wk	15.0	47	118	32.0	(3–10)	—	290
Term[d] (cord)	16.5 (13.5)	51 (42)	108 (98)	33.0 (30.0)	(3–7)	18.1 (9–30)[e]	290
1–3dy	18.5 (14.5)	56 (45)	108 (95)	33.0 (29.0)	(1.8–4.6)	18.9 (9.4–34)	192
2wk	16.6 (13.4)	53 (41)	105 (88)	31.4 (28.1)		11.4 (5–20)	252
1mo	13.9 (10.7)	44 (33)	101 (91)	31.8 (28.1)	(0.1–1.7)	10.8 (4–19.5)	
2mo	11.2 (9.4)	35 (28)	95 (84)	31.8 (28.3)			
6mo	12.6 (11.1)	36 (31)	76 (68)	35.0 (32.7)	(0.7–2.3)	11.9 (6–17.5)	
6mo–2 yr	12.0 (10.5)	36 (33)	78 (70)	33.0 (30.0)		10.6 (6–17)	(150–350)

2–6yr	12.5 (11.5)	37 (34)	81 (75)	34.0 (31.0)	(0.5–1.0)	8.5 (5–15.5)	(150–350)
6–12yr	13.5 (11.5)	40 (35)	86 (77)	34.0 (31.0)	(0.5–1.0)	8.1 (4.5–13.5)	(150–350)
12–18yr							
Male	14.5 (13)	43 (36)	88 (78)	34.0 (31.0)	(0.5–1.0)	7.8 (4.5–13.5)	(150–350)
Female	14.0 (12)	41 (37)	90 (78)	34.0 (31.0)	(0.5–1.0)	7.8 (4.5–13.5)	(150–350)
Adult							
Male	15.5 (13.5)	47 (41)	90 (80)	34.0 (31.0)	(0.8–2.5)	7.4 (4.5–11)	(150–350)
Female	14.0 (12)	41 (36)	90 (80)	34.0 (31.0)	(0.8–4.1)	7.4 (4.5–11)	(150–350)

Data from Forestier[1]; Oski[2]; Nathan[3]; Metoth[4]; and Wintrobe[5].

Hb, hemoglobin.

[a] Data are mean (–2SD).

[b] Data are mean (+2SD).

[c] Values are from fetal samplings.

[d] <1mo, capillary hemoglobin exceeds venous: 1hr – 3.6g difference; 5dy – 2.2g difference; 3wk – 1.1g difference.

[e] Mean (95% confidence limits).

TABLE 15.9
AGE-SPECIFIC LEUKOCYTE DIFFERENTIAL

Age	Total leukocytes[a] Mean (range)	Neutrophils[b] Mean (range)	%	Lymphocytes Mean (range)	%	Monocytes Mean	%	Eosinophils Mean	%
Birth	18.1 (9–30)	11 (6–26)	61	5.5 (2–11)	31	1.1	6	0.4	2
12hr	22.8 (13–38)	15.5 (6–28)	68	5.5 (2–11)	24	1.2	5	0.5	2
24hr	18.9 (9.4–34)	11.5 (5–21)	61	5.8 (2–11.5)	31	1.1	6	0.5	2
1wk	12.2 (5–21)	5.5 (1.5–10)	45	5.0 (2–17)	41	1.1	9	0.5	4
2wk	11.4 (5–20)	4.5 (1–9.5)	40	5.5 (2–17)	48	1.0	9	0.4	3
1mo	10.8 (5–19.5)	3.8 (1–8.5)	35	6.0 (2.5–16.5)	56	0.7	7	0.3	3
6mo	11.9 (6–17.5)	3.8 (1–8.5)	32	7.3 (4–13.5)	61	0.6	5	0.3	3
1yr	11.4 (6–17.5)	3.5 (1.5–8.5)	31	7.0 (4–10.5)	61	0.6	5	0.3	3
2yr	10.6 (6–17)	3.5 (1.5–8.5)	33	6.3 (3–9.5)	59	0.5	5	0.3	3
4yr	9.1 (5.5–15.5)	3.8 (1.5–8.5)	42	4.5 (2–8)	50	0.5	5	0.3	3
6yr	8.5 (5–14.5)	4.3 (1.5–8)	51	3.5 (1.5–7)	42	0.4	5	0.2	3
8yr	8.3 (4.5–13.5)	4.4 (1.5–8)	53	3.3 (1.5–6.8)	39	0.4	4	0.2	2
10yr	8.1 (4.5–13.5)	4.4 (1.5–8.5)	54	3.1 (1.5–6.5)	38	0.4	4	0.2	2
16yr	7.8 (4.5–13.0)	4.4 (1.8–8)	57	2.8 (1.2–5.2)	35	0.4	5	0.2	3
21yr	7.4 (4.5–11.0)	4.4 (1.8–7.7)	59	2.5 (1–4.8)	34	0.3	4	0.2	3

From Dallman[b].

[a]Numbers of leukocytes are × $10^3/mm^3$; ranges are estimates of 95% confidence limits; percents refer to differential counts.

[b]Neutrophils include band cells at all ages and a small number of metamyelocytes and myelocytes in the first few days of life.

TABLE 15.10
AGE-SPECIFIC COAGULATION VALUES

Coagulation tests	Preterm infant 30–36wk, day of life #1	Term infant, day of life #1	1–5yr	6–10yr	11–16yr	Adult
PT (sec)	15.4 (14.6–16.9)	13.0 (10.1–15.9)	11 (10.6–11.4)	11.1(10.1–12.1)	11.2 (10.2–12.0)	12 (11.0–14.0)
INR	—	—	1.0 (0.96–1.04)	1.0 (0.91–1.11)	1.02 (0.93–1.10)	1.10 (1.0–1.3)
aPTT (sec)	108 (80–168)	42.9 (31.3–54.3)	30 (24–36)	31 (26–36)	32 (26–37)	33 (27–40)
Fibrinogen (g/L)	2.43 (1.50–3.73)	2.83 (1.67–3.09)	2.76 (1.70–4.05)	2.79 (1.57–4.0)	3.0 (1.54–4.48)	2.78 (1.56–4.0)
Bleeding time (min)	—	—	6 (2.5–10)	7 (2.5–13)	5 (3–8)	4 (1–7)
Thrombin time (sec)	14 (11–17)	12 (10–16)	—	—	—	10
II (U/mL)	0.45 (0.20–0.77)	0.48 (0.26–0.70)	0.94 (0.71–1.16)	0.88 (0.67–1.07)	0.83 (0.61–1.04)	1.08 (0.70–1.46)
V (U/mL)	0.88 (0.41–1.44)	0.72 (0.43–1.08)	1.03 (0.79–1.27)	0.90 (0.63–1.16)	0.77 (0.55–0.99)	1.06 (0.62–1.50)
VII (U/mL)	0.67 (0.21–1.13)	0.66 (0.28–1.04)	0.82 (0.55–1.16)	0.85 (0.52–1.20)	0.83 (0.58–1.15)	1.05 (0.67–1.43)
VIII (U/mL)	1.11 (0.50–2.13)	1.00 (0.50–1.78)	0.90 (0.59–1.42)	0.95 (0.58–1.32)	0.92 (0.53–1.31)	0.99 (0.50–1.49)
vWF (U/mL)	1.36 (0.78–2.10)	1.53 (0.50–2.87)	0.82 (0.47–1.04)	0.95 (0.44–1.44)	1.00 (0.46–1.53)	0.92 (0.50–1.58)
IX (U/mL)	0.35 (0.19–0.65)	0.53 (0.15–0.91)	0.73 (0.47–1.04)	0.75 (0.63–0.89)	0.87 (0.59–1.22)	1.09 (0.55–1.63)
X (U/mL)	0.41 (0.11–0.71)	0.40 (0.12–0.68)	0.88 (0.58–1.16)	0.75 (0.55–1.01)	0.79 (0.50–1.17)	1.06 (0.70–1.52)
XI (U/mL)	0.30 (0.08–0.52)	0.38 (0.10–0.66)	0.97 (0.56–1.50)	0.86 (0.52–1.20)	0.74 (0.50–0.97)	0.97 (0.67–1.27)
XII (U/mL)	0.38 (0.10–0.66)	0.53 (0.13–0.93)	0.93 (0.64–1.29)	0.92 (0.60–1.40)	0.81 (0.34–1.37)	1.08 (0.52–1.64)
PK (U/mL)	0.33 (0.09–0.57)	0.37 (0.18–0.69)	0.95 (0.65–1.30)	0.99 (0.66–1.31)	0.99 (0.53–1.45)	1.12 (0.62–1.62)
HMWK (U/mL)	0.49 (0.09–0.89)	0.54 (0.06–1.02)	0.98 (0.64–1.32)	0.93 (0.60–1.30)	0.91 (0.63–1.19)	0.92 (0.50–1.36)

Data from Andrew[9,11].
HMWK, high-molecular-weight kininogen; PK, prekallikrein; VIII, factor VIII proccoagulant.

Continued

15

HEMATOLOGY

TABLE 15.10

AGE-SPECIFIC COAGULATION VALUES—cont'd

Coagulation tests	Preterm infant 30–36wk, day of life #1	Term infant, day of life #1	1–5yr	6–10yr	11–16yr	Adult
XIIIa (U/mL)	0.70 (0.32–1.08)	0.79 (0.27–1.31)	1.08 (0.72–1.43)	1.09 (0.65–1.51)	0.99 (0.57–1.40)	1.05 (0.55–1.55)
XIIIs (U/mL)	0.81 (0.35–1.27)	0.76 (0.30–1.22)	1.13 (0.69–1.56)	1.16 (0.77–1.54)	1.02 (0.60–1.43)	0.97 (0.57–1.37)
D-Dimer	—	—	—	—	—	Positive titer = 1:8
FDPs	—	—	—	—	—	Borderline titer = 1:25
						Positive titer = 1:50
Coagulation inhibitors						
ATIII (U/mL)	0.38 (0.14–0.62)	0.63 (0.39–0.97)	1.11 (0.82–1.39)	1.11 (0.90–1.31)	1.05 (0.77–1.32)	1.0 (0.74–1.26)
α_2-M (U/mL)	1.10 (0.56–1.82)	1.39 (0.95–1.83)	1.69 (1.14–2.23)	1.69 (1.28–2.09)	1.56 (0.98–2.12)	0.86 (0.52–1.20)
C_1-Inh (U/mL)	0.65 (0.31–0.99)	0.72 (0.36–1.08)	1.35 (0.85–1.83)	1.14 (0.88–1.54)	1.03 (0.68–1.50)	1.0 (0.71–1.31)
α_2-AT (U/mL)	0.90 (0.36–1.44)	0.93 (0.49–1.37)	0.93 (0.39–1.47)	1.00 (0.69–1.30)	1.01 (0.65–1.37)	0.93 (0.55–1.30)
Protein C (U/mL)	0.28 (0.12–0.44)	0.35 (0.17–0.53)	0.66 (0.40–0.92)	0.69 (0.45–0.93)	0.83 (0.55–1.11)	0.96 (0.64–1.28)
Protein S total (U/mL)	0.26 (0.14–0.38)	0.36 (0.12–0.60)	0.86 (0.54–1.18)	0.78 (0.41–1.14)	0.72 (0.52–0.92)	0.81 (0.60–1.13)
Fibrinolytic system						
Plasminogen (U/mL)	1.70 (1.12–2.48)	1.95 (+/− 0.35)	0.98 (0.78–1.18)	0.92 (0.75–1.08)	0.86 (0.68–1.03)	0.99 (0.7–1.22)
TPA (ng/mL)	—	—	2.15 (1.0–4.5)	2.42 (1.0–5.0)	2.16 (1.0–4.0)	4.90 (1.40–8.40)
α_2-AP (U/mL)	0.78 (0.4–1.16)	0.85 (+/− 0.15)	1.05 (0.93–1.17)	0.99 (0.89–1.10)	0.98 (0.78–1.18)	1.02 (0.68–1.36)
PAI (U/mL)	—	—	5.42 (1.0–10.0)	6.79 (2.0–12.0)	6.07 (2.0–10.0)	3.60 (0–11.0)

Data from Andrew[9,11].

α_2-AP, α_2-antiplasmin; α_2-AT, α_2-antitrypsin; α_2-M, α_2-macroglobulin; ATIII, antithrombin III; PAI, plasminogen activator inhibitor; TPA, total plasminogen activator.

TABLE 15.11

AGE-SPECIFIC RBC/IRON INDICATORS

RBC iron indicator	Term neonate	Infant (1–12mo)	Child	Adolescent	Adult
Erythrocyte sedimentation rate (ESR)	0–4mm/hr	—	4–20mm/hr	—	0–20mm/hr female; 0–10mm/hr male
Ferritin (ng/mL)	25–200	200–600 (1mo); 50–200 (2–5mo)	7–140 (6mo–15yr)	7–140 (6mo–15yr)	10–120 female; 20–250 male
Folate (serum) (ng/mL)	5–65	15–55	5–21	5–21	5–21
Folate (RBC) (ng/mL)	150–200	75–1000	>160	>160	140–628
Free erythrocyte protoporphyrin (FEP)	30–70µmol/mol heme; <30µg/dL whole blood	30–70µmol/mol heme; <30µg/dL whole blood	30–70µmol/mol heme; <30µg/dL whole blood	30–70µmol/mol heme; <30µg/dL whole blood	30–70µmol/mol heme; <30µg/dL whole blood
Haptoglobin (mg/dL)	5–50	25–185	25–185	25–185	25–185
Hemoglobin A_1C (%Hb)	5–7.5%	5–7.5%	5–7.5%	5–7.5%	5–7.5%
Hemoglobin F (fetal) (%Hb)	77 +/- 7% (1day); 77 +/- 6% (5day); 70 +/- 7% (3wk)	53 +/- 11% (6–9wk); 23 +/- 16% (3–4mo); 5 +/- 2% (6mo); 1.6 +/- 1% (8–11mo)	<2%	<2%	<2%
Hemopexin (mg/dL)	18% of maternal concentration	—	—	—	50–115
Iron (µg/dL)	100–250	40–100	50–120	—	>75 pregnant women; 50–170 female; 65–175 male
Methemoglobin (%Hb)	0–1.5%	0–1.5%	0–1.5%	0–1.5%	0–1.5%
TIBC (µg/dL)	150–250	200–400	250–500	300–600	250–425
Transferrin (mg/dL)	130–275	200–360	200–360	220–400	220–400
Vitamin B_{12} (pg/mL)	160–1300	200–900	200–900	130–800	200–835

From Painter[14], Saarinen[15], and Lockitch[16].

HEMATOLOGY 15

X. REFERENCES

1. Forestier F, Daffos F, Galactéros F, Bardakjian J, Rainaut M, Beuzard Y. Hematological values of 163 normal fetuses between 18 and 30 weeks of gestation. *Pediatr Res* 1986; **20:**342.

2. Oski FA, Naiman JL. *Hematological problems in the newborn infant.* Philadelphia: WB Saunders; 1982.

3. Nathan D, Oski FA. *Hematology of infancy and childhood.* Philadelphia: WB Saunders; 1981.

4. Matoth Y, Zaizov R, Varsano I. Postnatal changes in some red cell parameters. *Acta Paediatr Scand* 1971; **60:**317.

5. Wintrobe MM. *Clinical hematology.* Philadelphia: Lea & Febiger; 1981.

6. Dallman PR. In: Rudolph AM, ed. *Pediatrics,* 16th edn. New York: Appleton-Century-Crofts; 1977: 11787.

7. Dallman PR, Siimes MA. Percentile curves for hemoglobin and red cell volume in infancy and childhood. *J Pediatr* 1979; **94:**26.

8. Rosenberg RD, Bauer KA. New insights into hypercoagulable states. *Hosp Pract* 1986; **21(3):**131.

9. Andrew M, Paes B, Milner R, Johnston M, Mitchell L, Tollefsen DM, Powers P. Development of the human coagulation system in the full-term infant. *Blood* 1987; **70:**165-172.

10. Andrew M, Paes B, Milner R, Johnston M, Mitchell L, Tollefsen DM, Castle V, Powers P. Development of the human coagulation system in the healthy premature infant. *Blood* 1988; **72:**1651-1657.

11. Andrew M, Vegh P, Johnston M, Bowker J, Ofosu F, Mitchell L. Maturation of the hemostatic system during childhood. *Blood* 1992; **8:**1998-2005.

12. Schreiber GB, Busch MP, Kleinman SH, Korelitz JJ. The risk of transfusion-transmitted viral infections: the Retrovirus Epidemiology Donor Study. *N Engl J Med* 1996; **334:**1685-1690.

13. Oski F. Personal communication, 1993.

14. Painter PC, Cope JY, Smith JL. Reference information for the clinical laboratory. In: Burtis CA, Ashwood ER, eds. *Tietz' textbook of clinical chemistry,* 3rd edn. Philadelphia: WB Saunders; 1999.

15. Saarinen UM, Siimes MA. Developmental changes in serum iron, total iron-binding capacity, and transferrin saturation in infancy. *J Pediatr* 1977 **91:**875–877.

16. Lockitch G, Halstead AC, Wadsworth L, Quigley G, Reston L, Jacobson B. Age- and sex-specific reference intervals and correlation for zinc, copper, selinium, iron, vitamins A and E, and related proteins. *Clin Chem* 1988; **34:**1625–1628.

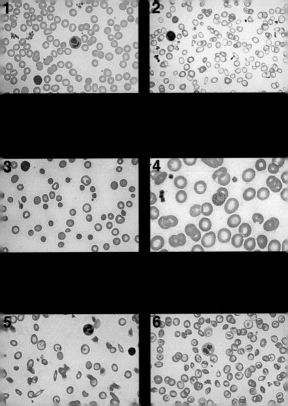

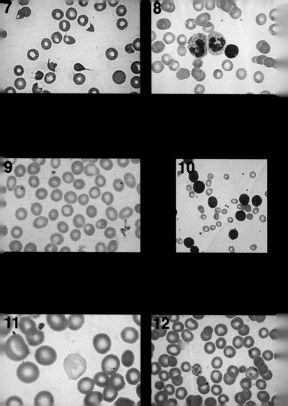

Plates begin opposite p. 330.

PLATE 1

Normal smear: Round RBCs with central pallor about one third of the cell's diameter, scattered platelets, occasional white blood cells.

PLATE 2

Iron deficiency: Hypochromic/microcytic RBCs, poikilocytosis, plentiful platelets, occasional ovalocytes, and target cells. Basophilic stippling may also be present, as in lead intoxication and β-thalassemia.

PLATE 3

Spherocytosis: Microspherocytes a hallmark (densely stained RBCs with no central pallor).

PLATE 4

Basophilic stippling as a result of staining of ribosomal complexes containing RNA throughout the cell; seen with heavy metal intoxication, thalassemia, pyrimidine 5′-nucleotidase deficiency, iron deficiency, and other states associated with ineffective erythropoiesis.

PLATE 5

HbSS disease: Sickled cells, target cells, hypochromic, poikilocytosis, Howell–Jolly bodies, nucleated RBCs common (not shown).

PLATE 6

HbSC disease: Target cells, 'oat cells,' poikilocytosis; sickle forms rarely seen.

PLATE 7

Microangiopathic hemolytic anemia: RBC fragments, anisocytosis, polychromasia, decreased platelets.

PLATE 8

Toxic granulations: Prominent dark blue primary granules; commonly seen with infection and other toxic states, such as Kawasaki's disease.

PLATE 9

Howell–Jolly body: Small, dense nuclear remnant in an RBC; suggests splenic dysfunction or asplenia.

PLATE 10

Leukemic blasts showing large nucleus:cytoplasm ratio.

PLATE 11

Polychromatophilia: Diffusely basophilic because of RNA staining; seen with early release of reticulocytes from the marrow.

PLATE 12

Intraerythrocytic parasites: Malaria.

15

HEMATOLOGY

IMMUNOLOGY

Pamela C. Schamber, MD

I. LABORATORY EVALUATION OF A SUSPECTED IMMUNODEFICIENCY (Table 16.1)

II. SELECTED PRIMARY IMMUNODEFICIENCY DISEASES (Table 16.2)

III. IMMUNE GLOBULIN (IVIG AND IMIG)

16

A. GENERAL INFORMATION

1. Separated from pooled human plasma by alcohol fractionation. IVIG then modified for IV administration.
2. Protein content is ≥95% IgG but contains trace amounts of IgA and IgM.
3. Standard dosing provides immediate antibody levels with a half-life of 3–4 weeks.

B. INTRAVENOUS IMMUNE GLOBULIN (IVIG)

1. **Availability:** As 5–12% solutions (50–120mg/mL).
2. **Indications**
   a. Antibody deficiency disorders (replacement therapy)
      1) Dosage: 300–400mg/kg IV per month.
      2) Determine optimal frequency and dose of IVIG by monitoring clinical response and IgG trough levels. (IgG trough levels ideally >300–400mg/dL over initial pretreatment level.)
   b. Idiopathic thrombocytic purpura (ITP)
      1) Initial therapy for acute ITP: 0.8–1.0g/kg IV in one or two doses.
      2) Alternatively for acute ITP: Prednisone (2mg/kg per day) or $Rh_0(D)$ immune globulin (see p. 739) may be added or substituted.
      3) Maintenance therapy for chronic ITP is individualized to the patient.
   c. Kawasaki's disease
      1) Recommended dosage: 2g/kg IV as a single dose over 10–12 hours or 400mg/kg daily on four consecutive days. Should be started within first 10 days of illness. Note: Should also include aspirin treatment.
      2) See p. 167.
   d. Pediatric HIV infection
      1) May be indicated in HIV-positive children with humoral immunodeficiency, including:
         a) Those with hypogammaglobulinemia.
         b) Those with recurrent serious bacterial infections.
         c) Those who fail to form antibodies to common antigens.
         d) Those at high risk for measles. *Text continued on p. 338*

TABLE 16.1

LABORATORY EVALUATION OF A SUSPECTED IMMUNODEFICIENCY

Suspected abnormality	Clinical findings	Initial tests	More advanced tests
Antibody	Sinopulmonary and systemic infections (pyogenic bacteria) Enteric infections (enterovirus, other viruses, *Giardia* sp.) Autoimmune disease (ITP, hemolytic anemia, IBD)	Immunoglobulin levels (IgG, IgM, IgA) Antibody titers to protein vaccines (diphtheria, tetanus) Antibody titers to polysaccharide vaccines (≥2year-old child) (pneumococcus)	B-cell enumeration Immunofixation electrophoresis IgG subclass levels
Cell-mediated immunity	Pneumonia (pyogenic bacteria, fungi, *Giardia* sp., *Pneumocystis carinii*, viruses) Gastroenteritis (viruses), *Cryptosporidium* sp., Dermatitis/mucositis (fungi)	Total lymphocyte counts HIV ELISA/Western blot Delayed-type hypersensitivity skin test (*Candida* sp., tetanus toxoid, mumps, *Trichophyton* sp.)	T-cell and subset enumeration (CD3, CD4, CD8) In vitro T-cell proliferation to mitogens, antigens, or allogeneic cells

Phagocytosis	Cutaneous infections, abscesses, lymphadenitis (staphylococci, enteric bacteria, fungi, mycobacteria)	WBC/neutrophil count and morphology	Nitroblue tetrazolium (NBT) test Chemotactic assay Phagocytic and bactericidal assay
Spleen	Bacteremia/hematogenous infection (pneumococci, other streptococci, Neisseria sp.)	Peripheral blood smear for Howell–Jolly bodies Hemoglobin electrophoresis (HbSS)	Technetium-99 spleen scan
Complement	Bacterial sepsis Autoimmune disease (lupus, glomerulonephritis)	CH_{50} (total hemolytic complement)	Alternative pathway assays Individual component assays

ITP, idiopathic thrombocytopenic purpura; IBD, inflammatory bowel disease; ELISA, enzyme-linked immunosorbent assay.

16

IMMUNOLOGY

TABLE 16.2

SELECTED PRIMARY IMMUNODEFICIENCY DISEASES

Disorder	Mode of inheritance	Functional deficiency	Characteristics
X-linked agammaglobulinemia	X-linked recessive	Antibody	Recurrent pyogenic infections (e.g., sinopulmonary)
Hyper-IgM syndrome	X-linked or autosomal recessive	Antibody and T cell	Recurrent pyogenic and opportunistic infections
Common variable immunodeficiency	Variable	Antibody and T cell	Recurrent sinopulmonary infections Opportunistic infections Autoimmune diseases
Severe combined immunodeficiency	X-linked or autosomal, recessive and sporadic	Antibody and T cell	Severe life-threatening pyogenic and/or opportunistic infections
Wiskott–Aldrich syndrome	X-linked recessive	Antibody and T cell	Thrombocytopenia Eczema Recurrent viral, bacterial, and fungal infections
Purine nucleoside	Autosomal recessive	T cell ± antibody	Recurrent viral, bacterial, and fungal infections Neurologic disorder

Disease	Inheritance	Component affected	Features
Ataxia telangiectasia	Autosomal recessive	Antibody and T cell	Progressive cerebellar ataxia Oculocutaneous telangiectasia Chronic sinopulmonary disease High incidence of malignancy
DiGeorge anomaly	Variable	T cell	Hypoparathyroidism Cardiac defects Abnormal facial features
Selective IgA deficiency	Sporadic	IgA immunoglobulin	Occasional susceptibility to recurrent infections Allergy, malignancy, autoimmune disease
Chronic granulomatous disease	X-linked or autosomal recessive	Phagocytic cells	Recurrent infections with catalase-positive bacteria (e.g., *Staphylococcus* spp., most Gram-negative rods) and fungi
Leukocyte adhesion deficiency	Autosomal recessive	Phagocytic cells Cytotoxic lymphocytes	Poor wound healing Frequent infections
Chédiak–Higashi syndrome	Autosomal recessive	Phagocytic cells Natural killer cells	Recurrent pyogenic infections Recurrent infections Partial oculocutaneous albinism

From Rosen[1] and Shyur[2].

16

IMMUNOLOGY

        2) Dose: 400mg/kg every 28 days.

        3) See *Red Book*[3] for other indications.

  e. Bone marrow transplantation

        1) May reduce incidence of infection and death; does not decrease graft-versus-host disease (GVHD).

        2) Dose: 500mg/kg on days −7 and −2 before transplant, then weekly through 90 days after transplant. Some experts measure IgG monthly thereafter.

  f. Low-birth-weight infants

        1) Not recommended for routine use in preterm infants to prevent late-onset infection; however, has proved beneficial in very-low-birth-weight (VLBW) (<1500g) infants (see *Report of the Committee on Infectious Diseases [Red Book]*[3]).

        2) Dose: Dosing and schedule vary. Dose, often 500mg/kg, is given each week or three times in first week of life and then each week. (Target IgG often 700mg/dL.)

  g. Parvovirus B19 infection

        1) Treatment of chronic parvovirus B19 infection in an immunodeficient patient appears to be effective and should be considered.

        2) Dose: 400 mg/kg per day for 5 days to 1g/kg per day for 2 days have been reported[4,5].

C. INTRAMUSCULAR IMMUNE GLOBULIN (IMIG)

1. Availability: As 16.5% solution (165mg/mL).

2. Indications

a. Hepatitis A prophylaxis (see pp. 356–357).

b. Measles prophylaxis (see pp. 364–366).

3. Precautions

a. IMIG preparations should never be given IV because they contain IgG aggregates (may cause anaphylactoid reaction).

b. Inject only into a large muscle mass.

c. No more than 5mL should be injected into one site. Max. 1–3mL per site for infants and young children.

D. SPECIFIC IMMUNE GLOBULINS

1. Hyperimmune globulins: These are prepared from donors known to have high antibody titers to antigens from specific sources.

2. Examples: Those used in infectious diseases include hepatitis B (HBIG), rabies (RIG), tetanus (TIG), varicella-zoster (VZIG), cytomegalovirus (CMV-IVIG), respiratory syncytial virus immune globulin (RSV-IVIG), and Rh_0(D) immune globulin (Rh_0[D]IVIG).

3. Exception: Palivizumab (Synagis) is a humanized monoclonal antibody against RSV.

E. ADVERSE REACTIONS TO BOTH IVIG AND IMIG

1. Systemic symptoms: Occur in 1–15% of patients.

a. High fever.
b. Hemodynamic changes (hypertension, hypotension, tachycardia).
c. Hypersensitivity reactions (urticaria, bronchospasm, anaphylaxis).
2. **IVIG:** May cause less serious systemic reactions (headache, myalgia, fever, chills, nausea, and vomiting), often related to infusion rate. Decreasing the rate of infusion can alleviate symptoms. Prophylaxis with antihistamines or IV hydrocortisone can prevent or reduce symptoms.
3. **Aseptic meningitis (IVIG only)**
4. **IMIG:** May cause local discomfort, bleeding, or acrodynia with repeated use.
5. **Immune globulin and all other blood products containing IgA:** Relatively contraindicated in patients with complete IgA deficiency because they may rarely develop anti-IgA antibodies, which can cause anaphylaxis. Because systemic reactions are very rare, routine screening for IgA deficiency is not recommended. Specific brands of IVIG with very low levels of IgA are available.

IV. IMMUNOLOGIC REFERENCE VALUES

A. **SERUM IgG, IgM, AND IgA LEVELS:** Mean (95% confidence interval [CI]) (Table 16.3).

TABLE 16.3

SERUM IgG, IgM, AND IgA LEVELS[a]

Age	IgG (mg/dL)	IgM (mg/dL)	IgA (mg/dL)
Cord blood (term)	1121 (636–1606)	13 (6.3–25)	2.3 (1.4–3.6)
1mo	503 (251–906)	45 (20–87)	13 (1.3–53)
2mo	365 (206–601)	46 (17–105)	15 (2.8–47)
3mo	334 (176–581)	49 (24–89)	17 (4.6–46)
4mo	343 (196–558)	55 (27–101)	23 (4.4–73)
5mo	403 (172–814)	62 (33–108)	31 (8.1–84)
6mo	407 (215–704)	62 (35–102)	25 (8.1–68)
7–9mo	475 (217–904)	80 (34–126)	36 (11–90)
10–12mo	594 (294–1069)	82 (41–149)	40 (16–84)
1yr	679 (345–1213)	93 (43–173)	44 (14–106)
2yr	685 (424–1051)	95 (48–168)	47 (14–123)
3yr	728 (441–1135)	104 (47–200)	66 (22–159)
4–5yr	780 (463–1236)	99 (43–196)	68 (25–154)
6–8yr	915 (633–1280)	107 (48–207)	90 (33–202)
9–10yr	1007 (608–1572)	121 (52–242)	113 (45–236)
Adult	994 (639–1349)	156 (56–352)	171 (70–312)

Adapted from Jolliff[6].
[a]Numbers in parentheses are the 95% CIs.

16

IMMUNOLOGY

B. **SERUM IgG SUBCLASS LEVELS:** Mean (95% CI) (Table 16.4).
C. **SERUM IgE LEVELS:** Geometric mean (95% CI)[8] (Table 16.5).
D. **LYMPHOCYTE ENUMERATION**
1. **T cells:** Normal values (5–95th percentile) for T cells in peripheral blood (Table 16.6).
2. **B cells:** Normal values (25–75th percentile)* for B cells in peripheral blood (Table 16.6).

---

*Values are 5–95th percentile for the adult data.

TABLE 16.4

SERUM IgG SUBCLASS LEVELS[a]

Age (yr)	IgG1 (mg/dL)	IgG2 (mg/dL)	IgG3 (mg/dL)	IgG4 (mg/dL)[b]
0–1	340 (190–620)	59 (30–140)	39 (9–62)	19 (6–63)
1–2	410 (230–710)	68 (30–170)	34 (11–98)	13 (4–43)
2–3	480 (280–830)	98 (40–240)	28 (6–130)	18 (3–120)
3–4	530 (350–790)	120 (50–260)	30 (9–98)	32 (5–180)
4–6	540 (360–810)	140 (60–310)	39 (9–160)	39 (9–160)
6–8	560 (280–1120)	150 (30–630)	48 (40–250)	81 (11–620)
8–10	690 (280–1740)	210 (80–550)	85 (22–320)	42 (10–170)
10–13	590 (270–1290)	240 (110–550)	58 (13–250)	60 (7–530)
13–adult	540 (280–1020)	210 (60–790)	58 (14–240)	60 (11–330)

Adapted from Schur[7].
[a]Numbers in parentheses are the 95% CIs.
[b]Ten percent of individuals appear to have absent IgG4 levels.

TABLE 16.5

SERUM IgE LEVELS[a]

Age	IgE (IU/mL)
<1day	0.22 (0.04–1.28)
6wk	0.69 (0.08–6.12)
3mo	0.82 (0.18–3.76)
6mo	2.68 (0.44–16.3)
9mo	2.36 (0.76–7.31)
1yr	3.49 (0.80–15.2)
2yr	3.03 (0.31–29.5)
3yr	1.80 (0.19–16.9)
4yr	8.58 (1.07–68.9)
7yr	12.89 (1.03–161.3)
10yr	23.66 (0.98–570.6)
14yr	20.07 (2.06–195.2)
17–85yr[b]	13.20 (1.53–114.0)

From Kjellman[8].
[a]Numbers in parentheses are the 95% CIs.
[b]Data from Zetterström[9].

TABLE 16.6

NUMBERS OF B AND T CELLS[a]

Age	CD3 (total T cells) (%)	CD4 (T-helper/inducer) (%)	CD8 (T-suppressor/cytotoxic) (%)	CD4/CD8 ratio	CD19 (B cells) (%)
Neonatal	0.6–5.0 (28–76)	0.4–3.5 (17–52)	0.2–1.9 (10–41)	1.0–2.6	0.04–1.1 (5–22)
1wk–2mo	2.3–7.0 (60–85)	1.7–5.3 (41–68)	0.4–1.7 (9–23)	1.3–6.3	0.6–1.9 (4–26)
2–5mo	2.3–6.5 (48–75)	1.5–5.0 (33–58)	0.5–1.6 (11–25)	1.7–3.9	0.6–3.0 (14–39)
5–9mo	2.4–6.9 (50–77)	1.4–5.1 (33–58)	0.6–2.2 (13–26)	1.6–3.8	0.7–2.5 (13–35)
9–15mo	1.6–6.7 (54–76)	1.0–4.6 (31–54)	0.4–2.1 (12–28)	1.3–3.9	0.6–2.7 (15–39)
15–24mo	1.4–8.0 (39–73)	0.9–5.5 (25–50)	0.4–2.3 (11–32)	0.9–3.7	0.6–3.1 (17–41)
2–5yr	0.9–4.5 (43–76)	0.5–2.4 (23–48)	0.3–1.6 (14–33)	0.9–2.9	0.2–2.1 (14–44)
5–10yr	0.7–4.2 (55–78)	0.3–2.0 (27–53)	0.3–1.8 (19–34)	0.9–2.6	0.2–1.6 (10–31)
10–16yr	0.8–3.5 (52–78)	0.4–2.1 (25–48)	0.2–1.2 (9–35)	0.9–3.4	0.2–0.6 (8–24)
Adult	0.7–2.1 (55–83)	0.3–1.4 (28–57)	0.2–0.9 (10–39)	1.0–3.6	0.1–0.5 (6–19)

From Comans-Bitter[10].

[a]Absolute counts (×10^9/L): 5–95th percentiles. Figures in parentheses are relative frequency 5–95th percentiles.

16

IMMUNOLOGY

E. **SERUM COMPLEMENT LEVELS:** Geometric mean (95% CI) (Table 16.7).

V. COMPLEMENT CASCADE (Fig. 16.1)

VI. COMPLEMENT DEFICIENCIES (Table 16.8)

TABLE 16.7

SERUM COMPLEMENT LEVELS[a]

Age	C3 (mg/dL)	C4 (mg/dL)
Cord blood (term)	83 (57–116)	13 (6.6–23)
1mo	83 (53–124)	14 (7.0–25)
2mo	96 (59–149)	15 (7.4–28)
3mo	94 (64–131)	16 (8.7–27)
4mo	107 (62–175)	19 (8.3–38)
5mo	107 (64–167)	18 (7.1–36)
6mo	115 (74–171)	21 (8.6–42)
7–9mo	113 (75–166)	20 (9.5–37)
10–12mo	126 (73–180)	22 (12–39)
1yr	129 (84–174)	23 (12–40)
2yr	120 (81–170)	19 (9.2–34)
3yr	117 (77–171)	20 (9.7–36)
4–5yr	121 (86–166)	21 (13–32)
6–8yr	118 (88–155)	20 (12–32)
9–10yr	134 (89–195)	22 (10–40)
Adult	125 (83–177)	28 (15–45)

Adapted from Jolliff[6].
[a]Numbers in parentheses are the 95% CIs.

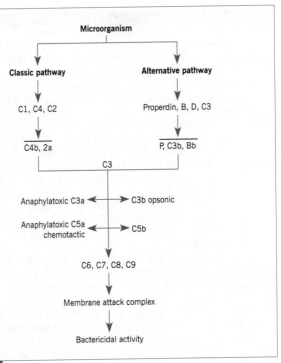

FIG. 16.1

Complement cascade. (From Oski[11].)

TABLE 16.8

COMPLEMENT DEFICIENCIES

Deficient component	Mode of inheritance	Characteristics
C1, C4, C2	Autosomal recessive	Lupus-like illness and glomerulonephritis
		Susceptible to pyogenic infections
C3	Autosomal recessive	Susceptible to pyogenic infections
		Lupus-like illness and glomerulonephritis
C5, C6, C7, C8, C9	Autosomal recessive	Susceptible to systemic *Neisseria* infections
Properdin	X-linked recessive	Susceptible to *Neisseria* and pyogenic infections
C1 esterase inhibitor	Autosomal dominant	Hereditary angioedema

From Stiehm[12].

16

IMMUNOLOGY

VII. REFERENCES

1. Rosen FS, Cooper MD, Wedgewood R. The primary immunodeficiencies. *N Engl J Med* 1995; **333(7):**431–440.
2. Shyur SD, Hill HR. Recent advances in the genetics of primary immunodeficiency syndromes. *J Pediatr* 1996; **129(1):**8–24.
3. American Academy of Pediatrics. *1997 Red book: report of the Committee on Infectious Diseases,* 24th edn. Elk Grove Village, IL: The Academy; 1997.
4. Fuller D, Moaven L, Spelman D, Spicer WJ, Wraight H, Curtis D, Leydon J, Doultree J, Locarnini S. Parvovirus B19 in HIV infection: a treatable cause of anemia. *Pathology* 1996; **28(3):**277–280.
5. Mathias RS. Chronic anemia as a complication of parvovirus B19 infection in a pediatric kidney transplant patient. *Pediatr Nephrol* 1997; **11(3):**355–357.
6. Jolliff CR, Cost KM, Stivrins PC, Grossman PP, Nolte CR, Franco SM, Fijan KJ, Fletcher LL, Shriner HC. Reference intervals for serum IgG, IgA, IgM, C3, and C4 as determined by rate nephelometry. *Clin Chem* 1982; **28:**126–128.
7. Schur PH. IgG subclasses: a review. *Ann Allergy* 1987; **58:**89–96,99.
8. Kjellman NM, Johansson SG, Roth A. Serum IgE levels in healthy children quantified by a sandwich technique (PRIST). *Clin Allergy* 1976; **6:**51–59.
9. Zetterström O, Johansson SG. IgE concentrations measured by PRIST in serum of healthy adults and in patients with respiratory allergy: a diagnostic approach. *Allergy* 1981; **36(8):**537–547.
10. Comans-Bitter WM, de Groot R, van den Beemd R, Neijens HJ, Hop WC, Groeneveld K, Hooijkaas H, van Dongen JJ. Immunophenotyping of blood lymphocytes in childhood: reference values for lymphocyte subpopulations. *J Pediatr* 1996; **130(3):**388–393.
11. Oski FA. *Principles and practice of pediatrics,* 2nd edn. Philadelphia: JB Lippincott; 1994.
12. Stiehm ER. *Immunologic disorders in infants and children,* 4th edn. Philadelphia: WB Saunders; 1996.

IMMUNOPROPHYLAXIS

Beth E. Ebel, MD, MSc, and
Amy B. Hirshfeld, MD

17

I. SOURCES OF INFORMATION

A. PRINTED SOURCES

1. American Academy of Pediatrics. *1997 Red Book: Report of the Committee on Infectious Diseases,* 24th edn. Elk Grove Village, IL: The Academy, 1997, including Sources of Vaccine Information (p. 1) and Directory of Telephone Numbers (p. 667). New edition published every 3 years.
2. Updated Recommended Childhood Vaccination Schedule is published in each January in *Pediatrics* and *Morbidity and Mortality Weekly Report*.
3. Current issues of *Morbidity and Mortality Weekly Report*.
4. Vaccine package inserts.

B. ELECTRONIC/TELEPHONE SOURCES

1. State Health Departments.
2. The Voice Information System from the Centers for Disease Control and Prevention (CDC) can provide telephone consultation and send printed material on vaccines. Phone: (800) 232-SHOT.
3. THE CDC home page on the World Wide Web: http://www.cdc.gov.

II. IMMUNIZATION SCHEDULES

A. RECOMMENDED CHILDHOOD IMMUNIZATION SCHEDULE
(Fig. 17.1)

B. CATCH-UP IMMUNIZATION SCHEDULES

1. **Lapsed immunizations**
   a. Resume immunization schedule as if the usual interval had elapsed.
   b. Repeating doses is not indicated.
2. **Catch-up immunization schedules** (Tables 17.1 and 17.2)
3. *Haemophilus influenzae* **type b (Hib):** For catch-up immunizations, see p. 356.

C. MINIMUM AGE FOR INITIAL VACCINATION AND MINIMUM INTERVALS BETWEEN DOSES OF VARIOUS VACCINES
(Table 17.3)

Age ▶ Vaccine ▼	Birth	1 mo	2 mo	4 mo	6 mo	12 mo	15 mo	18 mo	4–6 yr	11–12 yr	14–16 yr
Hepatitis B	Hep B	Hep B									
		Hep B				Hep B				Hep B	
Diphtheria, tetanus, pertussis[1]			DTaP	DTaP	DTaP		DTaP[1]		DTaP		Td
H. influenzae type b[2]			Hib	Hib	Hib[2]	Hib					
Polio[3]			IPV	IPV		Polio[3]			Polio		
Rotavirus[4]			Rv[4]	Rv[4]	Rv[4]						
Measles, mumps, rubella[5]							MMR		MMR[5]	MMR[5]	
Varicella[6]							Var			Var[6]	

[1] The fourth dose of DTaP may be administered as early as 12mo of age if 6mo have elapsed since the third dose and if the child is unlikely to return at age 15–18mo. Td is recommended at 11–12yr of age if at least 5yr have elapsed since the last dose of DTaP. Subsequent routine Td boosters are recommended every 10yr.

[2] If PRP-OMP is administered at 2 and 4mo of age, a dose at 6mo is not required. DTaP/Hib combination products should not be used for primary immunization in infants at 2, 4, or 6mo of age until FDA approved for these ages.

[3] The ACIP, AAP, and AAFP now recommend that the first two doses of poliovirus vaccine should be IPV. As of January 1999, the ACIP recommends a sequential schedule of two doses of IPV administered at ages 2 and 4mo, followed by two doses of OPV at 12–18mo and 4–6yr. Use of IPV for all doses is acceptable and is recommended for immunocompromised persons and their household contacts. OPV is no longer recommended for the first two doses of the schedule and is acceptable only for special circumstances: children of parents who do not accept the number of injections, late initiation of immunization that would require an unacceptable number of injections, and imminent travel to polio-endemic areas. OPV remains the vaccine of choice for mass immunization campaigns to control outbreaks caused by wild poliovirus.

[4] Rotavirus vaccine is shaded and italicized to indicate that health care providers may require time and resources to incorporate this new vaccine into practice. The first dose of Rv vaccine should not be administered before 6wk of age, and the minimum interval between doses is 3wk. The Rv vaccine series should not be initiated at 7mo of age or older, and all doses should be completed by the first birthday.

[5] The second dose of MMR is recommended routinely at 4–6yr of age but may be administered during any visit, provided at least 4wk have elapsed since the first dose. Those who have not previously received the second dose should complete the schedule by the 11–12yr-old visit.

[6] Varicella vaccine is recommended at any visit for susceptible children ≥1yr of age. Susceptible persons ≥13yr of age should receive two doses given at least 4wk apart.

FIG. 17.1

Recommended childhood immunization schedule,* United States, January–December 1999. Bars indicate range of recommended ages for immunization. Ovals indicate vaccines to be given if previous recommended doses were missed or given earlier than the recommended minimum age. (Adapted from Committee on Infectious Diseases[1].)

In July, 1999, the AAP temporarily suspended its recommendation for routine use of the rotavirus vaccine in infants to investigate a possible association with intussusception. Updated recommendations are expected in the autumn of 1999.

*From Joint Statement of the American Academy of Pediatrics (AAP) and the United States Public Health Service (PHS)—July 7, 1999, regarding *mercury/thimerosal* in vaccines: The PHS and AAP continue to recommend that all children should be immunized against the diseases indicated in the recommended immunization schedule. Given that the risks of not vaccinating children far outweigh the unknown and much smaller risk, if any, of exposure to thimerosal-containing vaccines over the first 6 months of life, clinicians and parents are encouraged to immunize all infants even if the choice of individual vaccine products is limited for any reason. *Thimerosal free vaccines are anticipated by late 1999 or early 2000.* (If thimerosal-free vaccines are not available,) for infants born to hepatitis B surface antigen (HbsAg)–negative women, . . . postpone the first dose of hepatitis B vaccine from birth until 2 to 6 months of age, when the infant is considerably larger. Preterm infants born to HbsAg-negative mothers should similarly receive hepatitis B vaccine but ideally not until they reach term gestational age and a weight of at least 2.5 kg. Because of the substantial risk of disease, there is no change in the recommendations for infants of HbsAg-positive mothers or of mothers whose status is not known.

TABLE 17.1

RECOMMENDED IMMUNIZATION SCHEDULES FOR CHILDREN <7 YEARS
NOT IMMUNIZED IN THE FIRST YEAR OF LIFE

Recommended time/age	Immunizations	Comments
First visit	DTaP, Hib, HBV, MMR, polio[a]	Hib not needed if normal child ≥5yr age.
Interval after first visit:		
1mo	DTaP, HBV, Var	—
2mo	DTaP, Hib, polio[a]	Second dose of Hib indicated only if first dose given at <15mo.
≥8mo	DTaP, HBV, polio[a]	Polio[a] and HBV are not given if the third doses were previously given.
4–6yr (at or before school entry)	DTaP, polio[a], MMR	DTaP not necessary if fourth dose given after fourth birthday. OPV not necessary if third dose given after fourth birthday.

Adapted from *1997 Red Book*[3]. See the current *Red Book* for details.
[a]IPV preferred; OPV acceptable if parents refuse the number of injections necessary to use IPV; see *2000 Red Book* for update.

17

IMMUNOPROPHYLAXIS

TABLE 17.2

RECOMMENDED IMMUNIZATION SCHEDULES FOR CHILDREN 7–12 YEARS
NOT IMMUNIZED IN THE FIRST YEAR OF LIFE

Recommended time/age	Immunizations	Comments
First visit	HBV, MMR, Td, polio[a]	—
Interval after first visit:		
2mo[b]	HBV, MMR, Var[a], Td, polio[a]	—
8–14mo[b]	HBV, Td, polio[a]	Polio, HBV not needed if third doses given earlier
11–12yr	Var[a], HBV, Td	HBV if third dose has not been given

Adapted from *1997 Red Book*[3].
[a]IPV preferred; OPV acceptable if parents refuse the number of injections necessary to use IPV; see *2000 Red Book* for update.
[b]Varicella vaccine can be administered to susceptible children any time after 12mo of age. Unimmunized children who lack a reliable history of chickenpox should be immunized before their thirteenth birthday. Children >12yr require two doses of varicella vaccine.

TABLE 17.3

MINIMUM AGE FOR INITIAL VACCINATION AND MINIMUM INTERVAL BETWEEN VACCINE DOSES, BY TYPE OF VACCINE

Vaccine	Minimum age for first dose[a]	Minimum interval from dose to dose		
		1 to 2[a]	2 to 3[a]	3 to 4
DTaP[b]	6wk	1mo	1mo	6mo
Hib (primary series)				
HbOC	6wk	1mo	1mo	2mo[c]
PRP-T	6wk	1mo	1mo	2mo[c]
PRP-OMP	6wk	1mo	2mo[c]	—
IPV/OPV	6wk	1mo	1mo	1mo[d]
MMR	12mo[e]	1mo	—	—
HBV	Birth	1mo	2mo[f]	—
Varicella	12mo	1mo[g]	—	—
Rotavirus	6wk	3wk	3wk	—

Adapted from *The Pink Book*[2].   1 month = at least 28 days.

[a]These minimum acceptable ages and intervals may not correspond with the optimal recommended ages and intervals for vaccination. See Fig. 17.1.

[b]The total number of doses of diphtheria and tetanus toxoids should not exceed six each before the seventh birthday. If the fourth dose is given after the fourth birthday, the fifth (booster) dose is not needed.

[c]The booster dose of Hib vaccine recommended after the primary vaccination series should be administered no earlier than 12mo of age.

[d]If the third dose is given after the fourth birthday, the fourth (booster) dose is not needed.

[e]Although the age for measles vaccination may be as young as 6mo in outbreak areas where cases are occurring in children <1yr of age, children initially vaccinated before the first birthday should be revaccinated at 12–15mo of age, and an additional dose of vaccine should be administered at the time of school entry or according to local policy. Doses of MMR or other measles-containing vaccine should be separated by at least 1mo.

[f]This final dose is recommended at least 4mo after the first dose and no earlier than 6mo of age.

[g]A second dose of varicella is indicated only in children ≥13yr.

III. IMMUNIZATION GUIDELINES

A. **VACCINE INFORMED CONSENT:** Vaccine information statements (VISs) can be obtained from local health departments, the CDC, the American Academy of Pediatrics (AAP), and vaccine manufacturers. For vaccines that do not currently have VISs, the CDC produces 'important information' statements.

B. **VACCINE ADMINISTRATION**

1. **Volume/dose:** Unless otherwise specified, all pediatric immunization doses are 0.5mL.

2. **Site:** See also p. 66 for administration technique. Preferred sites of administration of IM and SC vaccines follow:

a. Children ≤18 months old: Anterolateral thigh.

b. Toddlers: Anterolateral thigh or deltoid (deltoid preferred if large enough).

c. Older children: Deltoid preferred.

3. **Route**
a. IM: Deep into muscle to avoid tissue damage from adjuvants, usually with a 22–23G needle ⅞ inch (2cm) in length.
b. SC: Into pinched skinfold with a 25G needle ⅞ inch (2cm) in length.
4. **Simultaneous administration:** Routine childhood vaccines are safe and effective when administered simultaneously at different sites, generally 1–2 inches apart. Live viral vaccines (e.g., MMR and varicella) may be given simultaneously at different sites; otherwise the interval between administration should be >1 month.

C. **GENERAL CONTRAINDICATIONS TO VACCINE ADMINISTRATION**
1. Anaphylactic reaction to vaccine or vaccine constituent (see also sections on MMR [see pp. 364–365] and influenza [see p. 361] for specific guidelines).
2. Moderate or severe illness regardless of fever.
3. For special hosts, see pp. 349–352.

D. **MISCONCEPTIONS REGARDING VACCINE ADMINISTRATION:** Vaccines **may** be given despite the presence of the following:
1. Mild acute illness regardless of fever.
2. Low-grade fever.
3. Convalescent phase of illness.
4. Recent exposure to infectious disease.
5. Mild to moderate local reaction to previous dose of vaccine (soreness, redness, swelling).
6. Current antimicrobial therapy.
7. Prematurity (see also p. 352).
8. Malnutrition.
9. Allergy to penicillin or other antibiotic (except anaphylactic reaction to neomycin or streptomycin).
10. Pregnancy of mother or another household contact (exception: varicella vaccine may be deferred if there is a pregnant, varicella-susceptible household contact).
11. Breast-feeding.
12. Unimmunized household contact (exception: oral poliovirus vaccine [OPV] is contraindicated if there is an adult contact who has not been immunized against polio).

E. **EGG ALLERGIES**
1. MMR *can* be given to children with egg allergies without prior skin testing (see p. 365 for details).
2. Prior anaphylactic reaction to chicken or eggs *is a contraindication* to yellow fever and influenza vaccines.

IV. IMMUNOPROPHYLAXIS GUIDELINES FOR SPECIAL HOSTS

A. **IMMUNOCOMPROMISED HOSTS**
1. **Congenital immunodeficiency disorders:** See *1997 Red Book*[3] for details. In general:
a. Live bacterial and live viral vaccines are contraindicated.

17

IMMUNOPROPHYLAXIS

b. Inactivated poliovirus vaccine (IPV) should be used for the entire polio series.

c. Other inactivated vaccines should be given according to the routine schedule.

d. Immunoglobulin (IG) therapy may be indicated.

e. See p. 351 for recommendations for household contacts.

2. Known or suspected HIV disease

a. Inactivated vaccines (DTaP, Hib, HBV, Td [see Fig. 17.1, p. 346]) should be given as scheduled for routine immunizations.

b. Polio vaccine: IPV rather than OPV should be given to patients and household contacts.

c. MMR: Decision to immunize depends on degree of immunosuppression as defined in Table 18.3 (p. 387).

  1) Asymptomatic (class N) or mildly symptomatic (class A) patients with no evidence of immune suppression (category 1) or evidence of moderate immune suppression (category 2): Immunize at 12 months of age; administer the second dose as soon as 1 month later to ensure early seroconversion.

  2) Severely immunocompromised patients should not receive MMR.

d. Varicella vaccine should be considered in CDC class N1 or A1 and with CD4+ T-lymphocyte counts ≥25%. Give two doses 3 months apart.

e. Pneumococcal vaccine is recommended at 2 and 5 years.

f. Influenza: Immunize all patients at the start of the influenza season as early as 6 months of age and yearly thereafter.

3. Oncology patients (Table 17.4).

4. Functional or anatomic asplenia (including sickle cell disease)

a. Penicillin prophylaxis: Start at diagnosis. The appropriate time to discontinue therapy is controversial.

  1) In sickle cell anemia, one study supports discontinuation 1 year after second pneumococcal vaccine if no history of invasive pneumococcal disease.

  2) Continue indefinitely for patients with a history of invasive pneumococcal disease.

  3) Recommendations may change after licensure of the conjugate pneumococcal vaccine.

b. Pneumococcal vaccine

  1) Children <2 years at diagnosis: Give at 2 and 5 years.

  2) Children 2–10 years at diagnosis: Give at diagnosis and 3–5 years later. (Second dose should not be given before the fifth birthday.)

  3) People >10 years at diagnosis: Give at diagnosis and 5 years later.

c. Meningococcal vaccine at 2 years of age or at diagnosis if ≥2 years old.

d. Ensure that Hib series is completed; children ≥60 months who never received Hib immunization should receive one dose.

e. Children undergoing *elective* splenectomy should receive the

TABLE 17.4

IMMUNIZATION FOR ONCOLOGY PATIENTS[a]

Vaccine	Indications and comments
DTaP	Indicated for incompletely immunized children <7yr, even during active chemotherapy.
Td	Indicated 1yr after completion of therapy in children ≥7yr.
Hib	Indicated for incompletely immunized children if <7yr.
HBV	Indicated for incompletely immunized children.
Pneumococcus	Indicated for asplenic patients.
Meningococcus	Consider in asplenic patients.
IPV	Indicated for incompletely immunized children; IPV also recommended for all household contacts requiring immunization to reduce the risk of vaccine-associated polio.
MMR	Contraindicated until child is in remission and finished with all chemotherapy for 3–6mo. May need to reimmunize after chemotherapy if titers have fallen below protective levels.
Influenza	Defer in active chemotherapy. May give as early as 3–4wk after remission and off chemotherapy if during influenza season; peripheral granulocyte and lymphocyte counts should be >1000/mm^3. Should also be given to household contacts of children with cancer.
Varicella	Consider immunizing children who have remained in remission and have finished chemotherapy for >1yr, with absolute lymphocyte count of >700/mm^3 and platelet count of >100,000/mm^3 within 24hr of immunization. Check titers of previously immunized children to verify protective levels of antibodies.

[a]Immune reconstitution is slower for oncology patients who have received bone marrow transplants. Inactivated vaccines should be given 1yr after transplantation, and live vaccines should be deferred until 2yr after transplantation. Titers should be checked to document an adequate immune response.

pneumococcal and meningococcal vaccines (if ≥2 years) at least 2 weeks before surgery to ensure optimal immune response. If Hib series was previously completed, an additional dose is recommended at least 7–10 days before surgery.

B. **CORTICOSTEROID ADMINISTRATION:** Only **live** viral and **live** bacterial vaccines are potentially contraindicated. (See Table 17.5 for details.)

C. **CONTACTS OF IMMUNOCOMPROMISED HOSTS:** Immunize according to the routine childhood immunization schedule. Contacts should receive IPV rather than OPV. Varicella vaccine and a yearly influenza vaccine are recommended.

D. **PATIENTS TREATED WITH IG OR OTHER BLOOD PRODUCTS:** Defer MMR 3–11 months according to Table 3.37, p. 353, of the *1997 Red Book*[3]. Varicella vaccine should be deferred 9 months after RSV–IGIV and 5 months after all other blood products. OPV and rotavirus may be used without delay.

TABLE 17.5

LIVE VIRUS IMMUNIZATION FOR PATIENTS RECEIVING
CORTICOSTEROID THERAPY

Steroid dose	Recommended guidelines
Topical and inhaled therapy or local injection of steroids	Live virus vaccines may be given unless there is clinical evidence of immunosuppression. If suppressed, wait 1 month after cessation of therapy to give live vaccines.
Physiologic maintenance doses of steroids	No contraindication to live virus vaccines.
Low-dose steroids (<2mg/kg/day prednisone or equivalent, or <20mg/day if >10kg)	No contraindication to live virus vaccines.
High-dose steroids (≥2mg/kg/day prednisone or equivalent, or 20mg/day if >10kg)	
• Duration of therapy <14 days	May give live virus vaccines immediately after cessation of therapy.
• Duration of therapy ≥14 days	Do not give live virus vaccines until therapy has been discontinued for 1mo.
Children with immuno-suppressive disorders receiving steroid therapy	Live virus vaccines are contraindicated.

From *1997 Red Book*[3].

E. **PRETERM INFANTS:** Immunize according to chronologic age using regular vaccine dosage.
1. **Polio:** IPV, not OPV, should be used in the nursery to prevent nosocomial transmission of polio.
2. **HBV:** Initiation of HBV vaccine may be delayed for infants of HBsAg-negative mothers until the child is >2kg or 2 months of age, whichever is earlier. See footnote on p. 346.
3. **Influenza:** Give each fall to children >6 months of age with chronic lung disease. Household contacts should also receive influenza vaccine.
4. **Rotavirus:** May be given after discharge from hospital when at least 6 weeks old.

F. **PREGNANT WOMEN:** Live viruses are generally contraindicated during pregnancy. Influenza vaccine **should** be given to all women who will be >14 weeks' gestation during the influenza season. Influenza vaccine is considered safe at any stage of pregnancy. Pregnant women not immunized or incompletely immunized against tetanus should receive Td to prevent neonatal tetanus. When indicated, hepatitis A virus (HAV), HBV, and pneumococcal vaccines may be given to pregnant women.

TABLE 17.6

INDICATIONS FOR TETANUS PROPHYLAXIS

Prior tetanus toxoid doses	Clean, minor wounds		All other wounds	
	Tetanus vaccine	TIG	Tetanus vaccine	TIG
Unknown or <3	Yes	No	Yes	Yes
≥3, last <5yr ago	No	No	No	No[a]
≥3, last 5–10yr ago	No	No	Yes	No[a]
≥3, last >10yr ago	Yes	No	Yes	No[a]

Adapted from *1997 Red Book*[3].

TIG, tetanus immune globulin.

[a]Any child with HIV infection should receive TIG for any tetanus-prone wound regardless of vaccination status.

V. IMMUNOPROPHYLAXIS GUIDELINES FOR SPECIFIC DISEASES

A. DIPHTHERIA/TETANUS/PERTUSSIS VACCINES AND TETANUS IMMUNOPROPHYLAXIS

1. **Description**

a. DTaP: Diphtheria and tetanus toxoids combined with acellular pertussis vaccine; **preferred** formulation for children <7 years.

b. DTP: Diphtheria and tetanus toxoids combined with whole-cell pertussis vaccine; both local and systemic side effects are more common than with DTaP; acceptable alternative to DTaP for children <7 years.

c. DT: Diphtheria and tetanus toxoids without pertussis vaccine; use in children <7 years in whom pertussis vaccine is contraindicated.

d. Td: tetanus toxoid with one third to one sixth the dose of diphtheria toxoid of other preparations; use in individuals ≥7 years.

2. **Indications**

a. Routine: See Fig. 17.1.

b. Tetanus prophylaxis in wound management: See Table 17.6.

c. Unimmunized pregnant women: Two doses of Td 4 weeks apart; the second dose should be ≥2 weeks before delivery.

d. Pregnant women who have not completed a primary series: Give Td as soon as possible.

3. **Contraindications**

a. General contraindications

   1) Anaphylactic reaction to vaccine or vaccine constituent.

   2) Moderate or severe illness *regardless of fever*.

b. Contraindication to pertussis vaccine: Encephalopathy not attributable to another cause within 7 days of a prior dose of pertussis vaccine. Use DT for remaining doses in series.

Note: DTaP is not a substitute for DTP in children in whom there is a contraindication to pertussis vaccine.

4. **Precautions to pertussis vaccine:** The following adverse events **after a prior dose of pertussis vaccine** are now considered **precautions and not contraindications** to subsequent doses. Risks and benefits should be weighed before subsequent doses. DTaP is recommended if pertussis vaccine is given. Use DT to complete series if not giving pertussis vaccine.

a. Convulsion with or without fever within 3 days.

b. Persistent, inconsolable crying for ≥3 hours within 48 hours.

c. Collapse or shocklike state (hypotonic–hyporesponsive episode) within 48 hours.

d. Temperature ≥40.5°C not explained by another cause within 48 hours.

5. **Children with neurologic disorders**

a. Seizures

   1) Poorly controlled or new-onset seizures: Defer pertussis immunization until seizure disorder is well controlled and progressive neurologic disorder is excluded; then use DTaP and antipyretics for 24 hours after immunization.

   2) Personal or family history of febrile seizures: Not a contraindication; use DTaP and antipyretics for 24 hours after immunization.

b. Known or suspected progressive neurologic disorder: Defer pertussis immunization until diagnosis and treatment are established and neurologic condition is stable. Progressive disorders may merit permanent deferral of pertussis immunization. Reconsider pertussis immunization at each visit. Use DTaP if pertussis vaccine given; use DT if pertussis vaccine permanently deferred.

Note: Children <1 year with neurologic disorders necessitating temporary deferment of pertussis vaccine should not receive DT because the risk of diphtheria and tetanus is low in the first year of life. After the first birthday, initiate either DT or DTaP immunization as clinically indicated previously.

6. **Conditions under which pertussis vaccine can be given**

a. Minor adverse event or condition listed as 'precaution' (see above) after prior pertussis immunization.

b. Family history of minor adverse events after pertussis immunization, sudden infant death syndrome, or seizures.

7. **Precaution to tetanus vaccine:** Guillain–Barré syndrome within 6 weeks of a prior dose of tetanus vaccine; see *1997 Red Book*[3], p. 522.

8. **Vaccine side effects**

a. Minor side effects within 3 days

   1) DTaP: Erythema (26–39%), swelling (15–30%), pain (4–11%), fever >38.3°C (3–5%), anorexia (19–25%), vomiting (7–13%), drowsiness (40–47%), fussiness (14–19%).

   2) DTP: Erythema (73%), swelling (61%), pain (40%), fever >38.3°C

(16%), anorexia (35%), vomiting (14%), drowsiness (62%), fussiness (42%).

b. Moderate to severe side effects: Anaphylaxis (1/50,000), seizures (DTP, 1/1750; DTaP, rare), persistent crying >3 hours (DTP, 1%; DTaP, rare), hypotonic-hyporesponsive episode (DTP, 3.5–290/100,000; DTaP, rare), temperature ≥40.5°C (DTP, 0.3%; DTaP, rare).

9. **Vaccine administration:** DTP, DTaP, DT, and Td are all given in a dose of 0.5mL IM.

10. **Special considerations**

a. Pertussis exposure

  1) Immunize all unimmunized or partially immunized close contacts <7 years.

    a) Give fourth dose of DTaP if third dose given >6 months ago.

    b) Give booster dose of DTaP if last dose given >3 years ago.

    c) Continue or initiate schedule for all other children.

  2) Chemoprophylaxis for all household and other close contacts: treat with erythromycin to limit secondary transmission regardless of immunization status. Estolate preparation may be better tolerated (see p. 709). Azithromycin and clarithromycin may be effective in children who cannot tolerate erythromycin.

b. Pertussis outbreak: See *1997 Red Book*[3], p. 396.

c. Prophylaxis of tetanus in wound management

  1) Indications: See Table 17.6.

  2) Passive immunization

    a) Tetanus immune globulin (TIG): 250 U IM.

    b) Equine tetanus antitoxin (TAT) 3000–5000 U IM, *after sensitivity testing of patient* (See *1997 Red Book*[3], p. 42), may be substituted if TIG unavailable.

  3) Vaccine choice

    a) <7 years old

      i) DTaP. (DTP is an acceptable alternative.)

      ii) DT if pertussis contraindicated.

    b) ≥7 years old: Td.

Note: The total number of DT, DTaP, and DTP immunizations should not exceed six by the fourth birthday.[3]

B. *HAEMOPHILUS INFLUENZAE* TYPE B (HIB) VACCINE

1. **Description:** The four licensed vaccines consist of a capsular polysaccharide antigen (PRP) conjugated to a carrier. It is not necessary to use the same formulation for the entire series. Vaccines do not confer protection against the disease associated with the carrier (e.g., PRP-T does not protect against tetanus). Routine use of these vaccines has led to a 95% decline in invasive Hib disease in infants and young children.

a. PRP-OMP: Conjugated to outer membrane protein of *Neisseria meningitidis;* requires only two doses in primary series; children without prior DT/DTaP/DTP vaccine may respond better to PRP-OMP than to other formulations.

b. HbOC: Conjugated to mutant diphtheria toxin.

c. PRP-T: Conjugated to tetanus toxoid.

d. PRP-D: Conjugated to diphtheria toxoid; licensed for primary series only for children ≥15 months but may be used as a booster dose at ≥12 months.

2. Indications

a. Routine: See Fig. 17.1.

b. Children not immunized against Hib before 7 months of age: Give all doses 2 months apart (1 month acceptable to accelerate immunization). If initiating Hib immunization at 7–11 months, give three doses; at 12–14 months, give 2 doses; and at 15–59 months, give 1 dose. Immunization is not necessary for **normal** children ≥60 months.

c. Unimmunized children >15 months with underlying conditions predisposing to invasive Hib disease (e.g., IgG2 deficiency, HIV) require two doses of vaccine.

d. Children undergoing splenectomy may benefit from an additional dose 7–10 days before procedure even if series was previously completed.

e. Children with invasive Hib disease

1) Disease at age <24 months: Begin Hib immunization 1 month after acute illness and continue as if previously unimmunized.

2) Disease at age ≥24 months: No further Hib immunization.

Note: Consider immunologic workup for children who contract invasive Hib disease after completing the immunization series.

3. Contraindications

a. Anaphylactic reaction to vaccine or vaccine constituent.

b. Moderate or severe illness regardless of fever.

4. Side effects: Local pain, redness, and swelling in 25% of recipients; frequency of fever and irritability when Hib is given with DTaP are the same as for DTaP alone.

5. Vaccine administration: Dose 0.5mL IM; PRP-T may be given SC in patients with coagulation disorders.

6. Special considerations: Give prophylactic rifampin to selected household and child care contacts of children with invasive Hib disease; see p. 841 and *1997 Red Book*[3], p. 222, for details.

C. HEPATITIS A VIRUS (HAV) IMMUNOPROPHYLAXIS

1. Description: HAV vaccine is an inactivated adsorbed vaccine; two brands are available, both with pediatric and adult formulations; licensed only for persons >2 years.

2. Vaccine indications

a. Travelers to or residents of endemic areas.

b. Populations at increased risk, including Native Americans.

c. After exposure to HAV if future exposure is likely.

d. Military personnel.

e. Homosexual or bisexual men.
f. Users of illicit injection drugs.
g. Patients with chronic liver disease, including HBV or hepatitis C (HCV).
h. Persons at risk of occupational exposure.
i. Healthy people at the discretion of the physician.
j. Immunocompromised individuals may be immunized, although efficacy is not established in immunocompromised children.
k. Consider use in staff of institutions with ongoing or recurrent outbreaks.
l. Consider use in patients with hemophilia.

3. **Vaccine contraindications**
a. Anaphylactic reaction to vaccine or vaccine constituent.
b. Moderate or severe illness regardless of fever.

4. **Vaccine side effects:** Local reactions include induration, redness, swelling (18%); headache (12%); fever (6%); fatigue, malaise, anorexia, nausea (1–10%). No serious adverse events have been reported.

5. **Vaccine administration:** Dose and schedule (Table 17.7); give IM.

6. **Special considerations**
a. Preexposure immunoprophylaxis for travelers
   1) HAV vaccine is preferred for travelers >2 years old; a single dose usually provides adequate immunity if time does not allow further doses before travel.
   2) IG, given IM, is protective for up to 5 months; see Table 3.12 in *1997 Red Book*[3], p. 240 for dosing.
b. Postexposure immunoprophylaxis
   1) IG 0.02mL/kg IM is 80–90% effective in preventing symptomatic infection if given within 2 weeks of exposure. Maximum dose per site is 3mL for infants and small children and 5mL for large children and adults.
   2) Also give HAV vaccine if ≥ 3 years old and future exposure is likely. Studies suggest that HAV vaccine alone may be effective for post-exposure prophylaxis, but data are insufficient to recommend alone.

17

IMMUNOPROPHYLAXIS

TABLE 17.7

RECOMMENDED DOSAGES AND SCHEDULES FOR HAV VACCINES

Age (yr)	Vaccine	Antigen	Volume (mL)	No. of doses	Schedule
2–18	Havrix (SB)	720 ELU	0.5	2	Initial and 6–12mo later
	Vaqta (Merck)	25 U	0.5	2	Initial and 6–18mo later
≥19	Havrix (SB)	1440 ELU	1.0	2	Initial and 6–12mo later
	Vaqta (Merck)	50 U	1.0	2	Initial and 6–12mo later

Adapted from *1997 Red Book*[3].
SB, SmithKline Beecham; ELU, enzyme-linked immunoassay units; U, antigen units.

D. HEPATITIS B VIRUS [HBV] IMMUNOPROPHYLAXIS

1. Description

a. Hepatitis B immune globulin (HBIG): Prepared from plasma containing high-titer anti–hepatitis B surface antigen (HBsAg) antibodies and negative for antibodies to HIV and HCV. Dose: Infants, 0.5mL IM; older children, 0.06mL/kg IM.

b. HBV vaccine: Adsorbed HBsAg produced recombinantly. Different recombinant vaccines may be used interchangeably.

2. Vaccine indications

a. All infants (see Fig. 17.2 for infants of mothers who are HBsAg positive or indeterminate). See footnote on p. 346.

b. All children and adolescents not previously immunized.

c. Children at risk of acquiring HBV horizontally: Members of ethnic groups or immigrants from regions with high rates of HBV and household contacts of HBV carriers. Screen adoptees from regions with endemic HBV (e.g., Asia, Eastern Europe, Middle East, Africa).

d. High-risk lifestyle: Sexually active persons with more than one partner in 6 months, persons with a sexually transmitted disease (STD), sexual contacts of HBV carriers, sexually active homosexual or bisexual males, IV drug users.

e. Health care workers and others at risk of occupational exposure to blood.

f. Children and staff of residential institutions for the developmentally disabled; staff of nonresidential programs known to be attended by an HBV carrier.

g. Hemodialysis patients.

h. Patients with bleeding disorders receiving clotting factor concentrates.

i. International travelers to areas with endemic HBV.

j. Inmates of correctional facilities.

3. Vaccine contraindications

a. Anaphylactic reaction to vaccine, yeast, or another vaccine constituent.

b. Moderate or severe illness regardless of fever.

4. Vaccine side effects: Pain at injection site or fever >37.7°C in 1–6%.

5. Vaccine administration: See Table 17.8 for dose; give IM.

6. Special considerations

a. Management of neonates with positive or unknown maternal HBsAg status (Fig. 17.2), p. 360. See Table 19.1 on pp. 412–413 for following up on serologies.

b. HBV prophylaxis after percutaneous exposure to blood (Table 17.9).

c. Management of injuries from discarded needles in the community, see *1997 Red Book*[3], p. 120.

E. INFLUENZA VACCINE AND CHEMOPROPHYLAXIS

1. Vaccine description

a. Preparations

   1) Whole inactivated virus vaccine grown in eggs; not used in children <13 years.

TABLE 17.8

RECOMMENDED DOSE FOR HBV VACCINES

Patient group	Recombivax HB dose (mcg)[a]	Engerix-B dose (mcg)[b]
Up to 19yr	5	10
≥20yr	10	20
Patients undergoing dialysis and other immunosuppressed adults	40	40

Adapted from *1997 Red Book*[3].

[a]Recombivax HB is available from Merck & Co. in pediatric, adult, and dialysis patient formulations.
[b]Engerix-B is available from SmithKline Beecham in a single formulation.

TABLE 17.9

HBV PROPHYLAXIS AFTER PERCUTANEOUS EXPOSURE TO BLOOD

Exposed person	HBsAg status of source of blood		
	Positive	Negative	Unknown
Unimmunized	HBIG Start vaccine series	Start vaccine series	Start vaccine series
Immunized			
Known responder	No treatment	No treatment	No treatment
Known nonresponder	HBIG Start vaccine series	No treatment	If source known to be high risk, treat as if HBsAg positive
Response unknown	Test exposed person for anti-HBs If <10mIU/mL, give HBIG, reimmunize If ≥10mIU/mL, no treatment	No treatment	Test exposed person for anti-HBs If <10mIU/mL, reimmunize If ≥10mIU/mL, no treatment

Adapted from *1997 Red Book*[3].

    2) 'Split' vaccines: Licensed for children >6 months
      a) Subvirion: Inactivated virus vaccine grown in eggs with additional step of denaturing viral lipid membrane.
      b) Purified surface antigen vaccine.
    3) A nasally administered attenuated vaccine was in clinical trials at the time of publication and will likely become available in 2000.
  b. Protective response in 70–80% of hosts.
2. Vaccine indications
  a. Recommended for high-risk children
    1) Asthma and other chronic pulmonary diseases.
    2) Hemodynamically significant cardiac disease.
    3) Immunosuppressive disorders and therapy.

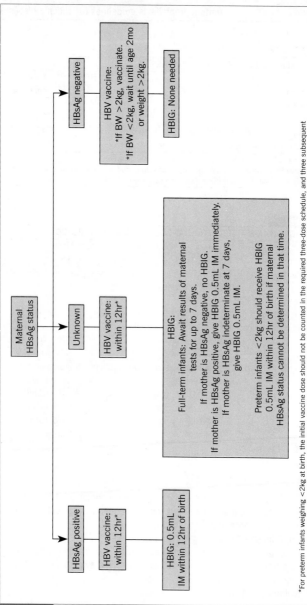

FIG. 17.2

Management of neonates born to mothers with unknown or positive HBsAg status. For mercury/thimerosal–containing vaccine, see footnote on p. 346. BW, birth weight. (Adapted from *1997 Red Book*[3].)

The text content within the figure:

Maternal HBsAg status

HBsAg positive

HBV vaccine: within 12hr*

HBIG: 0.5mL IM within 12hr of birth

Unknown

HBV vaccine: within 12hr*

HBIG:

Full-term infants: Await results of maternal tests for up to 7 days.
If mother is HBsAg negative, no HBIG.
If mother is HBsAg positive, give HBIG 0.5mL IM immediately.
If mother is HBsAg indeterminate at 7 days, give HBIG 0.5mL IM.

Preterm infants <2kg should receive HBIG 0.5mL IM within 12hr of birth if maternal HBsAg status cannot be determined in that time.

HBsAg negative

HBV vaccine:
*If BW >2kg, vaccinate.
*If BW <2kg, wait until age 2mo or weight >2kg.

HBIG: None needed

*For preterm infants weighing <2kg at birth, the initial vaccine dose should not be counted in the required three-dose schedule, and three subsequent doses are required (see *1997 Red Book*[3], p. 254).

TABLE 17.10			
INFLUENZA VACCINE DOSAGE AND SCHEDULE			
Age	Vaccine type	Volume (mL)	Number of doses
6–35mo	Split virus only	0.25	1 or 2[a]
3–8yr	Split virus only	0.5	1 or 2[a]
9–12yr	Split virus only	0.5	1
>12yr	Whole or split virus	0.5	1

Adapted from *1997 Red Book*[3].

[a]Two doses, at least 1 month apart, are recommended for children <9 years receiving influenza vaccine for the first time.

    4) HIV infection.

    5) Sickle cell anemia and other hemoglobinopathies.

    6) Diseases requiring long-term aspirin therapy.

b. Recommended for close contacts of high-risk children and adults

    1) Household contacts.

    2) Health care workers.

c. Consider immunization for other high-risk persons.

    1) Diabetes mellitus.

    2) Chronic renal disease.

    3) Chronic metabolic disease.

    4) Any underlying condition that may marginally compromise children.

    5) Pregnant women who will be ≥14 weeks' gestation during influenza season.

    6) International travel to areas with influenza outbreaks.

    7) Institutional settings, including colleges and other residential facilities.

d. Any child on parental request, if vaccine supply is adequate.

3. Contraindications

a. Anaphylactic reaction to vaccine, vaccine constituent, chicken, or eggs.

b. Moderate or severe illness regardless of fever.

4. Side effects

a. Fever 6–24 hours after immunization in children <2 years; rare in children >2 years.

b. Local reactions rare in children <13 years; 10% in children ≥13 years.

c. Side effects and immunogenicity are similar for whole and split-cell vaccines in children >12 years.

d. Guillain-Barré syndrome (GBS): New studies show a rate of 1–2 cases of GBS per million people immunized, about 10 times the baseline population risk.

5. Vaccine administration

a. Antigenic makeup varies from year to year; administer during the fall in preparation for winter influenza season.

b. Dosage and schedule (Table 17.10); give IM.

6. **Special considerations**
   a. Children receiving chemotherapy have poor seroconversion rates until chemotherapy is discontinued for 3–4 weeks and absolute neutrophil and lymphocyte counts are >1000/mm^3.
   b. Immunization may be delayed in patients on prolonged high-dose steroids (equivalent to 2mg/kg per day or 20mg/day of prednisone) until dose decreased, only if time allows before the influenza season.
   c. Chemoprophylaxis for influenza A
      1) Amantadine and rimantadine can effectively reduce symptoms and transmission of influenza (see pp. 623 and 841 for dosing).
      2) Indications
         a) High-risk children immunized after influenza is present in the community: Give for 2 weeks after immunization.
         b) Unimmunized individuals providing care to high-risk individuals.
         c) Immunodeficient individuals unlikely to have protective response to vaccine.
         d) Individuals at high risk for influenza infection with contraindication to vaccine.
      3) Chemoprophylaxis does not interfere with the immune response to the vaccine.
      4) Precaution: Neither drug has been adequately evaluated for safety and efficacy in children <12 months of age.

F. **LYME IMMUNOPROPHYLAXIS**
1. **Description:** Recombinant vaccine (rOspA) against the *Borrelia burgdorferi* outer surface protein A (OspA), an antigen expressed by the Lyme spirochete in the tick midgut. The tick ingests host antibody over 24–36 hours, killing the organism in the tick and aborting human infection.
2. **Indications for immunization**
   a. Currently licensed *only* for persons between 15 and 70 years of age.
   b. Highest rates of Lyme transmission occur in the Northeast and North Central United States, but geographic risk varies even within townships and counties. Practitioners should check with local public health authorities to identify areas of high risk for disease transmission.
   c. Current ACIP recommendations*:
      1) Vaccine should be considered for high-risk persons who reside, work, and play in high-risk or moderate-risk areas during the transmission season (typically April through July) **and** have frequent or prolonged exposure to tick habitats (woods, thick brush, overgrown grassy areas).
      2) Vaccine may be considered for moderate-risk persons who reside in high-risk to moderate-risk areas during the transmission season **and** who have tick exposure that is neither frequent nor prolonged. In

*Prevention of Lyme disease through active immunization: recommendations of the Advisory Committee in Immunization Practices (ACIP). US Department of Health and Human Services, Centers for Disease Control and Prevention, Atlanta, 1999.

these cases the vaccine is of uncertain benefit beyond that supplied by personal protection (long sleeves, N,N-diethyl-3-methylbenzamide (DEET) repellent, checking for and removing ticks).

3) Vaccine is **not** recommended for persons who do not reside, work, or play in high-risk areas **or** who do reside in such areas but have minimal or no exposure to tick habitats.

d. Vaccination should be considered for those with a history of previous uncomplicated Lyme arthritis who are at continued risk. Individuals with treatment-resistant Lyme arthritis should **not** be vaccinated (see below).

3. Contraindications

a. The rOspA vaccine is **not** recommended for the following groups because safety and efficacy has not been established:
   1) Children <15 years of age or adults >70 years of age.
   2) Pregnant women
   3) Persons with immunodeficiency, musculoskeletal disease (rheumatoid arthritis, joint pain, diffuse musculoskeletal pain, etc.), second- or third-degree heart block, chronic joint or neurologic illness related to Lyme disease.

b. Persons with treatment-resistant Lyme arthritis should not be vaccinated because this condition is associated with increased reactivity to the OspA antigen used in the vaccine.

4. Vaccine side effects:
Still under investigation. Pain at the injection site (24%); local redness and swelling (<2%); myalgias, influenza-like illness, fever or chills in ≤3%. Vaccine recipients more likely to report arthralgia or myalgia within 30 days after each dose of vaccine.

5. Vaccine administration

a. Dose 0.5mL (30mcg) recombinant Osp-A protein (rOspA) IM into deltoid.

b. Three doses given at 0, 1, and 12 months are recommended. For optimal protection, doses should be timed so that the second and third doses are given several weeks before the start of Lyme transmission season (usually in April).

c. Vaccine efficacy: For the LYMErix rOsp-A vaccine, protection against clinical Lyme disease was 49% after two doses and 76% after three doses. The duration of protective immunity is unknown, but data suggest that boosters beyond the third dose may be needed.

d. If Lyme vaccine is given with other vaccines, each should be given in a separate syringe at a separate injection site.

6. Special considerations

a. The risk of Lyme disease is greatly reduced by the use of tick repellants (DEET), protective clothing (long-sleeve shirts and long pants, tucking pant legs into socks), and checking for and removing ticks. Transmission of disease requires 24–48 hours of tick attachment.

17

IMMUNOPROPHYLAXIS

b. Early detection of Lyme disease is important, since timely and correct antibiotic therapy nearly always results in a prompt cure.

c. Care providers should be aware the vaccine-induced antibodies to OspA antigen routinely cause falsely positive ELISA results for Lyme disease. Careful interpretation of Western immunoblotting can usually discriminate between *B. burgdorferi* infection and rOspA immunization, since most patients do not develop anti-OspA antibodies after natural infection.

G. MEASLES/MUMPS/RUBELLA (MMR) IMMUNOPROPHYLAXIS

1. Description

a. MMR: Combined vaccine composed of live, attenuated viruses. Measles and mumps vaccines are grown in chick embryo cell culture; rubella vaccine is prepared in human diploid cell culture.

b. Monovalent measles vaccine, rubella vaccine, and measles/rubella (MR) formulations are available. Monovalent measles vaccine is recommended for infants 6–11 months for measles outbreak or exposure, but MMR can be substituted if monovalent vaccine is not available. Two doses of measles-containing vaccine are still required after 12 months of age.

c. IG: Intramuscular IG and intravenous IG (IGIV) preparations contain similar concentration of measles antibody.

2. Indications for immunization: MMR is recommended in most circumstances.

a. Routine (Fig. 17.1).

b. People are susceptible to measles unless they have documentation of physician-diagnosed measles, have laboratory evidence of immunity, had **two** doses of measles-containing vaccine after 12 months of age, or were born before 1957. Screen all individuals for susceptibility, especially if they are enrolling in post–high school institutions or have immunocompromised contacts, and immunize as follows:

   1) No prior measles immunization after 12 months of age: Two doses separated by 1 month.

   2) One prior measles immunization after 12 months of age: Reimmunize with one dose.

c. Measles postexposure prophylaxis (see p. 365 for details).

d. Control of school-based measles outbreaks: See *1997 Red Book*[3], p. 356.

e. People are considered susceptible to rubella unless they have documentation of one dose of rubella-containing vaccine or serologic evidence of immunity. Screen all women of child-bearing age for susceptibility at all health care encounters, including prenatal visits. If susceptible, immunize with one dose of MMR unless pregnant.

3. Contraindications to MMR, MR, and monovalent vaccine preparations

a. Anaphylactic reaction to prior MMR, MR, or monovalent immunization.

b. Anaphylactic neomycin or gelatin allergy.

c. Immunocompromised states (see pp. 349–350).

d. Moderate or severe illness regardless of fever.

e. Pregnant women or women considering pregnancy within 3 months.

f. Recent IG or blood product administration. See Table 3.37, p. 353, *1997 Red Book*[3].

4. Precautions for MMR, MR, and monovalent vaccine preparations

a. Hypersensitivity reaction after first dose of vaccine: Consider skin test or check antibody titers to see if a second dose is needed.

b. Children with a history of thrombocytopenia may develop transient thrombocytopenia after immunization, but the benefits often outweigh the risks.

5. Misconceptions: The following are **not contraindications** to MMR administration:

a. Anaphylactic reaction to eggs: Consider observing patient for 90 minutes after vaccine administration. Skin testing is not predictive of hypersensitivity reaction and therefore is not recommended.

b. Allergy to penicillin.

c. Exposure to measles.

d. History of seizures: There is a slightly increased risk of seizure after immunization. Parents should follow temperature and treat with antipyretics.

6. Vaccine side effects

a. Minor side effects 7–12 days after immunization: Fever to $\geq 39.4\,^\circ$C lasting 1–5 days (5–15%); transient rash (5%).

b. Moderate to severe side effects: Febrile seizures (rare); transient thrombocytopenia (1/25,000–1/40,000) 2–3 weeks after immunization; encephalitis and encephalopathy (<1/1 million).

7. Vaccine administration

a. Dose 0.5mL SC.

b. Immunize >2 weeks before planned administration of IG, such as for international travel.

c. MMR should not be given earlier than 5 months after standard dose or 6 months after high-dose IG administration.

d. Purified protein derivative (PPD) testing may be done on the day of immunization; otherwise postpone PPD 4–6 weeks due to suppression of response.

8. Special considerations

a. Measles postexposure immunoprophylaxis (see also *1997 Red Book*[3])

   1) Vaccine: Prevents disease if given within 72 hours of exposure; indicated for the following groups:

      a) Household contacts with one prior dose of vaccine (do not require IG).

      b) Susceptible nonhousehold contacts ≥ 6 months old.

      c) Susceptible siblings ≥ 6 months old of exposed persons.

      d) Infants 6–12 months old in an outbreak setting: Give monovalent measles vaccine or MMR if monovalent vaccine is unavailable.

2) Immune globulin (IG)
   a) Indications: Prevents or modifies disease if given within 6 days of exposure; indicated for the following groups:
      i) Infants <6 months old if mother is susceptible.
      ii) Unimmunized household contacts ≥6 months old. These contacts also receive the measles vaccine.
      iii) Immunocompromised individuals.
      iv) Susceptible pregnant women.
   b) Dosing
      i) Standard dose IG for children and pregnant women: 0.25mL/kg (max. 15mL) IM.
      ii) High-dose IG for immunocompromised children: 0.5mL/kg (max. 15mL) IM. Not required if IGIV received within 3 weeks before exposure.

b. Rubella postexposure immunoprophylaxis: IG may modify rubella disease but does not prevent congenital rubella syndrome; therefore not recommended for exposed pregnant women.

H. MENINGOCOCCUS IMMUNOPROPHYLAXIS

1. **Description:** Quadrivalent serogroup-specific vaccine made from purified capsular polysaccharide antigen from groups A, C, Y, and W-135. Immunogenicity of serogroup antigens varies with age of child. No vaccine is available for group B because of poor immunogenicity.

2. **Indications for immunization**
a. High-risk children ≥2 years of age
   1) Functional or anatomic asplenia.
   2) Terminal complement or properdin deficiencies.
   3) Consider reimmunization after 1 year if child <4 years at initial dose or after 5 years if child ≥4 years at initial dose.
b. Adjunct to postexposure chemoprophylaxis (see below).
c. Travelers to endemic or hyperendemic areas.
d. Community outbreak with serotype A, C, Y, or W-135.

3. **Contraindications**
a. Anaphylactic reaction to vaccine or vaccine constituent.
b. Moderate or severe illness regardless of fever.

4. **Precaution:** Vaccine safety has not been established in pregnant women, who should be immunized only if they face a high risk of infection.

5. **Side effect:** Localized erythema for 1–2 days occurs infrequently.

6. **Vaccine administration:** Dose is 0.5mL SC.

7. **Postexposure chemoprophylaxis**
a. Exposed persons
   1) Household, child care, and nursery school contacts.
   2) Potential contact with oral secretions of infected patient.
b. Antibiotic chemoprophylaxis should be given to exposed individuals within 24 hours of primary case diagnosis.

1) Rifampin is the drug of choice (see p. 841).
2) Ciprofloxacin may be given to persons >18 years (see p. 672).
3) Ceftriaxone may be more efficacious than rifampin in reducing nasal carriage when exposed to group A meningococci (see p. 663).
4) Sulfisoxazole may be used for sensitive isolates (see p. 856).

c. Carefully observe exposed persons for febrile illness and evaluate promptly if symptomatic; presumptive therapy for infection may be indicated pending cultures.

I. PNEUMOCOCCUS IMMUNOPROPHYLAXIS

1. Vaccine description

a. Purified capsular polysaccharide antigen from 23 serotypes of *Streptococcus pneumoniae*.

b. Effective against most serotypes causing bacteremia and meningitis; however, protection is not 100%, and fatal infection may still occur.

c. Not immunogenic in children <2 years.

d. Pneumococcal conjugate vaccines are being evaluated in clinical trials and will likely become available in 2000.

2. Indications for immunization

a. High-risk children ≥2 years of age, including those with the following:
1) Sickle cell disease.
2) Functional or anatomic asplenia.
3) Chronic renal failure or nephrotic syndrome.
4) Immunosuppression, including organ transplantation, drug therapy chemotherapy, leukemia, and lymphoma.
5) CSF leaks.
6) HIV infection.

b. Other groups for which immunization is indicated at ≥2 years.
1) Chronic cardiovascular, pulmonary, or liver disease.
2) Populations at high risk for invasive pneumococcal disease, including Alaskan Native and some other Native American populations.

c. Reimmunization
1) **Any** child <5 years old qualifying for pneumococcal vaccine: Reimmunize once 3–5 years after the first dose.
2) Children 5–10 years old in 'high-risk' group: Reimmunize once 3–5 years after the first dose.
3) Persons >10 years old in 'high-risk' groups: Reimmunize once after 5 years.

3. Contraindications

a. Anaphylactic reaction to vaccine or vaccine constituent.

b. Moderate or severe illness regardless of fever.

c. Generally defer during pregnancy because effect on the fetus is unknown; consider in mothers at high risk of severe pneumococcal disease.

4. Side effects: Pain and erythema at injection site (common); fever and myalgia (less common); severe systemic reactions such as anaphylaxis (rare).

5. **Vaccine administration**
a. Dose: 0.5mL SC or IM.
b. May be given concurrently with other vaccines.
c. Give vaccine 2 weeks or more before elective splenectomy, chemotherapy, radiotherapy, or immunosuppressive therapy; or give 3 months after chemotherapy or radiotherapy.

6. **Special considerations**
a. Passive immunoprophylaxis with IG is recommended for some children with congenital or acquired immune deficiencies.
b. Chemoprophylaxis: Penicillin 125mg PO BID if <5 year, 250mg PO BID if ≥5 years.
   1) Indicated in patients with functional or anatomic asplenia.
   2) Begin at diagnosis for patients with sickle cell disease.
   3) Duration of chemoprophylaxis is controversial.
      a) In sickle cell anemia, one study supports discontinuation 1 year after second pneumococcal vaccine if no history of invasive pneumococcal disease.
      b) Continue indefinitely for patients with a history of invasive pneumococcal disease.
      c) Recommendations may change after licensure of conjugate pneumococcal vaccines.

J. **POLIOMYELITIS IMMUNOPROPHYLAXIS**
1. **Description**
a. IPV: Trivalent enhanced-potency vaccine of formalin-inactivated poliovirus types 1, 2, and 3 grown in human diploid or Vero cells.
b. OPV: Trivalent vaccine of live attenuated poliovirus types 1, 2, and 3 grown in monkey kidney cells.

2. **Indications**
a. Routine: See Fig. 17.1. Give IPV-only schedule when there are contraindications to OPV (see below). The IPV-only schedule may become universally recommended in the future.
b. Unimmunized or partially immunized individuals who are at imminent risk of exposure to poliovirus. (Dose interval may be 4 weeks.)

3. **Contraindications**
a. General contraindications
   1) Anaphylaxis to vaccine or vaccine constituent.
   2) Moderate or severe illness, regardless of fever.
   3) Although there is no convincing evidence of adverse effects, immunization during pregnancy should be avoided for reasons of theoretical risk.
b. Contraindications to IPV: Anaphylaxis to streptomycin, polymyxin B, or neomycin.
c. Contraindications to OPV (IPV to be used unless specifically contraindicated)
   1) Immunodeficiency disorders.

2) Immunocompromised household contacts.

3) Incompletely immunized adult household contacts.

4) Patient ≥18 years and previously unimmunized.

4. **Side effects:** Risk of vaccine-associated paralytic poliomyelitis is 1/760,000 first doses of OPV without prior IPV; prior IPV reduces the risk by 75–90%.

5. **Vaccine administration**

a. IPV: Dose 0.5mL SC.

b. OPV: Dose 0.5mL PO; may repeat once if patient regurgitates dose within 10 minutes.

K. RABIES IMMUNOPROPHYLAXIS

1. **Description**

a. Human diploid cell vaccine (HDCV): Inactivated rabies virus grown in human diploid cell culture; IM (1mL/dose) and intradermal (0.1mL/dose) formulations are available.

b. Rhesus diploid cell vaccine, rabies vaccine adsorbed (RVA): Inactivated rabies virus grown in rhesus monkey fetal lung cell culture; adsorbed to aluminum salt; IM administration only (1mL/dose).

c. Human rabies immune globulin (RIG): Antirabies IG prepared from plasma from donors hyperimmunized with rabies vaccine.

2. **Indications for immunization**

a. Preexposure prophylaxis: Indicated for high-risk groups, including veterinarians, animal handlers, laboratory workers, children living in high-risk environments, those traveling to high risk areas, spelunkers.

   1) Three injections of vaccine on days 0, 7, and 21 or 28.

   2) For those taking chloroquine or related drugs, if HDCV is given, the IM formulation and route should be used.

   3) Follow antibody titers; give booster doses only if titers are nonprotective (see *1997 Red Book*[3], p. 442, for details).

b. Postexposure prophylaxis (see below).

3. **Contraindications**

a. Anaphylactic reaction to vaccine or vaccine constituent.

b. Moderate or severe illness regardless of fever.

Note: If a patient has a serious allergic reaction to HDCV, RVA may be used instead.

4. **Side effects (HDCV):** Local reactions (pain, erythema, swelling) in 25%, mild systemic reactions (headache, nausea, abdominal pain, muscle aches, dizziness) in 20%, neurologic illness similar to GBS or focal CNS disorder (1/150,000), immune complex–like reaction (generalized urticaria, arthralgia, arthritis, angioedema, nausea, vomiting, fever, and malaise) 2–21 days after immunization, rare in primary series, 6% after booster dose.

5. **Special considerations:** Postexposure prophylaxis.

a. General wound management

   1) Clean immediately with soap and water.

      2) Avoid suturing wound.

      3) Consider tetanus prophylaxis and antibiotics if indicated.

  b. Indications: Infectious exposures include bites, scratches, or contamination of open wound or mucous membrane with body fluid or brain tissue of the infectious animal.

Note: Report all patients suspected of rabies to public health authorities.

      1) Infectious exposures to domestic or wild animals (Table 17.11); consider immunization status of animal, prevalence of rabies, nature of attack.

      2) Infectious exposures to a human infected with rabies.

      3) Infectious exposure or casual contact with bat if infectious exposure cannot be ruled out (Table 17.11).

  c. Administration

      1) Vaccine and RIG should be given jointly except in previously immunized patients (no RIG required).

      2) Vaccine for postexposure prophylaxis

        a) Either IM HDCV or RVA may be used, particularly if patient has severe allergy to one type; do not use intradermal HDCV.

        b) Deltoid muscle except infants.

        c) Routine serologic testing not indicated.

        d) Unimmunized: 1mL IM on days 0, 3, 7, 14, and 28.

        e) Previously immunized: 1mL IM on days 0 and 3. Do not give RIG.

      3) RIG: Dose is 20 IU/kg. Infiltrate the wound with half of the dose; give remainder IM.

L. RESPIRATORY SYNCYTIAL VIRUS (RSV) IMMUNOPROPHYLAXIS

1. Description

  a. There is no vaccine available.

  b. Palivizumab (monoclonal RSV-IG): Humanized mouse monoclonal IgG to RSV, recombinantly produced for IM administration.

  c. Polyclonal RSV-IGIV: IG pooled from donors with high serum titers of RSV-neutralizing antibody, for IV administration. Provides some protection against other respiratory viruses.

2. Indications: Consider RSV immunoprophylaxis for the following:

  a. Infants and children <2 years with bronchopulmonary dysplasia (BPD) who require oxygen within the 6 months before the RSV season.

  b. Infants <32 weeks' estimated gestational age (EGA) at birth who do not have BPD may benefit from prophylaxis

      1) EGA ≤28 weeks: Consider until 12 months of age.

      2) EGA 29–32 weeks: Consider until 6 months of age.

  c. Children with severe immunodeficiency may benefit from RSV-IGIV, although its use has not been evaluated in randomized trials.

3. Contraindications: RSV-IGIV is contraindicated in cyanotic congenital heart disease. Palivizumab is also **not** recommended for children with cyanotic congenital heart disease. However, those with BPD or prematurity who meet the criteria and who also have asymptomatic

TABLE 17.11

RABIES POSTEXPOSURE PROPHYLAXIS

Animal type	Evaluation and disposition of animal	Postexposure prophylaxis recommendations
Dogs, cats, ferrets	Healthy and available for 10 days observation.	Do not begin prophylaxis unless animal develops symptoms of rabies.
	Rabid or suspected rabid.	Immediate immunization and RIG; euthanize animal and test brain.
	Unknown (escaped).	Consult public health officials.
Skunk, raccoon, bat, fox, most other carnivores, woodchuck	Regard as rabid unless (1) local area known to be free from rabies *or* (2) animal is euthanized and brain is negative for rabies by fluorescein antibody test.	Immediate immunization and RIG.
Livestock, rodent, rabbit	Consider individually.	Consult public health officials; these bites rarely require treatment.

Adapted from *1997 Red Book*[3].

Treatment may be discontinued if animal fluorescent antibody is negative, do not give RIG if patient previously immunized.

acyanotic heart disease (ventricular septal defect, patent ductus arteriosus) may benefit from palivizumab.

4. **Side effects**
a. Palivizumab: Local reaction, fever, rash, changes in LFTs, and symptoms of upper respiratory infections after administration were all comparable with placebo.
b. RSV-IGIV
   1) Fever in 6% (2% in placebo group).
   2) 15mL/kg fluid load; 8% of children with BPD required extra diuretics around the time of administration.
   3) Must defer MMR and varicella vaccines for 9 months after the last dose.
5. **Administration:** Give RSV-IGIV or palivizumab 1 month before the RSV season and then monthly during the RSV season. Consult the local health department for the optimal schedule.
a. Palivizumab: Dose 15mg/kg IM monthly.
b. Polyclonal RSV-IGIV: Dose 15mL/kg (750mg/kg) IV monthly.
6. **Efficacy:** Both palivizumab and RSV-IGIV have been shown to reduce the incidence of RSV-related hospitalization in children who are either <24 months old with BPD or <6 months old born at ≤35 weeks' gestation.

a. Palivizumab: 55% decrease compared with placebo, from 10.6% to 4.8%.
b. RSV-IGIV: 41% decrease compared with placebo, from 13.5% to 8%.
c. The two have not been directly compared.

M. ROTAVIRUS VACCINE (for update, see p. 346)

1. **Description:** Tetravalent live attenuated vaccine produced by reassortment with rhesus rotavirus; for oral administration.
2. **Indications:** Routine (Fig. 17.1).
3. **Contraindications**
a. Anaphylactic reaction to vaccine, monosodium glutamate, amphotericin B, aminoglycosides, or another vaccine constituent.
b. Acute vomiting or diarrhea; moderate or severe illness regardless of fever.
c. Immunocompromised hosts; however, their household contacts should be immunized.
d. Children born to HIV-positive women until the infant is shown to be HIV negative at ≥ 2 months of age.
e. Do not initiate first dose of series at ≥ 7 months of age, and all doses should be completed by the first birthday.
4. **Side effects**
a. Low-grade fever in 2–8% 3–5 days after immunization.
b. Loose stool frequency is comparable to that with placebo.
5. **Vaccine administration:** Dose is 2.5mL PO.
6. **Special considerations**
a. Aim to complete immunization series before rotavirus season, which starts in the fall in the Southwest United States and spreads across to the Northeast United States by winter.
b. Efficacy: 50–70% for all rotaviral disease; 70–90% protective against severe disease.
c. Limited data in preterm infants; may immunize after discharge from nursery if chronologic age is ≥ 6 weeks.
d. Consider immunizing children with chronic gastrointestinal disease (e.g., Hirschprung's disease, short gut syndrome, malabsorption syndromes), but data on efficacy and safety are not available.

N. VARICELLA IMMUNOPROPHYLAXIS

1. **Description**
a. Vaccine: Cell-free live attenuated varicella virus vaccine.
b. Efficacy: 70% against all disease, 95% against severe disease; annual prevalence in vaccinees followed for 7 years was 1–4% per year vs 7–8% per year for unimmunized children, and subsequent disease in immunized children was milder.
c. Varicella-zoster immune globulin (VZIG): Prepared from plasma-containing high-titer antivaricella antibodies, and negative for HBsAg and antibodies to HIV and HCV.
2. **Indications for immunization**
a. Routine (Fig. 17.1).

b. All persons >1 year not previously infected with chickenpox. Aim to immunize before the thirteenth birthday because two doses are needed after that time.

c. Serologic evaluation is optional before vaccination in healthy persons ≥13 years of age but unlikely to be cost effective. Children <13 years do not require serologic evaluation.

3. **Contraindications to immunization**

a. Anaphylactic reaction to vaccine, neomycin, or gelatin.

b. Moderate to severe illness regardless of fever.

c. Patients with altered immunity: See pp. 349–350.

d. Patients on salicylate therapy.

e. Pregnant women.

f. Recent blood product or IG administration. Defer 9 months after RSV-IVIG and 5 months after all other blood products.

4. **Misconceptions:** Vaccine may be given in the following circumstances:

a. Certain children with acute lymphoblastic leukemia in remission >1 year may be immunized. See *1997 Red Book*[3] for details.

b. Household contacts of immunocompromised hosts: Precautions are necessary only if a rash develops.

c. Household contacts of pregnant women: Consider deferring only if pregnant woman is known to be susceptible.

5. **Vaccine side effects**

a. Local reaction, 20–35%; fever 1–42 days after the immunization, 15% (comparable with placebo); varicelliform rash, 7–8%; zosterlike illness, 18 cases/100,000 person-years.

b. Vaccine rash often very mild, but patient may be infectious; reversion to wild-type virus has not been reported.

6. **Vaccine administration**

a. Dose: 0.5mL SC.

b. May give simultaneously with MMR; otherwise, allow at least 1 month between MMR and varicella vaccines.

c. Do not give for 5 months after VZIG; do not give concurrently.

d. Avoid salicylates for 6 weeks after vaccine administration (theoretical risk of Reye syndrome).

7. **Special considerations:** Postexposure prophylaxis.

a. Indications: VZIG should be administered within 96 hours of exposure to individuals who are at high risk for severe varicella **and** have had a significant exposure. Repeat VZIG Q3wk if ongoing or repeated exposure.

   1) Individuals at high risk for severe varicella

     a) Immunocompromised individuals without a history of varicella.

     b) Susceptible pregnant women.

     c) Newborn infant with onset of varicella in mother from 5 days before to 2 days after delivery (even if mother received VZIG during pregnancy).

17

IMMUNOPROPHYLAXIS

    d) Hospitalized preterm infant who was born at <28 weeks gestation or who weighs <1000g, regardless of maternal history.

    e) Hospitalized preterm infant who was born at ≥28 weeks gestation to a susceptible mother.

2) Significant exposures

    a) Household contact.

    b) Face-to-face indoor play.

    c) Onset of varicella in the mother of a newborn from 5 days before to 2 days after delivery.

    d) Hospital exposures: Roommate, face-to-face contact with infectious individual, visit by contagious individual, or intimate contact with person with active zoster lesions.

Note: For VZIG recipients, incubation period may be up to 28 days instead of 21 days.

b. Dosing of VZIG: 125 U (one vial) for each 10kg of body weight IM, max. 625 U, min. 125 U. Do not give IV. Local discomfort is common.

VI. REFERENCES

1. Committee on Infectious Diseases. American Academy of Pediatrics. Recommended childhood immunization schedule: United States, January–December 1999. *Pediatrics* 1999; **10**:1-4.

2. Atkinson W, Humiston S, Wolfe C, Nelson R. *Epidemiology and prevention of vaccine-preventable diseases,* 5th edn. Atlanta: National Immunization Program, Centers for Disease Control and Prevention; 1999.

3. American Academy of Pediatrics. *1997 red book: report of the Committee on Infectious Diseases,* 24th edn. Elk Grove Village, IL: The Academy; 1997.

INFECTIOUS DISEASES

Aklil Getachew, MD, and
Beth D. Kaufman, MD

I. FEVER WITHOUT LOCALIZING SIGNS (FWLS)

A. DEFINITIONS

1. **Fever:** Rectal temperature >38°C (>100.4°F).

Note: Serious life-threatening infections can be present in an infant without fever. Hypothermia (temperature <36°C [<96.8°F]) can be associated with serious infections in young infants.

2. **FWLS:** Acute (<5–7 days) febrile illness in which the etiology of the fever is not apparent after a careful history and physical examination.

3. **Occult bacteremia:** Infants and children who look well and have no source of fever detected by history or physical examination but who subsequently demonstrate bacteria in blood cultures obtained at the time of the illness.

4. **Toxic appearance:** *Toxicity* refers to the severity of a child's illness based on observation and physical examination. It has been used to describe a child who manifests signs of sepsis, including lethargy, poor perfusion, cyanosis, hypoventilation, and hyperventilation.

B. FWLS EVALUATION AND MANAGEMENT (Figs. 18.1 and 18.2): All infants and children who appear toxic should be admitted to the hospital; cultures should be obtained and parenteral antibiotics initiated. Figs. 18.1 and 18.2 represent suggested guidelines for the management of previously healthy, febrile infants. Actual practice may vary from institution to institution.

II. PERINATALLY ACQUIRED INFECTION

A. GROUP B STREPTOCOCCAL (GBS) INFECTIONS

1. **Presentation**

a. Early onset disease (<7 days old): Respiratory distress, apnea, shock, pneumonia, meningitis.

b. Late-onset disease (1 week–3 months): Bacteremia, meningitis, osteomyelitis, septic arthritis, cellulitis.

2. **Maternal intrapartum antibiotic prophylaxis (IAP):** Chemoprophylaxis regimen is with benzylpenicillin or clindamycin if penicillin allergic. Recommended for women with vaginal/anorectal screening cultures positive for GBS at 35–37 weeks' gestation or one or more of the following clinical risk factors:

18

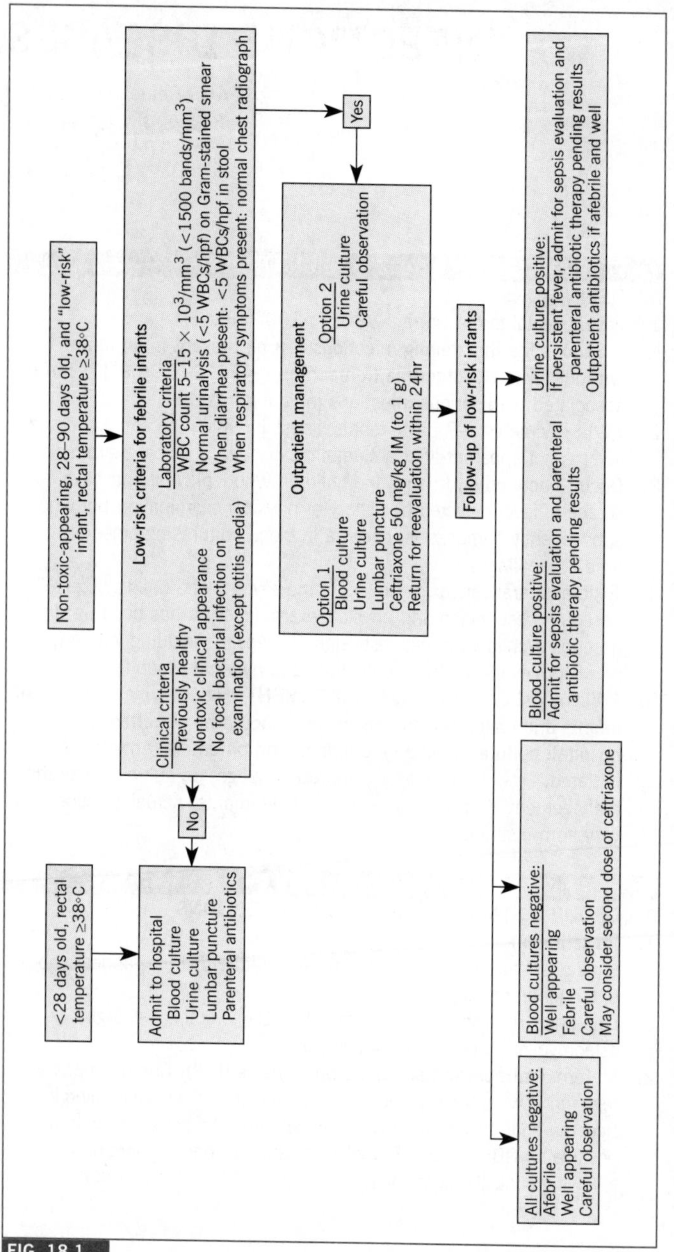
Non-toxic-appearing, 28–90 days old, and "low-risk" infant, rectal temperature ≥38∘C
Low-risk criteria for febrile infants
Clinical criteria
Previously healthy
Nontoxic clinical appearance
No focal bacterial infection on examination (except otitis media)
Laboratory criteria
WBC count 5–15 × 10³/mm³ (<1500 bands/mm³)
Normal urinalysis (<5 WBCs/hpf) on Gram-stained smear
When diarrhea present: <5 WBCs/hpf in stool
When respiratory symptoms present: normal chest radiograph
Yes
No
<28 days old, rectal temperature ≥38∘C
Admit to hospital
Blood culture
Urine culture
Lumbar puncture
Parenteral antibiotics
Outpatient management
Option 1
Blood culture
Urine culture
Lumbar puncture
Ceftriaxone 50 mg/kg IM (to 1 g)
Return for reevaluation within 24hr
Option 2
Urine culture
Careful observation
Follow-up of low-risk infants
All cultures negative:
Afebrile
Well appearing
Careful observation
Blood cultures negative:
Well appearing
Febrile
Careful observation
May consider second dose of ceftriaxone
Blood culture positive:
Admit for sepsis evaluation and parenteral antibiotic therapy pending results
Urine culture positive:
If persistent fever, admit for sepsis evaluation and parenteral antibiotic therapy pending results
Outpatient antibiotics if afebrile and well

FIG. 18.1

Algorithm for the management of a previously healthy infant <90 days of age with a fever without localizing signs. hpf, high power field.

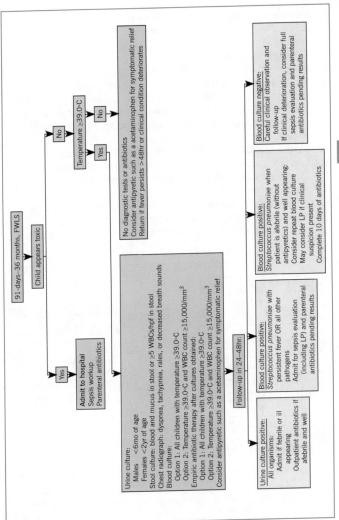

FIG. 18.2

Algorithm for the management of a previously healthy child 91 days–36 months of age with a fever without localizing signs. (Adapted from Baraff[1].)

    a. Previous infant with invasive GBS disease.
    b. GBS bacteriuria during this pregnancy.
    c. Delivery at <37 weeks' gestation.
    d. Ruptured membranes ≥18 hours.
    e. Intrapartum temperature ≥38°C (100.4°F).

  3. Management of neonates: Fig. 18.3 shows the management of neonates born to mothers receiving intrapartum prophylaxis for GBS.

  4. Treatment of neonatal GBS disease: Benzylpenicillin or ampicillin, plus an aminoglycoside. Duration of therapy depends on extent of disease.

B. OTHER CONGENITAL INFECTIONS 'TORCH': Toxoplasmosis, Other (syphilis, varicella-zoster, and parvovirus in this list), Rubella, Cytomegalovirus (CMV), and Herpes simplex/Hepatitis/HIV.

1. Toxoplasmosis

  a. Presentation: Maculopapular rash, generalized lymphadenopathy, hepatosplenomegaly, jaundice, thrombocytopenia, cerebral calcifications, chorioretinitis, hydrocephalus, microcephaly. May be asymptomatic.

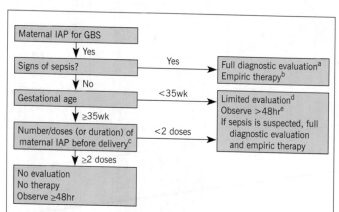

[a]Includes CBC and differential, blood culture, and chest radiograph if respiratory symptoms. A lumbar puncture is performed at the discretion of the physician.
[b]Duration of therapy will vary depending on results of blood culture and CSF findings (if obtained), as well as on the clinical course of the infant. If laboratory results and clinical course are unremarkable, duration may be as short as 48–72hr.
[c]Applies to penicillin or ampicillin chemoprophylaxis.
[d]CBC and differential, blood culture.
[e]Does not allow early discharge.
(From American Academy of Pediatrics, Committee on Infectious Diseases and Committee on Fetus and Newborn[2].)

FIG. 18.3

Empiric management of neonate born to a mother who received intrapartum antimicrobial prophylaxis (IAP) to prevent early onset GBS disease. This algorithm is a suggested but not an exclusive approach to management.

b. Transmission/diagnosis: Maternal infection (often acquired from an infected cat or undercooked meat) in the first trimester almost always leads to transmission of symptomatic disease; risk decreases with progression of gestation. Prenatal diagnosis is by detection of *Toxoplasma* IgM, IgA antibodies, or parasite in fetal blood. After birth, *Toxoplasma gondii* may be isolated from placental or cord tissue. *Toxoplasma* IgM, IgA, or IgG antibody persisting >12 months of age is also diagnostic.

c. Maternal treatment: Primary infection during gestation is treated with spiramycin.

d. Infant therapy: Symptomatic or asymptomatic congenital infection is treated with pyrimethamine and sulfadiazine for up to 1 year (see pp. 835 and 855).

2. Syphilis

a. Presentation: Stillbirth, intrauterine growth retardation (IUGR), hydrops fetalis, prematurity, hepatosplenomegaly, lymphadenopathy, osteochondritis, hemolytic anemia, mucocutaneous lesions, and thrombocytopenia.

b. For diagnosis, evaluation, and treatment of congenital syphilis, see pp. 392 and 396–398.

3. Varicella-zoster

a. Presentation: Limb atrophy and scarring (associated with fetal infections in the first or early second trimester), CNS and ocular symptoms, rash.

b. Diagnosis: Skin scrapings and serum immunoassays.

c. Maternal intervention: Acyclovir may be beneficial for varicella during pregnancy. Varicella-zoster immune globulin (VZIG) after exposure for susceptible women is recommended (see p. 373).

d. Infant therapy: VZIG immediately if maternal rash between 5 days before and 2 days after birth. Acyclovir if infant develops varicella.

4. Parvovirus B19 infection

a. Presentation: Severe anemia in utero, cardiac decompensation, hydrops fetalis, and stillbirth (associated with infection in the first or second trimester). May be asymptomatic.

b. Transmission/diagnosis: Infection transmission rate of 30%; diagnosis with polymerase chain reaction (PCR) or IgM antibody.

c. Maternal intervention: Intrauterine blood transfusion in selected cases.

d. Infant therapy: Supportive care.

5. Rubella

a. Presentation: Cataracts, retinopathy, cardiac anomalies, sensorineural deafness, meningoencephalitis, mental retardation, IUGR, hepatosplenomegaly, thrombocytopenia, purple rash ('blueberry muffin' appearance) of extramedullary hematopoiesis.

b. Diagnosis: Rubella-specific IgM (in the infant) or stable or increasing IgG levels for several months and culture.

18

INFECTIOUS DISEASES

c. Maternal treatment: Routine postexposure prophylaxis (PEP) with immune globulin is not recommended. Mothers not immune to rubella should be immunized after delivery, even if breast-feeding.

d. Infant therapy: Supportive care and isolation.

6. **CMV infection**

a. Presentation: IUGR, neonatal jaundice, purpura, thrombocytopenia, hepatosplenomegaly, microcephaly, intracerebral calcifications, chorioretinitis, mental retardation, sensorineural deafness. May be asymptomatic.

b. Diagnosis: CMV IgM; urine for CMV culture and early antigen between 2 days and 1 week of age.

c. Infant therapy: Treatment of the newborn with ganciclovir is under study.

7. **Herpes simplex**

a. Presentation: CNS disease, skin/eye/mouth (vesicles, keratitis), respiratory distress, sepsis. Initial symptoms of congenital herpes simplex infection can occur at birth or as late as 4–6 weeks of age.

b. Diagnosis: Culture of blood, urine, stool/rectum, CSF, conjunctivae, skin vesicles, nasopharynx, mouth; CSF PCR. All surface cultures should be obtained 48 hours after delivery of infant.

c. Maternal intervention: Screening by history and physical examination ± cesarean section ± acyclovir.

d. Infant therapy: Acyclovir (see *1997 Red Book*[3] for details).

8. **Hepatitis B**

a. Presentation: Infant of mother infected with hepatitis B—signs of hepatitis may appear.

b. Diagnosis: Chronic serum levels of hepatitis B surface antigen (HBsAg) (see pp. 412–413).

c. Maternal intervention: Screening and immunization.

d. Infant therapy: Hepatitis B immune globulin and immunization (see p. 360).

9. **HIV:** See Section IV, below.

III. COMMON PEDIATRIC INFECTIONS: GUIDELINES FOR INITIAL MANAGEMENT (Table 18.1)

A. **COMMON BACTERIAL INFECTIONS** (Table 18.1)

B. **COMMON FUNGAL INFECTIONS** (Table 18.2)

IV. HIV AND AIDS

For the most recent information on the diagnosis and management of children with HIV infection, check the recommendations at http://www.hivatis.org/.

A. **COUNSELING AND TESTING:** Legal requirements vary by state. Counseling should include informed consent for testing, implications of positive test results, and prevention of transmission. All pregnant

Text continued on p. 386

TABLE 18.1

COMMON PEDIATRIC INFECTIONS: GUIDELINES FOR INITIAL MANAGEMENT

Infectious syndrome	Usual etiology	Suggested empiric therapy	Suggested length of therapy/comments
Bacteremia (outpatient)	*Streptococcus pneumoniae, Haemophilus influenzae, Neisseria meningitidis, Escherichia coli, Salmonella*	Empiric: Ceftriaxone.	7–10 days (longer for some pathogens). Occult bacteremia with susceptible *S. pneumoniae* may be treated with amoxicillin if afebrile, well, and without focal complications.
Bites			
Human	Streptococci, *Staphylococcus aureus, Staphylococcus epidermidis,* anaerobes, *Eikenella corrodens*	PO: Amoxicillin/clavulanate. Alt: TMP/SMX + clindamycin. IV: Ampicillin/sulbactam	5–7 days. Cleaning, irrigation, and debridement most important. Assess tetanus immunization status, risk of hepatitis B and HIV. Antibiotic prophylaxis routinely used for human bites.
Dog/cat	Human bite pathogens plus *Pasteurella multocida*	Same.	7–10 days. Assess tetanus immunization status, risk of rabies. Antibiotic prophylaxis for all cat bites and selected dog bites.
Cellulitis	GAS, *Staphylococcus aureus*	PO: Dicloxacillin. Alt: Cephalexin. If penicillin allergic, clindamycin or macrolide. IV: Oxacillin. Alt: Clindamycin.	3 days after acute inflammation resolves (usually 7–10 days).
Conjunctivitis			
Neonatal	*Chlamydia trachomatis, Neisseria gonorrhoeae*	PO: Erythromycin, other macrolides. Ceftriaxone. Cefotaxime.	14 days. Topical ineffective in preventing pneumonia. Localized to eye: Single dose. Disseminated: 7 days of parenteral therapy.
Suppurative	*Streptococcus pneumoniae, Haemophilus influenzae,* S. aureus	Ophthalmic; Erythromycin or bacitracin/polymyxin B, or polymyxin B/TMP.	5 days. Ointments preferred for infants or young children and eyedrops for older children and adolescents.

Alt, Alternative; TMP/SMX, trimethoprin–sulfamethoxazole; GAS, group A streptococci; GBS, group B streptococci; Hib, *Haemophilus influenzae* type b.

Continued

TABLE 18.1

COMMON PEDIATRIC INFECTIONS: GUIDELINES FOR INITIAL MANAGEMENT—cont'd

Infectious syndrome	Usual etiology	Suggested empiric therapy	Suggested length of therapy/comments
Gastroenteritis			
Community acquired	Viruses, Escherichia coli	Antibiotic therapy rarely indicated.	Primary treatment: fluid and electrolyte replacement.
	Salmonella	Cefotaxime or ceftriaxone.	10–14 days for infants <6mo, toxicity or immunocompromised status. Antibiotics generally not indicated otherwise.
	Shigella	TMP/SMX. Alt: Cefixime.	5 days.
	Yersinia	TMP/SMX, aminoglycosides, cefotaxime, tetracycline (>8yr).	Usually no antibiotic therapy is recommended except with bacteremia, extraintestinal infections, or immunocompromised hosts.
Nosocomial	Clostridium difficile	Metronidazole.	7 days. Community organisms unlikely after 72hr of hospitalization.
Mastoiditis (acute)	Streptococcus pneumoniae, Streptococcus pyogenes, Staphylococcus aureus, Haemophilus influenzae	Oxacillin plus cefotaxime or ceftriaxone. Alt: Amoxicillin/clavulanic acid.	10 days.
Meningitis			
Neonate			
<1mo	GBS, Enterobacteriaceae, Listeria monocytogenes	Ampicillin and cefotaxime. Alt: Ampicillin and gentamicin.	14–21 days for GBS and Listeria. 21 days for Enterobacteriaceae (cefotaxime, aminoglycoside).
1–3mo	GBS, Streptococcus pneumoniae, Haemophilus influenzae, Neisseria meningitidis, Enterobacteriaceae	Ampicillin and cefotaxime.	10–14 days for S. pneumoniae, 7 days for N. meningitidis, 7–10 days for H. influenzae.

Infants >3mo and children	*Streptococcus pneumoniae*, *Neisseria meningitidis*, *Haemophilus influenzae*, neonatal pathogens	Cefotaxime or ceftriaxone. Vancomycin should be also added empirically for possible penicillin-resistant *Streptococcus pneumoniae*, until susceptibility is known.	Dexamethasone before antibiotics recommended for infants and children >6wk with Hib meningitis. Dexamethasone treatment is otherwise controversial. See *Red Book*[3] for chemoprophylaxis recommendations for contacts of meningococcal and Hib disease.
Orbital cellulitis	*Streptococcus pneumoniae*, *Haemophilus influenzae*, *Moraxella catarrhalis*, *Staphylococcus aureus*, GAS, anaerobes	Cefotaxime or ceftriaxone *plus* clindamycin.	10 days. Monitor for cavernous thrombosis.
Osteomyelitis	*Staphylococcus aureus*, GAS	Oxacillin. Alt: Clindamycin.	4–6wk.
<5yr	Add Hib	Add cefotaxime.	
Foot puncture	Add *Pseudomonas*	Add ceftazidime.	
Sickle cell disease	Add *Salmonella*	Add cefotaxime.	
Otitis media (acute)	*Streptococcus pneumoniae*, *Haemophilus influenzae* (nontypeable), *Moraxella catarrhalis*	Firstline: Amoxicillin, or high-dose amoxicillin (80mg/kg/day). Alt for penicillin allergy: Cefuroxime, azithromycin. Persistent otitis media: Amoxicillin/clavulanic acid, cefuroxime, or ceftriaxone (IM/IV).	5–10 days. For persistent otitis media (at 2–3 days' follow-up) despite antibiotic therapy, consider tympanocentesis (see p. 65). Short course 5–7 days for > 2yr old without language or hearing deficit.
Otitis externa (uncomplicated)	*Pseudomonas*, Enterobacteriaceae, *Proteus*	Eardrops: Polymyxin B/ neomycin/hydrocortisone. Alt: Ofloxacin drops.	7–10 days.

INFECTIOUS DISEASES

Continued

TABLE 18.1

COMMON PEDIATRIC INFECTIONS: GUIDELINES FOR INITIAL MANAGEMENT—cont'd

Infectious syndrome	Usual etiology	Suggested empiric therapy	Suggested length of therapy/comments
Periorbital cellulitis (preseptal)	Associated with sinusitis: See sinusitis	IV: Cefuroxime **or** Oxacillin + cefotaxime.	10–14 days.
	Associated with skin lesion: See cellulitis or oxacillin and cefotaxime.	PO: Amoxicillin/clavulanate.	
	PO: Amoxicillin/clavulanate.		
	Hematogenous (<2yr):		
	See bacteremia		
Pharyngitis	GAS	PO: Penicillin VK.	10 days.
		IM: Benzathine penicillin G ×1 dose.	TMP/SMX **not** effective.
		Alt: Erythromycin, cephalexin.	10 days.
Pneumonia			
Neonatal	*Escherichia coli,* GBS, *Staphylococcus aureus, Listeria monocytogenes*	Ampicillin + gentamicin or ampicillin + cefotaxime.	10–21 days. Blood cultures indicated. Effusions should be drained, Gram stain of fluid obtained.
3wk–4mo	*Chlamydia trachomatis*	Erythromycin. Alt: clarithromycin.	10 days.
Infant/child (6wk–4yr)			
Lobar	*Streptococcus pneumoniae*	IV: Cefuroxime, ceftriaxone, cefotaxime. PO: Amoxicillin. Alt: Clindamycin.	7–10 days.
Atypical	*Bordetella pertussis*	Erythromycin (estolate preparation preferred) or clarithromycin.	14 days. Chemoprophylaxis indicated for close contacts.
	Respiratory viruses	No antibiotics indicated.	
≥ 4yr			
Lobar	*Streptococcus pneumoniae*	IV: Cefuroxime, ceftriaxone, or cefotaxime PLUS PO/IV macrolide.	

Atypical	*Mycoplasma pneumoniae* or *Chlamydia pneumoniae*	PO: Amoxicillin. Alt: Erythromycin.	7–10 days.
		Clarithromycin.	5 days.
		Azithromycin.	3 days.
		Erythromycin, clarithromycin, azithromycin, or tetracycline (>8 yr).	14–21 days.
Septic arthritis			
<5yr	*Staphylococcus aureus*, GBS, Hib	See osteomyelitis.	3–4wk IV. May switch to PO after response.
>5yr	*Staphylococcus aureus*, GAS		Aspiration of affected joint recommended.
Adolescent	Add *Neisseria gonorrhoeae*	See p. 395.	
Sinusitis			
Acute	*Streptococcus pneumoniae*, *Haemophilus influenzae*, *Moraxella catarrhalis*	See otitis media.	10–14 days.
Chronic	Add *Staphylococcus aureus*, anaerobes	Amoxicillin/clavulanate.	21 days.
UTI			
Uncomplicated	*Escherichia coli*, *Proteus* Enterococci	IV: Cefotaxime **or** ampicillin and gentamicin. PO: TMP/SMX, cefixime.	5–14 days (cystitis vs pyelonephritis and age dependent).
Abnormal host/ urinary tract	Add *Pseudomonas*	Ceftazidime.	14–21 days. Parenteral until afebrile ×24 hr.
Ventriculoperitoneal shunt, infected	*Staphylococcus epidermidis*, *Staphylococcus aureus*, Enterobacteriaceae	Vamcomycin + cefotaxime or ceftriaxone. Add aminoglycoside for Enterobacteriaceae. Consider adding rifampin.	21 days. Shunt removal or revision may be necessary.

INFECTIOUS DISEASES

18

TABLE 18.2

COMMON COMMUNITY-ACQUIRED FUNGAL INFECTIONS

Disease	Usual etiology	Suggested therapy	Suggested length of therapy
Tinea capitis (ringworm of scalp)	*Trichophyton tonsurans, Microsporum canis*	Oral griseofulvin: Give with fatty foods. Fungal shedding decreased with 1–2.5% selenium sulfide shampoo. Alt: Terbinafine.	4–6wk or 2wk after clinical resolution.
Tinea corporis/pedis (ringworm of body/feet)	*Trichophyton rubrum, Trichophyton mentagrophytes, Microsporum canis*	Topical antifungal (miconazole, clotrimazole). Terbinafine.	4wk. 2wk.
Oral candidiasis (thrush)	*Candida albicans, Candida tropicalis*	Nystatin suspension or troches.	3 days after clinical resolution.
Candidal skin infections (intertriginous)	*Candida albicans*	Topical nystatin, miconazole, clotrimazole.	3 days after clinical resolution.

women should be offered counseling and testing so that they can make an informed decision regarding therapy aimed at reducing transmission to their infants.

B. DIAGNOSIS OF HIV IN CHILDREN

1. Infected child

a. Child <18 months is considered HIV infected if he or she:
  1) Has positive results on two separate determinations (excluding cord blood) from one or more of the following HIV detection tests:
    a) HIV culture.
    b) HIV PCR.
    c) HIV antigen (p24).
  2) Meets criteria for AIDS diagnosis based on 1987 AIDS surveillance case definition (from revision of the Centers for Disease Control and Prevention [CDC] surveillance case definition for AIDS[4]).
b. A child ≥18 months is considered HIV infected if he or she:
  1) Is HIV antibody positive by repeated reactive enzyme immunoassay (EIA) and confirmatory test (e.g., Western blot or immunofluorescence assay [IFA]).
  2) Meets any of the test criteria for a child <18 months.

2. Perinatally exposed child: A child is considered exposed when he or she does not meet the aforementioned criteria and who:

TABLE 18.3

1994 REVISED PEDIATRIC HIV CLASSIFICATION SYSTEM: IMMUNOLOGIC CATEGORIES BASED ON AGE-SPECIFIC CD4+ LYMPHOCYTE COUNT AND PERCENT

	Age of child		
	<12mo	1–5yr	6–12yr
Immunologic category	No./mcL (%)	No./mcL (%)	No./mcL (%)
1: No suppression	≥1500 (≥25)	≥1000 (≥25)	≥500 (≥25)
2: Moderate suppression	750–1499 (15–24)	500–999 (15–24)	200–499 (15–24)
3: Severe suppression	<750 (<15)	<500 (<15)	<200 (<15)

From Centers for Disease Control and Prevention[5].

a. Is HIV seropositive by EIA and confirmatory test (e.g., Western blot or IFA) and who is <18 months old at the time of the test.
b. Has unknown antibody status but was born to a mother known to be infected with HIV.

3. **Seroreverter:** A child who was born to an HIV-infected mother and who:

a. Has been documented as HIV antibody negative (i.e., two or more negative EIA tests performed at 6–18 months of age or one negative EIA test after 18 months of age) **or**
b. Has no other laboratory evidence of infection **and**
c. Has not had an AIDS-defining condition.

C. **PEDIATRIC HIV IMMUNOLOGIC CATEGORIES** (Table 18.3)
D. **GUIDELINES FOR PROPHYLAXIS AGAINST FIRST EPISODE OF OPPORTUNISTIC INFECTIONS** (Table 18.4)
E. **MANAGEMENT OF PERINATAL HIV EXPOSURE:** Recommendations provided are current at the time of publication; check the recent recommendations for most current therapy at http//www.hivatis.org/.

1. **Prophylactic regimen to reduce transmission:** Use of antiretroviral therapy during pregnancy, during delivery, and in the newborn dramatically reduces HIV transmission.

a. Pregnancy: The following regimen was shown to reduce transmission: zidovudine (ZDV) 100mg PO 5×/24hr initiated at 14–34 weeks' gestation and continued throughout pregnancy (established to be effective in women who do not otherwise have clinical indications for ZDV therapy). Many experts use 200mg PO TID or 300mg PO BID, extrapolated from data on other adult populations.
b. Labor: During labor, IV ZDV in a loading dose of 2mg/kg over 1 hour, followed by continuous infusion of 1mg/kg per hour until delivery.
c. Newborn: For the newborn, ZDV 2mg/kg per dose PO Q6hr for first 6 weeks of life, beginning 8–12 hours after birth.

2. **Ongoing management of indeterminate infants**

a. PCP prophylaxis with trimethoprim–sulfamethoxazole (TMP/SMX) should be initiated for all HIV-exposed infants at 4–6 weeks of life.

TABLE 18.4
PROPHYLAXIS FOR FIRST EPISODE OF OPPORTUNISTIC DISEASE IN HIV-INFECTED INFANTS AND CHILDREN

Pathogen	Indication	Preventive regimens	
		First choice	Alternatives
Strongly recommended as standard of care			
Pneumocystis carinii	HIV-infected or HIV-indeterminate infants 4–6wk→12mo of age HIV-infected children 1–5yr with CD4+ count <500mcL or CD4+ percent <15% HIV-infected children 6–12yr with CD4+ count <200mcL or CD4+ percent <15%	TMP/SMX 150/750mg/m²/day in 2 divided doses PO 3×/week on consecutive days. Acceptable alternative dosage schedules: Single dose PO 3×/week on consecutive days. 2 divided doses PO every day. 2 divided doses PO 3×/week on alternate days.	Aerosolized pentamidine (children ≥5yr) 300mg every month via Respirgard II nebulizer; dapsone (children ≥1mo) 2mg/kg (max. 100mg) PO every day; IV pentamidine 4mg/kg Q2–4wk.
Mycobacterium tuberculosis			
Isoniazid sensitive	Tuberculin skin test reaction ≥5mm **or** prior positive TST result without treatment **or** contact with case of active tuberculosis	Isoniazid 10–15mg/kg (max. 300mg) PO **or** IM every day × 12mo) **or** 20–30mg/kg (max. 900mg) PO BIW × 12mo.	Rifampin 10–20mg/kg (max. 600mg) PO or IV every day × 12mo.
Isoniazid resistant	Same as above; high probability of exposure to isoniazid-resistant tuberculosis	Rifampin 10–20mg/kg (max. 600mg) PO **or** IV every day × 12mo.	Uncertain.
Multidrug (isoniazid and rifampin resistant)	Same as above; high probability of exposure to multidrug-resistant tuberculosis	Choice of drug requires consultation with public health authorities.	None.

Mycobacterium avium complex	For children <1yr, CD4+ count <750/mcL 1–2yr, CD4+ count <500/mcL 2–6yr, CD4+ count <75/mcL ≥6yr, CD4+ count <50/mcL	Clarithromycin 7.5mg/kg PO BID (max. 500mg) **or** azithromycin 20mg/kg (max. 1200mg) PO once weekly.	Children <6yr: rifabutin 5mg/kg PO every day when suspension becomes available; children ≥ 6yr: rifabutin 300mg PO every day; azithromycin, 5mg/kg (max. 250mg) PO every day.
Varicella-zoster virus	Significant exposure to varicella with no history of chickenpox or shingles	VZIG 1 vial (1.25 mL)/10kg (max. 5 vials) IM, administered ≤96hr after exposure, ideally within 48hr.	None.
Generally recommended			
Toxoplasma gondii[a]	IgG antibody to *Toxoplasma* and severe immunosuppression	TMP/SMX 150/750mg/m²/day in 2 divided doses PO every day.	Dapsone (children ≥1mo): 2mg/kg or 15mg/m² (max. 25mg) PO every day **plus** pyrimethamine 1mg/kg PO every day **plus** leucovorin 5mg PO every 3 days.
Not recommended for most patients; indicated for use only in unusual circumstances			
Cryptococcus neoformans	Severe immunosuppression	Fluconazole 3–6mg/kg PO every day.	Itraconazole 2–5mg/kg PO Q12–24hr.
Histoplasma capsulatum	Severe immunosuppression, endemic geographic area	Itraconazole 2–5mg/kg PO Q12–24hr.	None.
Cytomegalovirus (CMV)[b]	CMV antibody positivity and severe immunosuppression	Children 6–12yr: Oral ganciclovir under investigation.	None.

From Centers for Disease Control and Prevention[6].

TMP/SMX, trimethoprim–sulfamethoxazole; BIW, twice a week.

[a]Protection against *Toxoplasma* is provided by the preferred anti-*Pneumocystis* regimens. Pyrimethamine alone probably provides little, if any, protection.

[b]Data on oral ganciclovir are still being evaluated; durability of effect is unclear. Acyclovir is not protective against CMV.

18

INFECTIOUS DISEASES

PCP prophylaxis should be continued until clinical status excludes HIV infection. For infected infants, refer to Table 18.4.

b. HIV diagnostic tests (DNA PCR or viral culture) should be obtained on the infant between birth and 2 weeks of life (cord blood should not be used), at 1–2 months, and again at 4–6 months to determine infection status. A positive test should be promptly repeated for confirmation of infection. If all tests are negative, the infant should be tested for HIV antibody at 12 and 18 months of age to document disappearance of the antibody.

c. Clinical monitoring: Infants should be evaluated at routine well-child visits for signs and symptoms of HIV infection. In addition to HIV diagnostic tests, the following monitoring tests are recommended: CBC and T-cell subsets at birth–2 weeks, 1–2 months, and 4–6 months. Any suspicious clinical or laboratory findings merit careful and close follow-up.

F. MANAGEMENT OF HIV INFECTED INFANTS AND CHILDREN

Note: Primary care physicians are encouraged to participate in the care and management of HIV-infected children in consultation with specialists who have expertise in the care of such children. Knowledge about antiretroviral therapy is changing, and in areas where enrollment into clinical trials is possible, it should be encouraged.

1. **Criteria for initiation of antiretroviral therapy**
a. Initiation of antiretroviral therapy depends on virologic, immunologic, and clinical status.
b. All HIV-infected infants <12 months of age, regardless of immunologic, virologic, or clinical status, should be started on antiretroviral therapy.
c. Antiretroviral therapy should be initiated in children with evidence of immune suppression as indicated by CD4+ lymphocyte absolute number or percentage in Immunologic Category 2 or 3 (Table 18.3).
d. Therapy should be initiated in any child with clinical symptoms related to HIV infection.
e. For asymptomatic HIV-infected children >1 year of age with normal immune status, consideration should be given to initiating therapy.

2. **Antiretroviral regimen:** For the most recent recommendations, refer to http://www.hivatis.org/. Data suggest the use of combination therapy for initial and ongoing therapy (except chemoprophylaxis in an exposed infant as previously listed; if an infant is identified as HIV infected while receiving prophylaxis, therapy should be changed to combination therapy). Refer to Table 31-11.

3. **Clinical and laboratory monitoring in HIV-infected children:** Immune status, viral load, evidence of HIV progression and drug toxicity should be monitored on a regular basis (about every 3 months). Careful attention to routine aspects of pediatric care, such as growth, development, and vaccines, is essential.

G. **IMMUNIZATIONS IN HIV-INFECTED OR HIV-EXPOSED INFANTS AND CHILDREN:** Specific guidelines are discussed on p. 350. In general, live viral (e.g., oral poliovirus vaccine [OPV]) and live bacterial (e.g., Bacillus Calmette–Guérin [BCG]) vaccines should not be given. The measles/mumps/rubella (MMR) vaccine and varicella vaccine may be administered under certain circumstances. Pneumococcal vaccine at 2 years of age and yearly influenza immunization, starting at 6 months of age, are also recommended.

V. SEXUALLY TRANSMITTED DISEASES (STDs)

Note: Patients diagnosed with any one STD should be tested for other STDs (e.g., syphilis) and pregnancy.

A. **PELVIC INFLAMMATORY DISEASE (PID)**
1. **Definition:** Spectrum of inflammatory disorders of the upper female genital tract (any combination of salpingitis, tuboovarian abscess, endometritis, and pelvic peritonitis).
2. **Etiology:** *Neisseria gonorrhoeae, Chlamydia trachomatis,* and microorganisms endogenous to the lower genital tract flora (e.g., anaerobes, *Haemophilus influenzae,* enteric Gram-negative rods, and *Streptococcus agalactiae*).
3. **Diagnostic criteria:** Minimal criteria (must have **all** of the following):
a. Lower abdominal tenderness.
b. Adnexal tenderness.
c. Cervical motion tenderness.
d. Absence of an established etiology other than PID.
4. **Additional criteria:** Presence of the following increases the specificity of the diagnosis:
a. Routine criteria
   1) Oral temperature >38.3°C.
   2) Abnormal cervical or vaginal discharge.
   3) Elevated erythrocyte sedimentation rate.
   4) Elevated C-reactive protein.
   5) Laboratory documentation of cervical infection with *N. gonorrhoeae* or *C. trachomatis.*
b. Elaborate criteria
   1) Histopathologic evidence of endometritis on endometrial biopsy.
   2) Tuboovarian abscess on sonography or other radiologic tests.
   3) Laparoscopic abnormalities consistent with PID.
5. **Criteria for hospitalization**
a. Surgical emergencies such as appendicitis cannot be excluded.
b. Presence of a tuboovarian abscess.
c. Pregnancy.
d. Immunodeficiency (e.g., HIV with low CD4 counts or immunosuppressive therapy).

18

INFECTIOUS DISEASES

    e. Inability to follow or tolerate an outpatient oral regimen.

    f. Severe illness, nausea and vomiting, or high fever.

    g. Failure to respond clinically to oral antimicrobial therapy.

    h. Clinical follow-up within 72 hours of starting antibiotic treatment cannot be arranged. (Many experts recommend hospitalizing adolescents because their ability to complete a therapeutic regimen as an outpatient may be unpredictable.)

6. Treatment[7] of PID

a. Inpatient parenteral treatment

    1) Regimen A: Cefoxitin 2g IV Q6hr or cefotetan 2g IV Q12hr **plus** doxycycline 100mg IV/PO Q12hr.

    2) Regimen B: Clindamycin 900mg IV Q8hr (15–40mg/kg per 24 hours Q8hr) **plus** gentamicin 2mg/kg IV/IM loading dose followed by 1.5mg/kg per dose Q8hr maintenance dose.

    3) These regimens should be continued for at least 24 hours after patients demonstrate substantial clinical improvement; then they should be followed with doxycycline 100mg PO Q12hr or clindamycin 450mg PO Q6hr to complete a total of 14 days of therapy.

b. Outpatient treatment

    1) Regimen A: Doxycycline 100mg PO BID ×14 days **plus** one of the following:

        a) Cefoxitin 2g IM ×1 dose plus probenecid 1g PO ×1 dose concurrently.

        b) Ceftriaxone 250mg IM ×1 dose.

        c) Another parenteral third-generation cephalosporin (e.g., ceftizoxime or cefotaxime).

    2) Regimen B (>18 years of age): Ofloxacin 400mg PO BID ×14 days **plus** clindamycin 450mg PO QID or metronidazole 500mg PO BID ×14 days.

B. THERAPY FOR CHLAMYDIA AND GONORRHEA FOR ILLNESSES OTHER THAN PID (Table 18.5)

C. CONGENITAL SYPHILIS

1. Testing during pregnancy: All pregnant women should be screened with a nontreponemal antibody test (Venereal Disease Research Laboratory [VDRL] test or rapid plasma reagin [RPR] test) early in pregnancy and preferably again at delivery. In areas of high prevalence and in patients considered at high risk, a test early in the third trimester is also indicated. Treat if there is evidence of infection and follow serologies to assess the effectiveness of therapy.

2. Evaluation of infants

a. No newborn should be discharged from the hospital without determining the mother's serologic status for syphilis. Testing of cord blood or infant serum is not adequate for screening.

TABLE 18.5

THERAPY FOR CHLAMYDIA AND GONORRHEA

Type or stage	Firstline drug and dosage	Alternatives
Chlamydia trachomatis infection		
Urethritis, cervicitis, or proctitis	Doxycycline 100mg PO BID ×7 days (if >9yr) **or** Azithromycin 1g PO ×1 dose	Erythromycin base 500mg PO QID ×7 days **or** Erythromycin ethylsuccinate 800mg PO QID ×7 days **or** Ofloxacin 300mg PO BID ×7 days (if >18yr)
Infection in pregnancy	Erythromycin base 500mg PO QID ×7 days **or** Amoxicillin 500mg PO TID ×7 days	Erythromycin base 250mg QID ×14 days **or** Erythromycin ethylsuccinate 400mg PO QID ×14 days, **or** Azithromycin 1g PO ×1 dose
Neonatal ophthalmia	Erythromycin base 50mg/kg/24hr PO or IV ÷6hr or QID ×14 days	Topical treatment is ineffective.
Neonatal pneumonia	Erythromycin base 50mg/kg/24hr PO or IV QID ×14 days	—
Gonorrhea[a]		
Newborns		
Sepsis, arthritis, meningitis, scalp abscess	Ceftriaxone 25–50mg/kg/24hr IV/IM Q24hr ×7 days (10–14 days if meningitis) **or** Cefotaxime 50mg/kg/24hr IV/IM Q12hr ×7 days (10–14 days if meningitis)	—

From Centers for Disease Control and Prevention[7].
[a]Therapy should include treatment for presumed concomitant chlamydial infection.

Continued

INFECTIOUS DISEASES **18**

TABLE 18.5

THERAPY FOR CHLAMYDIA AND GONORRHEA—cont'd

Type or stage	Firstline drug and dosage	Alternatives
Gonorrhea—cont'd		
Neonatal ophthalmia	Ceftriaxone 25–50mg/kg (max. 125mg) IV/IM ×1 dose plus saline irrigation **or** Cefotaxime 100mg/kg per dose IM/IV ×1 dose	All infants should receive silver nitrate, tetracycline, or erythromycin ointment instilled into each eye within 1hr of birth. Note: All infants with GC conjunctivitis should be evaluated for possible sepsis/disseminated disease and the need to be treated for a longer time.
Prepubertal children who weigh <100lb (45kg)		
Uncomplicated urethritis, vulvovaginitis, proctitis, or pharyngitis	Ceftriaxone 125mg IM ×1 dose	Spectinomycin 40mg/kg (max. 2g) IM ×1 dose.
Bacteremia, peritonitis, or arthritis	Ceftriaxone 50mg/kg/24hr (max. 1g) IM/IV Q24hr ×7–10 days	—
Children who weigh ≥100 lb (45kg) and ≥9yr		
Uncomplicated endocervicitis or urethritis	Ceftriaxone 125mg IM ×1 dose **or** Cefixime 400mg PO ×1 dose **or** Ciprofloxacin 500mg PO ×1 dose (if >18yr) **PLUS** Ofloxacin 400mg PO ×1 dose (if >18yr) **or** Azithromycin 1g PO ×1 dose **or** Doxycycline 100mg PO BID ×7 days	Spectinomycin 40mg/kg (max. 2g) IM ×1 dose.

Pharyngitis	Same as uncomplicated endocervicitis or urethritis therapy	—
PID	See p. 392	—
Disseminated gonococcal infections	Ceftriaxone 1g/24hr IV/IM Q24hr ×7 days	Cefotaxime or ceftizoxime 3g IV Q8hr ×7 days. For persons allergic to β-lactam drugs: Spectinomycin 2g IM Q12hr ×7 days **or** Ciprofloxacin 1g/24hr IV Q12hr **or** Ofloxacin 800mg IV Q12hr.
Bacteremia or arthritis	Ceftriaxone 50mg/kg/day (max. dose 2g) IM or IV Q24hr ×10–14 days	—

From Centers for Disease Control and Prevention[7].

    b. An infant should be evaluated for congenital syphilis if he or she is born to a mother who has a positive nontreponemal test, confirmed by a positive treponemal test, and who has one or more of the following:
       1) Was not treated.
       2) Had treatment but course was poorly documented.
       3) Received inadequate doses or duration of treatment.
       4) Was treated with nonpenicillin regimen (e.g., erythromycin).
       5) Was treated <1 month before delivery.
       6) Had insufficient serologic follow-up to ensure that she responded appropriately to treatment by demonstrating a fourfold or greater decrease in titers in 3 months after course of treatment.
    c. Further evaluation of infants with the preceding conditions should include:
       1) Physical examination (e.g., rash [vesicobullous], hepatomegaly, generalized lymphadenopathy, persistent rhinitis).
       2) Quantitative nontreponemal test on infant's serum. (Cord blood may give false-positive or false-negative results.)
       3) Examine CSF for protein, cell count, and VDRL test. CSF VDRL is specific but not sensitive. (Do not perform RPR and fluorescent treponemal antibody absorption [FTA-ABS] test on CSF.)
       4) Radiologic studies: Long bone films for diaphyseal periostitis, osteochondritis.
       5) If available, antitreponemal IgM antibody via a testing method recognized by the CDC either as a standard or provisional method.
       6) Other tests as clinically indicated (e.g., chest radiograph, CBC, LFTs).
3. Guide for interpretation of the syphilis serology of mothers and their infants[3] (Table 18.6)
4. Treatment of neonates with proven or possible congenital syphilis (Table 18.7): Follow nontreponemal serologic tests at 3, 6, and 12 months after treatment.
D. TREATMENT OF SYPHILIS (POSTNEONATAL) (Table 18.8)

VI. TUBERCULOSIS
A. RECOMMENDED TUBERCULOSIS TESTING
1. Tuberculin skin test recommendations[3]:BCG immunization is not a contraindication to tuberculin skin testing.
    a. Children for whom immediate skin testing is indicated
       1) Contacts of people with confirmed or suspected infectious tuberculosis (contact investigation); this includes children identified as contacts of family members or associates in jail or prison in the last 5 years.
       2) Children with radiologic or clinical findings suggesting tuberculosis.
       3) Children emigrating from endemic countries (e.g., Asia, the Middle East, Africa, Latin America).
       4) Children with travel histories to endemic countries and/or significant contact with indigenous people from such countries.

TABLE 18.6

GUIDE FOR INTERPRETATION OF THE SYPHILIS SEROLOGY
OF MOTHERS AND THEIR INFANTS

Nontreponemal test (e.g., VDRL, RPR, ART)		Treponemal test (e.g., MHA-TP, FTA-ABS)		
Mother	Infant	Mother	Infant	Interpretation[a]
−	−	−	−	No syphilis or incubating syphilis in the mother and infant
+	+	−	−	No syphilis in mother (false-positive nontreponemal test with passive transfer to infant)
+	+ or −	+	+	Maternal syphilis with possible infant infection; or mother treated for syphilis during pregnancy; or mother with latent syphilis and possible infection of infant[b]
+	+	+	+	Recent or previous syphilis in the mother; possible infection in infant
−	−	+	+	Mother successfully treated for syphilis before or early in pregnancy; or mother with Lyme disease, yaws, or pinta (i.e., false-positive serology)

Adapted from *1997 Red Book*[3].

ART, automated reagin test; MHA-TP, microhemagglutination test for *T. pallidum*.

[a]Table presents a guide and not the definitive interpretation of serologic tests for syphilis in mothers and their newborns. Other factors that should be considered include the timing of maternal infection, the nature and timing of maternal treatment, quantitative maternal and infant titers, and serial determination of nontreponemal test titers in both mother and infant.

[b]Mothers with latent syphilis may have nonreactive nontreponemal tests.

b. Children who should be tested annually for tuberculosis (initial tuberculin skin testing is at the time of diagnosis or circumstance, beginning as early as age 3 months).
   1) Children infected with HIV or living in a household with HIV-infected people.
   2) Incarcerated adolescents.
c. Children who should be tested every 2–3 years
   1) Children exposed to people who are HIV infected, homeless, residents of nursing homes, institutionalized adolescents or adults, users of illicit drugs, incarcerated adolescents or adults, and migrant farm workers. Foster children with exposure to adults in the preceding high-risk groups are included.

TABLE 18.7

TREATMENT OF NEONATES WITH PROVEN OR POSSIBLE CONGENITAL SYPHILIS

Clinical status	Antimicrobial therapy[a]
Proven or highly probable disease[b]	Aqueous crystalline penicillin G 50,000 U/kg/dose for the first week, then Q8hr for a total course of 10–14 days[c,d]
Asymptomatic, normal CSF and radiologic examination—maternal treatment history:	
• None, inadequate penicillin treatment,[e] undocumented, failed, or reinfected	Aqueous crystalline penicillin G IV for 10–14 days[c,d] (see dosing above) **or** Clinical, serologic follow-up and benzathine penicillin G 50,000 U/kg IM, single dose[f]
• Adequate therapy but given <1mo before delivery, mother's response to treatment not demonstrated by a fourfold decrease in titer of a nontreponemal serologic test or erythromycin therapy	Clinical, serologic follow-up and benzathine penicillin G 50,000 U/kg IM, single dose[f]

From *1997 Red Book*[3].
[a]See formulary (ch. 32) for further drug information.
[b]Proven or probable disease if:
 1) Physical or radiologic evidence of active disease.
 2) Infant's nontreponemal titer is at least four times higher than the mother's titer.
 3) CSF VDRL is reactive or CSF cell count and/or protein is abnormal.
 4) Positive antitreponemal IgM test.
 5) Placenta or umbilical cord is positive for treponemes organisms using specific fluorescent antibody staining.
[c]If more than 1 day of therapy is missed, the entire course should be restarted.
[d]Alternatively, some experts recommend procaine penicillin G 50,000 U/kg IM daily for 10–14 days, but CSF levels may be inadequate.
[e]Mother's penicillin dose unknown, undocumented, or inadequate **or** lack of fourfold or greater decrease in nontreponemal antibody titer in mother.
[f]Some experts recommend aqueous crystalline penicillin G as for proven or highly probably disease (see text). Other experts would follow the infant without giving antibiotic therapy if both clinical and serologic follow-up can be ensured.

 d. Children who should be considered for tuberculin skin testing at 4–6 and 11–16 years
  1) Children whose parents emigrated (with unknown tuberculin skin test status) from regions of the world with a high prevalence of tuberculosis; continued potential exposure by travel to endemic areas and/or household contact with people from the endemic areas (with unknown tuberculin skin status) should be indications for repeat tuberculin skin testing.

TABLE 18.8

TREATMENT FOR SYPHILIS (POSTNEONATAL)[a]

Type or stage	Firstline drug and dosage	Alternatives
Congenital syphilis (diagnosed >4wk of age)	Aqueous crystalline penicillin 200,000–300,000U/kg/24 hr IV Q6hr × 10–14 days	—
Early acquired syphilis of <1 year's duration	Benzathine benzylpenicillin 50,000U/kg (max. 2.4 × 10^6 U) IM × 1 dose	Tetracycline 500mg PO Q6hr × 14 days (for >8yr) **or** Doxycycline 4mg/kg/24hr (max. 200mg) PO Q12hr × 14 days (for >8yr).
Syphilis of >1 year's duration (late syphilis)	Benzathine benzylpenicillin 50,000U/kg per dose (max. 2.4 × 10^6U) IM every week ×3 successive weeks (Note: Must examine CSF to exclude asymptomatic neurosyphilis)	Tetracycline 500mg PO Q6hr × 28 days (for >8yr) **or** Doxycycline 4mg/kg/24hr (max. 200mg) PO Q12hr × 28 days.
Neurosyphilis	Aqueous crystalline benzylpenicillin 200,000–300,000U/kg/day IV Q4–6hr (max. 4 × 10^6U IV Q4hr) × 10–14 days; may be followed by benzathine penicillin 50,000U/kg/dose (max. 2.4 × 10^6 U) IM every week × 3wk	Aqueous procaine benzylpenicillin 2.4 × 10^6 U IM Q24hr × 10–14 days + probenecid 500mg PO Q6hr × 10–14 days; may be followed by benzathine penicillin 50,000U/kg/dose (max. 2.4 × 10^6 U) IM every week × 3wk. (If penicillin allergic, especially if <9yr, consider penicillin desensitization and administration in an appropriate setting. Also patient should be managed in consultation with a specialist.)

Adapted from *1997 Red Book*[3].
[a]Refer to p. 418 for diagnosis and collection techniques.

2) Children without specific risk factors who reside in high-prevalence areas; in general, a high-risk neighborhood or community does not mean that an entire city is at high risk; rates in any area of the city may vary by neighborhood or even from block to block. Physicians

should be aware of these patterns in determining the likelihood of exposure; public health officials or local tuberculosis experts should help clinicians identify areas that have higher tuberculosis rates.

e. Children at increased risk of progression of infection to disease: Those with other medical risk factors, including diabetes mellitus, chronic renal failure, malnutrition, and congenital or acquired immunodeficiencies, deserve special consideration. Without recent exposure, these people are not at increased risk of acquiring tuberculosis infection. Underlying immune deficiencies associated with these conditions would theoretically enhance the possibility for progression to severe disease. Initial histories of potential exposure to tuberculosis should be included for all such patients. If these histories or local epidemiologic factors suggest a possibility of exposure, immediate and periodic tuberculin skin testing should be considered. An initial Mantoux tuberculin skin test should be performed before initiation of immunosuppressive therapy in any child with an underlying condition that necessitates immunosuppressive therapy.

2. **Standard tuberculin test:** Mantoux test—5 tuberculin units (5TU) of purified protein derivative (0.1mL). *The tine test (MPT) is no longer recommended.*

a. Inject intradermally on volar aspect of forearm to form 6–10mm weal. All results (positive or negative) should be read at 48–72 hours by *qualified medical personnel.*

b. Definition of **positive** Mantoux skin test (regardless of whether BCG has been previously administered)
   1) Reaction ≥5mm
      a) Children in close contact with people who have known or suspected infectious cases of tuberculosis.
      b) Children suspected to have tuberculous disease based on chest radiographs or other clinical evidence of tuberculosis.
      c) Children with immunosuppressive conditions or HIV infection.
   2) Reaction ≥10 mm
      a) Children at increased risk of dissemination based on young age (<4 years) or other medical risk factors, including Hodgkin's disease, lymphoma, diabetes mellitus, chronic renal failure, and malnutrition.
      b) Children with increased environmental exposure
         i) Those born, or whose parents were born, in regions of the world where tuberculosis is highly prevalent.
         ii) Those who travel to high-prevalence regions.
         iii) Those frequently exposed to adults who are HIV infected, homeless, users of street drugs, medically indigent, residents of nursing homes, incarcerated, institutionalized, or migrant farm workers.
   3) Reaction ≥15mm: Children (≥4 years of age without any risk factors.

c. Cutaneous anergy skin tests for control are indicated only in patients with suspected or proven immunosuppression and in those with the possibility of disseminated disease.

B. DRUG THERAPY

1. Prophylaxis

a. Indications

   1) Children with positive tuberculin tests but no evidence of clinical disease.

   2) Recent contacts, especially HIV-infected contacts, of people with infectious tuberculosis, even if tuberculin test and clinical evidence are not indicative.

b. Recommendations (see individual drugs in formulary [ch. 29] for specific doses) (Table 18.9).

2. Treatment for active tuberculosis disease (for details, see *1997 Red Book*[3]) (Table 18.9).

VII. ISOLATION TECHNIQUES FOR SELECTED ILLNESSES

A. UNIVERSAL PRECAUTIONS

Note: Use universal/standard precautions during all patient encounters to reduce the risk of transmission of blood-borne pathogens and to reduce the risk of transmission of pathogens from moist body substances. Minimize contact with blood, all body fluids, mucous membranes, and nonintact skin of all patients as follows.

1. **Handwashing:** After touching blood, all body fluids, and contaminated items; after gloves are removed; and between patients.

2. **Gloves:** Wear gloves when touching blood, all body fluids, mucous membranes, nonintact skin, and contaminated items. Change gloves between tasks and procedures on the same patient after contact with material that may contain a high concentration of microorganisms.

3. **Gown:** Wear a gown to protect skin and prevent soiling of clothing during procedures that are likely to generate splashes.

4. **Mask, eye protection, faceshield:** Wear during procedures that are likely to generate splashes.

5. **Needles and sharps:** Do not recap needles; dispose of needles only in needle containers.

B. TRANSMISSION-BASED PRECAUTIONS: Designed for patients documented with or suspected to be infected with pathogens for which additional precautions beyond **standard precautions** are necessary to interrupt transmission (Table 18.10).

1. **Airborne transmission** (e.g., *Mycobacterium tuberculosis,* rubeola, varicella-zoster, or disseminated zoster).

2. **Droplet transmission:** Invasive *H. influenzae* infection; invasive *Neisseria meningitidis* infection; diphtheria (respiratory); *Mycoplasma pneumoniae* infection; pertussis, plague (pneumonic); streptococcal pharyngitis, pneumonia, or scarlet fever in infants and young children; adenovirus infection; influenza; mumps; parvovirus B19 infection; rubella.

18

INFECTIOUS DISEASES

TABLE 18.9

RECOMMENDED TREATMENT REGIMENS FOR DRUG-SUSCEPTIBLE TUBERCULOSIS IN INFANTS, CHILDREN, AND ADOLESCENTS

Infection or disease category	Regimen[a]	Remarks
Asymptomatic infection (positive skin test, no disease)	Prophylaxis	If daily therapy is not possible, therapy twice a week may be used for 6–9mo. HIV-infected children should be treated for 12mo. Also indicated for contacts of people with infectious tuberculosis, even if tuberculin test is negative, including all children <4yr with household TB contacts.
Isoniazid susceptible	6–9mo of isoniazid Q24hr	
Isoniazid resistant	6–9mo of rifampin Q24hr	Repeat TST 12wk after contact with TB is broken; if negative (in normal host), may discontinue prophylaxis; if positive (and no evidence of TB disease), complete prophylactic regimen.
Isoniazid/rifampin resistant[a]	Consultation with a tuberculosis specialist	For management of neonates born to mothers with evidence of TB infection, see *1997 Red Book*[3].
Pulmonary	**6mo regimens**	
	2mo of isoniazid, rifampin, and pyrazinamide Q24hr, followed by 4mo of isoniazid and rifampin daily **or**	If possible drug resistance is a concern, another drug (ethambutol or streptomycin) is added to the initial three-drug therapy until drug susceptibilities are determined.
	2mo of isoniazid, rifampin, and pyrazinamide daily, followed by 4mo of isoniazid and rifampin twice a week	Drugs can be given 2 or 3 times/wk under direct observation in the initial phase if nonadherence is likely.

	9mo alternative regimens (for hilar adenopathy only): 9mo of isoniazid and rifampin Q24hr **or** 1mo of isoniazid and rifampin Q24hr, followed by 8mo of isoniazid and rifampin twice a week	Regimens consisting of 6mo of isoniazid and rifampin Q24hr, and 1mo of isoniazid and rifampin Q24hr, followed by 5mo of isoniazid and rifampin twice a week, have been successful in areas where drug resistance is rare.
Extrapulmonary: meningitis, disseminated (miliary), bone/joint disease	2mo of isoniazid, rifampin, pyrazinamide, and streptomycin once a day, followed by 10mo of isoniazid and rifampin Q24hr (12mo total) **or** 2mo of isoniazid, rifampin, pyrazinamide, and streptomycin Q24hr, followed by 10mo of isoniazid and rifampin twice a week (12mo total)	Streptomycin is given with initial therapy until drug susceptibility is known. For patients who may have acquired tuberculosis in geographic areas where resistance to streptomycin is common: capreomycin (15–30mg/kg/day) or kanamycin (15–30mg/kg/day) may be used instead of streptomycin.
Other (e.g., cervical lymphadenopathy)	See Pulmonary.	

From *1997 Red Book*[3].

[a]Duration of therapy is longer in HIV-infected persons, and additional drugs may be indicated.

INFECTIOUS DISEASES

18

TABLE 18.10

TRANSMISSION-BASED PRECAUTIONS FOR HOSPITALIZED PATIENTS[a]

Category of precautions	Single room	Masks	Gowns	Gloves
Airborne	Yes, with negative air-pressure ventilation	Yes	No	No
Droplet	Preferred[b]	Yes, for those close to patient	No	No
Contact	Preferred[b]	No	Yes	Yes

Adapted from 1997 Red Book3.
[a]These recommendations are in addition to those for standard precautions for all patients.
[b]Preferred but not required. Cohorting of children infected with the same pathogen is acceptable.

3. **Contact transmission:** Multidrug-resistant bacteria (e.g., VRE, MRSA); *Clostridium difficile* infection in diapered and/or incontinent patients; *Escherichia coli* 0157:H7 infection in diapered and/or incontinent patients; *Shigella* infection in diapered and/or incontinent patients; hepatitis A infection in diapered and/or incontinent patients; rotavirus infection in diapered and/or incontinent patients; respiratory syncytial virus infection in infants and young children; parainfluenza virus infection in infants and young children; enterovirus infection in infants and young children; diphtheria (cutaneous), herpes simplex virus cutaneous infection; impetigo; major (noncontained) abscesses, cellulitis, or ducubitus; pediculosis (lice); scabies; *Staphylococcus aureus* cutaneous infection; herpes zoster, disseminated or in immunocompromised patients; conjunctivitis, viral and/or hemorrhagic; viral hemorrhagic fevers (Ebola, Lassa, or Marburg).

VIII. EXPOSURES TO BLOOD-BORNE PATHOGENS AND POSTEXPOSURE PROPHYLAXIS (PEP)

A. HIV

1. **Risk of occupational transmission of HIV**

a. Needlesticks: 3 infections for every 1000 exposures (0.3%). The risk is greater when the exposure involves a larger volume of blood and/or higher titer of HIV, as in a deep injury, visible blood on the device causing the injury, a device previously used in the source patient's vein/artery, or a source patient in the late stages of HIV infection.

b. Mucous membrane exposure: ≤1 infection for every 1000 exposures. The risk may be higher when the exposure involves a larger volume of blood and a higher titer of HIV, prolonged skin contact, extensive surface area of exposure, or skin integrity that is visibly compromised.

2. **Prophylaxis**

a. Optimally, PEP should be initiated within 1–2 hours of exposure.

b. Zidovudine (AZT) has been widely used as a PEP. In a CDC case study, it was associated with a 79% decrease in risk of seroconversion after percutaneous (needlestick) exposure to HIV.

c. Use of AZT alone as a PEP is no longer recommended. For most recent recommendations refer to CDC guidelines or Web site.

B. **HEPATITIS B:** Recommendations for hepatitis B prophylaxis after percutaneous exposure to blood that contains (or might contain) HBsAg (see Table 17.9, p. 359).

IX. LYME DISEASE

A. PRESENTATION

1. **Early localized disease:** Clinical manifestations between 3 and 32 days after tick bite—erythema migrans (annular rash at site of bite, target lesion with clear or necrotic center), fever, headache, myalgia, malaise.

2. **Early disseminated disease:** Some 3–10 weeks after the tick bite—secondary erythema migrans with multiple, smaller target lesions, cranioneuropathy (especially facial nerve palsy), systemic symptoms as previously listed, and lymphadenopathy; <1% may develop carditis with heart block or aseptic meningitis.

3. **Late disease:** Intermittent, recurrent symptoms 2–12 months from initial tick bite—pauciarticular arthritis affecting large joints (7% of those untreated), peripheral neuropathy, encephalopathy.

B. **TRANSMISSION:** Disease is caused by spirochete *Borrelia burgdorferi.* Inoculation occurs via a deer tick, *Ixodes scapularis* or *Ixodes pacificus.* After a bite from an infected deer tick, the spirochete disseminates systemically through the blood and lymphatics. Of note, transmission of *B. burgdorferi* from infected ticks requires a prolonged time (24–48 hours) of tick attachment. Lyme disease is endemic in New England, has a high occurrence on the East coast, but has been reported in 48 states. April to October is the peak season.

C. **DIAGNOSIS:** Most cases of Lyme disease can be diagnosed clinically by the characteristic erythema migrans rash or arthritis. Serologic confirmation of diagnosis is with immunoassays for *B. burgdorferi*–specific IgM, which peaks at 3–6 weeks after disease onset and with *B. burgdorferi*–specific IgG, which rises weeks to months after symptoms appear and persists. False-positive results of these assays are frequent as a result of cross-reactivity with viral infections, other spirochetal infections (except syphilis), and autoimmune diseases. Western blot assays should be used to confirm positive results. Lyme disease-specific antibodies can be isolated from CSF in patients with CNS involvement.

D. **TREATMENT:** Therapy depends on the stage of disease. Antibiotic prophylaxis is not routinely recommended for ticks attached <24–48 hours. For early localized disease, doxycycline for 14–21 days is the treatment of choice for patients ≥8 years of age. Amoxicillin is recommended for younger children. Early disseminated and late-onset disease can both be treated by the same oral regimen as early disease but for an extended period of 21–28 days. Of note, when facial palsy

18

INFECTIOUS DISEASES

is present, therapy is effective only at preventing late stages of disease and does not affect the duration of paralysis. Disease resulting in carditis, persistent or recurrent arthritis (>2 months), and/or meningitis or encephalitis should be treated with a parenteral regimen of either ceftriaxone or penicillin for 14–21 days.

X. INFECTIOUS DISEASES IN INTERNATIONALLY ADOPTED CHILDREN

1. **Screening tests for infectious diseases in internationally adopted children[8]** (summarized by William Moss, MD, MPH)
a. Complete blood count with differential.
b. Hepatitis B surface antigen, hepatitis B surface antibody, and hepatitis B core antibody.
c. Hepatitis C antibody.
d. Syphilis serology (RPR).
e. ELISA for antibodies to HIV-1 and HIV-2 and HIV PCR.
f. Mantoux skin test for tuberculosis.
g. Stool examination for ova and parasites.

XI. REFERENCES

1. Baraff LK et al. Practice guidelines for management of infants and children 0 to 36 months of age with fever without source. *Pediatrics* 1993; **92:**5-9.
2. American Academy of Pediatrics, Committee on Infectious Diseases and Committee on Fetus and Newborn. Revised guidelines for prevention of early-onset group B streptococcal (GBS) infection. *Pediatrics* 1997; **99:**493.
3. American Academy of Pediatrics. *1997 red book: report of the Committee on Infectious Diseases,* 24th edn. Elk Grove Village, IL: The Academy; 1997.
4. Council of State and Territorial Epidemiologists; AIDS Program, Center for Infectious Diseases. Revision of the CDC surveillance case definition for acquired immunodeficiency syndrome. *MMWR* 1987; **36(suppl 1):**1S–15S.
5. Centers for Disease Control and Prevention. 1994 revised classification system for human immunodeficiency virus infection in children less than 13 years of age. *MMWR* 1994; **43(RR-12).**
6. Centers for Disease Control and Prevention. Guidelines for the prevention of opportunistic infections in persons infected with HIV. *MMWR* 1997; **46(RR-12).**
7. Centers for Disease Control and Prevention. Sexually transmitted diseases treatment guidelines. *MMWR* 1998; **47(RR-1).**
8. Hostetter MK, Iverson S, Thomas W, McKenzie D, Dole K, Johnson DE. Medical evaluation of internationally adopted children. *N Engl J Med* 1991; **325:**479–485.

MICROBIOLOGY

Beth D. Kaufman, MD
Aklil Getachew, MD

I. BACTERIA

A. RAPID MICROBIOLOGIC IDENTIFICATION OF COMMON AEROBIC BACTERIA AND YEAST

1. **Bacteria** (Fig. 19.1)
2. **Yeast**
a. Specimens containing yeast/fungi (e.g., nail or skin scrapings, biopsy specimens, fluid from tissues or lesions) placed in 10% KOH on a glass slide show hyphae, pseudohyphae, and other fungal elements under microscopy.
b. Germ tube screen of yeast (3 hours) for *Candida albicans*: all germ tube–positive cultures are *C. albicans*, but not all *C. albicans* are germ tube positive.

B. ANTIBIOTIC SENSITIVITIES

1. **Definitions**[1,2]
a. Minimum inhibitory concentration (MIC): The lowest bacteriostatic concentration of an antimicrobial agent that prevents visible growth after an 18–24-hour incubation period.
b. Minimum bactericidal concentration (MBC): The lowest concentration of antimicrobial that kills >99.9% of organisms as measured by subculturing to antibiotic-free media after 18–24-hour incubation.
c. Serum bactericidal test: The dilution of serum (from a patient receiving antibiotics) that kills >99.9% of the organism grown out of the patient's original culture.
2. **Common pitfalls:** Clinically significant, common discrepancies between in vitro (laboratory reported) and in vivo antibiotic sensitivity profiles.
a. Cephalosporins against staphylococci: If a staphylococcus is more than two dilutions more sensitive to a first-generation cephalosporin than to a 'staphylococcal penicillin' (e.g., oxacillin), suspect that the organism is methicillin-resistant *Staphylococcus aureus,* and consider using vancomycin rather than cephalosporins or other β-lactams[2].
b. Aminoglycosides against salmonellae: Despite in vitro susceptibility to aminoglycosides, salmonellae are not susceptible in vivo to this class of antibiotics[2].
c. The following organisms are inducibly resistant to all cephalosporins; therefore cephalosporins should not be used as **sole** treatment for these organisms outside the urinary tract. β-Lactamase inhibitors are potent inducers of resistance to cephalosporins in these organisms and should not be used[3].
   1) *Enterobacter* spp.
   2) *Citrobacter* spp.
   3) Indole-positive *Proteus* spp.

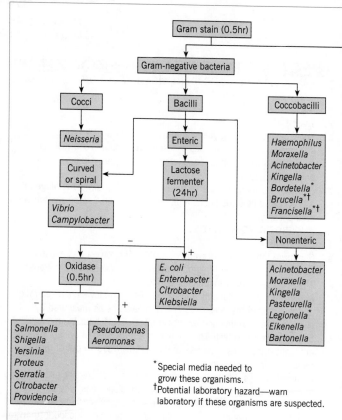

FIG. 19.1

Algorithms demonstrating identification of aerobic bacteria. Numbers in parentheses indicate the time required for the tests.

4) *Pseudomonas aeruginosa*

5) *Serratia* spp.

6) *Providencia* spp.

e. Susceptibility differences among *Pseudomonas* spp.: 'Oxidase-positive presumptive *Pseudomonas*' includes species with varying antibiotic sensitivities. Most species are resistant to aminoglycosides. Trimethoprim–sulfamethoxazole (TMP/SMX) is the drug of choice. *P. aeruginosa* is the exception because it is resistant to TMP/SMX despite in vitro sensitivity and is usually susceptible to aminoglycosides.

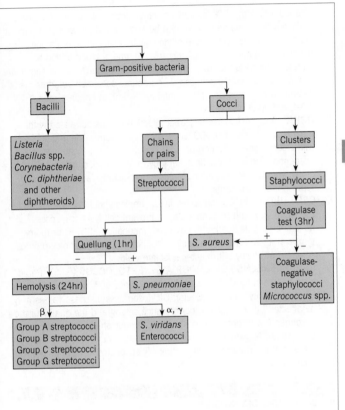

f. Coagulase-negative staphyloccoci (*Staphylococcus epidermidis*) are intrinsically resistant to clindamycin despite reported in vitro sensitivity.

g. Enterococci are intrinsically resistant to most antibiotic classes, requiring double-agent therapy for synergy. Recommended therapy is with vancomycin or a β-lactam such as ampicillin PLUS an aminoglycoside, specifically gentamicin or streptomycin. (Amikacin and tobramycin should be avoided.)

C. **BACTERIAL BLOOD CULTURES:** Proper specimen collection is essential to minimize contamination. Venipuncture site should be cleaned first with 70% isopropyl or ethyl alcohol. Tincture of iodine or 10% povidone–iodine should then be applied and allowed to dry for at least 1 minute. Blood culture bottle injection sites should also be disinfected, but with alcohol only. The volume of blood added to culture systems is the most important factor in improving the sensitivity of a blood culture. Guidelines for appropriate specimen volumes are 1–2mL in neonates, 2–3mL in infants, 3–5mL in children, and 10–20mL in adolescents[4].

D. URINE CULTURES: Urinary tract infection can be correlated with growth of either >100,000 isolated colonies from a 'clean catch' midstream urine specimen or >1000 colonies from a catheterized specimen, and with any bacterial growth from a specimen obtained by sterile suprapubic aspiration. Multiple organism isolates are likely to represent contaminants.

E. CSF CULTURES: Cerebrospinal fluid samples should be transported to the laboratory with minimal delay to prevent cell lysis or glucose utilization. If delay cannot be avoided, incubation at 37°C or room temperature will maximize bacterial isolation. Larger sample volumes correlate positively with bacterial isolate yield.

F. RAPID SCREENS FOR GROUP A STREPTOCOCCUS (GAS): Rapid tests to screen for GAS pharyngitis have about 90% sensitivity and 95% specificity reported (Becton Dickinson assay). These values may be affected by variations in performance setting and the quality of the specimen (swab *both* tonsils and the posterior pharyngeal wall; avoid other sites). Negative antigen detection tests should be confirmed by throat culture in those patients clinically suspected of having GAS pharyngitis.

II. VIRUSES

A. SEROLOGIC DIAGNOSIS

1. **Hepatitis** (Table 19.1)
2. **Hepatitis B virus (HBV)** (Fig. 19.2)
3. **Epstein–Barr virus (EBV)** (Fig. 19.3)

a. The heterophile agglutination antibody test or monospot can be used to confirm clinical diagnosis of acute disease. This test is not as sensitive for young children (<4 years) because they are more likely to be heterophile antibody negative, despite acute EBV infection. Negative monospot results can therefore be confirmed by viral capsid antigen immunoglobulin M (VCA-IgM) to rule out acute EBV.

b. Convalescent or past infection is indicated by the presence of VCA-IgG and/or antibody against Epstein–Barr nuclear antigen (EBNA).

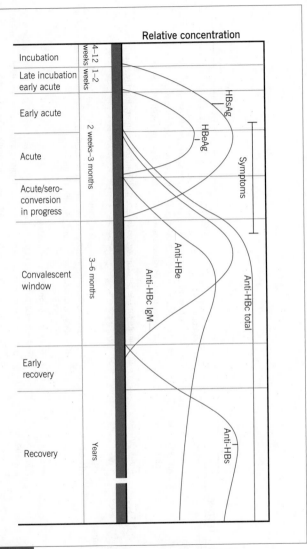

Relative concentration

Incubation	4–12 weeks	
Late incubation early acute	1–2 weeks	
Early acute		
Acute	2 weeks–3 months	
Acute/sero-conversion in progress		
Convalescent window	3–6 months	
Early recovery		
Recovery	Years	

HBsAg

HBeAg

Symptoms

Anti-HBe

Anti-HBc IgM

Anti-HBc total

Anti-HBs

FIG. 19.2

Serologic profile in the .75–85% of patients who develop acute type B hepatitis with complete resolution. Note that chronic HBV carriers will be persistently surface antigen (HBsAg) positive and surface antibody negative; they may also be persistently HBe antigen positive. See Table 19.1.

19

MICROBIOLOGY

TABLE 19.1

HEPATITIS PANEL TESTING

Type	Profile name	Markers	Purpose/comments
Diagnostic	Acute	HBsAg Anti-HBc IgM Anti-HAV IgM Anti-HCV	To differentiate among hepatitis B, A, and C viruses (HBV, HAV, HCV) in acute infection. Retest for anti-HCV if negative but history and/or clinical signs/symptoms suggest hepatitis C. Positive anti-HCV should be confirmed with HCV RIBA.
Screen	Hepatitis C	Anti-HCV HCV PCR	To evaluate for late seroconversion in recent HCV infection and to identify chronic HCV-infected individuals.
	Perinatal	HBsAg HBeAg	To identify HBsAg-positive pregnant women who may transmit hepatitis B to their newborn infants. If the HBsAg positive mother is HBeAg positive, her infant will have a 90% chance of acquiring chronic hepatitis B infection.
	Immunity	HBsAg Anti-HBc Anti-HBs	1. Test blood for infection with HBsAg. 2. Test exposed person for immunity with anti-HBc and anti-HBs (in particular, dialysis patients, health care workers, recipients of frequent transfusions, and illicit drug users). 3. Test sexual partners of individuals with acute or chronic HBV to identify infected contacts and/or candidates for immunization. 4. Test to determine if an individual is currently infected or has antibodies to HBV.

Monitor	Chronic hepatitis B	HBsAg HBeAg Anti-HBe	To evaluate for late seroconversion and/or disease resolution in known HBV carrier.
	Infant follow-up	HBsAg Anti-HBs	To monitor success of efforts to prevent perinatal transmission of HBV (obtain 1–3 months after completion of HBV series).
	Postvaccination	Anti-HBs	To ensure that immunity has been achieved after vaccination.
	Chronic Hepatitis C	Quantitative HCV PCR	To monitor viral load in known HCV carrier.

HBsAg, Hepatitis B surface antigen; Anti-HBc IgM, immunoglobulin M antibodies to HB core antigen; RIBA, recombinant immunoblot assay; PCR, polymerase chain reaction; HBeAg, HB core protein (e) antigen

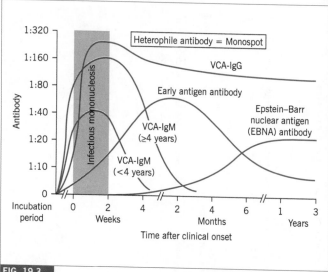

FIG. 19.3
Schematic representation of the development of antibodies to various EBV antigens in patients with infectious mononucleosis. The titers are geometric mean values expressed as reciprocals of the serum dilution. The minimum titer tested for antibodies to VCA and early antigen is 1:10, and for nuclear antigen is 1:25. The IgM response to VCA is divided because of the significant differences noted according to age of the patient. The heterophile antibody may persist for up to 18 months after the onset of clinical disease in 20% of cases. (From Sumaya[5] and Jenson[6].)

III. SELECTED SEXUALLY TRANSMITTED DISEASES
A. DIAGNOSTIC TECHNIQUES
1. *Chlamydia trachomatis*
a. Definitive diagnosis: Isolation in tissue culture; this is the only acceptable method when evaluating a child for sexual abuse. Specimen must include cells.
b. Presumptive diagnosis: Specimen from site of suspected infection sent for rapid detection of antigen through direct fluorescent staining using

monoclonal antibody (DFA), enzyme immunoassay (EIA), or DNA probe; these should not be used for testing rectal, vaginal, or urethral specimens from children because of fecal cross-contamination. DNA probes are not reliable for bloody specimens (e.g., during menstruation). Polymerase chain reaction (PCR) and ligase chain reaction (LCR) may be used to detect chlamydia in urine specimens.

c. Serologies are not generally available.

2. Gonorrhea

a. Definitive diagnosis: Direct culture is the only acceptable method in the context of a sexual abuse evaluation; specimens for *Neisseria gonorrhoeae* culture are inoculated immediately onto selective medium with CO_2 incubation before transport. Media include chocolate agar for cultures from sterile sites (joint, CSF) and more selective agars (e.g., Thayer–Martin) for cultures from nonsterile sites (urethra, cervix).

b. Presumptive diagnosis: Gram-negative intracellular diplococci on microscopic examination of smear. EIA and DNA probe of specimen from site of suspected infection. PCR and LCR may be used to detect gonorrhea in urine specimens.

3. Syphilis

a. Definitive diagnosis: Microscopic darkfield examination or DFA test of lesion exudate or tissue (not for oral or rectal sites).

b. Nontreponemal antibody tests (Venereal Disease Research Laboratories [VDRL], rapid plasma reagin [RPR]) are useful for screening, and titers are indicators of disease activity and effectiveness of therapy; false positives with EBV, tuberculosis, connective tissue disease, endocarditis, and IV drug use.

c. Serologic treponemal tests (fluorescent treponemal antibody absorbed [FTA-Abs], microhemagglutination–*Treponema pallidum* [MHA-TP]) are useful in determining a provisional diagnosis; false positives with other spirochetal diseases (e.g., Lyme disease). Reactive tests remain positive for life and are therefore not useful for identifying disease reinfection.

IV. APPROPRIATE TRANSPORT SYSTEMS ACCORDING TO SOURCE OF SPECIMEN (Table 19.2)

19

MICROBIOLOGY

TABLE 19.2

APPROPRIATE TRANSPORT SYSTEMS ACCORDING TO SOURCE OF SPECIMEN

Specimen	Transport system
Blood	Blood culture vials
Cerebrospinal fluid	Sterile screw-cap tube
Brain abscess	Anaerobic transport medium
Feces	Sterile screw-cap container
Rectal swab*	Swab transport system
Gastric lavage, duodenal aspirate	Sterile screw-cap container
Biopsied tissue	Sterile screw-cap container with preservative-free 0.85% NaCl
Conjunctival swab*	Prepare smears, directly inoculate media
Vaginal, anal swab*	Swab transport, GC transport system (see section III)
Sputum, BAL	Sputum trap, sterile screw-cap container
Lung aspirate, transtracheal aspirate	Anaerobic transport system or sterile screw-cap container
Throat, nasal, nasopharyngeal swab*	Swab transport system
Tympanocentesis fluid, sinus aspirate	Sterile screw-cap tube or anaerobic transport system
Pleural, peritoneal ascites fluid	Sterile screw-cap container or blood culture broth bottle; anaerobic transport system
Urine	Sterile screw-cap container
Wound, superficial, deep	Sterile screw-cap container and anaerobic transport system (do not inject into blood culture media)

Adapted from Christenson[4].

BAL, Bronchoalveolar lavage; GC, gonococcal.

*Commonly used swabs: Calcium alginate is toxic to *Neisseria gonorrhoeae*, herpes simplex, and ureaplasmas and may interfere with *Chlamydia* growth in media; cotton inhibits bacteria and *Chlamydia*; Dacron useful for viruses, group A streptococci, and *Chlamydia*.

V. REFERENCES

1. Nelson JD. *Pocket book of pediatric antimicrobial therapy*. Baltimore: Williams & Wilkins; 1995.
2. Mandell GL, Bennett JE, Dolin R. *Principles and practice of infectious disease*. New York: Churchill Livingstone; 1995.
3. Sanders WE, Sanders CC. Inducible β-lactamases: clinical and epidemiologic implications for use of newer cephalosporins. *Rev Infect Dis* 1988; **10**:830.
4. Christenson J. The clinician and the microbiology laboratory. In: Long S, Pickering LK, Prober CG, eds. *Principles and practice of pediatric infectious diseases*. Edinburgh: Churchill Livingstone; 1997: 1517.
5. Sumaya CV, Jenson HB. Epstein–Barr virus. In: Rose NR, et al, eds. *Manual of clinical laboratory immunolgy*, 4th edn. Washington, DC: American Society for Microbiology; 1992: 570.
6. Jenson HB, Baltimore RS. *Pediatric infectious diseases: principles and practices*. New York: Appleton & Lange; 1995: 571.

Diana C. Alexander, MD, MPH,
and Beverley Robin, MD

I. FETAL ASSESSMENT

A. MATERNAL α-FETOPROTEIN (AFP)

1. **Elevated (>2.5 multiples of the median):** Associated with incorrect gestational dating, neural tube defects, anencephaly, multiple pregnancy, Turner's syndrome, omphalocele, cystic hygroma, epidermolysis bullosa, and renal agenesis.
2. **Low (<0.75 multiples of the median):** Associated with underestimation of gestational age, intrauterine growth retardation (IUGR), and chromosomal trisomies (13, 18, 21).

B. FETAL ANOMALY SCREENING

1. **Routine ultrasound:** Performed on low-risk patients at 18–20 weeks gestation.
2. **Amniotic fluid volume (AFV) estimation**
   a. Oligohydramnios (<500mL): Associated with Potter's syndrome, renal or urologic abnormalities, lung hypoplasia, limb deformities, or premature rupture of membranes.
   b. Polyhydramnios (>2L): Suggestive of GI anomalies (gastroschisis, duodenal atresia, tracheoesophageal fistula, diaphragmatic hernia), CNS abnormalities (anencephaly, Werdnig–Hoffman syndrome), chromosomal trisomies, maternal diabetes, and cystic adenomatoid malformation of the lung.
3. **Fetal karyotyping** (Table 20.1).

C. FETAL MATURITY ASSESSMENT

1. **Menstrual history:** Most accurate determination of gestational age. Nägele's rule, based on a 28-day cycle, calculates expected date of confinement (EDC) as 9 months (280 days) plus 7 days from the last menstrual period.
2. **Ultrasound:** Crown–rump length obtained between 6 and 12 weeks predicts gestational age ±3–4 days. After 12 weeks, the biparietal diameter is accurate within 10 days, and beyond 26 weeks accuracy diminishes to ±3 weeks.
3. **Growth:** Expected birth weight (50th percentile) by gestational age is as follows: 24wk—700g; 26wk—900g; 28wk—1100g; 30wk—1350g; 32wk—1650g; 34wk—2100g; 36wk—2600g; 38wk—3000g.
4. **Fetal lung maturity:** Lecithin (L), the active component of surfactant, is present in amniotic fluid in increasing amounts throughout gestation, compared with constant levels of sphingomyelin (S).
   a. L:S ratio: >2:1 indicates fetal lung maturity in nondiabetic pregnancies. L/S ratio is generally 1:1 at 31–32 weeks gestation, and 2:1 by 35 weeks gestation.

20

b. Phosphatidyl glycerol (PG): Late-appearing surfactant component. Risk of respiratory distress syndrome (RDS) is <0.5% if PG is present in the amniotic fluid. Excellent indicator of lung maturity in nondiabetic pregnancies.

TABLE 20.1

METHODS FOR FETAL KARYOTYPING

	Amniocentesis	Chorionic villus sampling
Method	20–30mL amniotic fluid is withdrawn under ultrasound guidance; results delayed as tissue culture of amniocytes required to provide sufficient sample for analysis	Transcervical: Flexible catheter advanced under ultrasound guidance, small placental segment aspirated Transabdominal: Chorionic villi obtained via needle aspiration though the abdominal wall; results available quickly as mitotically active cells are sampled
Indications	Detects chromosomal abnormalities, metabolic disorders, neural tube defects	Detects chromosomal abnormalities and metabolic disorders; cannot detect neural tube defects or measure AFP
Gestational age performed	16–18 weeks gestation	8–11 weeks gestation
Complications	Pregnancy loss (<0.5%), chorioamnionitis (<1/1000), leakage of amniotic fluid (1/300), fetal injury (primarily superficial scars/dimpling of the skin)	Pregnancy loss (0.5–2%), maternal infection, increased risk of fetomaternal hemorrhage, fetal limb and jaw malformation

D. ANTEPARTUM FETAL MONITORING

1. **Nonstress test (NST):** Fetal heart rate (FHR) is monitored with the mother at rest. In a normal, reactive NST, FHR increases >15 beats per minute (bpm) for >15 seconds at least twice in 20 minutes. Reactivity can be absent in fetuses <30 weeks gestation because of CNS immaturity.
2. **Biophysical profile:** 30-minute ultrasound examination of five biophysical assessments: NST, AFV, fetal breathing, fetal movements/tone, and heart rate. Each parameter is scored as 2 (if normal) or 0 (if abnormal). Total scores of 8–10 are reassuring.

E. INTRAPARTUM FETAL MONITORING

1. FHR monitoring

a. Normal baseline FHR: 120–160 bpm. Mild bradycardia: 100–120 bpm.

b. Normal beat-to-beat variability: Deviation from baseline of >6 bpm. Absence of variability is <2 bpm from baseline.

c. Early decelerations: Begin with the onset of contractions. The heart rate reaches the nadir at the peak contraction, and returns to baseline as the contraction ends. Occur secondary to changes in vagal tone after brief hypoxic episodes or head compression and are benign.

d. Variable decelerations: Represent umbilical cord compression and have no uniform temporal relationship to the onset of the contraction. They are considered severe when the heart rate drops <60 bpm for ≥60 seconds with slow recovery to baseline.

e. Late decelerations: Occur after the peak of contraction, persist after the contraction stops, and show a slow return to baseline. Result from uteroplacental insufficiency and indicate fetal distress.

II. NEWBORN RESUSCITATION AND DELIVERY ROOM MANAGEMENT

A. NALS ALGORITHM FOR NEONATAL RESUSCITATION (Fig. 20.1)

B. ENDOTRACHEAL TUBE (ETT) SIZE (Table 20.2)

C. MECONIUM DELIVERY (Fig. 20.2): For infants with meconium in the amniotic fluid, the mouth, pharynx, and nose should be suctioned before delivery of the thorax. Depressed infants or those who have passed thick, particulate meconium should have residual meconium removed from the hypopharynx via suctioning under direct visualization. This should occur before drying and stimulating the infant. After intubation, a meconium aspirator attached to wall suction is connected to the endotracheal tube to suction the lower airway. Intubation of very active, meconium-stained babies remains controversial.

20

NEONATOLOGY

TABLE 20.2

ETT SIZE BY WEIGHT AND GESTATIONAL AGE

Weight (g)	Gestational age (wk)	ETT size (mm)
<1000	<28	2.5
1000–2000	28–34	3.0
2000–3000	34–38	3.5
>3000	>38	3.5–4.0

From Bloom[1].

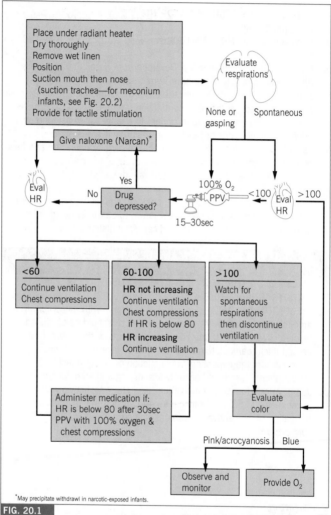

FIG. 20.1

Overview of resuscitation in the delivery room. HR, heart rate; PPV, positive-pressure ventilation. (Adapted from Bloom[1].)

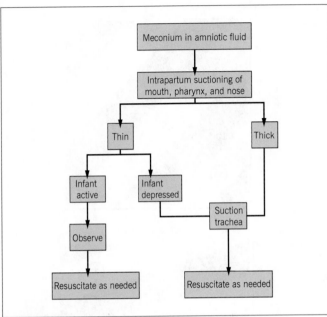

FIG. 20.2

Algorithm for management of meconium delivery.

TABLE 20.3

APGAR SCORES

Score	0	1	2
Heart rate	Absent	<100 bpm	>100 bpm
Respiratory effort	Absent, irregular	Slow, crying	Good
Muscle tone	Limp	Some flexion of extremities	Active motion
Reflex irritability (nose suction)	No response	Grimace	Cough or sneeze
Color	Blue, pale	Acrocyanosis	Completely pink

Data from Apgar[3].

III. NEWBORN ASSESSMENT

A. **VITAL SIGNS:** Average heart rate and respiratory rate are 120–160 bpm and 40–60 breaths/min respectively. Arterial blood pressure is related to birth weight and gestational age (see pp. 171–172).

B. **THERMOREGULATION** (Fig. 20.3)

C. **APGAR SCORES** (Table 20.3): Assessed at 1 and 5 minutes and may be repeated at 5-minute intervals for depressed infants.

20

NEONATOLOGY

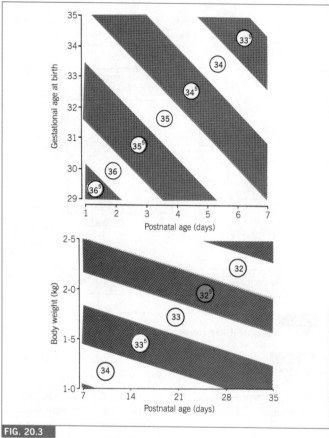

FIG. 20.3

Neutral thermal environmental temperatures. (Adapted from Sauer[2].)

D. **GESTATIONAL AGE**
1. **Anterior lens vessel examination:** Using an ophthalmoscope, focus on the anterior lens to estimate gestational age (Fig. 20.4).
2. **Neuromuscular and physical maturity (Ballard score):** The Ballard score is most accurate when performed between 12 and 20 hours of age (Fig. 20.5).
a. Neuromuscular maturity.
   1) Posture: Observe infant quiet and supine. Score 0 for arms, legs extended; 1 for starting to flex hips and knees, arms extended; 2 for

| Grade 4 | Grade 3 | Grade 2 | Grade 1 |
| 27–28wk | 29–30wk | 31–32wk | 33–34wk |

FIG. 20.4

Anterior lens vessels. (Adapted from Hittner[4].)

stronger flexion of legs, arms extended; 3 for arms slightly flexed, legs flexed and abducted; and 4 for full flexion of arms, legs.

2) Square window: Flex hand on forearm enough to obtain fullest possible flexion without wrist rotation. Measure angle between the hypothenar eminence and the ventral aspect of the forearm.

3) Arm recoil: With infant supine, flex forearms for 5 seconds, fully extend by pulling on hands, then release. Measure the angle of elbow flexion to which the arms recoil.

4) Popliteal angle: Hold infant supine with pelvis flat, thigh held in the knee–chest position. Extend leg by gentle pressure and measure the popliteal angle.

5) Scarf sign: With baby supine, pull infant's hand across the neck toward the opposite shoulder. Determine how far the elbow will go across. Score 0 if elbow reaches opposite axillary line; 1 if past midaxillary line; 2 if past midline; and 3 if elbow unable to reach midline.

6) Heel-to-ear maneuver: With baby supine, draw foot as near to the head as possible without forcing it. Observe distance between foot and head, and degree of extension at the knee. Knee is free and may be down alongside abdomen.

b. Physical maturity.

c. Maturity rating: Add scores for neuromuscular maturity and physical maturity assessments.

IV. MANAGEMENT OF THE PRETERM INFANT

A. FLUID AND ELECTROLYTE MANAGEMENT

1. **Insensible water loss:** Preterm infants experience increased insensible losses through the skin because of increased surface area per unit body mass and immaturity of the skin (Table 20.4).

2. **Water requirements** (Table 20.5)

Neuromuscular maturity sign	Score							Record score here
	-1	0	1	2	3	4	5	
Posture 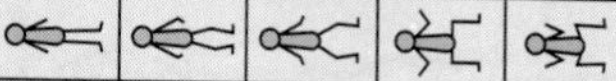								
Square window (wrist) 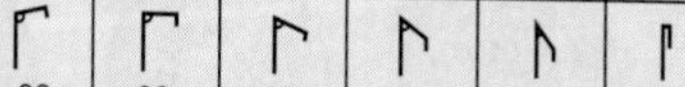	>90°	90°	60°	45°	30°	0°		
Arm recoil 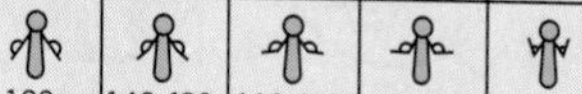		180°	140–180°	110–140°	90–110°	<90°		
Popliteal angle 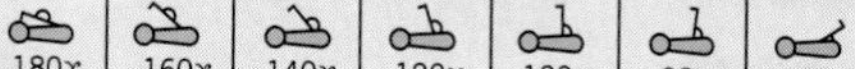	180°	160°	140°	120°	100°	90°	<90°	
Scarf sign 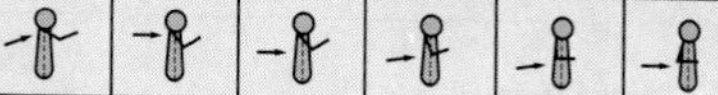								
Heel to ear 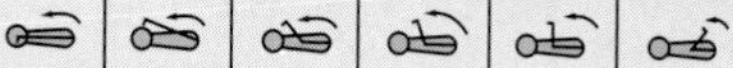								

TOTAL NEUROMUSCULAR MATURITY SCORE

Physical maturity

Physical maturity sign	Score							Record score here
	-1	0	1	2	3	4	5	
Skin	Sticky, friable, transparent	Gelatinous, red, translucent	Smooth, pink, visible veins	Superficial peeling and/or rash, few veins	Cracking, pale areas, rare veins	Parchment, deep cracking, no vessels	Leathery, cracked, wrinkled	
Lanugo	None	Sparse	Abundant	Thinning	Bald areas	Mostly bald		
Plantar surface	Heel–toe: 40–50mm: -1 <40mm: -2	>50mm, no crease	Faint red marks	Anterior transverse crease only	Creases anterior two thirds	Creases over entire sole		
Breast	Imperceptible	Barely perceptible	Flat areola, no bud	Stippled areola, 1–2mm bud	Raised areola, 3–4mm bud	Full areola, 5–10mm bud		
Eye/ear	Lids fused: loosely: -1 tightly: -2	Lids open, pinna flat, stays folded	Sl. curved pinna, soft, slow recoil	Well-curved pinna, soft but ready recoil	Formed and firm, instant recoil	Thick cartilage, ear stiff		
Genitals (male)	Scrotum flat, smooth	Scrotum empty, faint rugae	Testes in upper canal, rare rugae	Testes descending, few rugae	Testes down, good rugae	Testes pendulous, deep rugae		
Genitals (female)	Clitoris prominent and labia flat	Prominent clitoris and small labia minora	Prominent clitoris and enlarging minora	Majora and minora equally prominent	Majora large, minora small	Majora cover clitoris and minora		

TOTAL PHYSICAL MATURITY SCORE

Score		Maturity rating															Gestational age (weeks)
Neuromuscular ___		Score	-10	-5	0	5	10	15	20	25	30	35	40	45	50		By dates ___
Physical ___		Weeks	20	22	24	26	28	30	32	34	36	38	40	42	44		By ultrasound ___
Total ___																	By exam ___

FIG. 20.5

Neuromuscular and physical maturity (New Ballard Score). (Adapted from Ballard[5].)

TABLE 20.4

ESTIMATES OF INSENSIBLE WATER LOSS AT DIFFERENT BODY WEIGHTS

Body weight (g)	Insensible water loss (mL/kg/day)
<1000	60–70
1000–1250	60–65
1251–1500	30–45
1501–1750	15–30
1751–2000	15–20

Data from Veille[6].

TABLE 20.5

WATER REQUIREMENTS OF NEWBORNS

Birthweight (g)	Water requirements (mL/kg/24 hr) by age		
	1–2 days	3–7 days	7–30 days
<750	100–250	150–300	120–180
750–1000	80–150	100–150	120–180
1000–1500	60–100	80–150	120–180
>1500	60–80	100–150	120–180

Adapted from Taeusch[7].

3. **Electrolyte requirements:** Common electrolyte abnormalities include hyponatremia, hypernatremia, hypokalemia, hyperkalemia, and hypocalcemia.
a. Sodium: None required in the first 72 hours of life unless serum sodium <135mEq/L without evidence of volume overload. After 72 hours the sodium requirement is generally 2–3mEq/kg per 24 hours for term infants and 3–5mEq/kg per 24 hours for preterm infants.
b. Potassium: Added to fluids after adequate urinary output is established and serum level <4.5mEq/L. Potassium requirements are generally 1–2.5mEq/kg per day.
B. **GLUCOSE REQUIREMENTS[1]:** Preterm neonates require approximately 5–6mg/kg per min of glucose to maintain euglycemia (40–100mg/dL). Term neonates require about 3–5mg/kg per min of glucose to maintain euglycemia. Formula to calculate rate of glucose infusion:

Glucose (mg/kg/min) =
$$\frac{(\% \text{ Glucose in solution} \times 10) \times (\text{Rate of infusion per hour})}{60 \times \text{Weight (kg)}}$$

1. **Hypoglycemia:** Serum blood glucose <40mg/dL in a term or preterm infant. Ensure that venous sample confirms bedside testing, assess for symptoms, and calculate glucose delivery to infant.
a. Differential diagnosis: Insufficient glucose delivery, decreased glycogen stores, increased circulating insulin (infant of diabetic mother, maternal drugs, Beckwith–Wiedemann syndrome, tumors), endocrine/metabolic disorders, sepsis, hypothermia, polycythemia, asphyxia, shock.

TABLE 20.6

GUIDELINES FOR THE TREATMENT OF NEONATAL HYPOGLYCEMIA

Plasma glucose (mg/dL) (venous sample)	Asymptomatic or mildly symptomatic	Symptomatic
35–45	Breastfeed or give formula or D_5W by nipple/gavage.	IV glucose (D_5–$D_{12.5}W$) at 4–6mg/kg/min.
25–34	IV glucose (D_5–$D_{12.5}W$) at 6–8mg/kg/min.	IV glucose D_5–$D_{12.5}W$ at 6–8mg/kg/min.
<25	Minibolus of 2mL/kg ($D_{10}W$) and continue at a rate to provide 6–8mg/kg/min.	

Adapted from Cornblath[8].

[a]Changes in infusion rates should not exceed 2mg/kg per min per change.

[b]If blood glucose <25mg/dL and IV access is not available, give glucagon 0.1mg/kg per dose (max. 1mg) IM/SC every 30 minutes. Not effective in small–for-gestational-age babies.

b. Management (Table 20.6).

c. Follow-up blood glucose should be documented every 30–60 minutes during therapy until normal values have been established.

2. Hyperglycemia: Serum blood glucose >125mg/dL in term infants and >150mg/dL in preterm infants. Assess glucose delivery and presence of glucosuria.

a. Differential diagnosis: Excess glucose administration, sepsis, hypoxia, hyperosmolar formula, transient neonatal diabetes mellitus, medications.

b. Evaluation: Serum glucose, CBC with differential, blood cultures, urine dipstick with urine culture, electrolytes, and insulin level if warranted.

V. NUTRITION AND GROWTH OF THE NEONATE

A. GROWTH RATES: After approximately 10 days of life, expected weight gain in growing, stable infants is 15–20g/kg per day for preterm infants and 10g/kg per day for full-term infants in a thermoneutral environment.

B. CALORIC REQUIREMENTS: To maintain weight: 50–75kcal/kg per day. Adequate growth requires 100–120kcal/kg per day in term, 115–130kcal/kg per day for preterm, and up to 150kcal/kg per day for very-low-birth-weight infants. These caloric requirements presume healthy children in a thermoneutral environment.

C. MINERAL REQUIREMENTS: Preterm infants have high calcium, phosphorus, sodium, and vitamin D requirements and require special preterm formulas or breast milk fortifier. Fortifier should be added to breast milk only after the second week of life.

1. **Calcium:** Supplementation is recommended for infants weighing <1000g to provide 150–200mg/kg per day of calcium until a weight of 1500–2000g is achieved.
2. **Iron:** Enterally fed preterm infants require elemental iron supplementation of 2mg/kg per day after 4–8 weeks of age.
D. **TOTAL PARENTERAL NUTRITION** (see pp. 516–517)

VI. RESPIRATORY DISEASES
A. RESPIRATORY DISTRESS SYNDROME (RDS)

1. **Summary:** Type II alveolar cells synthesize and secrete pulmonary surfactant, a phospholipid protein mixture that decreases surface tension and prevents alveolar collapse. It is produced in increasing quantities from 32 weeks gestation. Factors that accelerate lung maturity include maternal hypertensive states, sickle cell disease, narcotic addiction, IUGR, and prolonged rupture of membranes.
2. **Incidence:** 60% in infants <30 weeks gestation without steroids and decreases to 35% for those who have received antenatal steroids. Between 30 and 34 weeks gestation, 25% in untreated infants and 10% in those who have received full steroid treatment. For infants >34 incidence is 5%.
3. **Risk factors:** Prematurity, maternal diabetes, cesarean section without antecedent labor, perinatal asphyxia, second twin, previous infant with RDS.
4. **Clinical presentation:** Respiratory distress worsens during the first few hours of life, progresses over 48–72 hours, and subsequently improves. Recovery is accompanied by brisk diuresis. Classically, on chest x-ray, film lung fields have a 'reticulogranular' pattern that may obscure the heart border.
5. **Management**
a. Support ventilation and oxygenation.
b. Surfactant therapy (see formulary [ch. 29] for dosing).
   1) 'Rescue' therapy: Administration of surfactant to infants with diagnosed RDS.
   2) 'Prophylactic' therapy: Administration of surfactant immediately after delivery. May be more effective than rescue therapy in infants <26 weeks' gestation.
6. **Intrauterine acceleration of fetal lung maturation:** Maternal administration of steroids antenatally has been shown to decrease neonatal morbidity and mortality. In particular, the risk of RDS is decreased in babies born >24 hours and <7 days after maternal steroid administration (see ch. 31).

20

NEONATOLOGY

B. PERSISTENT PULMONARY HYPERTENSION OF THE NEWBORN (PPHN)

1. **Etiology:** Idiopathic or secondary to conditions leading to increased pulmonary vascular resistance. Most commonly seen in term or postterm infants, infants born via cesarean section, and infants with a history of fetal distress and low Apgar scores. Usually presents within 12–24 hours of birth. Accounts for up to 2% of all neonatal ICU admissions.

a. Physiologic conditions associated with PPHN
   1) Vasoconstriction secondary to hypoxemia and acidosis (neonatal sepsis).
   2) Interstitial pulmonary disease (meconium aspiration syndrome).
   3) Hyperviscosity syndrome (polycythemia).

b. Anatomic anomalies
   1) Pulmonary hypoplasia either primary or secondary to congenital diaphragmatic hernia or renal agenesis.

2. **Diagnostic features**

a. Severe hypoxemia (Pao_2 <35–45mmHg in 100% O_2) disproportionate to radiologic changes.

b. Structurally normal heart with right-to-left shunt at foramen ovale or ductus arteriosus; decreased postductal oxygen saturations compared with preductal values. Difference of at least 7–15mmHg between preductal and postductal Pao_2 is significant.

c. Must distinguish from cyanotic heart disease. Infants with heart disease will have an abnormal cardiac examination and show little to no improvement in oxygenation with hyperventilation.

3. **Principles of therapy:**

a. Consider transfer to a tertiary care center

b. Minimal handling and limited invasive procedures. Sedation and paralysis of intubated babies may be necessary.

c. Maintenance of systemic blood pressure with reversal of right-to-left shunt via volume expanders and/or inotropes.

d. Optimize oxygen-carrying capacity.

e. Broad-spectrum antibiotics.

f. Mild hyperventilation to induce respiratory alkalosis (Pco_2 in low 30s) or bicarbonate infusion to induce metabolic alkalosis with pH 7.55–7.60. Both may improve oxygenation. Avoid severe hypocapnea (Pco_2 <25), which can be associated with myocardial ischemia and decreased cerebral blood flow. Hyperventilation may result in barotrauma, which predisposes to chronic lung disease. Consider high-frequency ventilation.

g. Nonselective vasodilator therapy (tolazoline) has been used with inconsistent benefits, and significant risks include systemic hypotension and GI bleeding. A selective pulmonary vasodilator, nitric oxide, appears to be more promising but is not yet FDA approved.

h. Consider extracorporeal membrane oxygenation (ECMO) if infant has severe cardiovascular instability, if oxygenation index (OI) >40, or if alveolar–arterial diffusion gradient ($AaDo_2$) is ≥610 for 8 hours.

$$OI = \frac{\text{Mean airway pressure} \times Fio_2 \times 100}{Pao_2 \text{ (postductal)}}$$

$AaDo_2 = Fio_2 \times (760 - 47mmHg) - Pao_2 - Paco_2$

i. Mortality: Depends on the etiology, but overall mortality rates in North American centers approximate 30–40%.

C. CYANOSIS: DIFFERENTIAL DIAGNOSIS AND MANAGEMENT IN THE NEWBORN

1. **Clinical assessment:** Evaluation for respiratory distress, heart murmur, differential cyanosis, persistent vs intermittent cyanosis.

2. **Differential diagnosis of cyanosis in the newborn**
a. Respiratory diseases:
   1) Lung parenchymal disease: RDS, transient tachypnea of the newborn, pneumonia, meconium aspiration.
   2) Air leak syndrome.
   3) Congenital defects: Diaphragmatic hernia, pulmonary hypoplasia.
   4) PPHN.
   5) Choanal atresia.
b. Cardiac diseases
   1) Cyanotic heart lesions: Transposition of the great arteries, total anomalous pulmonary venous return, Ebstein's anomaly, tricuspid atresia, pulmonic stenosis, tetralogy of Fallot.
   2) Severe congestive heart failure (CHF).
c. CNS diseases
   1) Periventricular/intraventricular hemorrhage (IVH).
   2) Meningitis.
   3) Primary seizure disorder.
   4) Congenital myopathies.
d. Other disorders
   1) Polycythemia/hyperviscosity syndrome.
   2) Methemoglobinemia.
   3) Hypothermia, hypoglycemia, sepsis.
   4) Shock.
   5) Respiratory depression as a result of maternal medications (magnesium sulfate, opiates).

3. **Evaluation:** Note central vs peripheral cyanosis, degree of respiratory effort, hyperoxia test, preductal and postductal ABGs or pulse oximetry to assess for right-to-left shunt, CBC with differential, serum glucose, transillumination of chest for possible pneumothorax, chest radiograph, ECG, echocardiography as necessary.

VII. APNEA

A. DEFINITION: Respiratory pause >20 seconds or a shorter pause associated with cyanosis, pallor, hypotonia, or bradycardia <100 bpm. In preterm infants, apneic episodes may be central (no diaphragmatic activity), obstructive (upper airway obstruction), or mixed central and obstructive. Common causes of apnea in the newborn are listed in Fig. 20.6.

B. INCIDENCE: Apnea occurs in most infants <28 weeks, approximately 50% of infants 30–32 weeks, and <7% of infants 34–35 weeks gestation. Usually resolves by 34–36 weeks postconceptual age but may persist after term in infants born at ≤25 weeks gestation.

C. MANAGEMENT

1. Consider pathologic causes for apnea.
2. Pharmacotherapy with theophylline, aminophylline, caffeine, or doxapram (see formulary [ch. 29] for dosing).
3. Continuous positive-airway pressure or mechanical ventilation (see pp. 537–538 for details).

VIII. BRADYCARDIA WITHOUT CENTRAL APNEA

A. DIFFERENTIAL DIAGNOSIS: Obstructive apnea, mechanical airway obstruction, gastroesophageal reflux (GER), increased intracranial pressure (ICP), increased vagal tone (defecation, yawning, rectal stimulation, placement of nasogastric tube), electrolyte abnormalities, heart block (Fig. 20.6).

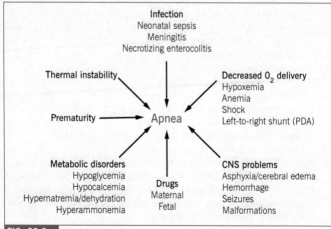

FIG. 20.6

Causes of apnea in the newborn. (From Klaus[9].)

IX. UNCONJUGATED HYPERBILIRUBINEMIA IN THE NEWBORN
(see Table 20.7)

A. **PHYSIOLOGIC INCREASES IN BILIRUBIN:** During the first 3–4 days of life, infants' serum bilirubin increases from cord bilirubin levels of 1.5mg/dL to 6.5 ± 2.5mg/dL. The maximum rate of increase in bilirubin for otherwise normal infants with nonhemolytic hyperbilirubinemia is 5mg/dL per 24 hours or 0.2mg/dL per hour. Visible jaundice or a total bilirubin concentration >10mg/dL on the first day of life is outside the normal range and suggests a potentially pathologic cause. Infants <37 weeks gestation tend to have maximum serum indirect bilirubin levels 30–50% higher compared with term infants. Treatment guidelines for preterm infants differ from those for term infants (see Table 20.8).

B. **EVALUATION**

1. **Maternal prenatal testing:** ABO and Rh(D) typing and serum screen for isoimmune antibodies.

2. **Infant or cord blood:** Evaluation of blood smear, direct Coombs' test, blood type, and Rh typing if mother has not had prenatal blood typing or she is blood type O or Rh negative.

C. **MANAGEMENT**

1. **Term newborn** (Table 20.7): Intensive phototherapy should produce a decline of the total serum bilirubin (TSB) level of 1–2mg/dL within 4–6 hours. The TSB level should continue to fall and remain below the threshold level for exchange transfusion. If this does not occur, it is considered a failure of phototherapy.

2. **Preterm newborn** (Table 20.8): Bilirubin levels may significantly increase in the infant who is 34–36 weeks gestation weighing >2500g, and who is breast-feeding.

3. **Neonatal exchange transfusion:** See p. 321 for volume calculations.

Note: CBC, reticulocyte count, peripheral smear, bilirubin, Ca, glucose, total protein, infant blood type, and Coombs' test should be performed on preexchange sample of blood because they are of no diagnostic value on postexchange blood. If indicated, save preexchange blood for serologic or chromosome studies.

a. Sensitized cells or hyperbilirubinemia[11]

1) Crossmatch donor blood against maternal serum for first exchange and against postexchange blood for subsequent exchanges.

2) Use type O-negative (low titer), irradiated blood; may use infant's type if no chance of maternal-infant incompatibility. Blood should be stored at room temperature, either fresh or ≤48 hours old, and anticoagulated with ACD or CPD unless infant is acidotic or hypocalcemic.

3) Make infant NPO during and at least 4 hours after exchange. Empty stomach if infant was fed within 4 hours of procedure.

4) Follow vital signs, blood sugar, and temperature closely; have resuscitation equipment ready.

20

NEONATOLOGY

TABLE 20.7

MANAGEMENT OF UNCONJUGATED HYPERBILIRUBINEMIA IN THE TERM NEWBORN

Age (hr)	Consider phototherapy	Phototherapy	Exchange transfusion if intensive phototherapy fails	Exchange transfusion and intensive phototherapy
≤24	—	—	—	—
25–48	≥12 (170)[a]	≥15 (260)	≥20 (340)	≥25 (430)
49–72	≥15 (260)	≥18 (310)	≥25 (430)	≥30 (510)
>72	≥17 (290)	≥20 (340)	≥25 (430)	≥30 (510)

TSB level (mg/dL)

Data from American Academy of Pediatrics, Provisional Committee for Quality Improvement and Subcommittee on Hyperbilirubinemia[10].

[a]Values in parentheses are mcmol/L.

TABLE 20.8

GUIDELINES FOR THE USE OF PHOTOTHERAPY
IN PRETERM INFANTS <1 WEEK OF AGE[a]

Weight (g)	Phototherapy	Consider exchange transfusion
500–1000	5–7	12–15
1000–1500	7–10	15–18
1500–2500	10–15	18–20
>2500	>15	>20

[a]Bilirubin values in milligrams per deciliter.

5) Prepare and drape patient for sterile procedure.
6) Insert umbilical artery and vein catheters as per pp. 51–54. During the exchange, blood is removed through the umbilical artery catheter and infused through the venous catheter. If unable to pass an arterial catheter, use a single venous catheter.
7) Prewarm blood in quality-controlled blood warmer if available; do not improvise with a water bath.
8) Exchange 15mL increments in vigorous full-term infants, smaller volumes for smaller, less stable infants. Do not allow cells in donor unit to form sediment.
9) Withdraw and infuse blood 2–3mL/kg per minute to avoid mechanical trauma to patient and donor cells.
10) Give 1–2mL of 10% calcium gluconate solution IV slowly for ECG evidence of hypocalcemia (prolonged QTc intervals). Flush tubing with NaCl before and after calcium infusion. Observe for bradycardia during infusion.
11) To complete double-volume exchange, transfuse 160mL/kg for full-term infant and 160–200mL/kg for preterm infant.
12) Send last aliquot withdrawn for Hct, smear, glucose, bilirubin, potassium, Ca^{++}, and type and crossmatch.

b. Complications
1) Cardiovascular: Thromboemboli or air emboli, thromboses, dysrhythmias, volume overload, cardiorespiratory arrest
2) Metabolic: Hyperkalemia, hypernatremia, hypocalcemia, hypoglycemia, acidosis
3) Hematologic: Thrombocytopenia, DIC, overheparinization, transfusion reaction
4) Infectious: Hepatitis, HIV, bacteremia
5) Mechanical: Injury to donor cells (especially from overheating), vascular or cardiac perforation, blood loss

D. MODES OF PHOTOTHERAPY AND SUGGESTIONS FOR USE:
Fiberoptic blanket is a useful adjunct to overhead phototherapy but may be inadequate as a sole modality for treating significant hyperbilirubinemia.

20

NEONATOLOGY

TABLE 20.9

MODIFIED BELL'S STAGING CRITERIA FOR NEC

Stage	Systemic signs	Intestinal signs	Radiologic signs	Treatment
I: Suspected				
A	Temperature instability, apnea, bradycardia	Elevated pregavage residuals, mild abdominal distention, occult blood in stool	Normal or mild ileus	NPO, antibiotics × 3 days
B	Same as IA	Same as IA + gross blood in stool	Same as IA	Same as IA
II: Definite				
A: Mildly ill	Same as IA	Same as IB + absent bowel sounds, abdominal tenderness	Ileus, intestinal pneumatosis	NPO, antibiotics × 7–10 days
B: Moderately ill	Same as IA + mild metabolic acidosis, mild thrombocytopenia	Same as IB + mild absent bowel sounds, definite abdominal tenderness, abdominal cellulitis, right lower quadrant mass	Same as IIA + portal vein gas with or without ascites	NPO, antibiotics × 14 days
III: Advanced				
A: Severely ill, bowel intact	Same as IIB + hypotension, bradycardia, respiratory acidosis, DIC, neutropenia	Same as IB and II + signs of generalized peritonitis, marked tenderness, and distention of abdomen	Same as IIB + definite ascites	NPO, antibiotics × 14 days, fluid resuscitation, inotropic support, ventilator therapy, paracentesis
B: Severely ill, bowel perforated	Same as IIIA	Same as IIIA	Same as IIB + pneumoperitoneum	Same as IIA + surgery

From Walsh[12].
DIC, disseminated vascular coagulation; NPO, nothing by mouth.

X. POLYCYTHEMIA

A. **DEFINITION:** Venous hematocrit >65% confirmed on two con-secutive samples. May be falsely elevated when sample obtained by heelstick.

B. **ETIOLOGY:** Delayed cord clamping; twin–twin transfusion; maternal-fetal transfusion; intrauterine hypoxia; trisomy 13, 18, or 21; Beckwith–Wiedemann syndrome; maternal gestational diabetes; neonatal thyrotoxicosis; and congenital adrenal hyperplasia.

C. **CLINICAL FINDINGS:** Plethora, respiratory distress, cardiac failure, tachypnea, hypoglycemia, irritability, lethargy, seizures, apnea, jitteriness, poor feeding, thrombocytopenia, hyperbilirubinemia.

D. **COMPLICATIONS:** Hyperviscosity predisposes to venous thrombosis and CNS injury. Hypoglycemia may result from increased erythrocyte utilization of glucose.

E. **MANAGEMENT:** Partial exchange transfusion for symptomatic infants with isovolemic replacement of blood with isotonic fluid. Blood is exchanged in 10–20mL increments to reduce hematocrit (Hct) to <55.

Volume of blood (mL) =

$$\frac{\text{Hct (measured)} - \text{Hct (desired)} \times \text{Birth weight (kg)} \times 90}{\text{Hct (measured)}}$$

XI. NECROTIZING ENTEROCOLITIS (NEC) (Table 20.9)

A. **DEFINITION:** Serious intestinal inflammation and injury thought to be secondary to bowel ischemia and immaturity.

B. **INCIDENCE:** More common in preterm infants (3–4% of infants <2000g) and African–American infants. No gender predominance.

C. **RISK FACTORS:** Prematurity, asphyxia, hypotension, polycythemia/hyperviscosity syndrome, umbilical vessel catheterization, exchange transfusion, bacterial/viral pathogens, enteral feeds, patent ductus arteriosus (PDA), CHF, RDS, in utero cocaine exposure.

XII. INTRAVENTRICULAR HEMORRHAGE (IVH)

A. **DEFINITION:** Intracranial hemorrhage usually arising in the germinal matrix and periventricular regions of the brain.

B. **INCIDENCE:** Approximately 30–40% of infants weighing <1500g; 50–60% of infants weighing <1000g. Highest incidence in first 72 hours of life, 60% within 24 hours, 85% within 72 hours, <5% after 1 week postnatal age.

C. **DIAGNOSIS AND CLASSIFICATION:** Ultrasonography is used in the diagnosis and classification of IVH. Routine screening is indicated in infants <32 weeks gestational age.

1. **Grade I:** Hemorrhage in germinal matrix only.

2. **Grade II:** IVH without ventricular dilatation.

3. **Grade III:** IVH with ventricular dilatation (30–45% incidence of motor/intellectual impairment).

4. **Grade IV:** IVH with periventricular hemorrhagic infarct (60–80% incidence of motor/intellectual impairment).

20

NEONATOLOGY

D. PROPHYLAXIS: Maintain acid–base balance and avoid fluctuations in blood pressure. Pharmacologic prophylaxis includes indomethacin for prevention of severe hemorrhage.

E. OUTCOME: Infants with grade III and IV hemorrhages have a higher incidence of neurodevelopmental handicap and an increased risk of posthemorrhage hydrocephalus.

XIII. PERIVENTRICULAR LEUKOMALACIA

A. DEFINITION AND ULTRASOUND FINDINGS: Ischemic necrosis of periventricular white matter characterized by CNS depression within first week, and ultrasound findings of cysts ± ventricular enlargement caused by cerebral atrophy.

B. INCIDENCE: More common in preterm infants, but also occurs in term infants; 3.2% in infants <1500g.

C. ETIOLOGY: Primarily ischemia/reperfusion injury, hypoxia, acidosis, hypoglycemia, acute hypotension, low cerebral blood flow.

D. OUTCOME: Commonly associated with cerebral palsy ± sensory/intellectual deficit[9].

XIV. RETINOPATHY OF PREMATURITY (ROP)

A. DEFINITION: Interruption of the normal progression of retinal vascularization.

B. ETIOLOGY: Exposure of the immature retina to high oxygen concentrations can result in vasoconstriction and obliteration of the retinal capillary network, followed by vasoproliferation. Risk is greatest in the most immature infant.

C. ZONES OF THE RETINA (Fig. 20.7)

D. STAGES OF ROP (Table 20.10)

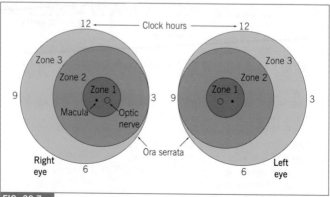

FIG. 20.7
Zones of the retina.

TABLE 20.10

STAGES OF ROP

Stage	Signs
Stage 1	Demarcation line separates avascular from vascularized retina.
Stage 2	Ridge forms along demarcation line.
Stage 3	Extraretinal, fibrovascular proliferation tissue forms on ridge.
Stage 4	Retinal detachment.
Plus disease	Posterior tortuosity and engorgement of blood vessels that may be present at any stage.
Prethreshold	Zone 1, any stage. Zone 2, stage 2 and plus disease. Zone 2, stage 3.
Threshold	A level of severity at which the risk of blindness predicted approaches 50%; five contiguous or eight total 30° sectors of stage 3 in zone 1, or zone 2 with plus disease.

From Ben-Sira[13].

XV. PATENT DUCTUS ARTERIOSUS (PDA)

A. **DEFINITION:** Failure of the ductus arteriosus to close in the first few days of life or reopening after functional closure typically results in left-to-right shunting of blood once pulmonary vascular resistance (PVR) has decreased. If the PVR remains high, blood may be shunted right to left, resulting in hypoxemia (see p. 428).

B. **ETIOLOGY:** Most often related to hypoxia and immaturity. Term infants with PDA usually have structural defects in the walls of the ductal vessel.

C. **INCIDENCE:** Up to 60% in preterm infants weighing <1500g, higher in those <1000g. Present in 60–70% of infants with congenital rubella syndrome. Female:male ratio is 2:1. Obligatory PDA is found in 10% of infants with congenital heart disease.

D. **CLINICAL PRESENTATION:** Small shunt through a PDA can be asymptomatic. Large left-to-right shunt results in CHF and failure to thrive.

1. **Physical signs of left-to-right shunt through a PDA:** Can include hyperdynamic precordium with prominent apical impulse, wide pulse pressure, bounding arterial pulses, and increased oxygen requirement. Murmur of PDA is classically described as continuous with a machinery or humming quality heard best at the second left interspace and radiating to the left clavicle or toward the apex. The murmur is often associated with a thrill. With increased PVR, the diastolic component may be quiet or absent, as is frequently the case in preterm infants.

E. **DIAGNOSIS:** Can be made clinically with echocardiographic confirmation. Radiograph may show prominent pulmonary artery with increased intrapulmonary vascular markings. Heart size may be normal or enlarged, depending on the degree of left-to-right shunting, with splaying of the carinal angle representing left atrial enlargement. Similarly, ECG may be normal or reflect left ventricular or biventricular hypertrophy, depending on degree of shunting.

F. **MANAGEMENT:** Fluid restriction and diuretics to treat CHF and mechanical ventilation when indicated. Indomethacin may be used in symptomatic infants, but it should be used with caution in infants with poor renal function (high serum creatinine and low urine output), renal/GI bleeding, sepsis, or NEC. Follow urine output, creatinine level, and platelet count. Surgical ligation may be necessary if medical treatment fails.

XVI. NEONATAL SEPSIS

See p. 375.

XVII. REFERENCES

1. Bloom RS. *Textbook of neonatal resuscitation.* Elk Grove Village, IL: AHA/AAP Neonatal Resuscitation Program Steering Committee; 1994.
2. Sauer PJJ, Dane HJ, Visser HK. New standards for neutral thermal environment of healthy very low birthweight infants in week one of life. *Arch Dis Child* 1984; **59:**18–22.
3. Apgar V. A proposal for new method of evaluation of the newborn infant. *Anesth Analg* 1953; **32:**260.
4. Hittner H, Hirsch NJ, Rudolph AJ. Assessment of gestational age by examination of the anterior vascular capsule of the lens. *J Pediatr* 1977; **91:**455–458.
5. Ballard JL, Khoury JC, Wedig K, Wang L, Eilers-Walsman BL, Lipp R. New Ballard Score, expanded to include extremely premature infants. *J Pediatr* 1991; **119:**417–423.
6. Veille JC. AGA infants in a thermoneutral environment during the first week of life. *Clin Perinatol* 1988; **15:**863.
7. Taeusch W, Ballard RA, eds: *Schaffer and Avery's diseases of the newborn,* 6th edn. Philadelphia: WB Saunders; 1991.
8. Cornblath M. In: Donn SM, Fisher CW, eds. *Risk management techniques in perinatal and neonatal practice.* Armonk, NY: Futura; 1996.
9. Klaus MH, Fanaroff AA. Care of the high-risk neonate, 4th edn. Philadelphia: WB Saunders, 1993.
10. American Academy of Pediatrics, Provisional Committee for Quality Improvement and Subcommittee on Hyperbilirubinemia. Practice parameter: management of hyperbilirubinemia in the healthy term newborn. *Pediatrics* 1994; **94(4 Pt 1):**558–565.
11. From Kitterman JA et al. Catheterization of umbilical vessels in newborn infants. *Pediatr Clin North Am* **17:**895–912, 1970.
12. Walsh MC, Kliegman RM, Fanaroff AA. Necrotizing enterocolitis: a practitioner's perspective. *Pediatr Rev* 1988; **9:**225.
13. Ben-Sira I et al. *Pediatrics* 1984; **74:**127.

NEPHROLOGY

Manaji M. Suzuki, MD

I. URINALYSIS

'Liquid biopsy of the urinary tract': Evaluate specimen within 1 hour after void, ideally collecting the first morning void.

A. **COLOR** (Table 21.1)

B. **TURBIDITY:** Can be normal; most often the result of crystal formation at room temperature. Uric acid crystals form in acidic urine, and phosphate crystals form in alkaline urine. Cellular material and bacteria can also cause turbidity.

C. **SPECIFIC GRAVITY**

1. **Hydrometer/urinometer:** Requires at least 15mL of urine at room temperature. Device must be free floating in the sample.

2. **Refractometer:** Requires only one drop of urine. Based on the principle that the refractive index (RI) of a solution is related to the content of dissolved solids present. The RI varies with, but is not identical to,

---

TABLE 21.1

ETIOLOGIES OF ABNORMAL URINE COLOR

Red

Beets, blackberries, deferoxamine (with elevated serum iron), doxorubicin, food coloring, hemoglobin, phenazopyridine (acid urine), phenolphthalein (laxatives, alkaline urine), phenothiazines, phenytoin, porphyrins, pyrvinium pamoate, red blood cells, red diaper syndrome (nonpathogenic *Serratia marcescens*), urates (brick dust syndrome)

Yellow–brown

Antimalarials (pamaquine, primaquine, quinacrine), B-complex vitamins, bilirubin, carotene, cascara, metronidazole, nitrofurantoin, sulfasalazine (alkaline urine), sulfonamides

Brown–black

Hemosiderin, homogentisic urine (alkaptonuria), melanin (especially in alkaline urine), myoglobin, old blood, quinine, rhubarb

Burgundy

Porphyrins (old urine)

Deep yellow

Riboflavin

Orange

Phenazopyridine, rifabutin, rifampin, urates, warfarin

Blue–green

Amitriptyline, biliverdin (obstructive jaundice), blue diaper syndrome (familial disorder characterized by hypercalcemica, nephrocalcinosis, indicanuria), doxorubicin, indomethacin, methylene blue, *Pseudomonas,* urinary tract infection (rare), riboflavin

specific gravity. The refractometer measures RI but is calibrated for specific gravity. Glucose, abundant protein, and iodine-containing contrast materials can give falsely high readings.

D. pH: Estimated using indicator paper or dipstick. To improve accuracy, use freshly voided specimen and pH meter. Can be inappropriately high with hypokalemia.

E. PROTEIN

1. **Tests for protein:** Significant proteinuria, as determined by the following tests, should be confirmed by a 24-hour collection.

   a. *Dipstick:* Easiest method. Detects only albumin. Significant if ≥1 + (30mg/dL) on two of three random samples 1 week apart when the urine specific gravity is <1.015 or if ≥2 + (100mg/dL) on similarly collected urine when the specific gravity is >1.015. False positives can occur with highly concentrated alkaline urine (pH >8), gross hematuria, pyuria, bacteriuria, and quaternary ammonium cleansers (e.g., antiseptics, chlorhexidine, or benzalkonium). False negatives can occur with very dilute or acidic urine (pH 4.5) and nonalbumin proteinuria, which can be detected by sulfasalicylic acid.

   b. *Protein/creatinine ratio[1]:* Determine ratio of protein (mg/dL) and creatinine (mg/dL) concentrations in a randomly collected spot urine during normal ambulation. The normal urinary protein: urinary creatinine (Upr:Ucr) is <0.2 in older children and <0.5 during the first few months of life. A Upr:Ucr ratio >1.0 is highly suspicious of nephrotic range proteinuria. All aberrant ratios should be confirmed with a 24-hour urine collection for proteinuria.

   c. *24-hour urine collection* (see p. 450).
      1) Most accurate method[2].
      2) Normal: ≤4mg of protein/m^2 per hour; abnormal: 4–40mg/m^2 per hour; nephrotic range: ≥40mg/m^2 per hour.[2]

2. **Types of proteinuria** (Fig. 21.1)

3. **24-hour urine protein excretion in children of different ages** (Table 21.2)

4. **Suggested evaluation of proteinuria[2]**

   a. *Laboratory studies:* Blood electrolytes, blood urea nitrogen (BUN), serum creatinine, protein, cholesterol, hepatitis B surface antigen, and hepatitis C antibody, quantitative immunoglobulins, spot Upr:Ucr ratio.

   b. *Fractionated 24-hour urine collection* if orthostatic proteinuria suspected
      1) Have patient wake up at 8am, void completely, and then discard the urine.
      2) Begin collecting all voided urine from this point into container #1. The patient should attempt to void at 4pm and add the urine to container #1.

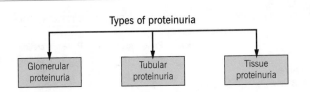

Types of proteinuria

- Glomerular proteinuria
- Tubular proteinuria
- Tissue proteinuria

A. GLOMERULAR

1. Transient proteinuria: Most common in children. Associated with exercise, stress, dehydration, postural changes, cold exposure, fever, seizures, congestive heart failure, and vasoactive drugs. Serial urine tests should be negative for protein.

2. Orthostatic proteinuria: Common, not associated with renal pathology. Repeat measure of excreted urinary protein in recumbent position should be negative. Rarely exceeds 1g/dy (see Table 21.2).

3. Proteinuria secondary to glomerulopathies
a. Primary glomerular disease: Minimal change disease, focal segmental glomerulonephritis, membranous glomerulonephritis, IgM nephropathy, IgA nephropathy.
b. Secondary glomerular disease: medications (NSAIDs, captopril, lithium, etc.), postinfectious (poststreptococcal, hepatitis B, chronic shunt infections, subacute bacterial endocarditis), infectious (bacterial, fungal, viral), neoplastic (solid tumors, leukemia), multisystem (systemic lupus erythematosus, Henoch-Schönlein purpura, sickle cell disease), reflux nephropathy, congenital nephrotic syndrome.

B. TUBULAR

1. Overload proteinuria: Occurs when excessive amount of low-molecular-weight proteins overwhelms the tubular reabsorption capacity (e.g., light chains: multiple myeloma; lysozyme: monocytic and myelocytic leukemias; myoglobin: rhabdomyolysis; hemoglobin: hemolysis).

2. Tubular dysfunction or disorders: Occurs when normal amounts of low-molecular-weight proteins (e.g., amino acids) are not adequately reabsorbed because of damaged or dysfunctional tubular cells (Fanconi's syndrome, Lowe's syndrome, reflux nephropathy, cystinosis, drugs/heavy metals [mercury, lead, cadmium, outdated tetracyclines]), ischemic tubular injury, and renal hypoplasia/dysplasia.

C. TISSUE
1. Acute inflammation of urinary tract
2. Uroepithelial tumors

FIG. 21.1
Types of proteinuria.

TABLE 21.2

24-HOUR URINE PROTEIN EXCRETION IN CHILDREN OF DIFFERENT AGES

Age	Protein concentration (mg/L)	Protein excretion (mg/24hr)	Protein excretion (mg/24hr per m² BSA)
Premature (5–30days)	88–845	29 [14–60]	182 [88–377]
Full-term	94–455	32 [15–68]	145 [68–309]
2–12mo	70–315	38 [17–85]	109 [48–244]
2–4yr	45–217	49 [20–121]	91 [37–223]
4–10yr	50–223	71 [26–194]	85 [31–234]
10–16yr	45–391	83 [29–238]	63 [22–181]

From Cruz[3].

3) All urine voided from 4pm until bedtime should be collected in container #2. The patient should void completely before retiring and add the urine to container #2.

4) Collect the remainder of the urine from bedtime until 8am in container #3. The patient should void at 8am because this may be the only urine in container #3. It is important that the patient does not ambulate before this void.

5) Record the specific gravity and measure protein concentration for the urine in each container. The diagnosis of orthostatic proteinuria is confirmed if samples #1 and #2 have significant proteinuria, whereas the urine in container #3 yields no significant protein. Yearly follow-up recommended with urinalysis and microscopic examination, timed quantitative urine protein evaluation or Upr:Ucr ratio, and measurement of BP and serum creatinine. If additional evidence of disease develops, referral to a pediatric nephrologist is indicated.

c. Measurement of complement C3 and C4; ASO (antistreptolysin-O); ANA (antinuclear antibody); ESR; double-stranded DNA.

d. Renal ultrasonography (and other radiologic studies as indicated).

e. Referral to a pediatric nephrologist.

f. Consider HIV testing.

Note: Asymptomatic patients should have dipstick/urinalysis repeated two or three times before extensive evaluation is started (Fig. 21.2). Negative repeat tests indicate transient/isolated proteinuria, and only routine medical care is necessary.

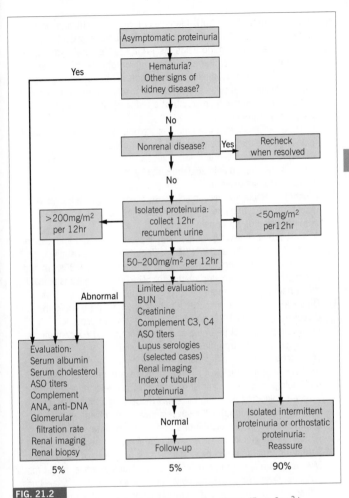

Asymptomatic proteinuria

Hematuria?
Other signs of
kidney disease?

Yes

No

Nonrenal disease? → Yes → Recheck
when resolved

No

Isolated proteinuria:
collect 12hr
recumbent urine

>200mg/m² ← | → <50mg/m²
per 12hr | per12hr

50–200mg/m² per 12hr

Abnormal

Limited evaluation:
BUN
Creatinine
Complement C3, C4
ASO titers
Lupus serologies
(selected cases)
Renal imaging
Index of tubular
proteinuria

Evaluation:
Serum albumin
Serum cholesterol
ASO titers
Complement
ANA, anti-DNA
Glomerular
filtration rate
Renal imaging
Renal biopsy

Isolated intermittent
proteinuria or orthostatic
proteinuria:
Reassure

Normal

Follow-up

5%   5%   90%

21

NEPHROLOGY

FIG. 21.2
Suggested evaluation of proteinuria in asymptomatic patients. (From Cruz[3].)

F. **SUGARS:** Normally, urine does not contain sugars. Glucosuria is
   suggestive but not diagnostic of diabetes mellitus or proximal renal
   tubular disease (see p. 451). The presence of other reducing sugars
   can be confirmed by chromatography.
1. **Dipstick:** Easiest method but only detects glucose. False negatives
   occur with high levels of ascorbic acid (used as preservative in
   antibiotics) in urine.

2. **Clinitest tablet** (Ames Co.): Identifies all reducing substances in urine, including reducing sugars (glucose, fructose, galactose, pentoses, lactose), amino acids, ascorbic acid, chloral hydrate, chloramphenicol, creatinine, cysteine, glucuronates, hippurate, homogentisic acid, isoniazid, ketone bodies, nitrofurantoin, oxalate, TPN, penicillin, salicylates, streptomycin, sulfonamides, tetracycline, and uric acid. Since sucrose is not a reducing sugar, it is not detected by Clinitest.

G. **KETONES:** Except for trace amounts, ketonuria suggests ketoacidosis, usually from either diabetes mellitus or catabolism induced by inadequate intake. Neonatal ketoacidosis may occur with a metabolic defect, such as propionic acidemia, methylmalonic aciduria, or a glycogen storage disease.

1. **Dipstick:** Detects acetoacetic acid best, acetone less well; does not detect β-hydroxybutyrate. False positives may occur after phthalein administration or with phenylketonuria.

2. **Acetest tablet** (Ames Co.): Detects only acetoacetic acid and acetone.

H. **HEMOGLOBIN/MYOGLOBIN/RBCs:** Centrifuged urine usually contains fewer than 5 RBCs/hpf. Significant hematuria is 5–10 RBCs/hpf and corresponds to a Chemstrip reading of 50 RBCs/hpf or Labstix reading 'trace hemolyzed' or 'small'.

1. **Dipstick:** Positive with intact RBCs, hemoglobin, and myoglobin; can detect as few as 3–4 RBCs/hpf. False positives can occur with the presence of bacterial peroxidases, high ascorbic acid concentrations, and Betadine (i.e., from fingers of medical staff).

2. **Microscopy:** Used to differentiate hemoglobinuria or myoglobinuria from hematuria (intact RBCs). In addition, examination of RBC morphology by phase contrast microscopy may help to localize the source of bleeding. Dysmorphic small RBCs suggest a glomerular origin, whereas normal RBCs suggest lower tract bleeding.

3. **Differentiation of hemoglobinuria and myoglobinuria**

a. *History:* Hemoglobinuria is seen with intravascular hemolysis or in hematuric urine that has been standing for an extended period. Myoglobinuria is seen in crush injuries, vigorous exercise, major motor seizures, fever and malignant hyperthermia, electrocution, snakebites, ischemia, some muscle and metabolic disorders, and some infections such as influenza.

b. *Laboratory studies:* Clinical laboratories may use many techniques to measure hemoglobin or myoglobin directly. Other laboratory data may also be used to identify the source of urinary pigment indirectly. For example, in nephropathy from myoglobinuria, the BUN:creatinine ratio is low (creatinine is released from damaged muscles) and CPK is high.

4. **Suggested evaluation of persistent hematuria** (Fig. 21.3)[1,2,4–6]

a. Examination of urine sediment, urine dipstick for protein, urine culture, sickle cell screen, urine calcium:creatinine ratio, family history, medication history, and audiology screen if indicated.

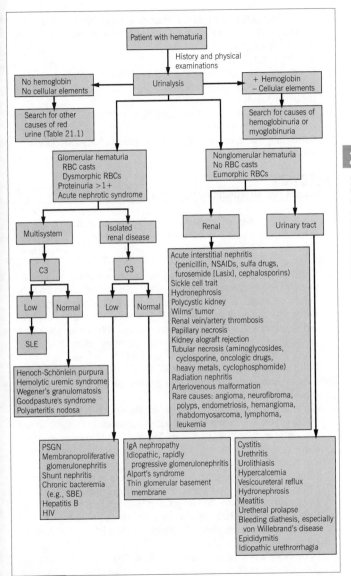

21

FIG. 21.3

A diagnostic strategy for hematuria. SLE, Systemic lupus erythematosus; SBE, subacute bacterial endocarditis; PSGN, poststreptococcal glomerulonephritis.

b. Serum electrolytes, BUN, serum creatinine, serum total protein and albumin, CBC with smear, immunoglobulins, and hepatitis serologies; consider testing for HIV.
c. ASO titers, C3, C4, ANA.
d. Renal ultrasonography and other indicated radiologic studies.
e. Referral to a pediatric nephrologist.

I. **BILIRUBIN/UROBILINOGEN**
1. **Dipstick:** Measures each individually. Both are normally present in the urine in only very small amounts.
2. **Correlating the results of both tests** can provide helpful diagnostic information (Table 21.3).

TABLE 21.3

URINALYSIS FOR BILIRUBIN/UROBILINOGEN

	Normal	Hemolytic disease	Hepatic disease	Biliary obstruction
Urine urobilinogen	Normal	Increased	Increased	Decreased
Urine bilirubin	Negative	Negative	±	Positive

J. **SEDIMENT:** Using light microscopy, unstained, centrifuged urine can be examined for formed elements, including casts, cells, and crystals. Centrifuge 10mL for 5 minutes, then decant 9mL of supernatant. Resuspend sediment in remaining 1mL of urine. Place drop on glass slide; use coverslip. Best results with subdued light. Focus particularly on the edge of coverslip because formed elements collect there. See Plates 1–12 for illustration of urine sediment[7,8].

K. **SCREENING TESTS FOR URINARY TRACT INFECTIONS (UTIs)**
Note: All tests must be confirmed with a urine culture.
1. Dipstick[12]
a. *Nitrite test:* Detects nitrites produced by the reduction of dietary nitrates by urinary Gram-negative bacteria (especially *Escherichia coli*, *Klebsiella,* and *Proteus* spp.). A positive test is virtually diagnostic of bacteriuria. False negatives can occur with inadequate dietary nitrates, insufficient time for bacterial proliferation or conversion of nitrates to nitrites (requires 4–6 hours), inability of bacteria to reduce nitrates to nitrites (many Gram-positive organisms such as *Enterococcus* as well as *Mycobacterium* spp. and fungi), and large volumes of dilute urine.
b. *Leukocyte esterase test:* Detects esterases released from broken-down leukocytes. This is therefore an indirect test for WBCs that may or may not be present with a UTI.
2. **Urine Gram stain:** Used to screen for UTIs. One organism/hpf in uncentrifuged urine represents at least 10^5 colonies/mL.
3. Suggested evaluation of UTIs[13]
Note: These recommendations are *suggestions* and vary from institution to institution and physician to physician. Use them together with the routinely practiced guidelines of your institution.

TABLE 21.4

URINE CULTURE: INTERPRETATION IN DIAGNOSIS OF A UTI

Method of collection	Quantitative culture: UTI present
Suprapubic aspiration	Growth of urinary pathogens in any number (the exception is up to 2–3×10^3 CFU/mL of coagulase-negative staphylococci)
Catheterization	Febrile infants or children usually have $\geq 50 \times 10^3$ CFU/mL of a single urinary pathogen, but infection may be present with counts from 10×10^3 to 50×10^3 CFU/mL
Midstream clean catch, voided	Symptomatic patients usually have $\geq 10^5$ CFU/mL of a single urinary tract pathogen
Midstream clean catch, voided	Asymptomatic patients: at least two specimens on different days with $\geq 10^5$ CFU/mL of the same organism

From Hellerstein[13].
CFU/mL, Colony-forming units per milliliter.

a. *History:* Voiding history (stool/urine) in toilet-trained children, sexual intercourse, sexual abuse, masturbation, pinworms, prolonged baths, evaluation of growth curve, and family history for vesicoureteral reflux/recurrent UTIs.

b. *Physical examination:* Abdominal examination for flank masses, bowel distention, evidence of impaction, meatal stenosis/circumcision in males, vulvovaginitis or labial adhesions in females, neurologic examination of lower extremities, perineal sensation/reflexes, rectal/sacral examination.

c. *Laboratory studies:* Urinalysis with microscopic examination and urine culture (Table 21.4).

    If suggestive of UTI, check BUN/creatinine and blood pressure to assess renal function indirectly. Some experts recommend repeating urine culture in 48–72 hours after initiation of antibiotic therapy for test of cure. Some experts recommend repeating urine culture at 1, 3, 6, and 12 months, and then yearly in prepubertal children secondary to high incidence of recurrence[14].

d. *Imaging studies*[15]: Imaging children with first documented UTI should be pursued in all boys, in girls <5 years, and in older girls with pyelonephritis or recurrent infections. Referral to a pediatric urologist is also recommended if studies reveal obstructive lesion, high-grade (IV or V) (Fig. 21.4) vesicoureteral reflux (VUR), or progressive DMSA or VCUG changes on follow-up studies.

   1) Abdominal radiograph: Indicated for checking stool pattern or if suspicious for spinal dysraphism.

   2) Renal sonography: A noninvasive/nonionizing evaluation for gross structural defects, lesions that are obstructive, positional abnormalities, and renal size/growth. Repeat in 1 year for evaluation of size/growth or resolution of obstructive lesion.

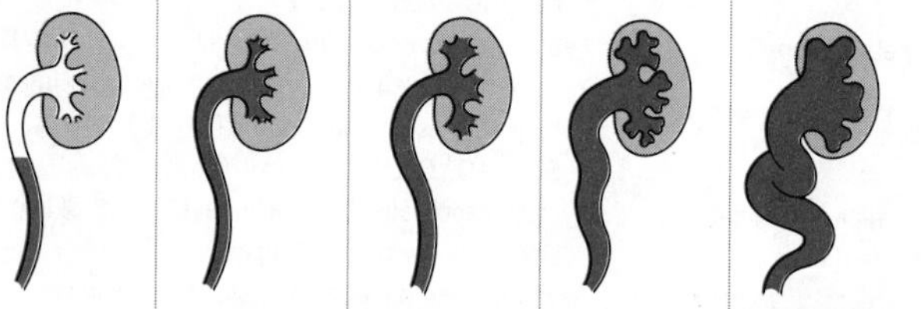

Grade I	Grade II	Grade III	Grade IV	Grade V
Ureter only	Ureter, pelvis, calyces; no dilatation, normal calyceal fornices	Mild or moderate dilatation and/or tortuosity of ureter; mild or moderate dilatation of the pelvis, but no or slight blunting of the fornices	Moderate dilatation and/or tortuosity of the ureter; mild dilatation of renal pelvis and calyces; complete obliteration of sharp angle of fornices, but maintenance of papillary impressions in majority of calyces	Gross dilatation and tortuosity of ureter; gross dilatation of renal pelvis and calyces; papillary impressions are no longer visible in majority of calyces

FIG. 21.4

International classification of vesicoureteral reflux. (Adapted from Rushton[15] and International Reflux Committee[16].)

3) *Voiding cystourethrography (VCUG):* Perform when asymptomatic and cleared of bacteriuria. Indicated in all boys, girls <5 years and those >5 years with recurrent or febrile UTIs. Repeat in 1 year if initial study is positive. May be substituted with radionucleotide cystography (RNC), which has 1/100th the radiation exposure of a VCUG and increased sensitivity for transient reflux. Does not visualize urethral anatomy, is not sensitive for low-grade reflux, and cannot grade reflux.

4) *DMSA:* Tc 99m DMSA normally taken up by renal tubules; defects on DMSA image indicates tubular defects. Indicated in patients with an abnormal VCUG or renal sonography, in patients with history of normal urinary tract/asymptomatic bacteriuria and fever, prenatally diagnosed VUR, and in neonates/infants secondary to high incidence of hematologic spread and difficult examination. Repeat in 4 months if initial study is positive.

5) *DTPA/MAG-3:* May also be used for indications given above for DMSA use. Provides quantitative assessment of renal function and

drainage of dilated collecting system, as in cases of hydronephrosis in absence of VUR.

e. *Treatment:* Should be based on urine culture and sensitivies if possible.

1) *Cystitis:* Conventional therapy for uncomplicated lower tract UTI is for 7–10 days, especially for children <5 years. Recent studies have also shown short (3–5 days) courses of antibiotic therapy to be effective in clearance of infection for acute uncomplicated UTIs in females >5 years and adolescents (with known normal renal function). Repeat urine culture after 48–72 hours of treatment for test of cure. Continue prophylactic dose antibiotics until radiologic evaluation has been performed.

2) *Pyelonephritis*[15]:

a) Nontoxic/clinically stable children and infants >3 months of age can be treated as outpatients as long as compliance is not an issue. It is reasonable to initiate therapy with 1–2 days of a long-acting, third-generation cephalosporin IM followed by 10–14 days of oral antibiotics and prophylaxis until evaluated and urine culture/sensitivities are known.

b) Toxic children and infants <3 months should be considered candidates for immediate hospitalization and parenteral therapy. Parenteral antibiotic therapy should be continued for 10–14 days in neonates, although outpatient therapy to complete a full 10–14 day course can be substituted in patients >2 months of age when afebrile and clinically stable for 24–48 hours as long as compliance is ensured[15].

3) *Asymptomatic bacteriuria:* Defined by bacteria in urine in an afebrile patient without pyuria. Antibiotics are not necessary if voiding habits and urinary tract are normal. Prophylaxis may be necessary in patients with bacteriuria and voiding dysfunction. DMSA may be helpful in differentiating pyelonephritis vs fever and coincidental bacteriuria.

4) *Suggested indications for prophylactic antibiotics*[15]

a) VUR of any grade until resolution (surgically or spontaneously) (Fig. 21.4).

b) Frequent recurrences of lower UTIs (>3 times per year), especially when associated with underlying bladder instability or abnormal voiding patterns. In conjunction with prophylactic therapy, correction of voiding disorder or constipation should also be carried out.

c) Neonates diagnosed with hydronephrosis antenatally until appropriately evaluated[17].

d) Children <2 years for 6 months after acute episode of pyelonephritis secondary to high risk of reinfection with or without VUR[18].

e) Consider in neonates and infants <1 year who present with febrile UTI and/or DMSA changes.

f) Children with UTI awaiting radiologic evaluations.

21

NEPHROLOGY

5) Nonsurgical management of VUR[15]: Amoxicillin recommended in first 2 months of life, otherwise TMP-SMX (trimethoprim–sulfamethoxazole) or nitrofurantoin (Macrodantin) with urine cultures every 4 months and when febrile. There is no need to discontinue antibiotics before screening urine culture. Change antibiotic therapy if patient has breakthrough UTIs while on prophylactic regimen. Repeat VCUG in 12–18 months to determine resolution of VUR. Surgical correction is indicated in children >2 years with high-grade reflux (IV–V) and children with breakthrough pyelonephritis (especially with DMSA changes) while on prophylaxis.

II. RENAL FUNCTION TESTS

A. TESTS OF GLOMERULAR FUNCTION

1. Creatinine clearance (Ccr)

a. *Timed urine specimen:* Standard measure of glomerular filtration rate (GFR); closely approximates inulin clearance in the normal range of GFR. When GFR is low, Ccr is greater than inulin clearance. Inaccurate in children with obstructive uropathy.

   Method: Collect urine over any time period; record interval to the nearest minute. Have patient empty bladder (discard specimen) before beginning the collection. Collect all urine during the time interval, including urine voided at the end of the collection period. If the patient's renal function is stable, draw blood sample for serum creatinine once during the test period. (If function is changing rapidly, draw the blood sample at the beginning and end of the period and use the average.)

$$Ccr \ (mL/min/1.73m^2) = (U \times [V/P]) \times 1.73/BSA$$

Note: U (mg/dL), urinary creatinine concentration; V (mL/min), total urine volume (mL) divided by the duration of the collection (min) (24 hours = 1440 minutes); P (mg/dL), serum creatinine concentration (may average two levels); BSA (m^2), body surface area.

b. *Estimated GFR from plasma creatinine:* Useful when a timed specimen cannot be collected; correlates well with standard GFR for children with relatively normal body habitus. If habitus is markedly abnormal, more standard methods of measuring GFR must be used.

$$Estimated \ GFR \ (ml/min/1.73m^2) = kL/Pcr$$

Note: k, proportionality constant; L, height (cm); Pcr, plasma creatinine (mg/dL) (Table 21.5).

2. Glomerular function as determined by nuclear medicine scans (see p. 574).

a. Normal values of GFR (measured by inulin clearance) (Table 21.6).

B. TESTS OF TUBULAR FUNCTION

1. Proximal tubule

a. *Proximal tubule reabsorption:* The proximal tubule is responsible for the reabsorption of electrolytes, glucose, and amino acids. Studies to

21

NEPHROLOGY

TABLE 21.5

PROPORTIONALITY CONSTANT FOR CALCULATING GFR

	k values
Low birth weight during first year of life	0.33
Term AGA during first year of life	0.45
Children and adolescent girls	0.55
Adolescent boys	0.70

From Schwartz[19].
AGA, Appropriate for gestational age.

TABLE 21.6

NORMAL VALUES OF GFR

Age	GFR - mean (ml/min/1.73m^2)	Range (ml/min/1.73m^2)
Neonates <34wk gestational age		
2–8days	11	11–15
4–28days	20	15–28
30–90days	50	40–65
Neonates >34wk gestational age		
2–8days	39	17–60
4–28days	47	26–68
30–90days	58	30–86
1–6mo	77	39–114
6–12mo	103	49–157
12–19mo	127	62–191
2yr–adult	127	89–165

From Holliday[20].

determine proximal tubular function compare urine and blood levels of specific compounds arriving at a percent tubular reabsorption (Tx):

$$Tx = 1 - \frac{Ux/Px}{Ucr/Pcr} \times 100\%$$

Note: Ux, concentration of compound in urine; Px, concentration of compound in plasma; Ucr, concentration of creatinine in urine; Pcr, concentration of creatinine in plasma. This formula is also used for amino acids, electrolytes, calcium, and phosphorus.

b. *Glucose reabsorption:* The glucose threshold is the plasma glucose concentration at which significant amounts of glucose appear in the urine. The presence of glucosuria must be interpreted in relation to simultaneously determined plasma glucose concentration. If the plasma glucose concentration is <120mg/dL, and glucose is present in the urine, this implies incompetent tubular reabsorption of glucose and proximal renal tubular disease. (For discussion of normal values and further studies of proximal tubule function consult Holliday et al[20].)

TABLE 21.7

AGE-ADJUSTED CALCIUM/CREATININE RATIOS

Age	Ca^{2+}/Cr ratio (mg/mg ratio) (95th percentile for age)
<7mo	0.86
7–18mo	0.6
19 mo–6yr	0.42
Adults	0.22

From Sargent[21].

TABLE 21.8

BIOCHEMICAL AND CLINICAL CHARACTERISTICS OF THE VARIOUS TYPES OF RTA

	Distal type 1	Type 1 with HCO_3^- wasting	Proximal type 2	Hyperkalemic type 4
At subnormal (HCO_3^-)[a]				
Minimal urine pH	>5.5	>5.5	<5.5	<5.5
TA and NH_4^+ excretion	↓	↓	nl or ↓	↓
Urinary citrate excretion	↓	↓	↑	?
Plasma K^+ concentration	nl or ↓	nl or ↓	Usually ↓	↑
Renal K^+ clearance	>20%	>20%	>20%	<20%
Urine anion gap[b]	Positive	Positive	Positive or ? negative	Positive
At normal (HCO_3^-)				
TA and NH_4^+ excretion	↓	↓	↓	↓
Fractional HCO_3^- excretion	3–5%	5–10%	>15%	1–15%
Urinary citrate excretion	nl	nl	↑	?
Plasma K^+ concentration	nl	nl	nl or ↓	nl or ↑
U-B Pco_2 (mmHg)[c]	<20	<20	>20	<20
Therapeutic alkali requirement (mEq/kg per day)	1–3	5–10	5–20	1–5
Osteomalacia	Rare	Rare	Frequent	Absent
Nephrocalcinosis/ nephrolithiasis	Common	Common	Rare	Absent

From Holliday[20].

TA, Titratable acid; nl, normal.

[a]Plasma bicarbonate concentration.

[b]Urine anion gap = [Na] + [K+] − [Cl] (based on urine electrolytes).

[c]Urine Pco_2 minus blood Pco_2. During bicarbonate loading, when urine pH >blood pH.

c. *Urine calcium:* Hypercalciuria is seen with RTA (renal tubular acidosis), vitamin D intoxication, hyperparathyroidism, steroids, immobilization, excessive calcium intake, and loop diuretics. It may be idiopathic (associated with hematuria and renal calculi). Diagnosis is as follows:
   1) 24-hour urine: Calcium >4mg/kg per 24 hours.
   2) Spot urine: Determine Ca^{2+}:Cr ratio. It is recommended that an abnormally elevated spot urine Ca^{2+}:Cr ratio be followed up with a 24-hour urine calcium determination (Table 21.7).
d. *Bicarbonate reabsorption (proximal RTA):* The majority of bicarbonate reabsorption occurs in the proximal tubule. Abnormalities in reabsorption lead to type II RTA. These patients have high fractional excretion of bicarbonate in their urine at normal serum bicarbonate levels. However, they can acidify their urine when faced with metabolic acidosis. (Table 21.8).

2. Distal tubule

a. *Urine acidification (distal RTA):* A urine acidification defect should be suspected when random urine pH values are >6 in the presence of moderate systemic metabolic acidosis. Acidification defects should be confirmed by simultaneous venous or arterial pH, plasma bicarbonate concentration, and pH meter (not dipstick) determination of the pH of fresh urine.
b. *Types of RTA* (Table 21.8).
c. *Urine concentration*[22]: A random urine specific gravity of 1.023 or more indicates intact concentrating ability within the limits of clinical testing; no further tests are indicated. A first-voided specimen after an overnight fast is adequate to test concentrating ability. (For more formal testing, see water deprivation test on p. 224.)

III. OLIGURIA

Urine output <300mL/m^2 per 24 hours, or <0.5mL/kg per hour in children and <1.0mL/kg per hour in infants.

A. BUN/CR RATIO (both in mg/dL)[10]

1. **Normal ratio:** 10–20; suggests intrinsic renal disease in the setting of oliguria.
2. **>20:** Suggests dehydration, prerenal azotemia, or GI bleeding.
3. **<5:** Liver disease, starvation, inborn error of metabolism.

B. LABORATORY DIFFERENTIATION OF OLIGURIA (Table 21.9)

IV. ACUTE DIALYSIS

A. INDICATIONS

1. **Metabolic or fluid derangements:** Not controlled by aggressive medical management alone. Generally accepted criteria include the following, although a nephrologist should always be consulted:
a. Volume overload with evidence of pulmonary edema or hypertension, which is refractory to therapy.

21

NEPHROLOGY

TABLE 21.9

LABORATORY DIFFERENTIATION OF OLIGURIA

Test	Prerenal oliguria >1mo	Prerenal oliguria Neonates	Low output failure >1mo	Low output failure Neonates	ADH secretion All ages
Urine sodium	<20	(<40)	(>40)	(>40)	>40
Specific gravity	≥1.020	(≥1.015)	<1.010	(<1.015)	>1.020
Osmolality (mOsmol/L)	>500	(>400)	<350	(<400)	>500
Urine/plasma osmolality ratio	>1.3	—	<1.3	—	>2
Urea nitrogen	>20	—	<10	—	>15
Creatinine	>40	(>20)	<20	(<15)	>30
RFI[a]	<1	(<3)	>1.0	(>3.0)	>1.0
FE (Na)[b]	<1	(<2.5)	>1	(>3.0)	Close to 1

Adapted from Rogers[23].

ADH, Antidiuretic hormone.

[a]RFI (renal failure index) = $(UNa \times 100)/UCr \times PCr$.

[b]FE (Na) (fractional excretion of sodium) = $(UNa/PNa)/(UCr/PCr) \times 100$.

b. Hyperkalemia >6.0mEq/L if hypercatabolic or >6.5mEq/L despite conservative measures.
c. Metabolic acidosis with pH <7.2 or HCO_3^- <10.
d. BUN >150; lower if rising rapidly.
e. Neurologic symptoms secondary to uremia or electrolyte imbalance.
f. Calcium/phosphorus imbalance (e.g., hypocalcemia with tetany or seizures in the presence of a very high serum phosphate).

2. **Dialyzable toxin or poison** (e.g., lactate, ammonia, alcohol, barbiturates, ethylene glycol, isopropanol, methanol, salicylates, theophylline).

B. **TECHNIQUES[23]**

1. **Peritoneal dialysis (PD):** Requires catheter to access the peritoneal cavity. May be used acutely as well as chronically, as in continuous ambulatory or continuous cycling peritoneal dialysis.

2. **Hemodialysis (HD):** Requires placement of special vascular access devices. May be the method of choice for certain toxins (e.g., ammonia, uric acid, or poisons) or when there are contraindications to peritoneal dialysis.

3. **Continuous arteriovenous hemofiltration/hemodialysis (CAVH/D) and continuous venovenous hemofiltration/hemodialysis (CVVH/D):** CAVH and CVVH are therapies with the primary goal of the continuous generation of a plasma ultrafiltrate. Indications include fluid management, renal failure with profound hemodynamic instability, electrolyte disturbance(s), and intoxication with substances that are freely filtered across the particular ultrafiltration

TABLE 21.10

PD vs HD vs CAVH/CVVH

	PD	HD	CAVH/CVVH
BENEFITS			
Fluid removal	+	+ +	+ +
Urea and creatinine clearance	+	+ +	+
Potassium clearance	+ +	+ +	+
Toxin clearance	+	+ +	+
COMPLICATIONS			
Abdominal pain	+	−	−
Bleeding	−	+	+
Decreased cardiac output	+	+	+
Disequilibrium	−	+	−
Electrolyte imbalance	+	+	+
Need for heparinization	−	+	+
Hyperglycemia	+	−	−
Hypotension	+	+ +	+
Hypothermia	−	−	+
Infection (other than peritonitis)	−	+	+
Inguinal hernia	+	−	−
Lactic acidosis	Possible	−	Possible
Neutropenia	−	+	−
Pancreatitis	+	−	−
Peritonitis	+	−	−
Protein loss	+ +	−	−
Respiratory compromise	+	Possible	−
Thrombocytopenia	−	+	−
Vessel thrombosis	−	+	+

Adapted from Rogers[23].

21

NEPHROLOGY

membrane utilized. CAVH and CVVH can be helpful in the management of oliguric patients who are in need of better nutritional support, postoperative cardiac patients, and patients with septicemia. These therapies also require special vascular access devices.

C. **PD, HD AND CAVH/CVVH** (Table 21.10)

V. CHRONIC HYPERTENSION

Note: For management of acute hypertension, see p. 11.

A. **DEFINITION:** See Tables 7.1 and 7.2.

1. **Normal BP:** Systolic and diastolic BP <90% for age, sex, height, and weight.

2. **High normal BP:** Average systolic and/or diastolic BP between 90% and 95% for age, sex, height, and weight.

3. **Significant hypertension:** The average of three separate systolic and/or diastolic blood pressures >95% for age, sex, height, and weight.

4. **Severe hypertension:** The average of three systolic and/or diastolic blood pressures >99% for age, sex, height, and weight.

B. **CAUSES OF HYPERTENSION IN NEONATES, INFANTS, AND CHILDREN** (Table 21.11)

C. **EVALUATION OF CHRONIC HYPERTENSION**[24–26]

1. **Rule out causes:** Rule out 'factitious' causes of hypertension (improper cuff size or measurement technique, i.e., manual vs Dynamap), 'nonpathologic' causes of hypertension (fever, pain, anxiety, muscle spasm), and iatrogenic mechanisms (medications and excessive fluid administration).

2. **History and physical examination:** Headache, blurred vision, history of UTIs, family history of renal dysfunction/hypertension, pitting edema, dyspnea on exertion, jugular venous distention; or displaced point of maximal impact (PMI).

3. **Laboratory studies:** Urinalysis with microscopic evaluation, urine culture, serum electrolytes, CBC, creatinine, BUN, calcium, uric acid, cholesterol, and plasma renin level.

TABLE 21.11

CAUSES OF HYPERTENSION BY AGE GROUP

Age	Cause	
	Most common	Less common
Neonates/infants	Renal artery thrombosis after umbilical artery catheterization	Bronchopulmonary dysplasia
		Medications
	Coarctation of the aorta	Patent ductus arteriosus
	Renal artery stenosis	Intraventricular hemorrhage
1 to 10 yr	Renal parenchymal disease	Renal artery stenosis
	Coarctation of aorta	Hypercalcemia
		Neurofibromatosis
		Neurogenic tumors
		Pheochromocytoma
		Mineralocorticoid ↑
		Hyperthyroidism
		Transient hypertension
		Hypertension induced by immobilization
		Sleep apnea
		Essential hypertension
		Medications
11 yr to adolescence	Renal parenchymal disease	All diagnoses listed above
	Essential hypertension	

Modified from Sinaiko[24].

4. **Imaging:** Renal ultrasonography, including Doppler and other imaging studies as indicated (echocardiography, renal arteriography).
5. Consider toxicology screen, hCG (human chorionic gonadotropin), thyroid function tests, urine catecholamines, plasma and urinary steroids.
6. Refer any patient with significant hypertension to pediatric nephrologist.

D. **TREATMENT OF HYPERTENSION**
1. **Nonpharmacologic:** Aerobic exercise, salt restriction, smoking cessation, and weight loss. Indicated in patients with systolic BP and/or diastolic BP >90%.
2. **Pharmacologic:** Indicated in patients with significant hypertension (especially diastolic hypertension) or accelerated hypertension.
3. **Parenteral:** Acute hypertensive crisis.

E. **ANTIHYPERTENSIVE MEDICATIONS FOR CHRONIC HYPERTENSIVE THERAPY** (Table 21.12)

21

NEPHROLOGY

TABLE 21.12

ANTIHYPERTENSIVE MEDICATIONS

Calcium channel blockers: Act on vascular smooth muscles
  Benefits: Renal perfusion/function minimally affected; ideal for posttransplant hypertension, especially in association with CSA use; ideal in low renin/volume-dependent hypertension
  Nifedipine: No effect on cardiac conduction; available in short- and long-acting form; variable GI absorption and sublingual route may cause precipitous drop in BP
  Verapamil: Depresses cardiac pacemaker, inhibits cyclosporin metabolism
  Amlodipine: Once-daily dose, tasteless, odorless, easily made into suspension with 90% GI absorption

ACE inhibitors (captopril, enalapril): Block angiotensin I → angiotensin II
  Benefits: Decreases proteinuria while preserving renal function; ↑potency and duration in neonatal and infantile renal function; ↓ pulmonary vascular resistance and mean arterial pressure with little ↓ in heart rate
  Side effects: elimination dependent on creatinine clearance; causes hyperkalemia; contraindicated in compromised renal perfusion and in pregnancy; associated with rash, cough, angioedema, and marrow depression

Diuretics
  Thiazides: Effective in primary hypertension; not effective when GFR <50% of normal; side effects: hypokalemia, hypercalcemia, hyperuricemia, hyperlipidemia
  Furosemide/bumetanide: Useful in renal failure; bumetanide known to have 40× more diuretic activity than furosemide, but varies with patient/route; side effects: hypokalemia, hyponatremia, ototoxicity (high-dose IV)
  K⁺ sparing: Spironolactone, triamterene, amiloride; modest antihypertensive medication; antiandrogenic effects

Modified from Hospital for Sick Children[27], Sinaiko[28], and Khattak[29].

Continued

TABLE 21.12

ANTIHYPERTENSIVE MEDICATIONS—cont'd

β Blockers

> **Benefits**: ↓ heart rate, ↓ cardiac output, ↓ renin release
>
> **Side effects**: May exacerbate underlying collagen vascular disease or Raynaud's disease; may cause exaggerated hypoglycemic response in diabetes mellitus and suppress hypoglycemic symptomatology; may cause nightmares, confusion, agitation, depression; contraindicated in persons with congestive heart failure, reactive airways disease, or pulmonary insufficiency
>
> > **Selective β_1 blockers**: Metoprolol, atenolol
> >
> > **Nonselective β blockers**: Propranolol, nadolol (once-daily dosing)

α_1 **Blockers** (prazosin): Block vasoconstriction

> **Benefits**: Effective in patients with renal failure, distorted lipid profile, Raynaud's disease/ collagen vascular disease
>
> **Side effects**: Nausea, palpitations, worsening of narcolepsy, dizziness/syncope

Combined α and β blocker: Labetalol (↓ peripheral resistance, ↓ heart rate) extremely potent; postural hypotension; can be used in hypertensive crisis

Centrally acting α stimulators (clonidine, α-methyldopa): Stimulates brain stem α_2 receptors → peripheral adrenergic drive

> **Benefits**: ↓ Intraocular pressure, ↓ opiate withdrawal, effective in renal failure, less hyponatremia and orthostatic symptomatology
>
> **Side effects**: Dry mouth, sedation/agitation, constipation, sudden withdrawal → rebound hypertension

Vasodilators (hydralazine, nitroprusside, minoxidil): Direct action on vascular smooth muscle. Very potent, used in hypertensive crisis; reflex ↑ heart rate, Na^+ and H_2O retention, therefore combine with diuretics/β blockers

Modified from Hospital for Sick Children[27], Sinaiko[28], and Khattak[29].

VI. REFERENCES

1. Roy III S. Hematuria. *Pediatr Ann* 1996; **2(5)**:284.
2. Norman ME. An office approach to hematuria and proteinuria. *Pediatr Clin North Am* 1987; **34**:545.
3. Cruz C, Spitzer A. When you find protein or blood in urine. *Contemp Pediatr* 1998; **15(9)**:89.
4. Feld L, Waz W, Perez L, Joseph D. Hematuria: an integrated medical and surgical approach. *Pediatr Clin North Am* 1997; **44**:1191.
5. Cilento B, Stock J, Kaplan G. Hematuria in children: a practical approach. *Urol Clin North Am* 1995; **22**:43.
6. Fitzwater D, Wyatt R. Hematuria. *Pediatr Rev* 1994; **15**:102.
7. Henry JB. *Clinical diagnosis and management by laboratory methods.* Philadelphia: WB Saunders; 1984.

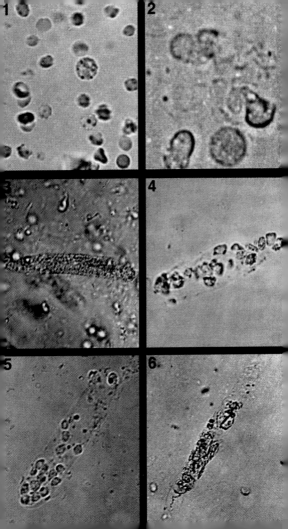

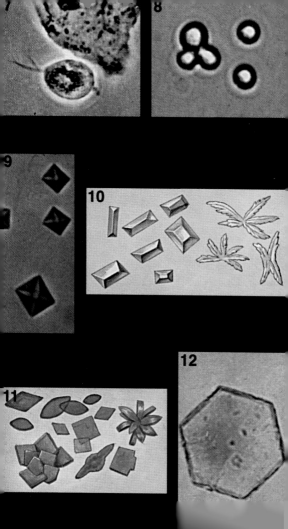

Plates begin opposite p. 458.

PLATE 1
Red blood cells and white blood cells. (From ROCOM[9].)

PLATE 2
White blood cells with bacteria in an infected urine specimen. (From Birch[10].)

PLATE 3
Fine granular cast. (From ROCOM[9].)

PLATE 4
White blood cell cast (seen in intrinsic renal diseases such as pyelonephritis and glomerulonephritis). Note discernible nuclei and cell boundaries. (From ROCOM[9].)

PLATE 5
Red blood cell cast. Note distinct and uniformly spheric shape of erythrocyte. (From ROCOM[9].)

PLATE 6
Epithelial cast (present in tubular disease). (From ROCOM[9].)

PLATE 7
Trichomonas vaginalis. (From ROCOM[9].)

PLATE 8
Budding yeast forms. (From ROCOM[9].)

PLATE 9
Calcium oxalate crystals. (From ROCOM[9].)

PLATE 10
Phosphate crystals. (From Netter[11].)

PLATE 11
Urate crystals. (From Netter[11].)

PLATE 12
Crystine crystal (indicative of cystinuria). (From ROCOM[9].)

21

NEPHROLOGY

8. Greenhill A, Gruskin AB. Laboratory evaluation of renal function. *Pediatr Clin North Am* 1976; **23**:661.

9. ROCOM. Urine under the microscope, 1975.

10. Birch DF et al. *A color atlas of urine microscopy*. London: Chapman & Hall Medical; 1994.

11. Netter FH, Shapter RK, Yonkman FF. *The CIBA collection of medical illustrations*, 1973; **6**:80.

12. Feigin RD, Cherry JD. *Pediatr Infect Dis* 1992; **483**.

13. Hellerstein S. Urinary tract infections: old and new concepts. *Pediatr Clin North Am* 1995; **42**:1142.

14. Todd J. Management of urinary tract infections: children are different. *Pediatr Rev* 1995; **16**:5.

15. Rushton H. Urinary tract infections in children: epidemiology, evaluation and management. *Pediatr Clin North Am* 1997; **44**:5.

16. International Reflux Committee. Medical versus surgical treatment of primary vesicoureteral reflux. *Pediatrics* 1981; **67**:392.

17. Belman A. Vesicouretal reflex. *Pediatr Clin North Am* 1997; **44**:5.

18. Hellerstein S. Urinary tract infections: old and new concepts. *Pediatr Clin North Am* 1995; **42**:6.

19. Schwartz GJ, Brion LP, Spitzer A. The use of plasma creatinine concentration for estimating glomerular filtration rate in infants, children, and adolescents. *Pediatr Clin North Am* 1987; **34**:571.

20. Holliday MA et al. *Pediatric nephrology*. Baltimore: Williams & Wilkins; 1994.

21. Sargent JD et al. Normal values for random urinary calcium to creatinine ratios in infancy. *J Pediatr* 1993; **123**:393.

22. Edelmann CM Jr, Barnett HL, Stark H, Boichis H, Soriano JR. A standardized test of renal concentrating capacity in children. *Am J Dis Child* 1967; **114**:639.

23. Rogers MC. *Textbook of pediatric intensive care*. Baltimore: Williams & Wilkins; 1992.

24. Sinaiko A. Hypertension in children. *N Engl J Med* 1996; **335**:26.

25. Rocella E et al. *Pediatrics* 1996; **98**:4.

26. Sadowski R, Falkner B. Hypertension in pediatric patients. *Am J Kidney Dis* 1996; **27**:3.

27. Hospital for Sick Children. *The HSC handbook of pediatrics*. 9th edn. St Louis: Mosby; 1997.

28. Sinaiko A. Treatment of hypertension in children. *Pediatr Nephrol* 1994; **8**:603.

29. Khattak S, Rogan JW, Saunders EF, Theis JG, Arbus GS, Koren G. Efficacy of amlodipine in pediatric bone marrow transplant patients. *Clin Pediatr* 1998; **37**:31.

NEUROLOGY

Jessica Sessions, MD

I. GENERAL PRINCIPLES

1. **Neurologic diagnosis:** Based almost completely on history; the remainder is based on physical examination and additional testing.
2. **Assessment:** Clear formulation of the problem that needs to be addressed:
   a. Parts of the nervous system involved: Brain, spinal cord, neuromuscular system.
   b. Onset and time course of the process: Acute and progressive, intermittent, chronic and static, or chronic and progressive.
   c. Need for urgency vs specificity of intervention.
3. **Differential diagnosis:** Includes trauma, tumor, infection, intoxication, epilepsy, endocrine abnormality, demyelination, developmental dysgenesis, or inflammatory/immune, vascular, psychogenic, metabolic degenerative processes.
4. **Neurologic emergencies:** See pp. 13–16.

II. NEUROLOGIC EXAMINATION

A. **GENERAL PHYSICAL EXAMINATION:** Note clues to genetic syndromes or malformations, especially head circumference, skull deformities, craniofacial dysmorphic features, ocular anomalies, malformation of the spine, neurocutaneous lesions; systemic signs of infection or other organ disease; signs of large molecular storage disease such as visceromegaly, corneal opacities, and dysostosis multiplex.

B. **MENTAL STATUS:** Alertness, attention, behavior, language, orientation, memory, abstraction, judgment (see p. 585).

C. **CRANIAL NERVES** (Table 22.1)

D. **MOTOR:** Must evaluate relative to developmental norms, quality and functionality of movement.

1. **Muscle bulk**
2. **Tone:** High, normal, low.
   a. Axial tone: Observe posture while patient is supine, sitting, and standing and during vertical and horizontal suspension (infants).
   b. Limb tone: Assess resting posture and resistance to passive range of motion.
   c. Note anatomic distribution of abnormalities, quality (rigid, spastic, cogwheel), and variability with voluntary activity and sleep. Tone varies with wakefulness and voluntary purposeful movement.
      1) Least resistance to passive movement.

TABLE 22.1

CRANIAL NERVES

Function/region	Cranial nerve	Test/observation
Olfactory	I	Smell (e.g., coffee, vanilla, peppermint)
Vision	II	Acuity, fields, color, fundus
Pupils	II, III, sympathetics	Shape, size, reaction to light, accommodation
Eye movements and eyelids	III, IV, VI	Range and quality of eye movements, saccades, pursuits, nystagmus, ptosis
Sensation	V	Corneal reflexes, facial sensation
Muscles of mastication	V	Clench teeth
Facial strength	VII	Observe degree of expression of emotions, eye or lip closure strength
Hearing	VIII	Localize voice, attend to finger rub
Mouth, pharynx	VII, IX, X, XII	Swallowing, speech quality (nasal deficits in labial, lingual, or palatal sound production), symmetric palatal elevation, tongue protrusion
Head control	XI	Head position and movement, shoulder shrug

    2) Stiffness with active skills.

    3) Regional increases in tone suggesting cortical dysfunction: Adducted thumbs, limited hand supination, equinus of feet.

3. Strength: Observe and describe activity such as rising from the floor. Quantify (e.g., distance of broad jump, time to run 30 feet, time to climb stairs)[1]:

a. 0/5: No movement.

b. 1/5: Palpable tightening only.

c. 2/5: Full range of movement in a gravity-neutral plane.

d. 3/5: Full range of movement against gravity but not resistance.

e. 4/5: Subnormal strength (against resistance).

f. 5/5: Normal strength (against resistance).

4. Movement quality and functionality: Assess spontaneity, speed, accuracy, and smoothness of purposeful tasks, all relative to developmental norms.

a. Pyramidal tract dysfunction may occur with only subtle degrees of weakness: Diminished spontaneous movement, slowing of fine repetitive movements (finger tapping), lack of postural persistence, loss of complex sequences of movement (writing, self-feeding).

b. Note posture and mobility skills relative to developmental norms.

c. Note involuntary movements: Tremor, dystonia, chorea, athetosis, tics, myoclonus.

E. DEEP TENDON REFLEXES: Most helpful in localizing other abnormalities, especially in the presence of weakness or asymmetry.

Isolated abnormalities of reflexes, in the setting of normal strength and coordination, have little significance. Combined with weakness, brisk reflexes indicate upper motor neuron disorder; absent reflexes reflect lower motor neuron or neuromuscular junction disorder. In muscle disease, reflexes may be diminished but are usually detectable. Selective reflex drop-out can help localize a spinal cord or root lesion (Table 22.2).

F. **SENSORY:** Primary disorders of sensation are rare in children, but the following tests may be useful in anatomic localization:
1. **Spinal cord dysfunction of discrete pathways** (Figs. 22.1 and 22.2)

TABLE 22.2

MUSCLE STRETCH REFLEXES

Reflex	Biceps	Brachioradialis	Triceps	Knee	Ankle
Site	C5, C6	C5, C6	C7, C8	L(2, 3)4	L5–S2

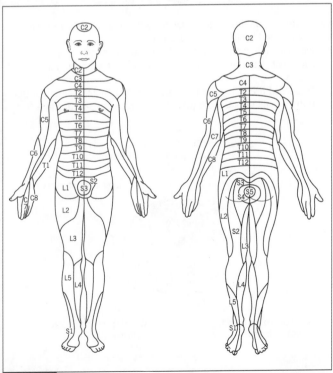

FIG. 22.1
Dermatomes. (From Athreya[2].)

a. Anterior cord: Pain and temperature sensation.
b. Posterior cord: Romberg's test, vibratory and joint position sense.
2. **Transverse spinal cord dysfunction:** Especially of concern if abnormal bowel or bladder function; use pinprick to identify level of impairment.
3. **Syringomyelia:** Evaluate for decreased pain or temperature sensitivity bilaterally, with preserved proprioception at the level of the syrinx and preserved function below.
4. **Polyneuropathy:** Look for proximal > distal gradient of loss of sensations, especially vibratory, pinprick.
5. **Mononeuropathies:** Pinprick to localize area of anesthesia to territories of specific peripheral nerves.
G. **COORDINATION:** Evaluate general coordination while watching activities such as throwing a ball, dressing, playing video games. Test rapid alternation and repetitive movements, finger to nose, heel to shin, walking and running.

III. HEADACHES

A. **DIFFERENTIAL DIAGNOSIS OF SYMPTOMATIC HEADACHE**

Note: Symptomatic headache is due to serious intracranial or systemic disease, and benign headache is not.
1. **Increased intracranial pressure (ICP):** Trauma, hemorrhage, tumor, hydrocephalus, pseudotumor cerebri, abscess, arachnoid cyst, cerebral edema.
2. **Decreased ICP:** After ventriculoperitoneal (VP) shunt, lumbar puncture (LP), or cerebrospinal fluid (CSF) leak from basilar skull fracture.

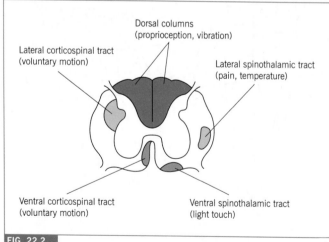

FIG. 22.2
Spinal pathways.

3. **Meningeal inflammation:** Meningitis, leukemia, subarachnoid or subdural blood.
4. **Vascular:** Vasculitis, arteriovenous malformation, hypertension, cerebrovascular accident.
5. **Bone, soft tissue:** Referred pain from scalp, eyes, ears, sinuses, nose, teeth, pharynx, cervical spine, temporomandibular joint.
6. **Infection:** Influenza, malaria, Lyme disease, encephalitis, etc.

B. **DIFFERENTIAL DIAGNOSIS OF CHRONIC BENIGN HEADACHE**
1. Migraine (with or without aura)
2. Tension
3. **Psychogenic:** Conversion disorder, malingering.
4. **Secondary to sleep deprivation** (e.g., in overweight children with sleep apnea) **or chronic hypoxia.**

C. **EVALUATION**
1. **History and physical:** Differentiate symptomatic from chronic, benign headaches. Careful general, neurologic, and fundoscopic examinations. Note localization/pain characteristics, duration, associated symptoms, and ameliorating factors. See Table 22.3.
2. **Studies**
a. Computed tomography (CT)/magnetic resonance imaging (MRI): Focal neurologic findings, increased ICP, atypical or progressive pattern, seizures, sudden severe headache.
b. LP: Fever, infection, pseudotumor, subarachnoid hemorrhage.
3. **Warning signs:** Pain that awakens child from sleep, increases in morning with rising or with Valsalva's maneuver; headache associated with emesis, neurologic signs, changes in chronic pattern, no family history of migraine, and altered mental status (change in mood/personality/school performance).

Note: The classic headache secondary to subarachnoid hemorrhage (SAH) is acute, severe, continuous, and generalized—classically the

TABLE 22.3	
HEADACHES	
Symptomatic	Benign
Rapid escalation (days, weeks)	Intermittent with headache-free periods, wax and wane over months and years
Unremitting	
Profoundly incapacitating ("worst headache of my life")	Stereotypical attacks, no escalation in a progressive manner
Early morning or overnight onset	Daytime onset, relieved by sleep
Early morning nausea and vomiting	Neurologic deficits rare, and transient in form of migraine aura (10–20min)
Progressive deterioration in function	
Altered consciousness	Intact consciousness during headache
New persistent localizing neurologic deficit	Normal neurologic examination except during transient aura
Papilledema	Normal fundus on examination

NEUROLOGY

22

'first and worst' headache. It may be associated with nausea, emesis, meningismus, focal neurologic symptoms, and loss of consciousness. If SAH is suspected, CT without contrast is the preferred method of evaluation, then LP (if CT negative) to rule out xanthochromia (develops approximately 12 hours after event). Send tubes 1 and 4 for cell counts and xanthochromia. With SAH, there is a persistently high red blood cell count and xanthochromia. The red blood cell count should significantly decline if not SAH.

D. MIGRAINE HEADACHE

1. **Characteristics:** Chronic recurrent, throbbing/pulsatile, relieved by sleep; triggered by stress, caffeine, diet, menses; hereditary predisposition. Associated symptoms: Nausea, vomiting, abdominal pain, photophobia, sensitivity to noise.

2. **Classification**

a. With aura: 'Classic,' often frontotemporal, unilateral (may have associated neurologic complications). Aura is a 20–30-minute focal neurologic deficit immediately preceding the headache.

b. Without aura: 'Common,' often bifrontal.

3. **Complications (rare):** Paresthesias, visual field cuts, aphasia, hemiplegia, ophthalmoplegia, vertigo, ataxia, confusion.

4. **Treatment:** includes reassurance and education[1].

a. Acute symptomatic: Dark and quiet room, sleep, acetaminophen, nonsteroid antiinflammatory drugs, antiemetics (e.g., metoclopramide), ergotamine, sumatriptan succinate, isometheptene (Midrin), sedative/analgesic combinations (see formulary [ch. 29]).

b. Prophylaxis (if frequency >3–4/month or interference with school)
   1) Avoid triggers/stress, improve general health with good diet (restrictive of certain 'migraine-causing' foods), aerobic exercise, regular sleep.
   2) Explore issues of secondary gain/role of pain in family's relationships, counseling, or biofeedback.
   3) Consider medications such as propranolol, verapamil valproate, cyproheptadine, antidepressants[3].

IV. PAROXYSMAL EVENTS

Transient alterations in neurologic function, which may or may not be seizures.

A. DIFFERENTIAL DIAGNOSIS OF RECURRENT EVENTS THAT MIMIC EPILEPSY IN CHILDHOOD (Table 22.4)

B. EVALUATION OF PAROXYSMAL EVENTS

1. **History:** Description, time course, and setting of event; change in level of consciousness, urinary incontinence, tongue biting; history of illness, trauma, medication, toxins, fever; presence of postictal period, past history or family history of similar events.

2. **Physical examination:** Mental status, behavior, asymmetry, paralysis, trauma, cardiac abnormalities, phakomatosis, dysmorphisms,

TABLE 22.4
DIFFERENTIAL DIAGNOSIS OF RECURRENT EVENTS
THAT MIMIC EPILEPSY IN CHILDHOOD

Event	Differentiation from epilepsy
Pseudoseizure (psychogenic seizure)	No EEG changes except movement artifact during event; movements thrashing rather than clonic; brief/absent postictal period
Paroxysmal vertigo (toddler)	Patient frightened and crying; no loss of awareness; staggers and falls, vomiting, dysarthria
GER in infancy, childhood	Paroxysmal dystonic posturing associated with meals (Sandifer's syndrome)
Breath–holding spells (18mo–3yr)	Loss of consciousness and convulsion always provoked by an event that makes child cry
Syncope	Loss of consciousness with onset of vertigo and clouded or tunnel vision; slow collapse to floor; triggered by postural change, heat, emotion, etc.
Cardiogenic syncope	Abnormal ECG (e.g., prolonged QT, atrioventricular block, other arrhythmias exercise a possible trigger; episodic loss of consciousness without consistent convulsive movement
Cough syncope	Prolonged cough spasm during sleep in asthmatic, leading to loss of consciousness, often with urinary incontinence
Paroxysmal kinesiogenic choreoathetosis	Generally occurs on rising; movements not accompanied by change in alertness
Shuddering attacks	Brief shivering spells with continued awareness
Night terrors (male, 4–6yr)	Brief nocturnal episodes of terror without typical convulsive movements
Rages (male, 6–12yr)	Provoked and goal-directed anger
Tics/habit spasms	Involuntary nonrhythmic repetitive movements not associated with impaired consciousness, suppressible
Narcolepsy/sleep apnea	Sudden loss of tone secondary to cataplexy emotional trigger; no postictal state or loss of consciousness; EEG with recurrent REM sleep attacks
Migraine (confusional)	Headache or visual changes that may precede attack; family history of migraine; EEG with regional area of slowing during attack

From Murphy[4].
EEG, electroencephalography; GER, gastroesophageal reflux; ECG, electrocardiography; REM, rapid eye movement.

developmental assessment. Consider hyperventilation to precipitate absence seizure (pinwheel for younger children).

3. **Studies:** Depending on clinical scenario, consider glucose, sodium, potassium, calcium, magnesium, blood urea nitrogen (BUN), creatinine, complete blood count, toxicology screen, blood pressure

TABLE 22.5

OUTLINE OF THE INTERNATIONAL CLASSIFICATION OF EPILEPTIC SEIZURES

I. Partial seizures (seizures with focal onset)
  A. Simple partial seizures (consciousness unimpaired)
    1. With motor signs
    2. With somatosensory or special sensory symptoms
    3. With autonomic symptoms or signs
    4. With psychic symptoms (higher cerebral functions)
  B. Complex partial seizures (consciousness impaired)
    1. Starting as simple partial seizures
      (a) Without automatisms
      (b) With automatisms
    2. With impairment of consciousness at onset
      (a) Without automatisms
      (b) With automatisms
  C. Partial seizures evolving into secondarily generalized seizures
II. Generalized seizures
  A. Absence seizures: Brief lapse in awareness without postictal impairment
     (Atypical absence seizures may have the following: Mild clonic, atonic, tonic,
     automatism, or autonomic components.)
  B. Myoclonic seizures: Brief, repetitive, symmetric muscle contractions (loss of tone)
  C. Clonic seizures: Rhythmic jerking; flexor spasm of extremities
  D. Tonic seizures: Sustained muscle contraction
  E. Tonic–clonic seizures
  F. Atonic seizures: Abrupt loss of muscle tone
III. Unclassified epileptic seizures

From Committee on Classification and Terminology of the International League Against Epilepsy[6].

(supine and upright), electroencephalography (EEG) ± video monitoring, electrocardiography, head CT, MRI, LP, tilt table, and sleep study.

C. SEIZURE DISORDERS

1. **Seizure:** Paroxysmal discharge of cortical neurons resulting in alteration of function (motor, sensory, cognitive).
2. **Epilepsy:** Two or more seizures not precipitated by a known cause (i.e., fever). See Tables 22.5 and 22.6 for further classification.
3. **Status epilepticus:** Prolonged or recurrent seizures lasting >30 minutes without the patient regaining consciousness. See pp. 15–16 for details of management.
4. **Etiology:** Acquired cortical defect (stroke, neoplasm, infection, trauma), inborn error of metabolism, congenital brain malformation, neurocutaneous syndrome, neurodegenerative disease, toxins/drugs, electrolyte disturbances, idiopathic.
5. **Diagnosis:** Establish etiology (cryptogenic vs symptomatic) and seizure type. Seizure type (e.g., primary generalized or primary partial) generally determines treatment.

TABLE 22.6

OUTLINE OF THE INTERNATIONAL CLASSIFICATION OF EPILEPSIES AND EPILEPTIC SYNDROMES

1 Localization-related (focal, partial) epilepsies and syndromes

1.1 Idiopathic (age-related onset): *No known underlying cause*

Benign childhood epilepsy with centrotemporal spikes: Onset 3–13 yr; awakened from sleep with unilateral tonic–clonic contractions of face, paresthesias of tongue/cheek; occasional clonic seizures of ipsilateral upper extremity; associated with normal development and spontaneous resolution by age 20

Childhood epilepsy with occipital paroxysms

1.2 Symptomatic: *Secondary to suspected CNS disorder*

Syndromes characterized by seizures based on anatomic localization, clinical features, precipitating factors (e.g., temporal lobe epilepsies, frontal lobe epilepsies)

1.3 Cryptogenic: *Unknown but presumed symptomatic*

2 Generalized epilepsies and syndromes

2.1 Idiopathic (with age-related onset), e.g.,

Benign neonatal familial convulsions

Childhood absence epilepsy (onset 3–6yr)

Juvenile myoclonic epilepsy: Onset 12–18 years with hallmark myoclonic jerks on awakening from sleep; stress, alcohol, and sleep deprivation can precipitate

Epilepsy with seizures precipitated by specific events

2.2 Cryptogenic or symptomatic

West syndrome (infantile spasms) (see p. 473)

Lennox–Gastaut syndrome: Onset 1–8 years with mixed seizure type, usually refractory to medication; associated with mental retardation

Epilepsy with myoclonic absences

2.3 Symptomatic

2.3.1 Nonspecific cause

Early myoclonic encephalopathy

2.3.2 Specific syndromes

Epileptic seizures complicating disease states

3 Epilepsies and syndromes undetermined whether focal or generalized

3.1 With both generalized and focal seizures

Neonatal seizures (see p. 473)

Acquired epileptic aphasia (Landau–Kleffner syndrome)

3.2 Without unequivocal generalized or focal features

4 Special syndromes

4.1 Situation-related seizures

Febrile convulsions (see p. 470)

Isolated seizures

Seizures related to acute metabolic or toxic event

Modified from the Commission on Classification and Terminology of the International League Against Epilepsy[5].

22

NEUROLOGY

6. **Studies**
a. Head CT is often of little use in the clinical management of seizures, but it can detect mass lesions, acute hemorrhage, hydrocephalus, and calcifications secondary to congenital disease such as cytomegalovirus infection.
b. Brain MRI should be obtained in children with complex partial seizures, focal neurologic deficits, or complex seizures increasing in frequency or intensity, and in adolescents with new-onset seizures. Can also detect migrational defects.
c. EEG used in conjunction with history and examination can be helpful, but routine interictal EEGs are abnormal in only 60% of patients. Prolonged EEG monitoring with video, or studies done with sleep deprivation/photic stimulation, may be more informative but are rarely needed. See Table 22.7 for some characteristic EEG findings.
7. **Treatment:** Epilepsy should be treated only when clinical events are recurrent and convincing.
a. Educate parents and patient regarding how to live with epilepsy. Review first aid and cardiopulmonary resuscitation. Base activity limitations on type, frequency, and timing of seizures, as well as age, compliance, and other diagnoses. Recommend that the child participate in activities but needs supervision during bath/swimming. Know driver's license laws in the state. Advocate teacher/school awareness. Assess child's behavior and school performance on each visit. Refer parents to guide by Freeman[7].
b. Pharmacotherapy (Table 22.8): Individualize. Weigh the risk of more seizures without therapy against the risk of treatment side effects plus more seizures despite therapy. Monotherapy may reduce complications; polytherapy increases risks of complications/side effects.
c. Therapeutic drug monitoring should be done at the start of therapy, when a new drug is added or stopped, if seizures are uncontrolled, if toxicity is suspected, or to assess compliance. Drug levels should be checked at regular intervals.

D. **SPECIAL SEIZURE SYNDROMES**
1. **Febrile seizure[9]:** Brief, generalized, symmetric, tonic–clonic seizure associated with a febrile illness, but without any CNS infection or neurologic cause. Possible etiology is lowered seizure threshold in immature brain in association with febrile illness. Genetic predisposition has been noted.
a. Incidence: 3–5% of children, 6 months to 5 years of age.
b. Evaluation: History of event and physical examination assessing high-risk, 'complex' features: Onset more than 24 hours after onset of fever, duration >15 minutes, focality, two discrete episodes within 24 hours, abnormal neurologic examination. Consider further evaluation if any one of these is present. Also include evaluation of source of fever. See Fig. 22.3.

TABLE 22.7
CHARACTERISTIC EEG FINDINGS

Condition	EEG findings
Absence seizures	Generalized 3Hz/sec spike and slow-wave discharge complexes
BECTS	Centrotemporal sharp waves superimposed on normal background activity
JME	Fast spike and wave discharges with multiple spike-and-wave pattern on arousal (enhanced by photic stimulation)
Lennox–Gastaut syndrome	Generalized sharp- and slow-wave complexes, 'slow spike-and-wave complexes'
Infantile spasms	Hypsarrhythmia
Complex partial seizure	Sharp waves or spike discharge in anterior temporal frontal lobe, or multifocal spikes

From Freeman[7].
BECTS, benign epilepsy with centrotemporal spikes (also called *benign rolandic epilepsy*); JME, juvenile myoclonic epilepsy.

TABLE 22.8
ANTICONVULSANT MEDICATIONS[a]

Seizure type	Firstline	Secondline
Partial (focal EEG changes at onset of seizure)		
Simple	CBZ, PHT, VPA	PHB, PRM
Complex		
Generalized (generalized EEG spikes at outset of seizure)		
GTC	VPA, PHT or CBZ	PHB, PRM
Absence	ESX	VPA
Myoclonic	VPA, BZD	ESX, PRM
Tonic, atonic	VPA, BZD	ESX, ACTH
Infantile spasms	ACTH	VPA, NTA, vigabatrin, lamotrigine, surgery

Modified from Chokrovery[8].
CBZ, carbamazepine; PHT, phenytoin; VPA, valproic acid; PHB, phenobarbital; PRM, primidone; GTC, generalized tonic–clinic; ESX, ethosuximide; BZD, benzodiazepine; ACTH, adrenocorticotropic hormone; NTA, nitrazepam.
[a]See formulary (ch. 29) for doses and side effects.
Ketogenic diet may be helpful in the management of intractable tonic and/or clonic and myoclonic seizures.

c. Treatment: None indicated for simple febrile seizures unless frequent recurrence disrupts normal functioning. Educate parents about benign nature of events, timely use of antipyretics, and basic first aid for seizures. Most of the time, prophylactic antiepileptic drug is not indicated, and parents should understand and believe that it is a benign disorder not requiring treatment. Prescription for rectal

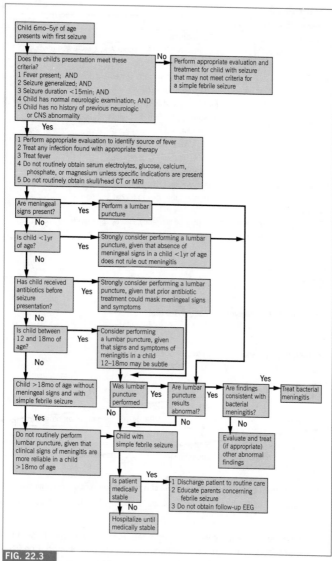

FIG. 22.3

Guidelines for febrile seizure evaluation. (From AAP subcommittee[9].)

diazepam may be helpful as a prophylactic measure, although respiratory depression is a rare side effect.

d. Outcome

1) Risk of recurrence is 30% after first febrile seizure, 50% after second episode up to age 5 years, then declines to near zero. Recurrence risk greater with younger age (<1 year) and with family history.

2) Risk of epilepsy: 2%. Increased in children with two or more of the following: Complex febrile seizures, previously abnormal development, family history of nonfebrile seizures.

2. **Neonatal seizure[10]:** Various paroxysmal behaviors or electrical events. May be tonic, myoclonic, clonic, or subtle (blinking, chewing, bicycling, apnea) because of CNS immaturity.

a. Etiologies of neonatal seizure: Almost all are symptoms of acute brain disorder. Hypoxic ischemic encephalopathy (35–42%); intracranial hemorrhage/infarction (15–20%); CNS infection (12–17%); CNS malformation (5%); metabolic (e.g., hypoglycemia, hypocalcemia, pyridoxine deficiency, toxins) (3–5%); other (5–20%).

b. Evaluation: Rapid search for acute cause. Assess clinical encephalopathy, basic laboratory screens (including glucose, calcium sodium, magnesium, and toxicology screen), LP, head CT, EEG. and sepsis workup. Prolonged or repeated EEG often needed because clinical electrical dissociation is common.

c. Treatment: Treat underlying disorder. Prevent secondary hypoxic–ischemic or metabolic complications. Treat acute symptomatic recurring seizures quickly using combined clinical and EEG end-points. Maintain anticonvulsants for sufficient period of time for acute cause to subside (days to weeks); for most acute symptomatic seizures, drugs can be safely stopped before discharge from nursery. See Table 22.9 for medical management of neonatal seizures.

3. **Infantile spasms[13]:** Head nodding with flexion or extension of the trunk and extremities, often in clusters during drowsiness or awakening. May be triggered by unexpected stimuli. EEG may show hypsarrhythmia. Usual onset after 2 months, peak onset 4–6 months. MRI/CT indicated.

a. Etiologies

1) Symptomatic (67%): CNS malformation, any acquired infantile brain injury, tuberous sclerosis.

2) Cryptogenic (33%): Associated with better outcome, less mental retardation.

b. Treatment: Controversial. Adrenocorticotropic hormone 150 units/m^2 per day IM divided Q12hr for 2–11 weeks, then slow taper, repeat as required. Options include valproic acid, benzodiazepine (clonazepam), or ketogenic diet. New experimental therapies include vigabatrin, lamotrigine, topiramate (Topamax), and surgery.

TABLE 22.9

TREATMENT OF NEONATAL SEIZURES

Establish airway, ensure oxygenation and circulation.	—
Treat metabolic abnormalities:	
Hypoglycemia	5–10mg/kg IV bolus (10% or 15% dextrose) or 2–4mL/kg D_{50} IV bolus followed by 8–10mg/kg/min IV drip as required.
Hypocalcemia	200 mg/kg calcium gluconate repeated Q5–6hr over first 24hr.
	If magnesium low, 0.2mg/kg IM.
Treat with medications:	
Phenobarbital	20mg/kg loading dose IV; additional boluses of 5–10mg/kg IV up to 30–50mg/kg. (Maintenance 3–4mg/kg/day.) If this fails, addition of phenytoin and/or a benzodiazepine.
Phenytoin	15–20mg/kg IV at 1mg/kg/min with cardiac monitoring.
Diazepam	0.5mg/kg IV; may give 0.3–0.8mg/kg/hr IV.
Lorazepam	0.05–0.1mg/kg IV over 2–5 min.
Pyridoxine	50–500mg pyridoxine IV during seizure with concurrent EEG monitoring in patients with refractory neonatal seizures; afterward, 50–100mg/day suggested.

Modified from Scher[11].

c. Outcome: Often poor, correlates best with underlying brain pathology. Of cryptogenic cases, 30–70% may have good outcome with treatment.

V. HYDROCEPHALUS

A. **DIAGNOSIS:** Assess increasing head circumference, misshapen skull, frontal bossing, bulging large anterior fontanelle, separated sutures with cracked pot sign, increased ICP (sunset sign, increased tone/reflexes), and developmental delay. Obtain head CT if increase in head circumference crosses percentiles or if patient is symptomatic. Differentiate hydrocephalus from megalencephaly or hydrocephalus ex vacuo.

B. **TREATMENT**

1. Medical[14]

a. Acute increase of ICP (see p. 13 for emergency management).

b. Slowly progressive hydrocephalus: The following medications may be effective in children 2 weeks–10 months of age with slowly progressive communicating hydrocephalus:

1) Acetazolamide: PO or IV: 20mg/kg per day ÷ Q8hr up to 100mg/kg per day. Max. 2g/24 hours.
2) Furosemide: 1mg/kg per 24 hours PO or IV divided Q8hr.
3) Polycitra: Titrate to maintain bicarbonate >18mEq/L and normal Na^+ and K^+. Usual dose is 2–4mEq/kg per 24 hours.

2. **Surgical:** Ventriculoperitoneal (VP) CSF shunting.

a. Shunt types: VP shunts are used most commonly. Ventriculoatrial/pleural shunts are associated with cardiac arrhythmias, pleural effusions, and higher rates of infection.

b. Shunt components: Typically a shunt is composed of three parts: Proximal tubing, a flushing device with a one-way valve, and a distal tube.

c. Shunt complications: Shunt dysfunction may be caused by infection, obstruction (clogging or kinking), disconnection, and migration of proximal and distal tips.

C. MANAGEMENT OF ACUTE SHUNT OBSTRUCTION OR INFECTION

1. **Evaluate shunt integrity:** Obtain shunt series (skull, neck, chest, and abdominal radiographs) to look for kinking or disconnection. Obtain head CT to evaluate shunt position, ventricular size, and evidence of increased ICP.

2. **Test shunt function:** Consider depressing bulb and allow it to refill. Decreased bulb depression phase may be caused by distal shunt obstruction or a stiffened bulb. Poor refill suggests obstruction at the ventricular end, or excessive ventricular decompression. Reasons not to depress bulb would include uncertainty of proximal tubing position and suspected slit ventricles.

3. **Percutaneous shunt drainage:** This procedure should be performed by a neurosurgeon; however, if a neurosurgeon is unavailable or the patient's condition is rapidly deteriorating, a percutaneous shunt drainage may be performed by any physician familiar with the procedure.

a. Cleanse the area over the shunt bulb using aseptic technique.

b. Insert a long-nose, 25G butterfly needle into the flushing device through the bulb diaphragm into the proximal chamber. A stopcock attached to the butterfly tubing may help prevent air from entering the ventricular system. Measure the fluid pressure, and remove the minimum amount of fluid needed to achieve symptomatic relief.

c. If blockage at the ventricular end is suspected and the patient's condition continues to deteriorate, insert a spinal needle (up to 18G) through the burr hole through which the shunt was placed, and direct it toward the lateral ventricles. (Aim spinal needle toward contralateral ear.) Measure the pressure and remove the minimal amount of fluid necessary for decompression.

d. Send CSF for culture, cell count and differential, glucose, and protein.

22

NEUROLOGY

VI. ENCEPHALOPATHY[15]

A. **DEFINITION:** Diffuse brain disorder characterized by two of the following: Altered state of consciousness, altered cognition/personality, and seizures. A global encephalopathy can be gradual or abrupt and is secondary to several different categories of insults. Brainstem function is usually intact.

B. **TYPES**

1. **Toxic/metabolic:** Consider exogenous toxins, including lead; both accidental and purposeful ingestion are the most common. Also consider endogenous toxins (urea, ammonia, metabolic acidosis, glucose) that could signify a genetic or metabolic disorder, organ failure, or endocrine disease. Use examination, environmental history (heavy metal exposure, pesticides, and medications at home), and laboratory abnormalities/toxicity screens.

2. **Infectious:** Meningoencephalitis has multiple viral/bacterial etiologies.

a. Presentation: Acute, nonspecific preceding illness. Headache, hyperesthesia, irritability/lethargy, meningeal irritation (nausea, vomiting, photophobia, meningismus). Exanthemata common.

b. History: This should include exposure to ill contacts, animals/pets/ticks, travel.

c. Laboratory/diagnostic studies: With viral disease, expect CSF pleocytosis (initial polymorphonuclear shift but majority of mononuclear cells on another LP), normal to high protein, normal glucose, negative Gram stain. Culture CSF for viral, bacterial, and even mycobacterial, fungal, and protozoan/parasite if relevant. Nasopharyngeal and rectal swabs and urine specimen for viral cultures. MRI helpful to evaluate for demyelination. EEG showing temporal periodic lateralized epileptiform discharges can be diagnostic for herpes encephalitis.

d. Treatment: Usually self-limited but symptomatic support helpful. IV antibiotics while ruling out bacterial causes. Acyclovir should be used if herpes suspected. Complications of disease include cerebral edema, seizures, fluid/electrolyte abnormalities, hyperthermia, respiratory and cardiovascular collapse.

3. **Noninfectious/other:** Malignancy, collagen vascular disease (systemic lupus erythematosus), ischemia, hypertension, AIDS, Leigh's disease, trauma. Include erythrocyte sedimentation rate, thyroid studies, liver enzyme tests, electrolytes, BUN, NH_3, and prothrombin time/partial thromboplastin time. Consider CT of head and then LP to evaluate for infection or hemorrhage if CT and laboratory tests are negative.

VII. BRAIN DEATH CRITERIA

Many sets of criteria have been proposed for the determination of brain death. Most agree that the irreversible loss of function of both cerebral hemispheres and the brainstem constitutes brain death. Table 22.10 represents some accepted guidelines used in determining brain death in

TABLE 22.10
BRAIN DEATH CRITERIA

Prerequisites

Irreversible lesion/event

Known etiology of lesion/event

Hemodynamically stable and normothermic during observation

No drugs of sedation or neuromuscular blockade

Physical examination

Coma; no response to sound, light, or deep pain (Glasgow Coma Scale <8)

No spontaneous movement or posturing, flaccid tone

Absent brainstem reflexes:

    Pupillary light reflex

    Corneal reflex

    Oculocephalic reflex[a]

    Oculovestibular reflex[b]

    Oropharyngeal (gag) reflex

    Facial grimace with nasopharyngeal stimulus gag

Apnea (established by formal testing)[c]

Period of observation

No definite consensus; period ranges from 6–48hr; may be specific to age group

Corroboratory tests

Cerebral angiography

EEG

Radioisotope cerebral blood flow study

Transcranial Doppler ultrasonography

Adapted from Rogers[15].

[a]*Oculocephalic reflex:* When the patient's head is turned rapidly from the midline to the lateral gaze position, the eyes should remain straight ahead in a normal patient ("doll's eyes").

[b]*Oculovestibular reflex:* With an intact tympanic membrane and the head elevated 30 degrees, up to 120mL of ice water is gently introduced over several minutes into the ear canal. In awake patients with an intact brainstem, nystagmus is produced with slow eye deviation toward the cold stimulus and a rapid nystagmus in the opposite direction. As cerebral hemisphere disease develops, the fast component disappears with tonic deviation of the eyes toward the cold stimulus. As metabolic depression continues to severe levels or in the presence of brainstem damage, the caloric reflex is abolished.

[c]*Apnea* defined as no spontaneous respirations with carbon dioxide stimulus (no breaths in 15min or until PCO_2 rises to 60mmHg) while 100% passive oxygenation is occurring.

the pediatric patient. Controversy exists on the period of observation in different ages as well as the need for or use of corroborative testing.

VIII. NEUROMUSCULAR DISORDERS

A. **DISORDERS OF THE MOTOR UNIT:** These are disorders of the peripheral nerve (motor neuron + its axon), the neuromuscular junction, and the muscle fibers innervated by the neuron.

1. **Myopathy:** Proximal/girdle weakness, muscle wasting. Deep tendon reflexes preserved or decreased; elevated creatine phosphokinase.

TABLE 22.11

TYPICAL ELECTRODIAGNOSTIC FINDINGS

Myopathy

Normal nerve conduction velocity

Short muscle action potential

Acute spontaneous activity in myositis

Demyelinating neuropathy

Slowing of nerve conduction velocity

Conduction block (drop of 50% in muscle action potential with proximal stimulation)

No spontaneous activity in weak muscles

Relative preservation of distal evoked amplitude

Axonopathy

Normal/mildly slowed nerve conduction velocity

Normal/mildly prolonged distal motor latencies

Distal spontaneous activity

Long duration, reduced muscle action potential

Motor neuron disease

Sensory nerves spared

Widespread acute spontaneous activity

Multiple points of motor conduction block

From Younger[16].

2. **Neuropathy:** Distal weakness; deep tendon reflexes generally lost; sensory abnormalities common.

B. **ELECTRODIAGNOSTIC STUDIES:** These can be used to investigate myopathy, a disorder of neuromuscular transmission, motor neuron disease, and peripheral neuropathy. See Table 22.11.

1. **Nerve conduction studies:** Nerve conduction velocity (NCV).

a. Surface electrodes are used to measure motor and sensory nerve conduction.

b. A nerve is stimulated at two points, and the latency is recorded between nerve stimulus and muscle contraction.

c. Useful in distinguishing demyelination (reduced NCV) from axonal degeneration of the peripheral nerve (reduced amplitude) and from muscular disorders (normal NCV).

d. Sensory NCV useful with hereditary sensory and autonomic neuropathies.

2. **Electromyography (EMG)**

a. Needle electrode inserted into muscle belly; action potentials recorded in different states of contraction.

b. The number of motor unit discharges as well as the amplitude (shape) of each discharge can be abnormal.

c. Duration of discharge more important than amplitude in myopathy.

d. More useful in evaluating lower motor neuron disease, in which denervation can be differentiated from myopathic involvement.

e. Spontaneous fibrillation potentials can be seen after denervation, hyperkalemic paralysis, botulism, muscular dystrophy, and some myopathies.

3. Muscle biopsy

a. Most informative test to distinguish a neurogenic from a myopathic etiology of weakness.

b. Helpful for diagnosing specific myopathy/enzyme deficiency.

C. SELECTED DISORDERS OF NEUROMUSCULAR TRANSMISSION

1. Myasthenia gravis

a. Often an autoimmune disorder resulting from the motor endplate being less responsive to the release of acetylcholine.

b. Characterized by fluctuating weakness of ocular, facial, neck, oropharyngeal, and limb muscles. In infant, poor head control and difficulty feeding (transient neonatal vs congenital).

c. Rapid fatigue of muscles characteristic. (Upward gaze for 30–90 seconds produces progressive ptosis.)

d. EMG: Decremental response of muscle action potential (MAP) noted with 3/second repetitive nerve stimulation, until refractory to further stimulation. Results reversed with cholinesterase inhibitor (i.e., edrophonium chloride).

e. Motor NCV normal.

2. Botulism

a. Ingestion of food containing toxin of *Clostridium botulinum*. Infantile form often associated with release of toxin from *C. botulinum* colonizing the intestinal tract after spore ingestion.

b. Involvement of the CNS with facial weakness, weak suck, loss of gag reflex. Hypotonia and weakness can lead to respiratory failure.

c. Abnormally low-amplitude MAP after supramaximal stimulation. With repetitive stimulation at rates of 20Hz, a 100–200% increase in MAP amplitude occurs, indicating a presynaptic neuromuscular junction defect.

d. Normal NCV.

e. Diagnosis: Botulinum toxin from blood or stool.

3. Guillain–Barré syndrome (acute acquired inflammatory polyneuropathy)

a. Postinfectious polyneuropathy causes demyelination in motor neuron (can affect sensory function or rarely, axonal loss).

b. Ascending, symmetric weakness. Bulbar involvement possible (e.g., Miller-Fischer variant).

c. Deep tendon reflexes lost early.

d. CSF (diagnostic) reveals elevated protein and low cell count (cytoalbuminemic dissociation).

e. Motor NCVs greatly reduced.

f. EMG: Acute denervation of muscle.

g. Treatment includes IV immune globulin. Consider plasma exchange therapy with bulbar involvement, loss of independent ambulation, or respiratory failure. Observation/stabilization. Check functional vital capacity, negative inspiratory force (respiratory compromise), and blood pressure frequently (autonomic dysfunction).

IX. REFERENCES

1. Medical Research Council (MRC). Strength Rating Scale.
2. Athreya BH, Silverman BK. *Pediatric physical diagnosis.* Norwalk, CT: Appleton-Century-Crofts; 1985.
3. Singer H, Rowe S. Chronic recurrent headaches in children. *Pediatr Ann* 1992; **21(6):**369.
4. Murphy JV, Dehkharghani F. Diagnosis of childhood seizure disorder. *Epilepsia* 1994; **35(suppl 2):**S7–S17.
5. Committee on Classification and Terminology of the International League Against Epilepsy. Proposal for revised clinical and electroencephalographic classification of epileptic seizures. *Epilepsia* 1981; **22(4):**490–501.
6. Committee on Classification and Terminology of the International League Against Epilepsy. Classification of epilepsia: its applicability and practical value of different diagnostic categories. *Epilepsia* 1996; **38(11):**1051–1059.
7. Freeman J. *Seizures and epilepsy in childhood: a guide to parents,* 2nd edn. Baltimore: Johns Hopkins University Press; 1997.
8. Chokrovery S, ed. *Management of epilepsy.* Boston: Butterworth-Heinemann; 1996.
9. AAP subcommittee. Practice parameter: the neurodiagnostic evaluation of the child with a first simple febrile. *Pediatr* 1996; **97(5):**772.
10. Freeman JM. What have we learned from febrile seizures? *Pediatr Ann* 1992; **21(6):**355.
11. Scher MS. Seizures in the newborn infant: diagnosis, treatment and outcomes. *Clin Perinatol* 1997; **24(4):**735–772.
12. Swaiman KF. *Principles and practice of pediatric neurology.* St Louis: Mosby; 1995.
13. Shinnar S, Gammon K, Bergman EW Jr, Epstein M, Freeman JM. Management of hydrocephalus in infancy: use of acetazolamide and furosemide to avoid cerebrospinal fluid shunts. *J Pediatr* 1985; **107(1):**31–37.
14. Behrman RE, Kliegman RM, Arvin AM. *Nelson textbook of pediatrics,* 15th edn. Philadelphia: WB Saunders; 1996.
15. Rogers M, ed. *Textbook of pediatric intensive care,* 3rd edn. Baltimore: Williams & Wilkins; 1996.
16. Younger DS, Gordon PH. Diagnosis in neuromuscular diseases. *Neurol Clin* 1996; **14(1):**135–150.

NUTRITION

Jeanne Cox, MS, RD

I. ASSESSMENT OF NUTRITIONAL STATUS

A. ELEMENTS OF NUTRITIONAL ASSESSMENT

1. **Medical history and physical examination** (medical diagnosis, clinical symptoms of nutritional deficiencies).
2. **Dietary evaluation** (feeding history, current intake).
3. **Laboratory findings** (comparison to age-based norms).
4. **Anthropometric measurements** (weight, length/height, head circumference, skinfolds); data are plotted on growth charts according to age and compared with a reference population.

23

B. PROTEIN–ENERGY MALNUTRITION (PEM)

1. **Classification of PEM** (Table 23.1)
2. **Characteristics of severe PEM** (Table 23.2)

C. EVALUATION OF OBESITY (Table 23.3)

1. **Evaluation of obesity is based on body mass index (BMI):**

$$BMI = \frac{(\text{Weight in kg})}{(\text{Height in meters})^2}$$

a. Children whose BMI is >85% are at risk of becoming overweight.
b. Children whose BMI is >95% are overweight.
c. New growth charts that include BMI/age are in press.

TABLE 23.1

CLASSIFICATION OF PEM

$\text{Acute PEM} = \dfrac{\text{Child's actual weight (kg)}}{\text{50th percentile weight/height (kg)}}$	90–100% normal 80–90% mild 70–80% moderate <70% severe
$\text{Chronic PEM} = \dfrac{\text{Child's actual height (cm)}}{\text{50th percentile height for age (cm)}}$	95–100% normal 90–95% mild 85–90% moderate <85% severe

From Waterlow[1].

TABLE 23.2

CHARACTERISTICS OF SEVERE PEM

Marasmus	**Energy and protein malnutrition**
	Weight for length <70% of 50th percentile weight/height
	Absence of subcutaneous fat
	Generalized muscular wasting
	Retardation of linear growth
	Hair is sparse, thin, dry, and lacks sheen
	Apathetic with look of anxiety
	Normal serum proteins
Kwashiorkor	**Predominantly protein malnutrition**
	Weight for length normal to slightly low
	Linear growth normal to slightly retarded
	Subcutaneous fat preserved
	Soft, pitting edema
	Skin lesions, erythema, epidermis peels off in large scales
	Distended abdomen
	Hepatomegaly
	Hair is brittle, discolored, dry, easily pluckable
	Apathetic and irritable
	Hypoalbuminemia, low hematocrit

TABLE 23.3

EVALUATION FOR OBESITY IN CHILDREN AND ADOLESCENTS IN THE UNITED STATES USING BMI (kg/m^2)

Age (yr)	At risk of overweight (85%ile BMI)		Overweight (95%ile BMI)	
	Males	Females	Males	Females
5	17.2	16.9	18.3	18.5
6	17.4	17.2	19.0	19.3
7	17.8	17.9	20.0	20.4
8	18.6	18.9	21.5	21.7
9	19.7	20.1	23.1	23.0
10	20.9	21.4	24.6	24.5
11	21.9	22.6	25.7	26.1
12	22.6	23.6	26.5	27.5
13	23.2	24.4	27.1	28.6
14	23.7	24.9	27.8	29.3
15	24.5	25.2	28.7	29.6
16	25.4	25.5	29.8	29.9
17	25.9	25.9	30.1	31.3

Adapted from Rosner[2].

II. ESTIMATING ENERGY NEEDS

A. **AVERAGE ENERGY NEEDS:** Several methods can be used for estimating energy needs. The most frequently used method is the average energy allowance from the Recommended Energy Intake for Age (Table 23.4).

B. **ADJUSTMENTS TO ENERGY NEEDS:** For children who have decreased energy needs secondary to neurologic impairment, or increased needs secondary to injury, sepsis, or increased motor activity, the resting energy expenditure (REE) (Table 23.4) can be used with the addition of factors for activity, injury, and disease.

1. **Calculation of total daily energy needs using REE method:**

Total daily energy needs (kcal/kg per day) = REE (kcal/kg/day) + REE (kcal/kg per day) × [Maintenance + Injury + Activity factors]

2. **Factors[5]**
- Maintenance: 0.2
- Activity: 0.1–0.25
- Fever: 0.13 per °C >38°
- Simple trauma: 0.2
- Multiple injuries: 0.4
- Burns: 0.5–1
- Growth: 0.5

Example: 10-year-old boy with multiple injuries from motor vehicle accident and temperature of 39°C.

REE + REE × (Maintenance + Activity + Fever + Injuries + Growth)
= 40kcal/kg per day +
     40kcal/kg per day × (0.2 + 0.1 + 0.13 + 0.4 + 0.5)
= 40kcal/kg per day + (40kcal/kg per day) (1.33)
= 40kcal/kg per day + 53kcal/kg per day
= 93kcal/kg per day

C. **CATCH-UP GROWTH REQUIREMENT FOR MALNOURISHED INFANTS AND CHILDREN**

1. **Calculations of energy needs for a malnourished child to catch up to expected growth parameters[6]:**

Catch-up energy needs (kcal/kg per day) =

$$\frac{\left[\begin{array}{c}\text{Average energy allowance}\\\text{for chronologic age (kcal/kg per day)}\end{array}\right] \times \left[\begin{array}{c}\text{50th percentile}\\\text{weight/height (kg)}\end{array}\right]}{\text{Actual weight (kg)}}$$

23

NUTRITION

TABLE 23.4

RECOMMENDED ENERGY INTAKE FOR AGE

	Age (yr)	REE[a] (kcal/kg/day)	Average energy needs	
			(kcal/kg/day)	(kcal/day)
Infants	0.0–0.5	53	108	650
	0.5–1.0	56	98	850
Children	1–3	57	102	1300
	4–6	48	90	1800
	7–10	40	70	2000
Males	11–14	32	55	2500
	15–18	27	45	3000
Females	11–14	28	47	2200
	15–18	25	40	2200
Pregnancy	1st trimester			+0
	2nd & 3rd trimesters			+300
Lactation				+500

Adapted from Food Nutrition Board[3].

[a]Resting energy expenditure, based on Food and Agricultural Organization (FAO) equations.

III. RECOMMENDED DIETARY ALLOWANCES (Tables 23.5 and 23.6)

A. VITAMINS (Table 23.5)

B. MINERALS (Table 23.6)

TABLE 23.5

RECOMMENDED DIETARY ALLOWANCES[a]—VITAMINS

Category	Age (yr)	Weight[b] (kg)	(lb)	Height[b] (cm)	(in)	Protein (g)	Fat-soluble vitamins					Water-soluble vitamins					
							Vitamin A (IU)[c]	Vitamin D (IU)[d]	Vitamin E (IU)[e]	Vitamin K (mcg)	Vitamin C (mg)	Thiamin (mg)	Riboflavin (mg)	Niacin (mgNE)[f]	Vitamin B$_6$ (mg)	Folate (mcg)	B$_{12}$ (mcg)
Infants	0.0–0.5	6	13	60	24	13	1250	300	3	5	30	0.3	0.4	5	0.3	25	0.3
	0.5–1.0	9	20	71	28	14	1250	400	4	10	35	0.4	0.5	6	0.6	35	0.5
Children	1–3	13	29	90	35	16	1333	400	6	15	40	0.7	0.8	9	1.0	50	0.7
	4–6	20	44	112	44	24	1667	400	7	20	45	0.9	1.1	12	1.1	75	1.0
	7–10	28	62	132	52	28	2333	400	7	30	45	1.0	1.2	13	1.4	100	1.4
Males	11–14	45	99	157	62	45	3333	400	10	45	50	1.3	1.5	17	1.7	150	2.0
	15–18	66	145	176	69	59	3333	400	10	65	60	1.5	1.8	20	2.0	200	2.0
	19–24	72	160	177	70	58	3333	400	10	70	60	1.5	1.7	19	2.0	200	2.0
Females	11–14	46	101	157	62	46	2667	400	8	45	50	1.1	1.3	15	1.4	150	2.0
	15–18	55	120	163	64	44	2667	400	8	55	60	1.1	1.3	15	1.5	180	2.0
	19–24	58	128	164	65	46	2667	400	8	60	60	1.1	1.3	15	1.6	180	2.0
Pregnant						60	2667	400	10	65	70	1.5	1.6	17	2.2	400	2.2
Lactating	1st 6 mo					65	4333	400	12	65	95	1.6	1.8	20	2.1	280	2.6
	2nd 6 mo					62	4000	400	11	65	90	1.6	1.7	20	2.1	260	2.6

Adapted from Food Nutrition Board[3].

[a],[b] See footnotes in Table 23.6.

Conversion factors for IU:

[c]Vitamin A: mcg RE/0.3 = IU, where RE is retinol equivalent.

[d]Vitamin D: 40 × mcg cholecalciferol = IU.

[e]Vitamin E: as RRR-α-tocopherol.

[f]NE (niacin equivalent) is equal to 1mg niacin or 60mg dietary tryptophan.

TABLE 23.6

RECOMMENDED DIETARY ALLOWANCES[a]—MINERALS

Category	Age (yr)	Weight[b] (kg)	Weight[b] (lb)	Height[b] (cm)	Height[b] (in)	Calcium (mg)	Phosphorus (mg)	Magnesium (mg)	Iron (mg)	Zinc (mg)	Iodine (mcg)	Selenium (mcg)
Infants	0.0–0.5	6	13	60	24	400	300	40	6	5	40	10
	0.5–1.0	9	20	71	28	600	500	60	10	5	50	15
Children	1–3	13	29	90	35	800	800	80	10	10	70	20
	4–6	20	44	112	44	800	800	120	10	10	90	20
	7–10	28	62	132	52	800	800	170	10	10	120	30
Males	11–14	45	99	157	62	1200	1200	270	12	15	150	40
	15–18	66	145	176	69	1200	1200	400	12	15	150	50
	19–24	72	160	177	70	1200	1200	350	10	15	150	70
Females	11–14	46	101	157	62	1200	1200	280	15	12	150	45
	15–18	55	120	163	64	1200	1200	300	15	12	150	50
	19–24	58	128	164	65	1200	1200	280	15	12	150	55
Pregnant						1200	1200	320	30	15	175	65
Lactating	1st 6 mo					1200	1200	355	15	19	200	75
	2nd 6 mo					1200	1200	340	15	16	200	75

Adapted from Food Nutrition Board[3].

[a]The allowances, expressed as average daily intakes over time, are intended to provide for individual variations among most normal persons as they live in the United States under usual environmental stresses. Diets should be based on a variety of common foods in order to provide other nutrients for which human requirements have been less well defined.

[b]Weights and heights of Reference Adults are actual medians for the United States population of the designated age, as reported by NHANES II. The median weights and heights of those under 19 years of age are from Hamill[4]. The use of these figures does not imply that the height-to-weight ratios are ideal.

IV. VITAMIN–MINERAL SUPPLEMENTATION FOR BREASTFED INFANTS

A. VITAMIN D

1. 400IU per day is recommended for breastfed infants, especially those who are deeply pigmented or have limited sunlight exposure. Generally an ADC multivitamin such as Tri-Vi-Sol or Vi-Daylin ADC can be used (see Table 23.17).

B. FLUORIDE

1. Supplementation is not needed during the first 6 months of life. Thereafter 0.25mg is recommended for the exclusively breastfed infant. See p. 720 for complete fluoride recommendations.

C. IRON

1. For exclusively breastfed infants, approximately 1 mg/kg per day is recommended after 4–6 months of age, preferably from iron-fortified cereal or elemental iron if sufficient cereal is not consumed.

V. ENTERAL NUTRITION (Tables 23.7 to 23.17)

23

NUTRITION

TABLE 23.7

CLASSIFICATION OF FORMULAS BY CARBOHYDRATE

	Lactose	Sucrose and glucose polymers	Glucose polymers	Minimal carbohydrate
Common ingredient names		See glucose polymers	Glucose polymers Maltodextrins Corn syrup solids Modfied tapioca starch	
Comments	Requires lactase enzyme for digestion Contraindicated in galactosemia	Requires sucrase enzyme for digestion (see also glucose polymers)	Easily digested For individuals with lactose malabsorption	For severe carbohydrate intolerance
Infants	Enfamil Enfamil 22[a] Enfamil AR Enfamil Premature Carnation Follow-up Carnation Good Start Neosure[a] Similac Similac PM 60/40 Similac Special Care	Alimentum Alsoy Isomil Isomil DF (Fiber) Portagen	Isomil SF Lactofree Neocate Nutramigen Pregestimil ProSobee Similac Lactose Free	MJ3232A RCF

Toddlers and young children	Next Step[a]	Compleat Pediatric[b] Kindercal (Fiber) Neocate One Plus Next Step Soy Nutren Junior PediaSure (also w/Fiber) Peptamen Junior ProPeptide for Kids Resource Just for Kids	Vivonex Pediatric L-Emental Pediatric
Older children and adolescents	Carnation Instant Breakfast Scandishake	All other formulas in Table 23.13	Criticare HN Deliver 2.0 Glucerna Isocal Jevity (fiber) L-Emental L-Emental Plus Peptamen PropPeptide Tolerex Vivonex TEN Vivonex Plus

[a]Also contains glucose polymers.
[b]Also contains fruit and vegetable purees.

23

NUTRITION

TABLE 23.8

CLASSIFICATION OF FORMULAS BY PROTEIN

	Cow's milk	Soy	Hydrolysate	Free amino acids
Common ingredient names	Cow's milk protein Nonfat milk Demineralized whey Reduced mineral whey Sodium, calcium, magnesium caseinate Casein	Soy protein Soy protein isolate	Casein hydrolysate Hydrolyzed whey, meat, and soy	—
Comments	Requires normal protein digestion and absorption	Requires normal protein digestion and absorption Not recommended for premature infants or those with cystic fibrosis	For individuals with protein allergy and/or malabsorption	For individuals with severe protein allergy and/or severe protein malabsorption
Infants	Enfamil Enfamil 22 Enfamil AR Follow-up Lactofree Neosure Portagen Enfamil Premature Similac Similac PM 60/40 Similac Special Care Similac Lactose Free	Alsoy Follow-up Soy Isomil Isomil DF ProSobee RCF	Alimentum Good Start Nutramigen Pregestimil MJ3232A	Neocate

Toddlers and young children	Compleat Pediatric[a] Resource Just for Kids Kindercal Next Step Nutren Junior PediaSure	Next Step Soy	Peptamen Junior Pro-Peptide for Kids	Vivonex Pediatric Neocate One Plus EleCare L-Emental Pediatric
Older children and adolescents	All other formulas in Table 23.13	Ensure[b] Ensure with Fiber[b] Isocal[b] Osmolite[b] Promote[b] Sustacal[b] Boost High-Protein[b] Boost with Fiber[b]	Criticare HN Peptamen Vital HN ProPeptide	Tolerex Vivonex TEN Vivonex Plus L-Emental L-Emental Plus

[a]Blenderized protein diet of meat, vegetables, and fruit.
[b]Also contains cow's milk.

23

NUTRITION

TABLE 23.9

CLASSIFICATION OF FORMULAS BY FAT

	Long-chain triglycerides		Medium-chain and long-chain triglycerides
Common ingredient names	Safflower oil Soy oil Palm olein Coconut oil	Sunflower oil Corn oil Canola oil Butterfat	Medium-chain triglycerides (MCT oil) Fractioned coconut oil
Comments	Requires normal fat digestion and absorption		For individuals with fat malabsorption Bile digestion not required Absorbed directly into portal circulation

Infants	Alsoy
	Enfamil
	Enfamil AR
	Carnation
	  Follow-up
	Carnation
	  Follow-up
	  Soy
	Carnation Good
	  Start
		Isomil (all)
		Lactofree
		Neocate
		Nutramigen
		ProSobee
		RCF
		Similac
		Similac PM
		  60/40
		Similac Lactose
		  Free
			Alimentum
			Enfamil Premature
			Enfamil 22
			Pregestimil
			Portagen
			Neosure
			Similac Special
			  Care

Toddlers and young children	Next Step
	Compleat
	  Pediatric
	Toddler's Best
			Resource Just
			  For Kids
			Kindercal
			Neocate One Plus
			Nutren Junior
			PediaSure
			L-Emental Pediatric
			Peptamen Junior
			Vivonex Pediatric

Older children and adolescents	Carnation Instant
	  Breakfast
	Ensure
	Ensure with Fiber
	Ensure Plus
	Glucerna
		Nepro
		Pulmocare
		Scandishake
		Suplena
		Boost Plus
		Boost
		  High-Protein
		Boost with
		  Fiber
			Deliver 2.0 Osmolite
			Isocal Promote
			Jevity Respalor
			Lipisorb Traumacal
			Nutren 2.0 Ultracal
			Nutrivent

TABLE 23.10

INFANT FORMULA ANALYSIS (PER LITER)

Formula	kcal/mL (kcal/oz)	Protein g (% kcal)	Carbohydrate g (% kcal)	Fat g (% kcal)	Na (mEq)	K (mEq)	Ca (mg)	P (mg)	Fe (mg)	Osmolality (mOsm/kg water)	Suggested uses
Alimentum (Ross)	0.67 (20)	19 (11) Casein hydrolysate Cystine, Tyr, Trp Methionine	69 (41) Sucrose 67% Modified tapioca starch	38 (48) MCT oil (50%) Safflower oil (40%) Soy oil (10%)	13	20	709	507	12	370	Infants with food allergies, protein or fat malabsorption
Alsoy (Carnation)	0.67 (20)	19 (11) Soy Isolate Methionine	75 (44) Sucrose Maltodextrin	36 (45) Soy oil	10	20	709	412	12	200	Infants with allergy to cow's milk, lactose malabsorption, galactosemia
Enfamil [w/Fe] (Mead Johnson)	0.67 (20)	14 (9) Nonfat milk Demineralized whey	73 (43) Lactose	36 (48) Palm olein (45%) Soy oil (20%) Coconut oil (20%) HO Sun oil (15%)	8	19	530	360	5 [12.5]	300	Infants with normal GI tract

23

NUTRITION

Continued

TABLE 23.10

INFANT FORMULA ANALYSIS (PER LITER)—cont'd

Formula	kcal/mL (kcal/oz)	Protein g (% kcal)	Carbohydrate g (% kcal)	Fat g (% kcal)	Na (mEq)	K (mEq)	Ca (mg)	P (mg)	Fe (mg)	Osmolality (mOsm/kg water)	Suggested uses
Enfamil AR (Mead Johnson)	0.67 (20)	16.7 (10) Nonfat milk Demineralized whey	73 (44) Lactose (57%) Rice starch (30%) Maltodextrins (13%)	34 (46) Palm olein (45%) Soy oil (20%) Coconut oil (20%) HO sun oil (15%)	11	18	520	353	12	230	When a thickened feeding is desired
Enfamil 24 [w/Fe] (Mead Johnson)	0.8 (20)	17 (9) Nonfat milk Whey	88 (43) Lactose	43 (48) Palm olein (45%) Soy oil (20%) HO Sun oil (15%)	10	22	630	430	6 [15]	360	Infants with normal GI tract requiring additional calories
Enfamil Premature Formula 20 [w/Fe] (Mead Johnson)	0.67 (20)	20 (12) Demineralized whey Nonfat milk	75 (44) Corn syrup solids Lactose	35 (44) MCT oil (40%) Soy oil Coconut oil	11	18	1120	560	1.7 [12]	260	Preterm infants
Enfamil Premature Formula 24 [w/Fe] (Mead Johnson)	0.8 (24)	24 (12) Demineralized whey Nonfat milk	9 (44) Corn syrup solids Lactose	41 (44) MCT oil (40%) Soy oil Coconut oil	14	21	1340	670	2 [15]	310	Preterm infants

Enfamil 22 with iron (Mead Johnson)	0.73 (22)	20.6 (11) Nonfat milk Demineralized whey	79 (43) Corn syrup solids Lactose	39 (48) HO sun oil Soy oil MCT oil Coconut oil	11	20	890	490	13	—	Preterm infants after hospital discharge until goal catch-up growth
Evaporated milk formula[a]	0.69 (21)	28 (16) Cow's milk	75 (43) Lactose Corn syrup	33 (43) Butterfat	20	33	1130	870	2	—	Infants with normal GI tract; need vitamin C and iron supplement
Follow-up (Carnation)	0.67 (20)	18 (10) Nonfat milk	89 (53) Corn syrup (43%) Lactose (37%)	28 (37) Palm olein (47%) Soy oil (26%) Coconut oil (21%) HO saff oil (6%)	11	23	912	608	13	328	Infants 4–12 months with normal GI tract
Follow-up Soy (Carnation)	0.67 (20)	21 (12) Soy isolate Methionine	81 (48) Maltodextrin Sucrose	29 (40) Palm olein (47%) Soy oil (26%) Coconut oil (21%) HO saff oil (6%)	12	20	912	608	12	200	Infants 4–12 months with allergy to cow's milk, lactose malabsorption, galactosemia
Good Start (Carnation)	0.67 (20)	16 (10) Hydrolyzed whey	74 (44) Lactose Maltodextrins	3.5 (46) Palm olein (47%) Soy oil (26%) Coconut oil (21%) HO saff oil (6%)	7	17	432	243	10	265	Infants with normal GI tract

a13 ounces evaporated whole milk 119 ounces water 12 tbsp corn syrup.

Continued

TABLE 23.10
INFANT FORMULA ANALYSIS (PER LITER)—cont'd

Formula	kcal/mL (kcal/oz)	Protein g (% kcal)	Carbohydrate g (% kcal)	Fat g (% kcal)	Na (mEq)	K (mEq)	Ca (mg)	P (mg)	Fe (mg)	Osmolality (mOsm/kg water)	Suggested uses
Isomil (Ross)	0.67 (20)	17 (10) Soy isolate Methionine	70 (41) Corn syrup Sucrose	37 (49) Soy oil Coconut oil	13	19	709	507	12	230	Infants with allergy to cow's milk, lactose malabsorption, galactosemia
Isomil DF (Ross)	0.67 (20)	18 (11) Soy isolate Methionine	68 (40) Corn syrup Sucrose Soy fiber	37 (49) Soy oil Coconut oil	13	19	709	507	12	240	Short-term management of diarrhea; contains fiber
Lactofree (Mead Johnson)	0.67 (20)	14 (9) Milk protein isolate	7 (43) Corn syrup solids	36 (48) Palm olein (45%) Soy oil (20%) Coconut oil (20%) HO Sun (15%)	9	19	550	370	12	200	Infants with lactose malabsorption
MJ3232A (Mead Johnson)	0.42 (12.6)	19 (17) Casein hydrolysate Cystine, Tyr, Trp	28 (25) Tapioca starch CHO selected by physician	28 (57) MCT oil (85%) Corn oil (15%)	13	19	630	420	13	250	Infants with severe CHO intolerance (CHO must be added)

Product	kcal/mL (kcal/oz)	Protein g (%) / Source	Carbohydrate g (%) / Source	Fat g (%) / Source						mOsm	Indications
Neocate (Scientific Hospital Supply)	0.69 (21)	20 (12) Free amino acids	78 (47) Corn syrup solids	32 (41) Safflower oil, Coconut oil, Soy oil	8	16	826	620	10	342	Infants with severe food allergies
Nutramigen (Mead Johnson)	0.67 (20)	19 (11) Casein hydrolysate, Cystine, Tyr, Trp	74 (44) Corn syrup solids, Modified cornstarch	34 (45) Palm olein (45%), Soy oil (20%), Coconut oil (20%), HO Sun oil (15%)	14	19	640	430	13	320	Infants with food allergies
Portagen (Mead Johnson)	0.67 (20)	24 (14) Na caseinate	78 (46) Corn syrup solids, Sucrose	32 (40) MCT oil (85%), Corn oil (15%)	16	22	640	470	13	230	Infants with fat malabsorption
Pregestimil (Mead Johnson)	0.67 (20)	19 (11) Casein hydrolysate, Cystine, Tyr, Trp	69 (41) Corn syrup solids (60%), Modified cornstarch (20%), Dextrose (20%)	38 (48) MCT oil (55%), Corn oil (20%), Soy oil (12.5%), HO Saff oil (12.5%)	11	19	640	430	13	320	Infants with food allergies, protein or fat malabsorption
ProSobee (Mead Johnson)	0.67 (20)	20 (12) Soy isolate, Methionine	73 (42) Corn syrup solids	37 (48) Palm olein (45%), Soy oil (20%), Coconut oil (20%), HO Sun oil (15%)	10	21	710	560	12	200	Infants with allergy to cow's milk, lactose malabsorption, galactosemia

Continued

23

NUTRITION

TABLE 23.10

INFANT FORMULA ANALYSIS (PER LITER)—cont'd

Formula	kcal/mL (kcal/oz)	Protein g (% kcal)	Carbohydrate g (% kcal)	Fat g (% kcal)	Na (mEq)	K (mEq)	Ca (mg)	P (mg)	Fe (mg)	Osmolality (mOsm/kg water)	Suggested uses
RCF[a] (Ross) [w/Fe]	0.4 (12)	20 (20) Soy isolate	— Selected by physician	36 (80) Soy oil Coconut oil	13	19	709	507	12	—[a]	Infants with severe CHO intolerance (CHO must be added) Modified for ketogenic diet
Similac [w/Fe] (Ross)	0.67 (20)	14 (8) Nonfat milk Whey protein	73 (43) Lactose	36 (49) Soy oil Coconut oil HO saff oil	7	18	527	284	1.5 [12]	300	Infants with normal GI tract
Similac 24 [w/Fe] (Ross)	0.8 (24)	22 (11) Nonfat milk	85 (42) Lactose	43 (47) Soy oil Coconut oil	12	27	726	565	1.8 [15]	380	Infants with normal GI tract requiring additional calories
Similac Lactose Free (Ross)	0.67 (20)	14.5 (9) Milk isolate	72.3 (43) Corn syrup solids Sucrose	36.5 (49) Soy oil Coconut oil	9	18.5	568	378	12	230	Infants with lactose malabsorption

Similac Neosure (Ross)	0.75 (22)	19 (10) Nonfat milk Whey	77 (41) Corn syrup solids (50%) Lactose (50%)	41 (49) MCT oil Soy oil Coconut oil HO saff oil	11	27	784	463	13	250	Preterm infants, after hospital discharge, until goal catch-up growth
Similac PM 60/40 (Ross)	0.67 (20)	15 (9) Whey Na caseinate	69 (41) Lactose	38 (50) Soy oil Coconut oil Corn oil	7	15	378	189	1.5	280	Infants who require lowered calcium and phosphorus levels
Similac Special Care 20 [w/Fe] (Ross)	0.67 (20)	18 (11) Nonfat milk Whey	72 (42) Corn syrup solids Lactose	37 (49) MCT oil Soy oil Coconut oil	13	22	1216	676	2.5 (12)	235	Preterm infants
Similac Special Care 24 [w/Fe] (Ross)	0.8 (24)	22 (11) Nonfat milk Whey	86 (42) Corn syrup solids Lactose	44 (49) MCT oil Soy oil Coconut oil	15	27	1452	806	3 [15]	280	Preterm infants

[a]Available as concentrated liquid. Nutrient values vary depending on amount of added carbohydrate (CHO) and water. A total of 12 fl oz of concentrated liquid with 15g CHO and 12 fl oz water yields 20kcal/fl oz formula with 68g CHO/L.

TABLE 23.11

HUMAN MILK AND FORTIFIERS ANALYSIS (PER LITER)

Formula	kcal/mL (kcal/oz)	Protein g (% kcal)	Carbohydrate g (% kcal)	Fat g (% kcal)	Na (mEq)	K (mEq)	Ca (mg)	P (mg)	Fe (mg)	Osmolality (mOsm/kg water)	Suggested uses
Human milk (mature)	0.69 (20)	9 (5) Human milk protein	73 (42) Lactose	42 (54) Human milk fat	8	13	280	147	0.4	286	Infants
Preterm human milk[a]	0.67 (20)	14 (8) Human milk protein	66 (40) Lactose	39 (52) Human milk fat	11	15	248	128	1.2	290	Preterm infants
Enfamil Human Milk Fortifier (per packet) (Mead Johnson)	3.5 (–)	0.15 (20) Whey protein concentrate Na caseinate	0.68 (76) Corn syrup solids	0.02 (3.9) From caseinate Lactose	0.08	0.1	23	11	0	—	Fortifier for preterm human milk
Similac Natural Care Human Milk Fortifier (Ross)	0.8 (24)	22 (11) Nonfat milk Whey protein concentrate	86 (42) Corn syrup solids Lactose	44 (47) MCT oil Soy oil Coconut oil	15	26.6	1694	935	3	280	Fortifier for preterm human milk
Preterm Human Milk + Similac Natural Care 75:25 ratio	0.7 (21)	16 (9) Human milk protein Nonfat milk Whey protein concentrate	71 (40) Lactose Corn syrup solids	40 (51) Human milk fat MCT oil Soy oil Coconut oil	12	18	610	330	1.65	288	Preterm infants

Product											
Preterm Human Milk + Similac Natural Care 50:50 ratio	0.74 (22)	18 (10) Human milk protein Nonfat milk Whey protein concentrate	71 (40) Lactose Corn syrup solids	41 (50) Human milk fat MCT oil Soy oil Coconut oil	13	21	971	531	2.1	285	Preterm infants
Preterm Human Milk + Similac Natural Care 25:75 ratio	0.77 (23)	19.9 (10) Nonfat milk Whey protein concentrate Human milk protein	81 (42) Lactose Corn syrup solids	43 (50) MCT oil Soy oil Coconut oil Human milk fat	14	24	1332	734	2.5	282	Preterm infants
Preterm Human Milk + Enfamil Human Milk Fortifier (1 pkt/50mL)	0.73 (22)	17.3 (9) Human milk protein Whey protein concentrate Na caseinate	79 (43) Lactose Corn syrup solids	39 (48) Human milk fat	12	16	688	348	1.2	350	Preterm infants
Preterm Human Milk + Enfamil Human Milk Fortifier (1 pkt/25mL)	0.78 (24)	20.5 (10) Human milk protein Whey protein concentrate Na caseinate	91 (46) Lactose Corn syrup solids	39 (44) Human milk fat	13	17	1166	561	1.2	410	Preterm infants

From Ross Products Division, Abbott Laboratories, Inc[7].
aComposition of human milk varies with maternal diet, stage of lactation, within feedings, diurnally, and among mothers.

23

NUTRITION

TABLE 23.12

TODDLER AND YOUNG CHILD FORMULA ANALYSIS (PER LITER)

Formula	kcal/mL (kcal/oz)	Protein g (% kcal)	Carbohydrate g (% kcal)	Fat g (% kcal)	Na (mEq)	K (mEq)	Ca (mg)	P (mg)	Fe (mg)	Osmolality (mOsm/kg water)	Suggested uses
Compleat Pediatric (Novartis)	1 (30)	38 (15) Meats Vegetables Na caseinate Ca caseinate	125 (50) Vegetables Fruit Hydrolyzed cornstarch	39 (35) HO sun oil Soy oil MCT oil	30	38	1000	1000	13	380	For those who desire a blenderized tube feeding
Cow's milk, whole	0.63 (19)	34 (22) Cow's milk	48 (31) Lactose	34 (49) Butterfat	22	40	1226	956	0.5	285	Children >1 year of age with normal GI tract
Elecare (Ross)	1 (30)	30 (15) Free L-amino acids	110 (44) Corn syrup solids	47.6 (42) HO, saff oil MCT oil Soy oil	19.6	38.4	1082	808	17	596	Children with malabsorption, protein allergy
Kindercal (contains fiber) (Mead Johnson)	1.06 (32)	34 (13) Na caseinate	135 (50) Maltodextrins (83%) Sucrose (17%)	44 (37) Canola oil (50%) HO sun oil (15%) Corn oil (15%) MCT oil (20%)	16	34	850	850	11	310	Tube feeding and oral supplement for children with normal GI tract
L-Emental Pediatric (GalaGen/ Nutrition, Medical)	0.8 (24)	24 (12) Free L-amino acids	130 (63) Maltodextrins Modified starch	24 (25) Soy oil MCT oil (68%)	17	31	970	800	10	360	Children with malabsorption, protein allergy

Neocate One Plus (Scientific Hospital Supply)	1 (30)	25 (10) Free amino acids	146 (58) Maltodextrins Sucrose	35 (32) MCT oil (35%) Safflower oil Canola oil	9	24	620	620	8	835	Children with malabsorption, protein allergy
Next Step (Mead Johnson)	0.67 (20)	17 (10) Nonfat milk	74 (45) Lactose Corn syrup solids	34 (45) Palm olein (45%) Soy oil (20%) Coconut oil (20%) HO sun oil (15%)	12	22	800	560	12	270	Toddlers with normal GI tract
Next Step Soy (Mead Johnson)	0.67 (20)	22 (13) Soy protein	79 (47) Corn syrup solids Sucrose	29 (40) Palm olein (45%) Soy oil (20%) Coconut oil (20%) HO sun oil (15%)	13	26	767	600	12	260	Toddlers with cow's milk allergy, galactosemia
Nutren Junior (also with fiber) (Clintec)	1 (30)	30 (12) Casein Whey	128 (51) Maltodextrins Sucrose Soy polysaccharides	42 (37) Soy oil Canola oil MCT oil	20	34	1000	800	14	350	Tube feeding and oral supplement for children with normal GI tract
PediaSure (also with fiber) (Ross)	1 (30)	30 (12) Na caseinate Whey protein	110 (44) Hydrolyzed corn-starch (70%) Sucrose (30%) (Soy fiber)	50 (44) HO saff oil (50%) Soy oil (30%) MCT oil (20%)	16.5	33.5	970	800	14	310	Tube feeding and oral supplement for children with normal GI tract

Continued

TABLE 23.12

TODDLER AND YOUNG CHILD FORMULA ANALYSIS (PER LITER)—cont'd

Formula	kcal/mL (kcal/oz)	Protein g (% kcal)	Carbohydrate g (% kcal)	Fat g (% kcal)	Na (mEq)	K (mEq)	Ca (mg)	P (mg)	Fe (mg)	Osmolality (mOsm/kg water)	Suggested uses
Peptamen Junior (Clintec)	1 (30)	30 (12) Hydrolyzed whey	138 (55) Maltodextrin Sucrose (flavored) Cornstarch	38.5 (33) MCT oil (60%) Soy oil Canola oil Lecithin	20	34	1000	800	14	260 (unflavored) 365 (flavored)	Children with malabsorption
ProPeptide for Kids (GalaGen/ Nutrition, Medical)	1 (30)	30 (12) Enzymatically hydrolyzed whey protein	137.5 (55) Maltodextrin Sucrose Cornstarch	38.5 (33) Medium- chain triglycerides (18.5%) Soy oil (22%) Canola oil (60%)	20	34	1000	800	14	360	Children with malabsorption
Resource Just for Kids (Novartis)	1 (30)	30 (12) Na caseinate Ca caseinate Whey protein concentrates	110 (44) Hydrolyzed cornstarch Sucrose	50 (44) HO Sun oil Soy oil MCT oil	17	33	1140	800	14	390	Tube feeding and oral supplement for children with normal GI tract
Vivonex Pediatric (Novartis)	0.8 (24)	24 (12) Free amino acids	130 (63) Maltodextrins Modified starch	24 (25) MCT oil (68%) Soy oil (32%)	17	31	970	800	10	360	Children with malabsorption, protein allergy

TABLE 23.13

OLDER CHILD & ADULT FORMULA ANALYSIS (PER LITER)

Formula	kcal/mL (kcal/oz)	Protein g (% kcal)	Carbohydrate g (% kcal)	Fat g (% kcal)	Na (mEq)	K (mEq)	Ca (mg)	P (mg)	Fe (mg)	Osmolality (mOsm/kg water)	Suggested uses
Carnation Instant Breakfast w/whole milk (Clintec)	1.2 (36)	53 (18) Cow's milk	161 (54) Lactose Maltodextrin Sucrose	34 (26) Butterfat	42	67	1632	1400	17	590	High-calorie supplement for patients with normal GI tract
Criticare HN (Mead Johnson)	1.06 (32)	38 (14) Hydrolyzed casein Amino acids	220 (81.5) Maltodextrin Modified corn-starch	53 (4.5) Safflower oil	27	34	530	530	9.5	650	Patients with malabsorption
Deliver 2.0 (Mead Johnson)	2 (60)	75 (15) Ca caseinate Na caseinate	200 (40) Corn syrup	102 (45) Soy oil (70%) MCT oil (30%)	35	43	1000	1000	18	640	Oral supplement or tube feeding for patients with fluid restriction or increased calorie needs
Ensure (Ross)	1.06 (32)	37 (14) Na caseinate Ca caseinate Soy protein	145 (55) Corn syrup (70%) Sucrose (30%)	37 (32) Corn oil	36	40	530	530	9.6	470	Oral supplement or tube feeding for patients with normal GI tract

Continued

23

NUTRITION

TABLE 23.13
OLDER CHILD & ADULT FORMULA ANALYSIS (PER LITER)—cont'd

Formula	kcal/mL (kcal/oz)	Protein g (% kcal)	Carbohydrate g (% kcal)	Fat g (% kcal)	Na (mEq)	K (mEq)	Ca (mg)	P (mg)	Fe (mg)	Osmolality (mOsm/kg water)	Suggested uses
Ensure Plus (Ross)	1.5 (45)	55 (15) Na caseinate Ca caseinate Soy protein	200 (53) Corn syrup Sucrose	53 (32) Corn oil	46	50	705	705	13	690	Oral supplement or tube feeding for patients with higher calorie needs, normal GI tract
Ensure with Fiber (Ross)	1.1 (33)	40 (15) Na caseinate Ca caseinate Soy protein	162 (55) Hydrolyzed corn-starch (58%) Sucrose (32%) Soy polysaccharide (10%)	37 (31) Corn oil	37	43	719	719	13	480	Oral supplement or tube feeding with fiber, normal GI tract
Glucerna (Ross)	1 (30)	42 (17) Na caseinate Ca caseinate	94 (33) Glucose polymers (53%) Soy polysaccharide (25%) Fructose (21%)	56 (50) HO saff oil (85%) Soy oil (15%)	40	40	704	704	13	375	Patients with impaired glucose tolerance, also contains fiber

Product		Protein g (%)	Carbohydrate g (%)	Fat g (%)							Indication
Isocal (Mead Johnson)	1.06 (32)	34 (13) Na caseinate Ca caseinate Soy protein	135 (50) Maltodextrin	44 (37) MCT oil (20%) Soy oil (80%)	23	34	630	530	10	270	Tube feeding for patients with normal GI tract
Jevity (Ross)	1.06 (32)	44 (17) Na caseinate Ca caseinate	152 (53) Hydrolyzed cornstarch Soy polysaccharide	36 (30) HO saff oil (50%) Canola oil (30%) MCT oil (20%)	40	40	909	758	14	300	Tube feeding with fiber, normal GI tract
L-Emental (GalaGen/ Nutrition, Medical)	1 (30)	38 (15) Free l-amino acids	205 (82) Maltodextrins	2.85 (2.5) Safflower oil	20	20	500	500	9	630	Patients with malabsorption, protein allergy
L-Emental Plus (Nutrition, Medical)	1 (30)	45 (18) Free l-amino acids	190 (76) Maltodextrins	6.7 (6) Soy oil	26	27	556	556	10	650	Patients with malabsorption, protein allergy
Lipisorb (Mead Johnson)	1.35 (40)	57 (17) Na caseinate Ca caseinate	161 (48) Maltodextrin Sucrose	57 (35) MCT oil (85%) Soy oil (15%)	59	43	850	850	15	630	Patients with fat malabsorption
Nepro (Ross)	2 (60)	70 (14) Ca caseinate Mg caseinate Na caseinate	215 (43) Hydrolyzed corn-starch (88%) Sucrose (12%)	96 (43) HO saff oil (90%) Soy oil (10%)	36	27	1373	686	19	635	Patients with renal failure undergoing dialysis

Continued

23

NUTRITION

TABLE 23.13

OLDER CHILD & ADULT FORMULA ANALYSIS (PER LITER)—cont'd

Formula	kcal/mL (kcal/oz)	Protein g (% kcal)	Carbohydrate g (% kcal)	Fat g (% kcal)	Na (mEq)	K (mEq)	Ca (mg)	P (mg)	Fe (mg)	Osmolality (mOsm/kg water)	Suggested uses
Nutren 2.0 (Clintec)	2 (60)	80 (16) K caseinate Ca caseinate	196 (39) Sucrose Corn syrup solids Maltodextrin	106 (45) MCT oil (75%) Canola oil Corn oil Soy oil Lecithin	57	49	1340	1340	24	720	Oral supplement or tube feedings for patients with fluid restriction or increased calorie needs
Nutrivent (Clintec)	1.5 (45)	68 (18) Ca caseinate K caseinate	100 (27) Maltodextrin Sucrose	95 (55) MCT oil (40%) Canola oil (43%) Corn oil (13%) Lecithin (4%)	50	42	1200	1200	18	330	Patients requiring higher percentage of calories from fat
Osmolite (Ross)	1.06 (32)	37 (14) Na caseinate Ca caseinate Soy protein	145 (55) Hydrolyzed cornstarch	38 (31) HO saff oil (50%) Canola oil (30%) MCT oil (20%)	28	26	530	530	9.5	300	Tube feeding for patients with normal GI tract

Product											
Peptamen (Clintec)	1 (30)	40 (16) Hydrolyzed whey	127 (51) Maltodextrin (88%) Hydrolyzed corn-starch (12%)	39 (33) MCT oil (67%) Sunflower oil (18%) Lecithin (6%) Milk fat (9%)	22	32	800	700	120	270	Patients with malabsorption
Promote (Ross)	1 (30)	63 (25) Na caseinate Ca caseinate Soy protein	130 (52) Hydrolyzed corn-starch (91%) Sucrose (9%)	26 (23) HO saff oil (50%) Canola oil (30%) MCT oil (20%)	40	51	960	960	14	330	Oral supplement or tube feeding for patients with increased protein needs
ProPeptide (unflavored) (GalaGen/ Nutrition, Medical)	1 (30)	40 (16) Hydrolyzed whey	127 (51) Maltodextrins Starch	39 (33) Sunflower oil (30%) MCT oil (70%)	22	32	800	700	14	270	Patients with malabsorption
Pulmocare (Ross)	1.5 (45)	63 (17) Na caseinate Ca caseinate	106 (28) Hydrolyzed corn-starch (46%) Sucrose (54%)	92 (55) Corn oil	57	44	1056	1056	19	465	Patient's requiring higher percentage of calories from fat
Respalor (Mead Johnson)	1.5 (45)	76 (20) Ca caseinate Na caseinate	148 (39) Corn syrup Sucrose	71 (41) Canola oil (70%) MCT oil (30%)	55	38	710	710	13	580	Patients requiring higher percentage of calories from fat

23

NUTRITION

Continued

TABLE 23.13
OLDER CHILD & ADULT FORMULA ANALYSIS (PER LITER)—cont'd

Formula	kcal/mL (kcal/oz)	Protein g (% kcal)	Carbohydrate g (% kcal)	Fat g (% kcal)	Na (mEq)	K (mEq)	Ca (mg)	P (mg)	Fe (mg)	Osmolality (mOsm/kg water)	Suggested uses
Scandishake w/ whole milk (Scandipharm)	2.5 (75)	50 (8) Cow's milk	292 (47) Lactose Maltodextrin Soy oil	125 (45) Coconut oil Safflower oil Palm oil	240	103	391	478	trace	1094	High-calorie supplement and for fat malabsorption
Suplena (Ross)	2 (60)	30 (6) Na caseinate Ca caseinate	255 (51) Hydrolyzed corn-starch (90%) Sucrose (10%)	96 (43) HO saff oil (90%) Soy oil (10%)	34	29	1385	728	19	600	Patients with renal failure not undergoing dialysis
Boost High Protein (Mead Johnson)	1 (30)	61 (24) Na caseinate Ca caseinate Soy protein	140 (55) Corn syrup Sucrose	23 (21) Partially hydrogenated soy oil	40	54	1010	930	17	650	Oral supplement or tube feeding for patients with increased protein needs
Boost Plus (Mead Johnson)	1.5 (45)	61 (16) Na caseinate Ca caseinate	190 (50) Corn syrup solids Sucrose	57 (34) Corn oil	37	38	850	850	15	670	Oral supplement or tube feeding for patients with high calorie needs, normal GI tract
Boost with Fiber (Mead Johnson)	1.06 (30)	46 (17) Na caseinate Ca caseinate Soy protein	140 (53) Maltodextrin Sucrose	35 (30) Corn oil	31	36	850	710	13	480	Oral supplement or tube feeding with fiber, normal GI tract

Product	kcal/mL (mL)	Protein g (%)	Carbohydrate g (%)	Fat g (%)						Osmolality	Indication
Tolerex (Novartis)	1 (30)	21 (8) Free amino acids	230 (91) Maltodextrin	1.5 (1) Safflower oil	20	31	560	560	10	550	Patients with malabsorption or severe food allergy
Traumacal (Mead Johnson)	1.5 (45)	82 (22) Na caseinate Ca caseinate	142 (38) Corn syrup Sucrose	68 (40) Soy oil (70%) MCT oil (30%)	51	36	750	750	9	560	Patients with increased protein and calorie needs
Ultracal (Mead Johnson)	1.06 (30)	44 (17) Na caseinate Ca caseinate	123 (46) Maltodextrin Soy fiber Oat fiber	45 (37) MCT oil (40%) Canola oil (60%)	40	41	850	850	15	310	Oral supplement or tube feeding with fiber, normal GI tract
Vital HN (Ross)	1 (30)	42 (17) Hydrolyzed whey, meat, and soy (87%) Free amino acids (13%)	185 (74) Hydrolyzed corn-starch (83%) Sucrose (17%) Lactose (<0.5%)	11 (9) Safflower oil (55%) MCT oil (45%)	25	36	667	667	12	500	Patients with malabsorption
Vivonex Plus (Novartis)	1 (30)	45 (18) Free amino acids	190 (76) Maltodextrin	6.7 (6) Soybean oil	27	28	560	560	10	650	Patients with malabsorption or severe food allergy
Vivonex TEN (Novartis)	1 (30)	38 (15) Free amino acids	210 (82) Maltodextrin	2.8 (3) Safflower oil	20	20	500	500	9	630	Patients with malabsorption or severe food allergy

CONCENTRATION OF INFANT FORMULAS[a]

Concentrates (40 cal/oz)		
Caloric concentration (cal/oz)	Concentrate (oz)	Water (oz)
20	13	13
24	13	8.5
26	13	7
28	13	5.5
30	**13**	**4.3**
Powder (40cal/scoop[b])		
Caloric concentration (cal/oz)	Powder (scoop)	Water (oz)
20	1	2
24	3	5
26	2	3
28	7	10
30	3	4

[a]Does not apply to Similac Neosure.
[b]1 scoop = ≈1tbsp.

COMMON CALORIC SUPPLEMENTS

	Component	Calories
	Protein	
	Casec	1g = 3.7kcal, 0.9g protein
		1tbsp = 17kcal, 4g protein
	Carbohydrate	
	Polycose	Powder: 3.8kcal/g
		8kcal/tsp
		Liquid: 2.0kcal/mL
		10kcal/tsp
	Fat	
	MCT oil	7.7kcal/mL
	Vegetable oil	8.3kcal/mL

TABLE 23.16

INFANT MULTIVITAMIN DROPS ANALYSIS (PER mL)

	Poly-Vi-Sol/(Flor) [with iron] Vi-Daylin (F) multi-vitamin [with iron]	Tri-Vi-Sol/(Flor) [with iron] Vi-Daylin/(F) ADC [with iron]	ADEK[a]
Vitamin A (IU)	1500	1500	1500
Vitamin D (IU)	400	400	400
Vitamin E (IU)	5	–	40
Vitamin C (mg)	35	35	45
Thiamin (mg)	0.5	–	0.5
Riboflavin (mg)	0.6	–	0.6
Niacin (mg)	8	–	6
Vitamin B_6 (mg)	0.4	–	0.6
Vitamin B_{12} (mcg)	2[b]	–	4
Iron (elemental) (mg)	[10]	[10]	–
Fluoride (mg)	(0.25)	(0.25)	–

[a]Also contains biotin 15mcg; pantothenic acid 3mg; zinc 5mg; β-carotene = to ~10,000 IU vitamin A.
[b]Poly-Vi-Sol only.

23

NUTRITION

TABLE 23.17
SELECTED MULTIVITAMIN TABLETS (ANALYSIS/TABLET)

	Multivitamins					Prenatal
	Flintstones Original Bugs Bunny Generic Poly-Vi-Sol/(Flor) Vi-Daylin/(F) [with iron]	Flintstones + Extra C Sunkist + Extra C Generic + C Bugs Bunny +Extra C	Centrum Jr	Flintstone Complete Generic Complete	ADEK	Natalins Rx Tablets Mynatal Rx Caplets Prenatal Rx Tablets
Vitamin A (IU)[a]	2500	2500	5000	5000	4000	4000
Vitamin D (IU)	400	400	400	400	400	400
Vitamin E (IU)	15	15	30	30	150	15
Vitamin K (mcg)	–	–	10	–	150	–
Vitamin C (mg)	60	250	60	60	60	80
Thiamin (mg)	1.05	1.05	1.5	1.5	1.2	1
Riboflavin (mg)	1.2	1.2	1.7	1.7	1.3	1.6
Niacin (mg)	13.5	13.5	20	20	10	17
Vitamin B_6 (mg)	1.05	1	2	2	1.5	4
Folate (mcg)	300	300	400	400	200	1000
Vitamin B_{12} (mcg)	4.5	4.5–5	6	6	12	2.5
Biotin (mcg)	–	–	45	40	50	30

Pantothenic acid (mg)	—	10	10	10	7
Calcium (mg)	—	108	100	—	200
Phosphorus (mg)	—	50	100	—	—
Iron (elemental) (mg)	[10–15]	18	18	—	60
Iodine (mcg)	—	150	150	—	—
Magnesium (mg)	—	40	20	—	—
Zinc (mg)	—	15	15	7.5	25
Copper (mg)	—	2	3	—	—
Manganese (mg)	—	1	—	—	—
Chromium (mcg)	—	20	—	—	—
Molybdenum (mcg)	—	20	—	—	—
β-Carotene (mg)	—	—	—	3	—
Fluoride	(0.25, 0.5, 1.0)	—	—	—	—

a Includes β-carotene.

VI. PARENTERAL NUTRITION (Tables 23.18 to 23.21)

TABLE 23.18

INITIATION AND ADVANCEMENT OF PARENTERAL NUTRITION

Nutrient	Initial dose	Advancement	Maximum
Glucose	5–10%	2.5–5%/day	12.5% peripheral 18mg/kg per min (max. rate of infusion)
Protein	1g/kg per day	0.5–1g/kg per day	3g/kg per day 10–16% of calories
Fat	0.5–1g/kg per day	0.5–1g/kg per day	4g/kg per day 0.17g/kg per hr (max. rate of infusion)

TABLE 23.19

DAILY PARENTERAL NUTRIENT RECOMMENDATIONS

Component	0–1 yr	1–7 yr	>7 yr
Energy (kcal/kg)	80–120	55–90	55–75
Protein (g/kg)	2–3	1.5–2.5	1.5–2.5
Sodium (mEq/kg)	3–4	2–4	2–4
Potassium (mEq/kg)	2–3	2–3	2–3
Magnesium (mEq/kg)	0.25–1	0.25–1	0.25–1
Calcium (mg/kg)	40–60	10–50	10–50
Phosphorus (mg/kg)	20–45	15–40	15–40
Zinc (mcg/kg)	400 (preterm) 100	100	100 max. 4mg/day
Copper (mcg/kg)	20	20	20 max. 1.5mg/day
Chromium (mcg/kg)	0.2	0.2	0.2 max. 15mg/day
Manganese (mcg/kg)	2–10	2–10	2–10 max. 0.8mg/day
Selenium (mcg/kg)	3	3	3 max. 40mg/day

Adapted from Committee on Nutrition of the AAP[8]; Kerner[9]; Collier[10]; and Cox[11].

TABLE 23.20

PARENTERAL MULTIVITAMIN FORMULATION[a]

	Pediatric (per 5mL)	Adult (per 10mL)
Ascorbic acid (mg)	80	100
Vitamin A (retinol), mg	0.7 (2300 IU)	1.0 (3285 IU)
Ergocalciferol (mcg)	10 (400 IU)	5 (200 IU)
Thiamin (mg)	1.2	3
Riboflavin (mg)	1.4	3.6
Vitamin B_6 (mg)	1	4
Niacin (mg)	17	40
Dexpanthenol (mg)	5	15
Vitamin E (mg)	7 (7 IU)	10 (10 IU)
Biotin (mcg)	20	60
Folic acid (mcg)	140	60
Vitamin B_{12} (mcg)	1	5
Vitamin K (mcg)	200	_[b]

[a]Note that iron is not a component of either formulation.
[b]Vitamin K is not a component of adult multivitamins.

TABLE 23.21

MONITORING SCHEDULE FOR PATIENTS RECEIVING PARENTERAL NUTRITION[a]

Variable	Initial period[b]	Later period[c]
GROWTH		
Weight	Daily	2 times/wk
Height	Weekly (infants)	Monthly[d]
	Monthly	
Head circumference (infants)	Weekly	Monthly[d]
Arm circumference	Monthly	Monthly
Skinfold thickness	Monthly	Monthly
LABORATORY STUDIES		
Electrolytes & glucose	Daily until stable	Weekly
BUN/creatinine	2 times/wk	Weekly
Albumin or prealbumin	Weekly	Weekly
Ca, Mg, P	2 times/wk	Weekly
ALT, AST, Alk P	Weekly	Weekly
Total & direct bilirubin	Weekly	Weekly
CBC	Weekly	Weekly
Triglycerides	With each increase	Weekly
Vitamins	—	As indicated
Trace minerals	—	As indicated

ALT, alanine transaminase; AST, aspartate transaminase; Alk P, alkaline phosphatase.
[a]For patients on long-term parenteral nutrition, monitoring every 2–4 weeks is adequate in most cases.
[b]The period before nutritional goals are reached or during any period of instability.
[c]When stability is reached, no changes in nutrient composition.
[d] Weekly in preterm infants.

VII. REFERENCES

1. Waterlow JC. Classification and definition of protein calorie malnutrition. *Br Med J* 1972; **3**:565.

2. Rosner B, Prineas R, Loggie J, Daniels SR. Percentiles for body mass index in US: children 5 to 17 years of age. *J Pediatr* 1998; **132**:211.

3. Food Nutrition Board, National Research Council. *Recommended dietary allowances*, 10th edn. Washington, DC: National Academy Press; 1989.

4. Hamill PVV, Drizd TA, Johnson CL, Reed RB, Roche AF, Moore WM. Physical growth: National Center for Health Statistics percentiles. *Am J Clin Nutr* 1979; **32**:607.

5. Seashore JH. Nutritional support of children in the intensive care unit. *Yale J Biol Med* 1984; **57**:111–132.

6. MacLean WC Jr, Lopez de Romaña G, Massa E, Graham GG. Nutritional management of chronic diarrhoea and malnutrition: primary reliance on oral feeding. *J Pediatr* 1980; **97**:316.

7. *Composition of feedings for infants and young children.* January 1999, Ross Products Division, Abbott Laboratories Inc.

8. Committee on Nutrition of the AAP. Commentary on parenteral nutrition. *Pediatrics* 1983; **73**:547.

9. Kerner JA. *Manual of pediatric nutrition*. New York: John Wiley & Sons; 1983.

10. Collier SB. Parenteral nutrition. In: Hendricks KM, Walker WA, eds. *Manual of pediatric nutrition*. Toronto: BC Decker; 1990.

11. Cox JH, Cooning SW. Parenteral nutrition. In: Queen PM, Lang CE, eds. *Handbook of pediatric nutrition*. Gaithersburg, Md; Aspen; 1993.

ONCOLOGY

David A. Jacobsohn, MD

I. INFECTIONS

A. FEVER AND NEUTROPENIA

1. **Definition:** Absolute neutrophil count (ANC) <500 or falling toward this and fever >38.3°C (orally), or 38.0°C when measured twice >4 hours apart in a 24-hour period. Patients who develop low-grade fever while on steroids or who appear ill also require similar evaluation.

2. **Management**

a. Hospital admission. No role for outpatient management. Patient should be urgently evaluated and admitted. Detailed H+P, including inspection of sites of recent procedures (BM, LP, biopsy), central line sites, perianal area (usually avoid digital rectal examination).

b. Laboratory tests: CBC with differential; blood culture from all central line lumens (the value of peripheral cultures is uncertain); electrolytes; blood type and screen; PT/aPTT if ill appearing; chest radiograph if respiratory symptoms or as baseline if a prolonged neutropenia is expected; abdominal radiograph if suspicious of typhlitis; urine, throat, stool surveillance cultures (bacterial, viral, fungal).

c. Antibiotic therapy

   1) Initially, select antibiotic with good Gram-negative (including *Pseudomonas*) and Gram-positive coverage (e.g., cefipime or piperacillin/tazobactam). Take account of local sensitivities. Select antibiotic that covers a previous blood culture isolate or an infectious focus.

   2) If patient appears ill, double cover for *Pseudomonas* (e.g., cefipime or piperacillin/tazobactam with an aminoglycoside).

   3) If blood culture turns positive, cover the particular organism but maintain broad Gram-positive and -negative coverage until neutropenia has resolved.

   4) If blood culture remains negative and patient afebrile, continue broad-spectrum coverage until early evidence of marrow recovery (e.g., ANC >200 and rising).

   5) Other antibiotic modifications

      a) If patient persistently febrile after 3 days, consider adding oxacillin or vancomycin (for better coverage of Gram-positive organisms), especially if central line infection suspected. Also consider broader Gram-negative coverage.

      b) Consider adding clindamycin or metronidazole (for better coverage of anaerobes), especially if enteric infection suspected.

      c) If persistently febrile or with a new fever 4–7 days into therapy, begin amphotericin B (0.5mg/kg per day IV) for empiric

24

519

antifungal coverage. Increase dose to 1.0mg/kg per day if fever persists 2 days after that. Consider 10mL/kg NS bolus before amphotericin dose to improve renal clearing. Consider chest and abdominal CT scans to rule out fungal abscess.

B. CENTRAL LINE INFECTIONS
1. Entry-site infections
a. Usually present with erythema, warmth, and purulent discharge at line site, although these signs may not be evident in a neutropenic patient.
b. Culture site and blood through all lumens of line; common site organisms are staphylococci, streptococci, and *Pseudomonas* spp.
c. Try oral antibiotics with staphylococcal coverage (e.g., cephalexin) if patient is not ill and not neutropenic. If not improved in 2–3 days, admit for IV antibiotics.
d. Intravenous antibiotics if patient is neutropenic. Broad-spectrum antibiotic (e.g., cefipime or piperacillin/tazobactam) with oxacillin or nafcillin is indicated.
e. Most lines with entry-site infection can be salvaged.
2. Tract infections or positive blood cultures
a. Tract infections present with erythema, warmth, and discharge along the entire line tract.
b. Culture site (if involved) and blood through all lumens of line.
c. A 2- to 3-day trial of IV antibiotics. Use broad antibiotic coverage (e.g., cefipime/oxacillin) while awaiting sensitivities. Minimize use of vancomycin to prevent vancomycin-resistant enterococcus (VRE).
d. Daily blood cultures from all lumens during therapy.
e. Remove line if no improvement in symptoms or if blood culture still positive after 2–3 days of antibiotic therapy.
f. If infection is associated with a venous clot, as evidenced by poor function and a dye study, removing the line is almost always necessary.
g. Additional positive blood cultures associated with fever in the future (particularly if it grows the same organism) is an indication for removing the line at that time.
h. Fungemia is an absolute indication for removing the line.
C. PULMONARY INFECTIONS
1. Differential diagnosis of respiratory distress with fever: Bacterial, viral, or fungal infection; acid-fast bacilli; *Mycoplasma; Legionella; Pneumocystis;* tumor; toxicity from chemotherapy/radiotherapy.
2. Management
a. Routine laboratory tests: Chest radiograph, surveillance cultures, herpes simplex virus (HSV) and cytomegalovirus (CMV) titers (including CMV early antigen), CMV culture, sputum for bacterial culture and *Pneumocystis*/fungal staining; consider chest CT with IV contrast.
b. Broad-spectrum antibiotic coverage, e.g., cefipime, high-dose trimethoprim–sulfamethoxazole (TMP-SMX) for presumptive PCP, and erythromycin for presumptive *Mycoplasma*.

c. Consider an early course of steroids for a patient with severe or rapidly worsening respiratory distress (particularly if suspicious of *Pneumocystis*). This is contraindicated if fungal disease is suspected.

d. If no improvement in 24–48 hours, diagnostic bronchoscopy or open-lung biopsy may be indicated before status deteriorates beyond point to tolerate procedure. Sensitivity of diagnostic bronchoalveolar lavage (BAL) for *Pneumocystis carinii* penumonia (PCP) is greatly diminished 24 hours after initiation of high-dose TMP-SMX.

D. ABDOMINAL INFECTIONS

1. Typhlitis: Inflammation of the bowel wall, usually localized to the cecum. Most common in patients treated for leukemia or lymphoma, especially when Ara-C is used.

a. Presentation: Right lower quadrant abdominal pain, nausea, fever, diarrhea. Abdominal radiograph may show pneumatoses, paucity of air, and/or bowel wall edema.

b. Management/diagnosis

   1) CT, MRI, or ultrasound to confirm diagnosis if necessary.

   2) Nothing by mouth, nasogastric tube to gravity.

   3) Laboratory tests: Chemistries, CBC with differential, PT/aPTT. Acidosis suggests infarcted/necrotic bowel.

   4) Aggressive fluid replacement.

   5) Correct coagulopathy, thrombocytopenia, and anemia as needed.

   6) Broad-spectrum antibiotics. Usually 'triples' are administered (e.g., ticarcillin/gentamicin/metronidazole).

   7) Surgical consultation is warranted, although intervention should be reserved for uncontrolled bleeding, perforation, shock, or severe peritonitis.

2. *Clostridium difficile* colitis (most common in patients recently treated with antibiotics)

a. Presentation: Nausea, abdominal pain, diarrhea.

b. Management

   1) Diagnosis by stool antigen test for *C. difficile* toxin.

   2) Treatment with oral/IV metronidazole or oral vancomycin.

3. Esophagitis: Most common in neutropenic patients who have received chemotherapy and/or mediastinal radiation.

a. Presentation: Retrosternal chest pain, odynophagia, upper GI bleeding, fever.

b. Differential: Includes *Candida*, HSV, CMV, reflux, perforation, chemical mucositis.

c. Management

   1) Initially treat empirically with H_2-receptor blocker, fluconazole $\pm$ acyclovir.

   2) Consider CT, upper GI contrast imaging, or esophagoscopy with biopsy if no improvement or if toxic.

24

ONCOLOGY

E. **PROPHYLAXIS** (see ch. 29 [formulary] for doses)

1. *Pneumocystis carinii*

a. TMP-SMX PO BID 3 days per week (preferred).

b. Dapsone PO QD.

c. Pentamidine once monthly IV infusion or aerosol.

(Administer one of above agents for all patients receiving chemotherapy and until 6 months after chemotherapy or 12 months after bone marrow transplantation [BMT]. Twice-weekly dosing of TMP-SMX recommended after BMT.)

2. **Antiviral**

a. Acyclovir in post-BMT period if patient or donor is HSV or CMV positive.

b. Acyclovir for patients with recurrent zoster, after chemotherapy.

3. **Antifungal**

a. Fluconazole for post-BMT patient until ANC recovery and off steroids (minimum of 28 days).

b. Consider amphotericin B IV for neutropenic patient with prior deep-tissue fungal infection.

4. **Antibacterial**

a. Consider including antibiotics in heparin flushes.

b. For chronic neutropenic patients (e.g., terminal patients with marrow disease) consider ciprofloxacin (age >12 years) and/or cephalexin.

c. Good dental care (especially pre-BMT).

d. Penicillin prophylaxis post-BMT (generally routine for the first month).

5. **Isolation practices**

a. Good handwashing for all health care professionals and everyone in contact with patient.

b. Neutropenic and post-BMT patients should consider wearing masks while in crowded areas.

c. Patients colonized with VRE need to be on contact isolation.

d. Patients with varicella-zoster virus (VZV) should be isolated from other patients for 28 days.

e. Varicella-zoster immune globulin (VZIG) should be administered to neutropenic patients within 4 days of exposure to VZV (if titers previously negative for VZV or if have lost titers post-BMT).

f. Patients with external catheters should avoid swimming in non-chlorinated and public pools and should change their dressing immediately afterward.

II. HEMATOLOGIC CARE AND COMPLICATIONS

A. **ANEMIA**

1. **Etiology:** Blood loss, chemotherapy, marrow infiltration, hemolysis.

2. **Management**

a. See p. 319 for specific details on packed red blood cell (pRBC) transfusions.

b. Generally, pRBC transfusions in cancer patients are not recommended until hematocrit falls below 20–22% or if patient is symptomatic.

c. Transfuse only irradiated pRBCs.

d. Use CMV-negative or leuko-filtered blood for CMV-negative patients; use leuko-filtered blood for those who may receive BMT in the future to prevent alloimmunization or those who have had nonhemolytic febrile transfusion reactions.

B. THROMBOCYTOPENIA

1. **Etiology:** Chemotherapy, marrow infiltration, consumptive coagulopathy, medications.

2. **Management**

a. See p. 320 for specific details on platelet transfusions.

b. Generally, strive to maintain platelet count above $10,000/mm^3$ unless clinically bleeding, febrile, or before procedure (e.g., lumbar puncture or IM injection requires $50,000/mm^3$). Consider maintaining platelet counts at higher levels for patients who have brain tumors or who have had brain surgery.

c. Transfuse only irradiated platelets.

d. Use CMV-negative or leuko-filtered platelets for CMV-negative patients; use leuko-filtered platelets for those who may receive BMT in the future or those who have had nonhemolytic febrile transfusion reactions.

e. Some patients become refractory to platelet transfusions because of alloimmunization. In these instances, attempt the following:
   1) HLA-matched platelet transfusion.
   2) Steroids (prednisone 2mg/kg per day, pretransfusion) or intravenous immune globulin (IVIG) (1g/kg).
   3) Amicar (aminocaproic acid) 100mg/kg per dose Q4–6hr, IV/PO, max. dose 30g/24hr. May help prevent bleeding in thrombocytopenic patients, especially at the time of procedures. Mechanism is antifibrinolysis.

C. HYPERLEUKOCYTOSIS

1. **Etiology:** In acute myeloid leukemia (AML) (especially M4 and M5) syndrome occurs with WBC as low as $100,000/mm^3$. Occurs in acute lymphoblastic leukemia (ALL) with WBC above $300,000/mm^3$.

2. **Presentation:** Hypoxia/dyspnea from pulmonary leukostasis, mental status changes, headaches, seizures, papilledema from leukostasis in cerebral vessels; occasionally, GI bleeding/abdominal pain, renal failure, priapism.

3. **Management**

a. Transfuse platelets as needed to keep count above $20,000/mm^3$ (reduce risk of intracranial hemorrhage).

b. Avoid RBC transfusions because they will raise viscosity (keep hemoglobin <10g/dL). If RBCs required, consider partial exchange.

c. Hydration, alkalinization, and allopurinol should be initiated (as discussed under tumor lysis syndrome).

24

ONCOLOGY

    d. Administer fresh frozen plasma (FFP) and vitamin K if patient is coagulopathic.

    e. Before cytotoxic therapy, consider leukopheresis to lower WBC count.

III. ONCOLOGIC EMERGENCIES[1,2]

A. TUMOR LYSIS SYNDROME

1. **Etiology:** Lysis of tumor cells before or during early stages of chemotherapy (especially Burkitt's lymphoma/leukemia, T cell ALL).

2. **Presentation:** Hyperuricemia, hypocalcemia, hyperkalemia, hyperphosphatemia, acidosis. Can lead to acute renal failure.

3. **Prevention/management**

    a. Hydration and alkalinization: D_5 0.2NS + 25–50mEq $NaHCO_3$ (without K^+) at two times maintenance rate. Keeping urine specific gravity <1.010 and pH 7.0–7.5 reduces risk of urate crystal formation. Reduce $NaHCO_3$ if pH >7.5 to avoid calcium phosphate precipitation.

    b. Allopurinol ($100mg/m^2$ per dose) Q8hr PO. Can load with $300mg/m^2$ PO.

    c. Check K^+, Ca^{2+}, P, and uric acid every 4–6 hours initially.

    d. Manage abnormal electrolytes as described in ch. 11. See pp. 453–454 for dialysis indications.

    e. Can consider stopping alkalinization soon after starting chemotherapy (if uric acid is normal).

B. SPINAL CORD COMPRESSION

1. **Etiology:** Extension of tumor into spinal cord.

2. **Presentation:** Back pain (localized/radicular), motor weakness, sensory loss, change in bowel/bladder function. Prognosis for recovery based on duration and level of disability at presentation.

3. **Management**

    a. With back pain and no neurologic abnormalities, may start dexamethasone 0.25–0.5mg/kg per day PO divided Q6hr and do spine MRI within 24 hours. **Be aware that steroids may prevent diagnosis of lymphoma; therefore plan diagnostic procedure as soon as possible.**

    b. With neurologic abnormalities: immediately start dexamethasone 2mg/kg per day IV divided Q6hr and emergent spine MRI.

    c. If cause of tumor known, emergent radiotherapy or chemotherapy is indicated for sensitive tumors; otherwise, emergent neurosurgery consultation is warranted.

    d. If cause of tumor unknown, surgery is indicated for decompressing spine.

C. INCREASED INTRACRANIAL PRESSURE

1. **Etiology:** Infratentorial brain tumor, ventricular obstruction.

2. **Diagnosis:** Head CT or MRI. MRI is more sensitive for diagnosis of posterior fossa tumors.

3. **Management**

a. See p. 13 for basic management.

b. If tumor identified, add dexamethasone 2mg/kg per day IV divided Q6hr.

c. Neurosurgical consultation.

D. CEREBROVASCULAR ACCIDENT

1. **Etiology:** Hyperleukocytosis, coagulopathy, thrombocytopenia, chemotherapy related (e.g., L-asparaginase-induced hemorrhage or thrombosis).

2. **Diagnosis/management**

a. Platelet transfusions, FFP as needed to replace factors (e.g., if depleted by L-asparaginase).

b. Brain CT scan with contrast, MRI, or magnetic resonance angiography (MRA) if venous thrombosis suspected.

c. Heparin acutely, followed by coumadin, for thromboses (if no venous hemorrhage is observed on MRI).

d. Avoid L-asparaginase.

E. RESPIRATORY DISTRESS/SUPERIOR VENA CAVA SYNDROME

1. **Etiology:** Hodgkin's disease, non-Hodgkin's lymphoma (e.g., lymphoblastic lymphoma), ALL (T lineage); germ cell tumors.

2. **Presentation:** Orthopnea, headaches, facial swelling, dizziness, plethora.

3. **Diagnosis:** Chest radiograph, CT/MRI to assess airway. Attempt diagnosis of malignancy (if not known) as least invasively as possible.

4. **Management**

a. Control airway.

b. Biopsy (e.g., bone marrow, pleurocentesis, lymph node biopsy) before therapy if patient can tolerate sedation or general anesthesia.

c. Empiric therapy: Radiotherapy, steroids, cyclophosphamide.

F. HEMORRHAGIC CYSTITIS

1. **Etiology:** Complication of cyclophosphamide or ifosfamide; BK virus infection post-BMT. Routine use of MESNA in conjunction with cyclophosphamide/ifosfamide has reduced the frequency and severity of this complication.

2. **Presentation:** Bloody urine or clots in the urine, dysuria.

3. **Management**

a. Vigorous hydration.

b. Stop cyclophosphamide/ifosfamide (although rarely occurs during administration).

c. Transfuse pRBCs and platelets as needed; correct coagulopathy.

d. Foley catheter and bladder irrigation to remove clots; cystoscopy and electrocoagulation or local chemical coagulation may be necessary if bleeding persists.

e. Norfloxacin or nalidixic acid may be helpful for BK virus–induced hemorrhagic cystitis.

24

ONCOLOGY

IV. PAIN TREATMENT IN CANCER PATIENTS

A. **TREAT UNDERLYING PROCESS AND CONTROL PAIN.**

B. **ANALGESICS:** Acetaminophen for mild pain (may mask fevers). May use codeine for moderate pain. Other opiates (e.g., morphine, hydromorphone, meperidine) for more severe pain.

C. **SPECIFIC ISSUES**

1. **Drugs to avoid:** Avoid aspirin and ibuprofen in patients with low platelet counts. Avoid ibuprofen *especially* with methotrexate due to a combined severe toxicity.

2. **Trilisate:** Useful NSAID with no platelet effects but can mask fevers.

3. **Mucositis:** Can be very painful; consider PCA (patient-controlled anesthesia).

4. **Adjuvant measures to pain medication**

a. Antianxiety medication (e.g., benzodiazepine).

b. Antidepressants (e.g., tricyclics) may change pain perception. Selective serotonin reuptake inhibitors may affect platelet function and may prolong the INR in persons taking coumadin.

c. Local anesthetics (e.g., epidural and celiac blocks).

d. Surgical treatment (e.g., cordotomy in a terminal patient).

e. Antiepileptic medications (e.g., carbamazepine, gabapentin) for postamputation 'phantom pain' or neurologic pain.

V. NAUSEA TREATMENT IN CANCER PATIENTS

1. **Etiology:** Usual cause is chemotherapy-induced nausea. Also suspect opiate therapy, GI/CNS radiotherapy, abdominal process, and CNS mass.

2. **Therapy:** Hydration plus one or more antinausea medications:

a. Ondansetron or granisetron: Usually first-line therapy. Patients may respond preferentially to one of these agents.

b. Diphenhydramine.

c. Dexamethasone: Especially helpful in brain tumor patients. See p. 687 for antiemetic dosing.

d. Lorazepam: also used as an adjunct antiemetic agent.

e. Metoclopramide: Especially helpful with brain tumor patients. Use diphenhydramine to reduce extrapyramidal symptoms (EPS).

f. Phenothiazines (promethazine, chlorpromazine). Use diphenhydramine to reduce EPS.

g. Droperidol can be used as continuous infusion.

h. Cannabinoids (e.g., dronabinol [Marinol] PO) can be helpful in resistant cases, especially in patients with large tumor burden.

VI. INITIAL EVALUATION FOR COMMON PEDIATRIC TUMORS

(See also local Pediatric Oncology Group [POG], Children's Cancer Group [CCG], or Children's Oncology Group [COG] protocols.)

A. **LEUKEMIA (AML/ALL):** Peripheral blood smear, CBC with differential, PT/aPTT, bone marrow smear, flow cytometry, DNA index (ALL only), karyotype, electrolytes, chemistry panel, amylase, blood type and screen, chest radiograph, echocardiogram and ECG, varicella titers, CMV titers, lumbar puncture (often with first intrathecal medications).

B. **LYMPHOMA (HODGKIN'S/NHL):** CBC with differential, chest radiograph, ESR (erythrocyte sedimentation rate), copper (Cu), lactate dehydrogenase (LDH), HIV test (if NHL), CT of chest/abdomen/ pelvis, bone marrow aspirate and biopsy, gallium scan, node biopsy.

C. **NEUROBLASTOMA:** CT of chest/abdomen/pelvis, bilateral bone marrow biopsies, bone scan, skeletal survey, urine for vanillylmandelic acid/homovanillic acid (VMA/HVA), CBC with differential, chemistry panel, ferritin. From tumor, send tissue for *N-myc,* DNA index (in infants), and karyotype. Consider MIBG scan.

D. **WILMS' TUMOR:** CT of abdomen/chest, chest radiograph, Doppler ultrasonography of inferior vena cava (IVC), urinalysis, CBC with differential, chemistry panel, including creatinine.

E. **BRAIN TUMORS:** MRI, biopsy (possibly stereotactic), CBC with differential, chemistry panel; alpha-fetoprotein (AFP) and human chorionic gonadotropin (β-hCG) (especially for suprasellar or pineal tumors). Some types (e.g., medulloblastoma) may require further metastatic workup (bone scan, bone marrow biopsy, and spine MRI for drop metastases).

F. **BONE TUMORS** (osteosarcoma/Ewing's/primitive neuroectodermal tumor (PNET)): Radiograph of specific bone, chest CT, bone scan, MRI of primary lesion, LDH, CBC, chemistry panel, bone marrow biopsy for Ewing's/PNET.

G. **SARCOMAS** (rhabdomyosarcoma/soft tissue sarcoma): Abdomen/chest CT, primary site CT or MRI, bone scan, bilateral bone marrow biopsies, lumbar puncture if cranial parameningeal primary, primary excision of tumor, CBC, chemistry panel, LDH.

H. **RETINOBLASTOMA:** Orbit/brain MRI (to exclude bilateral and pineal disease), examination under general anesthetic; lumbar puncture, bone marrow biopsy, and bone scan if invasion of optic nerve or orbit. Cytogenetics, fluorescence in situ hybridization (FISH) for chromosome 13 deletion.

I. **GERM CELL TUMORS:** Biopsy or resection of primary. CT of chest/abdomen/pelvis if malignant, AFP and β-hCG before resection, CBC, chemistry panel.

J. **HEPATOBLASTOMA/HEPATOCELLULAR CARCINOMA:** CT of chest/abdomen/pelvis, bone scan, AFP, β-hCG, CBC, chemistry panel. Biopsy or complete resection if possible.

24

ONCOLOGY

VII. REFERENCES

1. Kelly K, Lange B. Oncologic emergencies. *Pediatr Clin North Am* 1997; **44**:809.
2. Poplack D, Pizzo P. *Principles and practice of pediatric oncology*, 3rd edn. Philadelphia: Lippincott-Raven; 1997.

PULMONOLOGY

R. Skyler McCurley, MD

I. NORMAL RESPIRATORY RATES (Table 25.1)

TABLE 25.1

MEAN RESPIRATORY RATES ± 1 STANDARD DEVIATION

Age (yr)	Boys	Girls	Age (yr)	Boys	Girls
0–1	31±8	30±6	9–10	19±2	19±2
1–2	26±4	27±4	10–11	19±2	19±2
2–3	25±4	25±3	11–12	19±3	19±3
3–4	24±3	24±3	12–13	19±3	19±2
4–5	23±2	22±2	13–14	19±2	18±2
5–6	22±2	21±2	14–15	18±2	18±3
6–7	21±3	21±3	15–16	17±3	18±3
7–8	20±3	20±2	16–17	17±2	17±3
8–9	20±2	20±2	17–18	16±3	17±3

From Illif[1].

II. PULMONARY FUNCTION TESTS (PFTs)

Provide objective and reproducible measurements of airway function and lung volumes. Used to characterize disease, assess severity, and follow response to therapy.

A. **PEAK EXPIRATORY FLOW RATE (PEFR):** Maximum flow rate generated during a forced expiratory maneuver. Effort dependent, insensitive to small airway function. Useful in following the course of asthma and response to therapy. Compare a patient's PEFR to previous 'personal best' as well as normal predicted value (Table 25.2).

B. **SPIROMETRY:** Plot of airflow vs time. Measurements are made from a rapid, forceful, and complete expiration from total lung capacity (TLC) to residual volume (forced vital capacity maneuver). Often done before and after bronchodilators to assess response to therapy or after bronchial challenge to assess airway hyperreactivity. Can be performed reliably by most children aged 6 years and older.

1. **Forced vital capacity (FVC):** Maximum volume of air exhaled from the lungs after a maximum inspiration. Bedside measurement of vital capacity with a hand-held spirometer can be useful in confirming or predicting hypoventilation. FVC <15mL/kg may be an indication for ventilatory support.

2. **Forced expiratory volume in one second (FEV_1):** Volume exhaled during the first second of FVC maneuver. Single best measure of airway function.

3. **Forced expiratory flow (FEF$_{25-75}$):** Mean rate of airflow over the middle half of the FVC between 25% and 75% of FVC. Sensitive to small airway obstruction.

C. **LUNG VOLUMES:** Total lung capacity, functional residual capacity (FRC), and residual volume (RV) cannot be determined by spirometry and require determination by helium dilution, nitrogen washout, or body plethysmography (Fig. 25.1).

TABLE 25.2

PREDICTED AVERAGE PEAK EXPIRATORY FLOW RATES FOR NORMAL CHILDREN

Height (in)	PEFR (L/min)	Height (in)	PEFR (L/min)
43	147	56	320
44	160	57	334
45	173	58	347
46	187	59	360
47	200	60	373
48	214	61	387
49	227	62	400
50	240	63	413
51	254	64	427
52	267	65	440
53	280	66	454
54	293	67	467
55	307		

From Polger[2].

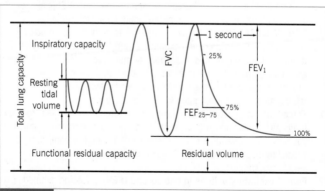

FIG. 25.1

Lung volumes. See text for abbreviations.

D. **FLOW–VOLUME CURVES:** Plot of airflow versus lung volume. Useful
   in characterizing different patterns of airway obstruction (Fig. 25.2).
E. **MAXIMAL INSPIRATORY AND EXPIRATORY PRESSURES:** Obtained
   by asking patient to inhale/exhale against fixed obstruction. Low
   pressures suggest neuromuscular problem or submaximal effort. An
   inspiratory pressure <20–25cmH$_2$O (negative inspiratory force, NIF)
   may be an indication for ventilatory support.

25

PULMONOLOGY

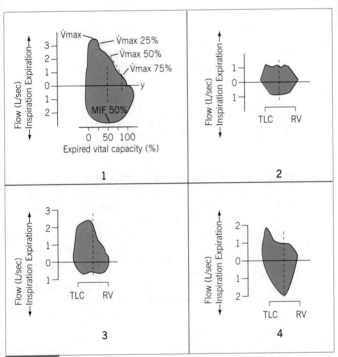

FIG. 25.2

Flow–volume curves. See text for abbreviations.

1. Normal flow–volume curve
2. **Fixed upper airway obstruction (tracheal stenosis):** Flattening of both inspiratory
   and expiratory phases.
3. **Variable extrathoracic obstruction (tracheomalacia, paralyzed vocal cords):**
   Flattened inspiratory phase as negative inspiratory pressure favors extrathoracic
   airway collapse.
4. **Variable intrathoracic obstruction (tumor):** Flattened expiratory phase as positive
   pleural pressure compresses trachea and increases resistance.

F. INTERPRETATION OF PFTs (Table 25.3)

TABLE 25.3

INTERPRETATION OF SPIROMETRY AND LUNG VOLUME READINGS

	Obstructive disease (asthma, cystic fibrosis)	Restrictive disease (interstitial fibrosis, scoliosis, neuromuscular)
Spirometry		
FVC^a	Normal or reduced	Reduced
$FEV_1{}^a$	Reduced	Reduced[d]
FEV_1/FVC^b	Reduced	Normal
FEF_{25-75}	Reduced	Normal or reduced[d]
$PEFR^a$	Normal or reduced	Normal or reduced[d]
Lung volumes		
TLC^a	Normal or increased	Reduced
RV^a	Increased	Reduced
RV/TLC^c	Increased	Unchanged
FRC	Increased	Reduced

[a]Normal range: ±20% of predicted.   [c]Normal range: 20±10%.
[b]Normal range: >85%.   [d]Reduced proportional to FVC.

III. PULMONARY GAS EXCHANGE

A. **ARTERIAL BLOOD GAS (ABG):** Used to assess oxygenation (Pao_2), ventilation ($\dot{V}$), $Paco_2$, and acid–base status (pH and HCO_3^-). Normal mean ABG values are shown in Table 25.4.

B. **VENOUS BLOOD GAS (VBG):** Peripheral venous samples are strongly affected by the local circulatory and metabolic environment. Can be used to assess acid–base status. Pco_2 averages 6–8mmHg higher than $Paco_2$, and pH is slightly lower.

C. **CAPILLARY BLOOD GAS (CBG):** Correlation with arterial sampling is generally best for pH, moderate for Pco_2, and worst for Po_2.

TABLE 25.4

NORMAL MEAN ABG VALUES

	pH	Pao_2 (mmHg)	$Paco_2$ (mmHg)	HCO_3^- (mEq/L)
Newborn (birth)	7.26–7.29	60	55	19
Newborn (24hr)	7.37	70	33	20
Infant (1–24mo)	7.40	90	34	20
Child (7–19yr)	7.39	96	37	22
Normal range (adult)	7.35–7.45	90–110	35–45	22–26

Adapted from Rogers[3].

D. ANALYSIS OF ACID–BASE DISTURBANCES

1. Estimate acid-base disturbance using nomogram (Fig. 25.3).
2. Approximate changes in pure acid–base disturbances
a. Pure respiratory acidosis (or alkalosis): 10mmHg rise (fall) in $Paco_2$ results in an average 0.08 fall (rise) in pH.
b. Pure metabolic acidosis (or alkalosis): 10mEq/L fall (rise) in HCO_3^- results in an average 0.15 fall (rise) in pH.
3. Determine primary disturbance and then assess for mixed disorder by calculating expected compensatory response (Table 25.5).

E. PULSE OXIMETRY

1. **Arterial oxygen saturation**: Noninvasive method of indirectly measuring arterial oxygen saturation (Sao_2). Uses light absorption characteristics of oxygenated and deoxygenated hemoglobin to estimate O_2 saturation.
2. **The oxyhemoglobin dissociation curve** (Fig. 25.4): This relates O_2 saturation to Pao_2. Increased hemoglobin affinity for oxygen (shift to the left) occurs with alkalemia, hypothermia, hypocapnia, decreased 2,3-diphosphoglycerate (2,3-DPG), increased fetal hemoglobin, and anemia. Decreased hemoglobin affinity for oxygen (shift to the right) occurs with acidemia, hyperthermia, hypercapnia, and increased 2,3-DPG.

25

PULMONOLOGY

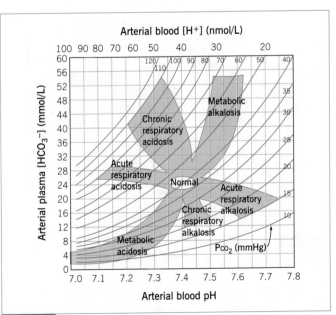

FIG. 25.3

Acid–base nomogram. (Adapted from Brenner[5].)

TABLE 25.5

CALCULATION OF EXPECTED COMPENSATORY RESPONSE

Disturbance	Primary change	pH	Expected compensatory response
Acute respiratory acidosis	↑Paco$_2$	↓pH	↑HCO$_3^-$ by 1mEq/L for each 10mmHg rise in Paco$_2$
Acute respiratory alkalosis	↓Paco$_2$	↑pH	↓HCO$_3^-$ by 1–3mEq/L for each 10mmHg fall in Paco$_2$
Chronic respiratory acidosis	↑Paco$_2$	↓pH	↑HCO$_3^-$ by 4mEq/L for each 10mmHg rise in Paco$_2$
Chronic respiratory alkalosis	↓Paco$_2$	↑pH	↓HCO$_3^-$ by 2–5mEq/L for each 10mmHg fall in Paco$_2$
Metabolic acidosis	↓HCO$_3^-$	↓pH	↓Paco$_2$ by 1–1.5 × fall in HCO$_3^-$
Metabolic alkalosis	↑HCO$_3^-$	↑pH	↑Paco$_2$ by 0.25–1 × rise in HCO$_3^-$

Adapted from Schrier[4].

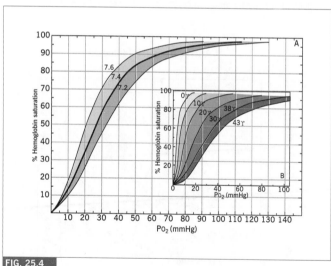

FIG. 25.4

Oxyhemoglobin dissociation curve. (Adapted from Lanbertsten[6].)

3. Important uses of pulse oximetry
a. Rapid and continuous assessment of oxygenation in acutely ill patients.
b. Monitoring of patients requiring oxygen therapy.
c. Assessment of oxygen requirements during feeding, sleep, and exercise.
d. Home monitoring of physiologic effects of apnea/bradycardia.
4. Limitations of pulse oximetry
a. Measures saturation (Sao_2) and not O_2 delivery to tissues. A marginally low saturation may be clinically significant in an anemic patient because a normal O_2 saturation does not ensure a normal O_2-carrying capacity (see p. 540).
b. Unreliable when detection of pulse signal is poor as a result of physiologic conditions (hypothermia, hypovolemia, shock) or movement artifact. The oximeter's pulse rate should match the patient's heart rate to achieve an accurate measurement.
c. Insensitive to hyperoxia ($Pao_2 > 100mmHg$) because of the sigmoid shape of the oxyhemoglobin curve.
d. Sao_2 artificially increased by carboxyhemoglobin levels >1–2% (chronic smokers, smoke inhalation).
e. Sao_2 artificially decreased by patient motion, intravenous dyes, such as methylene blue, and indocyanine green and opaque nail polish.
f. Sao_2 artificially increased or decreased by methemoglobin levels >1–2% (nitroglycerin ingestion), electrosurgical interference, or xenon arc surgical lamps.
g. Sao_2 reading often does not correlate with Pao_2 in sickle cell disease[7].
F. **CAPNOGRAPHY:** Measures CO_2 concentration of expired gas by infrared spectroscopy or mass spectroscopy. End-tidal CO_2 ($ETco_2$) correlates with $Paco_2$ (usually within 5mmHg of $Paco_2$ in healthy subjects). Can be used for demonstrating proper placement of endotracheal tube, continuous monitoring CO_2 trends in ventilated patients, and monitoring ventilation during polysomnography.
G. **DIFFUSING CAPACITY (DL_{CO}):** Measures gas transfer across alveolar–capillary membrane. Dilute CO is exposed to alveoli during a single breath, and the change in concentration indicates a rate of diffusion (mL/min/mmHg). The rate depends on area and permeability of alveolar–capillary membrane and hemoglobin concentration.

IV. OXYGEN DELIVERY SYSTEMS[8]
A. **NASAL CANNULA (NASAL PRONGS)**
1. Provides low-to-moderate O_2 concentrations (22–40%) at flow rates of 0.25–4 liters per minute (L/min).
2. High flow rates may be uncomfortable and cause dry mucous membranes, gastric distention, or headaches.
3. Fio_2 (inspired oxygen concentration) delivered is somewhat unpredictable depending on how much ambient air is entrained (influenced by age, inspiratory flow rate, and minute ventilation) during inspiration.

25

PULMONOLOGY

4. Mouth breathing is usually not a factor because O_2 can be entrained from the nasopharynx.

B. MASKS: Should be soft and pliable and clear so that regurgitation can be detected. Will increase dead space. If O_2 flow rate is not sufficient, CO_2 retention may occur.

1. Simple mask

a. Delivers Fio_2 of 35–55% at flow rates of 6–10L/min.

b. Fio_2 determined by O_2 flow rate supplied relative to inspiratory flow rate and tidal volume.

2. Partial rebreathing mask

a. Can deliver Fio_2 of 60–95% depending on inspiratory flow rate, tidal volume, and leaks.

b. Has reservoir bag but no valve system to prevent expired air from entering reservoir.

c. A collapsed reservoir bag indicates inadequate O_2 flow or a leak.

d. O_2 flow rates should be >6L/min to avoid CO_2 retention.

3. Nonrebreathing mask

a. Commonly used to deliver Fio_2 approaching 100%. Requires relatively tight seal with face and high rate of gas flow.

b. Has reservoir bag and one-way valve to prevent expired air from entering reservoir.

c. A collapsed reservoir bag indicates inadequate O_2 flow or a leak.

d. O_2 flow rates should be >6L/min to avoid CO_2 retention.

4. Venturi mask

a. Designed to deliver specific O_2 concentrations.

b. Especially useful in chronic lung disease where control of Fio_2 is crucial.

c. Based on Bernoulli principle where O_2 flows through a jet that entrains room air. Allows for predictable O_2 concentrations between 24% and 50%.

d. If back pressure develops on the jet, less room air may be entrained, and Fio_2 may increase unpredictably.

5. Tracheostomy mask

a. Provides a relatively controlled O_2 and humidity source.

b. Fio_2 not predictable unless Venturi circuit (same principle as a Venturi mask) is used. Fio_2 should be analyzed for each patient individually.

C. OXYGEN ENVIRONMENTS

1. Oxygen hoods/head boxes

a. Useful for patients who will not tolerate masks or cannulae (e.g., infants).

b. May achieve very high O_2 concentrations.

c. Flow rate must be sufficient to reduce CO_2 accumulation (usually >10L/min).

d. Disadvantages: An O_2 gradient may develop within the hood/box, and patients must be taken out for feeding and care.

2. **Oxygen tents**
a. May provide Fio_2 up to 50%.
b. Leaks are a major problem.
c. Flow rate must be sufficient to prevent CO_2 buildup.
d. Can be used to provide humidified air (croup or mist tent).
e. Disadvantages: Development of O_2 gradient, decreases in Fio_2 resulting from frequently entering the tent, and claustrophobia (may become a problem for older children). Sparks in or near the tent may be hazardous. Close monitoring of patient and apparatus is required.

V. MECHANICAL VENTILATION

25

PULMONOLOGY

A. **TYPES OF VENTILATORY SUPPORT**
1. **Volume limited**
a. Delivers a preset tidal volume to a patient regardless of pressure required.
b. Risk of barotrauma reduced by pressure alarms and pressure pop-off valves that limit peak inspiratory pressure (PIP).
2. **Pressure limited**
a. Gas flow is delivered to the patient until a preset pressure is reached and then held for the set inspiratory time (reduces the risk of barotrauma).
b. Useful for neonatal and infant ventilatory support (<10kg) where the volume of gas being delivered is small in relation to the volume of compressible air in the ventilator circuit, which makes reliable delivery of a set tidal volume difficult.
3. **High-frequency oscillatory ventilation (HFOV)**
a. High-amplitude and high-frequency pressure waveform generated in the ventilator circuit. Tidal volumes are less than dead space. Bias gas flow provides fresh gas at ventilator and maintains airway pressure.
b. Minimizes barotrauma, volutrauma, and oxygen toxicities.
B. **VENTILATOR PARAMETERS**
1. **Peak inspiratory pressure (PIP):** Maximum inspiratory pressure attained during the respiratory cycle.
2. **Positive end-expiratory pressure (PEEP):** Airway pressure maintained between inspiratory and expiratory phases (prevents alveolar collapse during expiration, decreasing work of reinflation and improving gas exchange).
3. **Rate (intermittent mandatory ventilation) or frequency (Hz):** Number of mechanical breaths delivered per minute, or rate of oscillations in HFOV.
4. **Inspired oxygen concentration (Fio_2):** Fraction of oxygen present in inspired gas.
5. **Inspiratory time (t_i):** Length of time spent in the inspiratory phase of the respiratory cycle.

6. **Tidal volume (TV):** Volume of gas delivered during inspiration.
7. **Power (ΔP):** Amplitude of the pressure waveform in HFOV.
8. **Mean airway pressure (MAP):** Average pressure over entire respiratory cycle.

C. **MODES OF OPERATION**
1. **Intermittent mandatory ventilation (IMV):** A preset number of breaths is delivered each minute. The patient can take breaths on his or her own, but the ventilator may cycle on during a patient breath.
2. **Synchronized IMV (SIMV):** Similar to IMV, but the ventilator synchronizes delivered breaths with inspiratory effort, and allows the patient to finish expiration before cycling on.
3. **Assist control (AC or AMV):** Every inspiratory effort by the patient triggers a ventilator-delivered breath at the set tidal volume. Ventilator-initiated breaths are delivered when the spontaneous rate falls below the backup rate.
4. **Pressure support ventilation (PSV):** Inspiratory effort opens a valve allowing airflow at a preset positive pressure. Patient determines rate and inspiratory time. May be used in combination with other modes of operation.
5. **Noninvasive positive-pressure ventilation (NIPPV):** Respiratory support provided through face mask.
a. Continuous positive airway pressure (CPAP): Delivers airflow (with set Fio_2) to maintain a set airway pressure.
b. Bilevel positive airway pressure: Delivers airflow to maintain set pressures for inspiration and expiration.

D. **INITIAL VENTILATOR SETTINGS**
1. **Volume limited**
a. Rate: Approximately normal range for age (Table 25.1).
b. Tidal volume: Approximately 10–15mL/kg.
c. Inspiratory time: Generally use I:E ratio of 1:2. More prolonged expiratory phases are required for obstructive diseases to avoid air trapping.
d. Fio_2: Selected to maintain targeted saturations and Pao_2.
2. **Pressure limited**
a. Rate: Approximately normal range for age (Table 25.1).
b. PEEP: Start with $3cmH_2O$ and increase as clinically indicated. (Monitor for decreases in cardiac output with increasing PEEP.)
c. PIP: Set at pressure required to produce adequate chest wall movement (approximate this using hand bagging and manometer).
d. Fio_2: Selected to maintain targeted saturations and Pao_2.
3. **High-frequency oscillatory**
a. Frequency: 10–15Hz for neonates.
b. Power: Select to achieve adequate chest wall movement.
c. MAP: $1–4cmH_2O$ higher than settings on a conventional ventilator.
d. Fio_2: Selected to maintain targeted saturations and Pao_2.

E. FURTHER VENTILATOR MANAGEMENT

1. **Follow patient closely** with serial blood gas measurements and clinical assessment. Adjust ventilator parameters as indicated (Table 25.6).
2. **Parameters predictive of successful extubation**
a. Normal $Paco_2$.
b. PIP generally <14–$16cmH_2O$.
c. PEEP <2–$3cmH_2O$ (infants) or $<5cmH_2O$ (children).
d. IMV <2–4 breaths per minute (infants); children may wean to CPAP.
e. Fio_2 $<40\%$ (maintaining Pao_2 >70).
f. Maximum negative inspiratory pressure >20–$25cmH_2O$.

TABLE 25.6

EFFECTS OF VENTILATOR SETTING CHANGES

Ventilator setting changes	Typical effects on blood gases	
	$Paco_2$	Pao_2
↑ PIP	↓	↑
↑ PEEP	↑	↑
↑ Rate (IMV)	↓	Min.↑
↑ I:E ratio	No change	↑
↑ Fio_2	No change	↑
↑ Flow	Min. ↓	Min.↑
↑ Power (in HFOV)	↓	No change
↑ MAP (in HFOV)	Min. ↓	↑

Adapted from Carlo[9].

25

PULMONOLOGY

VI. HOME APNEA MONITORING[10,11]

A. RECOMMENDED INDICATIONS

1. Infants with one or more severe apparent life-threatening event (ALTE).
2. Siblings of sudden infant death syndrome (SIDS) victim.
3. Symptomatic preterm infant: Preterm infants who continue to have pathologic apnea when they otherwise would be ready for discharge from the hospital.
4. Infants and young children with central hypoventilation.
5. Children <2 years old with tracheostomies.
6. Children with bronchopulmonary dysplasia requiring supplemental O_2.

B. MONITORING MAY BE CONSIDERED for infants with supplemental oxygen, ALTE not requiring CPR or vigorous stimulation, bronchopulmonary dysplasia not requiring supplemental O_2, metabolic disorders, substance-abusing mothers, and RSV-related apnea.

C. DISCONTINUATION CRITERIA

1. Decision should be based on infant's clinical condition (e.g., ability to tolerate stress) and age.
2. Decision is influenced by many variables, including medications and family anxiety level.
3. Should have no significant ALTE for at least 2–3 consecutive months.

4. Should have no significant cardiac or respiratory abnormalities detected by documented monitoring for at least 2–3 consecutive months.

VII. REFERENCE DATA

A. MINUTE VENTILATION ($\dot{V}_E$)

$$\dot{V}_E = \text{Respiratory rate} \times \text{Tidal volume}$$
$$V_E \times Paco_2 = \text{Constant (for volume-limited ventilation)}$$
$$\text{Normal TV} = 10\text{--}15mL/kg$$

B. HENDERSON–HASSELBACH EQUATION

$$pH = pK + \log\left(\frac{[HCO_3^-]}{a \times Paco_2}\right)$$

$$pK = 6.1 \text{ and } a = 0.0301$$

C. ALVEOLAR GAS EQUATION

$$PAo_2 = Pio_2 - (Paco_2/R)$$
$$Pio_2 = Fio_2 \times (PB - 47mmHg)$$

1. Pio_2 = Partial pressure of inspired $O_2 \cong 150mmHg$ at sea level on room air.
2. R = Respiratory exchange quotient (CO_2 produced/O_2 consumed) = 0.8.
3. $Paco_2$ = Partial pressure of alveolar $CO_2 \cong$ Partial pressure of arterial CO_2 ($Paco_2$).
4. PB = Atmospheric pressure = 760mmHg.
5. PAo_2 = Partial pressure of O_2 in the alveoli.

D. ALVEOLAR–ARTERIAL OXYGEN GRADIENT (A–a GRADIENT)

$$\text{A-a gradient} = PAo_2 - Pao_2$$

1. Obtain ABG measuring Pao_2 and $Paco_2$ with patient on 100% Fio_2 for at least 15 minutes.
2. Calculate the PAo_2 (see above) and then the A–a gradient.
3. The larger the gradient, the more serious the respiratory compromise. A normal gradient is 20–65mmHg on 100% O_2 or 5–20mmHg on room air.

E. OXYGEN CONTENT (Cao_2)

O_2 content of sample (mL/dL) =

$$(O_2 \text{ capacity} \times O_2 \text{ saturation [as decimal]}) + \text{Dissolved } O_2$$

1. O_2 capacity = Hemoglobin (g/dL) $\times$ 1.34.
2. Dissolved $O_2 = Po_2$ (of sample) $\times$ 0.003.
3. Hemoglobin carries more than 99% of O_2 in blood under standard conditions.

F. ARTERIOVENOUS O_2 DIFFERENCE ($AVDo_2$)

$$AVDo_2 = Cao_2 - C\bar{v}o_2 = \text{Arterial } O_2 \text{ content} - \text{Mixed venous } O_2 \text{ content}$$

1. Usually done after placing patient on 100% Fio_2 for 15 minutes.
2. Obtain ABG and mixed venous blood sample (best obtained from pulmonary artery catheter), and measure O_2 saturation in each sample.

3. Calculate arterial and mixed venous oxygen contents (see section E above) and then $AVDo_2$ (normal: 5mL/100dL).
4. Used in the calculation of O_2 extraction ratio.

G. O_2 EXTRACTION RATIO

$$O_2 \text{ extraction} = (AVDo_2/Cao_2) \times 100$$
Normal range 28–33%

1. Calculate $AVDo_2$ and O_2 contents (see sections E and F above).
2. Extraction ratios are indicative of the adequacy of O_2 delivery to tissues, with increasing extraction ratios suggesting that metabolic needs may be outpacing the oxygen content being delivered[3].

H. OXYGENATION INDEX (OI)

$$OI = \frac{\text{Mean airway pressure (cmH}_2\text{O}) \times \text{Fio}_2 \times 100}{\text{Pao}_2}$$

OI >35 for 5–6 hours is one criterion for ECMO (extracorporeal membrane oxygen) support.

I. INTRAPULMONARY SHUNT FRACTION ($\dot{Q}s/\dot{Q}t$)

$$\frac{\dot{Q}s}{\dot{Q}t} = \frac{(\text{A–a gradient}) \times 0.003}{(AVDo_2) + (\text{A–a gradient} \times 0.003)}$$

$\dot{Q}t$, cardiac output; $\dot{Q}s$, flow across right-to-left shunt.

1. Formula assumes blood gases obtained on 100% Fio_2.
2. Represents the mismatch of ventilation and perfusion and is normally <5%.
3. A rising shunt fraction (usually >15–20%) is indicative of progressive respiratory failure.

J. SWEAT CHLORIDE[12]

Normal (1wk–adult) <40 mmol/L
Patients with cystic fibrosis (CF) >60 mmol/L
(mmol/L = meq/L)

1. Sweat obtained through quantitative pilocarpine iontophoresis.
2. Results between 40–60 mmol/L require repeat testing or other tests for CF.
3. Normal levels (false negatives) may be found in patients with CF in the presence of edema and hypoproteinemia or inadequate sweat rate.
4. Elevated chloride levels may be from CF, untreated adrenal insufficiency, glycogen storage disease type I, fucosidosis, hypothyroidism, nephrogenic diabetes insipidus, ectodermal dysplasia, malnutrition, mucopolysaccharidosis, panhypopituitarism, or poor testing technique.

VIII. REFERENCES

1. Illif A, Lee V. *Child Dev* 1952; **23**:240.
2. Polger G, Promedhat V. *Pulmonary function testing in children: techniques and standards.* Philadelphia: WB Saunders; 1971.
3. Rogers M. *Textbook of pediatric intensive care,* 2nd edn. Baltimore: Williams & Wilkins; 1992.
4. Schrier RW. *Renal and electrolyte disorders*, 3rd edn. Boston: Little, Brown; 1986.
5. Brenner BM, Floyd CR Jr, eds. *The kidney*, vol. 1. Philadelphia: WB Saunders; 1991.
6. Lanbertsten CJ. Transport of oxygen, CO_2, and inert gases by the blood. In: Mountcastle VB, ed. *Medical physiology*, 14th edn. St Louis: Mosby; 1980.
7. Comber JT, Lopez BL. Examination of pulse oximetry in sickle cell anemia patients presenting to the emergency department in acute vasoocclusive crisis. *Am J Emerg Med* 1996; **14(1)**:16.
8. Burgess W, Chernick V. *Respiratory therapy in newborn infants and children.* New York: Thieme-Stratton; 1982.
9. Carlo WA, Chatburn RL. *Neonatal respiratory care,* 2nd edn. St Louis: Mosby; 1988.
10. *Infantile apnea and home monitoring.* NIH Consensus Statement 1986 Sep 29–Oct 1; **6(6)**:1.
11. Carroll JL, Marcus CL, Loughlin GM. Disordered control of breathing in infants and children. *Pediatr Rev* 1993; **14(2)**:51.
12. Soldin SJ, Hicks JM. *Pediatr reference ranges.* Washington, DC: AACC Press; 1995.

PSYCHIATRY

Geetha Subramaniam, MD, and
Jessica Sessions, MD

The psychiatric history and examination differs from a general pediatric assessment because it is necessary to include a psychiatric review of systems and a complete mental status examination. One needs to modify the content and style of interview to adapt to the different ages and capacities of the patients. The outline provided is applicable to all cases, with preschool age and younger children requiring additional assessments that take into consideration their stage of development.

I. PSYCHIATRIC HISTORY

With the exception of emergencies, the legal guardian has to consent to a psychiatric assessment and disposition. State laws may vary on how this is to be obtained.

A. **INFORMANTS:** Child, parents/caregivers, teachers, and other family members.

B. **HISTORY OF PRESENT ILLNESS**
- Elicit symptoms suggestive of all psychiatric disorders to make a differential diagnosis.
- Describe the onset, course, and severity of symptoms. Note settings where they occur.
- List precipitating and predisposing factors (stressors). Assess protective factors.
- Current treatments: Medications, therapy, providers. Response to treatment and compliance.

1. **Psychiatric review of symptoms**
a. Depression: Mnemonic (SIG E CAPS)—**S**leep changes; **I**nterest decline (hobbies, play activities); **G**uilt, worthlessness, hopelessness; **E**nergy changes (fatigue or hyperactivity); poor **C**oncentration; **A**ppetite changes; **P**sychomotor retardation or agitation; **S**uicidal ideations/attempt or wish to die. Also irritable or sad mood, temper outbursts, impaired social relationships worsening school performance, low self-esteem, chronic pain, menstrual irregularities, poor response to standard care for medical conditions.
b. Mania: Increased energy, racing thoughts, pressured speech, decreased need for sleep, increase in sexual behaviors, grandiosity, intense mood lability.

c. Attention deficit hyperactivity disorder (ADHD)
   1) Inattention: Often makes careless mistakes, is forgetful, is easily distracted, has difficulty sustaining attention in tasks, does not appear to listen, fails to finish schoolwork or chores, is disorganized, dislikes activities that require sustained attention, loses things.
   2) Impulsivity/hyperactivity: Often blurts out answers, has difficulty awaiting turn, interrupts others, fidgets, leaves seat, climbs excessively, is unable to play quietly, is often on the go, talks a lot.
d. Anxiety
   1) Separation issues: Experiences excessive distress when separation from significant adults is anticipated, worries about losing them, is reluctant to be alone, is reluctant to go to school, has recurrent somatic complaints, has nightmares, refuses to go to sleep alone, refuses sleep-overs.
   2) Generalized and phobic anxieties: Restlessness, tense feelings, need for repeated reassurance, sleep disturbances resulting from worries, somatic complaints, poor concentration, fear of social or performance situations, crying or tantrums in unfamiliar situations or in anticipation of them.
   3) Obsessive-compulsive: Recurrent and persistent thoughts, images, mental acts, or behaviors; beliefs that these acts prevent a dreaded event or reduce distress; rigidity in following rules.
   4) Posttraumatic stress symptoms: Reexperiences of the trauma (nightmares, repetitive play involving the themes of trauma), persistent avoidance of stimuli and generalized numbness (feelings of detachment, sense of foreshortened future, unable to express love/feelings), and symptoms of increased arousal (anger, exaggerated startle response, hypervigilance, poor sleep).
e. Psychosis: Auditory hallucinations (that come from outside the head), paranoia, loose associations, catatonic states, bizarre behaviors.
f. Defiant and conduct problems: Frequently refuses to comply with authority, blames others for problems, runs away, steals, initiates fights, gang membership, arrests, lack of remorse, truancy, fire-setting.
g. Substance use problems: Admits to alcohol or drug use, intoxication, peer group substance use, altered behaviors, or mental states uncharacteristic for the patient; possession of substances or paraphernalia; parental use and their attitude toward use; poor motivation; needle tracks.
h. Developmental delays: Delays in motor and speech milestones, inability to communicate needs, restricted interests, stereotypes (hand flapping, rocking, etc.), inability to engage in cooperative play, poor reciprocal social interactions (lack of eye contact), regression in growth.
i. Other: Eating problems; sadness or irritability in response to stressful events such as death of family member, friend, or pet; parental divorce or separation; change of residence; academic or athletic failure.

C. **PAST PSYCHIATRIC HISTORY:** Past episodes of illnesses, types of treatment, compliance and response, suicide attempts, abuse/neglect, legal problems, social service agency involvement.

D. **FAMILY HISTORY:** Obtain and draw a genogram. Elicit history of psychiatric and substance use disorders, learning disorders, medical illnesses, legal problems, and other problems among biologic family members. Assess family support and functional levels of caregivers.

E. **BIRTH AND DEVELOPMENTAL HISTORY:** Mother's pregnancy and labor, prenatal or postnatal complications, birth weight, feeding and sleep habits, delays in motor or language milestones, toilet training, temperament, ability to relate to caregivers.

F. **SCHOOL HISTORY:** Name of school, grade and level of education (regular vs special need), academic performance, attendance, behavior.

G. **PERTINENT MEDICAL HISTORY:** Head injury, seizures, surgeries, chronic medical illnesses and ability to cope with them, compliance with treatment, allergies to medications. Record menstrual and pregnancy history. Assess risk for HIV infection.

H. **SOCIAL HISTORY:** Ability to make and maintain friendships, makeup of peer groups (especially in adolescents), rejection by peers, romantic and sexual relationships, and risk-taking behaviors (e.g., high-risk sexual activity, defying curfew). Ask direct questions regarding sexual activity and sexually transmitted disease/pregnancy protection. The patient may be more forthcoming if interviewed without the parent/caregiver.

II. MENTAL STATUS EXAMINATION

A. **PHYSICAL APPEARANCE:** Describe grooming and hygiene, stature, head circumference, general health, observable facial or other deformities, tics, stereotypes, hearing, and vision.

B. **ATTITUDE TOWARD EXAMINER/INTERVIEW:** Observe for difficulty with separation from caregiver or indiscriminate attachments, and comment on eye contact, expression of hostility, distant or disinterested participation during the session. Describe play characteristics to include choice of toy, use of toy, cooperation and sharing with the examiner, and aggression, if present.

C. **MOTOR DEVELOPMENT/ACTIVITY:** Describe gait, gross motor skills (throwing, climbing), fine motor skills (grasp of objects, ability to use buttons, zippers, etc.), motor coordination, restlessness, motor retardation, and agitation.

D. **SPEECH/LANGUAGE:** Describe rate, tone, rhythm, vocabulary, articulation, and self-expression.

E. **MOOD/AFFECT:** Mood is a subjective state of mind (what the patient says)—Sad, mad, worried, elated, happy, irritable, angry or labile. Affect is observed by the examiner and is objective (e.g., bright, sad, anxious, angry, blunted or labile).

26

PSYCHIATRY

F. **CONTENT OF THOUGHT:** Inquire about obsessions, fears or worries, grief, fantasies, presence of delusions, visual and auditory hallucinations, ideas of reference.

G. **SUICIDE/HOMICIDE:** Elicit ideas, plans, attempts. Obtain reasons.

H. **FLOW OF THOUGHT:** Describe if goal directed, tangential, bizarre or with loose associations.

I. **ORIENTATION TO TIME, PLACE, PERSON, SITUATION:** If altered, do a Mini-Mental State Examination (MMSE) (Fig 26.1) to better determine whether an organic impairment such as delirium is the cause.

J **ATTENTION/CONCENTRATION:** Repeat digits forward and backward; do serial sevens (at least third-grade level), spell words forward and backward, or comment on the ability to focus during the interview.

K. **MEMORY:** Ask the patient to recall three objects in 5 minutes or past significant events, and dates.

L. **INTELLIGENCE:** Assess use of vocabulary, fund of knowledge. Use culturally and age-appropriate similarities or proverbs. Gesell's figures (see p. 204) provide a nonverbal assessment.

M. **MISCELLANEOUS:** Inquire about three wishes, future plans. Consider self-portrait, family drawings.

N. **INSIGHT AND JUDGMENT:** bility to perceive current situation and respond realistically.

III. FORMULATION AND DIAGNOSIS

A. Make a synopsis of pertinent findings (written in 3–5 sentences) summarizing the onset and course of the problems, including predisposing and precipitating factors, interventions, and outcome.

B. List clinical features to support the diagnoses on five axes from the fourth edition of *Diagnostic and Statistical Manual of Mental Disorders (DSM-IV*[1]*)* and *Diagnostic and Statistical Manual for Primary Care (DSM-PC)*[2]:

1. **Axis I:** Clinical psychiatric disorders and other conditions (e.g., abuse, neglect, bereavement).

2. **Axis II:** Mental retardation and/or personality disorders (one cannot diagnose a personality disorder before the age of 18, but if symptom criteria are met, consider the diagnosis of a personality trait). A diagnosis of mental retardation is made only if there is impairment in social adaptive functioning using a standardized test (e.g., Vineland Adaptive Behavior Scale).

3. **Axis III:** General medical conditions. Significant abnormal vital signs and laboratory results.

4. **Axis IV:** Psychosocial problems that impair self-esteem, family and peer relationships, and school performance.

5. **Axis V:** Global assessment of functioning (GAF) scored up to 100 based on *DSM-IV.*[1] GAF scale of zero indicates acute and most severe impairment, whereas a score of 100 indicates positive health.

Mini-Mental State
Examination (MMSE)

Date_____

Patient's Name_____

Maximum Score	Score	
		ORIENTATION
5	( )	What is the (year) (season) (date) (day) (month)?
5	( )	Where are we: (state) (county) (town or city) (hospital) (floor)?
		REGISTRATION
3	( )	Name 3 common objects (e.g., "apple," "table," "penny"). Take 1 second to say each. Then ask the patient to repeat all 3 after you have said them. Give 1 point for each correct answer. Then repeat them until he/she learns all 3. Count trials and record.
		Trials:
		ATTENTION AND CALCULATION
5	( )	Spell "world" backwards. The score is the number of letters in correct order (D___ L___ R___ O___ W___).
		RECALL
3	( )	Ask for the 3 objects repeated above. Give 1 point for each correct answer. (Note: Recall cannot be tested if all 3 objects were not remembered during registration.)
		LANGUAGE
2	( )	Name a "pencil" and "watch."
1	( )	Repeat the following: "No ifs, ands, or buts."
3	( )	Follow a 3-stage command: "Take a paper in your right hand, fold it in half, and put it on the floor."
1	( )	Read and obey the following: Close your eyes.
1	( )	Write a sentence.
1	( )	Copy the following design:

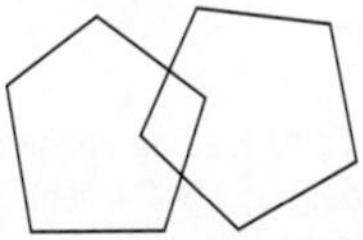

TOTAL
SCORE _____   No construction problem.

FIG. 26.1
Mini-Mental State Examination. (From Folstein[4] and Cockrell[5].)

IV. GENERAL PRINCIPLES OF TREATMENT PLANNING

A. TESTS

1. **Routine tests:** In most cases, order laboratory tests before initiating medication trials; also order them to rule out medical conditions that may interfere with treatment or that mimic psychiatric conditions.
   a. Chemistry panel (electrolytes, hepatic and renal function).
   b. CBC (anemia, leukemia).
   c. Lead levels in youths residing in older dwellings or inner city areas.
   d. Urine pregnancy tests in female patients of childbearing age.
   e. Thyroid screen (to rule out thyroid dysfunction).
   f. Urine toxic screen (for substance use).
   g. Liver function tests (for history of substance use, before and periodically during pemoline, divalproex sodium, or carbamazepine use).
   h. Renal function tests (before and periodically during lithium trial).
   i. Electrocardiography (ECG) (before stimulants, tricyclic antidepressants [TCAs], or lithium use and during maintenance).

2. **Specialized tests (in selected cases)**
   a. Brain scans (to rule out tumors, for history of birth injury, for head injury).
   b. Electroencephalograph (EEG) (e.g., to rule out temporal lobe seizures).
   c. Chromosomal analysis (for fragile X syndrome, in some cases of moderate to severe mental retardation, in pervasive developmental disorders).

3. **Psychologic tests:** Cognitive (e.g., Wechsler Intelligence Scale for Children [WISC-III]), academic (Woodcock Johnson-Revised [WJ-R]), and speech/language assessments. **Note: Deficits in these areas are often hidden and require probing questions and frequent consideration by the clinician when patients have other problems (e.g., reasons for referral are academic decline or failure, decline despite treatment).**

4. **Blood level monitoring:** Lithium, divalproex sodium, carbamazepine, imipramine, nortriptyline, and desipramine. Frequently during titration upward and regularly while on maintenance doses.

B. BRIEF DESCRIPTION AND MANAGEMENT OF EMERGENT AND NONEMERGENT CONDITIONS

1. **Emergent conditions**
   a. Suicide
      1) Prevalence rate: Third leading cause of death. 13/100,000 (completed suicides) in 15–24 year olds.
      2) Risk factors: Males, adolescent age, precipitating humiliating event or family crisis, substance use, affective and disruptive disorders, intent to die, access to weapons, planned attempt, lethal method, hopelessness, helplessness, impulsivity, prior attempt, negative family interactions, high parental stress, substance abuse.

3) Evaluation: Assess risk and protective factors, parental/caregiver functioning and supervision.
4) Management: Hospitalization to protect from imminent harm and to provide respite from stressful situations. Other interventions include structure, trust, rapport building, supportive therapy to reduce distress, cognitive behavioral therapy (CBT) to improve coping, and medications to treat underlying mood and anxiety disorders. Make certain that the patient receives follow-up psychiatric services.

b. Aggression/homicide/violence
  1) Prevalence rate: Homicide: second leading cause of death among 15–24 year olds.
  2) Risk factors
    a) General: Males, black race, early exposure to violence, physical abuse, lower socioeconomic status, overcrowding.
    b) Individual: History of being a loner, hopelessness, low self-esteem, impulsive and antisocial behaviors, paranoia, recent acts of violence, frequent thoughts with plan, access to a gun, use of substances or alcohol, presence of mood and anxiety disorders.
  3) Evaluation: Assess severity of risk, supervision available, family/caregiver functioning.
  4) Management: Emergent confinement if actively homicidal. When rapid tranquilization is indicated, consider the use of droperidol (Inapsine): 0.625–2.5mg IM. In less acute situations, refer for outpatient psychiatric services, consisting of group and family therapy, to control problem behaviors and improve coping skills. In addition, consider referrals for social skills training to decrease inappropriate social interactions, and medications to treat ADHD, mood or anxiety disorders. In some cases, lithium, carbamaz-epine, and antipsychotics may control aggression. Referral for substance abuse treatment is essential in known and suspected cases of use.

c. Alcohol/drug use problems
  1) Prevalence rate: 1997 Monitoring the Future Study—among high school seniors, 38.5% used marijuana, 5.5% used cocaine, 10.2% used stimulants, 8.4% used LSD, and 1.2% used heroin **in the past year.**
  2) Risk factors: Substance-abusing biologic parent, familial clustering of substance abuse, poor attention and planning problems, sensation seeking, negative peer influence, and lack of role models.
  3) Findings from history: May first present with problems caused by drug use; these problems include school failure, truancy, sudden changes in behaviors, frequent family conflicts, suicide attempts, motor vehicle accidents, sexually transmitted diseases, use of weapons, and arrests for fights, stealing, possession of drugs, and other criminal behaviors.

26

PSYCHIATRY

4) Mental status changes (intoxication and withdrawal): Agitation, aggression, irritability or euphoria, disorientation, decreased concentration, increased and loud speech to inability to talk, paranoia, hallucinations, suicidal ideations or attempts. Agitation and anxiety with stimulant (cocaine, PCP) intoxication or alcohol or benzodiazepine withdrawal. Lethargy and or stupor from opioid, alcohol, or sedative intoxication. Disorientation and inability to answer questions are common.

5) Physical examination findings
   a) Changes in vital signs (e.g., tachycardia, tachypnea, fever in stimulant intoxication, and alcohol or sedative withdrawal).
   b) Skin may show needle marks, scarring from tactile hallucinations secondary to cocaine use.
   c) Pupils may be pinpoint in opioid intoxication and dilated in stimulant use or opioid withdrawal. Conjunctival congestion in marihuana intoxication. Nystagmus in many types of intoxications.
   d) Chronic sinusitis or nasal septal perforation from intranasal use of cocaine. Rhinorrhea from opioid withdrawal.
   e) Cardiovascular changes such as tachycardia, arrhythmias, and chest pains in cocaine users.
   f) Tender right upper quadrant of abdomen may suggest hepatitis. Scleral icterus, jaundice.
   g) Genital examination for sexually transmitted diseases.

6) Evaluation
   a) Confront calmly, use direct questions, interview the adolescent separately. Self-administered screening instruments such as the Problem Oriented Screening Instrument for Teenagers (POSIT)[13] and Substance Abuse Subtle Screening Inventory—adolescent version (SASSI)[12].
   b) Urine toxicology and blood alcohol screens should be ordered with a low threshold of suspicion. Other laboratory tests such as CBC, liver enzymes analysis, rapid plasma reagin, hepatitis screening, and HIV testing.
   c) Females will require a pelvic examination and a Papanicolaou (Pap) smear.

7) Management: **Note—in the presence of comorbid psychiatric problems, drug use should be considered the primary problem.**
   a) Withdrawal from alcohol and sedatives is potentially life threatening and may require close attention to maintaining stable vital signs. Commonly, patients are well rehydrated, given thiamine and multivitamin supplements; if vital signs are unstable or the patient has a past history of withdrawal, use a benzodiazepine taper-down protocol to prevent seizures and delirium tremens.

b) Withdrawal from opioids requires detoxification with symptomatic use of nonopioid analgesics, clonidine, muscle relaxants, and antidiarrheals. It is generally not life threatening.

c) After detoxification, inpatient substance abuse treatment is indicated only in cases of failed outpatient treatment, a high-risk or substance-using family environment, and the need for treatment of comorbid medical or psychiatric treatments. In most cases, patients and their families should be referred to outpatient treatment programs emphasizing the participation of the family in the treatment process. In the case of delinquent patients, collaborate with the juvenile justice system to assess the appropriate level of care. For some of these patients, the court may order treatment.

26

PSYCHIATRY

d. Delirium
   1) Definition: A transient and reversible dysfunction of cerebral metabolism with an acute or a subacute onset presenting as fluctuations in consciousness, memory, orientation, hallucinations, and/or agitation.
   2) Causes: Mnemonic (I WATCH DEATH)—Infections, Withdrawal, Acute metabolic, Trauma, CNS pathology (e.g., hemorrhage, tumors, seizures, strokes), Hypoxia, Deficiencies (vitamin), Endocrinopathies, Acute vascular, Toxins, Heavy metals.
   3) Evaluation: Perform a MMSE (Fig. 26.1); assess mental and physical status, especially neurologic status; order laboratory and other relevant tests to determine etiology; and review medications.
   4) Management: The patient should be under close supervision at a medical setting to investigate and treat the identified cause. Frequent monitoring of vital signs and MMSEs are essential. Medications such as droperidol or haloperidol for agitation. Presence of familiar people, orientation guides (calendars, clocks), and reassurance help decrease anxiety.

e. Abuse/Neglect
   1) Prevalence: Exact incidence is unknown. Physical abuse estimated at 19/1000 between ages 3 and 17 years. Sexual abuse estimated to occur in 300,000 children in a 12-month period.
   2) Definitions: *Abuse* can be defined as intentional physical injury (physical), sexual contact (sexual), or chronic rejection of, hostility toward, or terrorizing (emotional) of the child. *Neglect* is defined as inadequate caregiving resulting from acts of omission of physical (nutrition), medical (discharge against medical advice), educational (permitting truancy several days a month), or emotional (exposure to chronic domestic violence) needs.
   3) Risk factors: Maternal depression or substance use, family history of violence. Incestuous families are socially isolated, and there is often a history of marital sexual difficulties.

4) Management: Assessment of the child in suspected abuse is often complex and requires an intimate knowledge of development and specialized training. A physical examination may provide signs of physical or sexual abuse. The safety of child is of prime importance. All states mandate reporting of suspected cases to state agencies. Treatment should also aim to prevent complications such as suicide, depression, anxiety, and posttrauma sequelae. The patient may need a referral for group and/or individual therapy. Parental treatment is directed toward reducing psychopathology and providing education to prevent repeated abuse.

2. Nonemergent conditions

a. ADHD

1) Prevalence: 3–5% of school-age children. Hyperactive/impulsive type is more common in males.

2) Diagnosis: *DSM-IV*[1] criteria for diagnosis require at least six of nine symptoms of inattention and/or at least six of the symptoms of hyperactivity and impulsivity, with a duration >6 months. Impairment must occur <7 years of age and be evident in two or more settings.

3) Evaluation: The diagnosis is clinical and is made based primarily on the parent and child interviews. Input from the school on learning, classroom behaviors, and attention needs to be integrated. Rating scales (e.g., Conners Parents and Teachers Rating Scales[3], Barkley's home/school situation questionnaires[17]) are used to measure the severity of symptoms at baseline and to monitor progress with treatment. Computerized tests (e.g., Continuous Performance Tests [CPTs]) may provide additional baseline and prognostic information.

4) Investigations: Vision and hearing evaluations. Serum lead levels. In relevant cases, exclude fragile X syndrome, phenylketonuria, etc. EEG, brain scans are indicated in cases with focal neurologic signs.

5) Management: Management of most cases (except mild cases with a positive and stable family environment) is best handled by a multimodal approach. The presence of comorbid psychiatric disorders, coexisting academic and cognitive deficits, patient strengths, and level of family functioning and support need to be considered for an effective treatment plan.

a) Pharmacotherapy: In most cases, psychostimulants (methylphenidate, dextroamphetamine, amphetamine [Adderall], and magnesium pemoline) are the first line of pharmacologic agents (Table 26.1). In case of side effects and poor response to more than two adequate stimulant trials, consider a consultation with a specialist for the possible use of other agents such as TCAs (nortriptyline, desipramine), bupropion, clonidine, and guanfacine hydrochloride (Table 26.1).

b) Psychosocial treatments

      i) Behavior modification: Several approaches (e.g., positive and negative contingencies, token economy) are used and can be used both at school and at home. They are ineffective in controlling inattention and hyperactivity disorders, especially if used alone.

      ii) Parent training: Usually includes education regarding behavior management, structuring the day to provide a routine, and giving clear instructions to the child as well as guides to developing positive peer relationships. This is often difficult for parents, and there are reports of noncompliance and problems with long-term maintenance.

      iii) Classroom accommodations: May recommend seating the patient in the front row of the class, use of rewards/contingencies, daily progress report to parents, smaller teacher:student ratios.

      iv) Social skills training: Usually done in group settings and may help with problem solving.

      v) Support: Organizations (e.g., Children and Adults with Attention Deficit/Hyperactivity Disorder [CHADD]) can be valuable in education, locating resources, referrals for services, etc.

b. Mood disorders

  1) Depression

    a) Major depressive disorder (MDD)

      i) Prevalence: 2% in children and 4–8% in adolescents. Gender ratio is equal in children, but male:female ratio is 1:2 in adolescents.

      ii) Diagnosis: *DSM-IV* diagnosis requires five of nine (SIG E CAPS [see p. 543]) symptoms to be present for 2 weeks. The natural course of each episode is approximately 7–9 months. The risk of recurrence is 20–60%. There is a 20–60% risk of developing bipolar disorder[10].

      iii) Risk factors: Female gender, adolescent age (compared with children), at least one parent with depression, poor academic performance, abuse or neglect, early parental death or separation, conflict-ridden family relationships, and rigid or harsh conscience.

    b) Dysthymic disorder

      i) Prevalence: 0.6–1.7% in children and 1.6–8% in adolescents.

      ii) Diagnosis: One-year duration of depressed or irritable mood with two of the following: poor appetite, poor sleep, fatigue, poor concentration, hopelessness, and low self-esteem. Duration of episode is often chronic, lasting 3–4 years. MDD may appear 2–3 years later (double depression).

26

PSYCHIATRY

    c) Evaluation (common for all depressive disorders): Based on a comprehensive psychiatric evaluation. Rating scales (e.g., Beck's Depression Inventory [BDI][7] or the Children's Depression Inventory (CDI])[6] may help assess severity and progress with treatment.

    d) Management (most features common to all depressive disorders)

      i) Treatment setting is selected based on need for safety, risk of suicide, severity of illness, and family support. Education and therapeutic alliance are best developed early in treatment.

      ii) Cognitive behavioral therapy is very effective in mild to moderate depression. Interpersonal and supportive therapy are also helpful in reducing the severity of symptoms.

      iii) Antidepressants (selective serotonin reuptake inhibitors [SSRIs], TCAs) should not be the only modality of treatment. SSRIs (fluoxetine, sertraline, paroxetine) have a safer side-effect profile and do not require ECG or blood level monitoring. Empirical data are limited in children and adolescents: Sertraline has been found to be superior to placebo in the treatment of MDD; in all but one controlled trial, TCAs were not found to be superior to placebo. Baseline ECG, vital signs, and weight are required before a trial with TCAs, and blood levels during maintenance are required. The risk of a lethal overdose of TCAs should be a factor influencing its selection. If the first choice of an antidepressant is not successful, consider changing to another antidepressant in the same class before changing to a medication in another class (e.g., SSRI to a TCA). If the latter is unsuccessful, consider augmentation strategies. At that stage, consider consultation with or transfer of care to a psychiatrist.

2) Bipolar disorder

    a) Prevalence: 20% of adult bipolar disorder patients report onset between 15 and 19 years. Lifetime prevalence for older adolescents is estimated at 1%. Childhood-onset bipolar disorder is being increasingly reported, but its incidence has not been well established.

    b) Diagnosis: A manic episode is characterized by a period of abnormal and persistently elevated or irritable mood lasting a week. During this period, one must have three of the following symptoms: grandiosity, decreased need for sleep, pressured speech, racing thoughts, distractibility, increased goal directed activity (school, sexual), and reckless activity. There are two types: Bipolar I requires at least one manic episode, and bipolar II requires both major depressive episode and hypomania.

   c) Evaluation: Medical conditions mimicking mania (e.g., drug intoxication/withdrawal, thyroid dysfunction, delirium) need to be excluded. Screen for cases of medication-induced mania caused by antidepressants, stimulants, corticosteroids, and bromocriptine.

   d) Management: Treatment of patients with this disorder is multimodal and is best handled by a mental health team. Medications such as lithium, divalproex sodium, and carbamazepine are indicated. Education, support, and insight-oriented therapy are necessary.

c. Anxiety disorders: One of the most prevalent illnesses in children and adolescents.

   1) Separation anxiety disorder: The core feature is an excessive and inappropriate concern regarding separation from attachment figures. Duration of symptoms >4 weeks. Onset age <18 years. Gender ratio is equal. School refusal and sleep problems are very common in these children.

      a) Evaluation: These patients should be screened for comorbid depression and other anxiety disorders. Multidimensional Anxiety Scale for Children (MASC)[8] and other rating scales should be used to assess the severity of symptoms.

      b) Management: Should begin with education of symptoms, clinical course, and outcome. CBT to facilitate separation and ensure rapid return to school. Psychodynamic and family therapy may help patient understand and diminish underlying fears and interrupt patterns of dysfunction. Medications such as SSRIs, TCAs, buspirone, and in some cases benzodiazepines may help reduce the symptoms of anxiety.

   2) Generalized anxiety disorder: Core issue is an excessive worry about school, activities, and/or the future. The presentation includes sleep and concentration difficulties, somatic complaints, restlessness, and irritability. Equal in both sexes as children, but after adolescence, more common in females.

      a) Evaluation and management: Similar to separation anxiety disorder.

   3) Social phobia: Anxiety regarding performance in peer settings and a fear of social situations. This may lead to crying, tantrums, and clinging to caregivers. Duration of symptoms >6 months.

      a) Evaluation and management: Similar to separation anxiety disorder.

   4) Selective mutism: Consistent failure (refusal) to speak in certain situations (most commonly at the school) despite adequate speech at other situations (especially the home). Duration of symptoms >1 month. Quite rare: Prevalence less than 1% of clinical population.

a) Evaluation: Rule out a language disorder, pervasive developmental and psychotic disorders.

b) Management: Behavior management using contingencies and token economy. SSRIs may be helpful in some cases.

5) Obsessive-compulsive disorder

a) Prevalence: 1–3% of adolescent community samples. Equal gender ratio in adolescents. Age of onset is usually in childhood and early adolescence. This disorder often persists for years.

b) Diagnosis: Most common obsessions (repeated and intrusive thoughts) are fear of contamination, obsessive doubting. Common compulsions (repetitive mental or physical acts) are washing, avoidance of contamination, checking, counting, touching, and arranging. They usually describe the need to be 'just right'. Compulsive acts temporarily reduce worry or tension. A special subgroup PANDAS (pediatric autoimmune neuropsychiatric disorders associated with streptococcal infections) have an abrupt onset of symptoms and require specialized assessment.

c) Evaluation: Clinical diagnosis based on interview but may be hidden, requiring the exploration of symptoms. Screen for comorbid depression (20–70%), anxiety disorders (30–50%), and tic disorders (up to 60%). These symptoms may also be seen in patients with eating disorders, pervasive developmental disorders, body dysmorphic disorders, and schizophrenia.

d) Management: Cognitive behavioral therapy is the psychotherapy of choice for obsessive-compulsive disorder. It involves exposing the patient to the anxiety-provoking thought and response prevention with homework assignments and education regarding the illness. Controlled studies have found that medications such as clomipramine, fluvoxamine, and fluoxetine can be effective in reducing the severity of symptoms.

6) Posttraumatic stress disorder (PTSD)

a) Prevalence: 34% of nonreferred urban youth exposed to community violence and 3–100% of at-risk children meet the full criteria for PTSD. Three factors have been found to influence the development of PTSD: Severity of trauma exposure, trauma-related parental distress, and temporal proximity to the traumatic event.

b) Diagnosis

i) Children are more likely to present with reenactment of the trauma in play, nightmares, social withdrawal, regression, new fears, or aggression. They may not meet the *DSM-IV*[1] criteria because of the complexity of the checklist requiring advanced language and cognitive skills.

ii) Adolescents may have the full symptomatology. *DSM-IV*[1] specifies three subtypes: acute (duration of symptoms ,3 months), chronic (duration >3 months), and delayed-onset (onset 6 months after the event).

c) Evaluation: Clinical interviews with direct questions to the child and caregivers. Screen for comorbid depression, substance abuse, and other anxiety disorders.

d) Management: Trauma-specific cognitive-behavioral therapy, psychodynamic therapy, group therapy, and family therapy are often considered the first line of therapy. Medications such as SSRIs, TCAs, and clonidine are often prescribed, but no data are available regarding their efficacy.

d. Eating disorders

1) Types

a) Anorexia nervosa: Is 8–12 times more common in females, rare in prepubertal years; may be one of two types: restricting or binge eating/purging. Typically, self-induced weight below 85% of expected (despite hunger for food), intense fear of fatness, and amenorrhea.

b) Bulimia nervosa: Usually follows anorexia. Characterized by overeating followed by self-induced vomiting or purging, and preoccupation with weight.

i) Evaluation: History, physical examination (hypothermia, bradycardia, hypotension, loss of subcutaneous fat). In cases of frequent vomiting, look for possible dental erosion, palatal trauma, subconjunctival hemorrhage, and metacarpal-phalangeal bruises.

ii) Management: Is multidisciplinary and should combine nutritional and psychologic approaches. It is very important to build rapport and gain the support of parents.

e. Bereavement/grief (especially secondary to the death of a parent or close relative): Patients wish to die, are sad, have sleep/appetite changes, and see or hear the dead person. The duration and expression of grief is highly variable but usually lasts <2 months. Children <5 years of age are likely to interpret death as sleep or a long journey. The 5–9 year olds better understand death but may not believe it can happen to them. Older children better accept that death is inevitable and is a universal occurrence.

1) Management: It is important to support the surviving parent in informing the child, providing a choice to attend and even help with the funeral, and encouraging reading on the subject. Since the very young compare death to a journey or long sleep, such an explanation should never be given because it can cause sleep problems. Bereavement is considered complicated if it lasts >6 months or presents with suicidal ideation, worthlessness, prolonged impaired functioning, and other hallucinations. Depression is the

most common complication in this setting, and it needs prompt attention.

f. Parental divorce/separation

1) Prevalence: 38% of all children born in the mid-1980s will face the divorce of their parents.

2) Risk factors for poorer outcome: Sudden or prolonged conflictual or hostile break-ups.

3) Evaluation: Preschool children may regress, yearn for the departed parent, and develop sleep problems. Prepubertal children may express anger, take sides, or develop school-related or peer problems. Adolescents may develop depression, anxiety, anger, or suicidal behaviors.

4) Management: Availability of mediation services through the courts is increasing. Disputed custody or visitations often impair the psychologic adjustment of the child to the new life situation. Family therapy needs to address the parent-child relationship. Parents may need to be educated about the psychologic impact of divorce on children. The child and the family should be screened for psychiatric disorders and treated appropriately. Support groups are often helpful.

V. PSYCHIATRY DRUG FORMULARY (Table 26.1)

TABLE 26.1

PSYCHIATRY DRUG FORMULARY

Agent	Suggested dose	Kinetics	Side effects/comments
STIMULANTS (ADHD TREATMENT)			
Methylphenidate (Ritalin) 5mg, 10mg, 20mg tabs	Starting dose: 2.5–5mg BID (breakfast/lunch) or 0.3mg/kg/dose. Increase 2.5–5 mg Qweek as needed. Max dose: 80mg/day Divided BID–QID.	Onset: within 30min Peak action: 1.9hr Duration: 4–6hr	Nervousness, insomnia, anorexia, weight loss/decreased growth velocity, tics, stomach aches, headaches. Use with caution in children with underlying seizure disorder. Contraindicated with MAOIs. Monitor height, weight, and blood pressure. Avoid caffeine and decongestants.
Methylphenidate sustained release (Ritalin SR) 20mg tabs	Starting dose: 20mg QD. Max dose 80mg/day.	Onset: 60–90min Peak action: 4.7hr Duration: 8hr	Do not crush or chew tablets. See comments for methylphenidate.
Dextroamphetamine (Dexedrine) 5mg, 10mg tabs	Starting dose 3–5yr: 2.5mg QD or 0.15mg/kg/dose. Adjust by 2.5–5mg Qweek. Starting dose: ≥6 yr: 5mg QD or BID. Increase by 5mg Qweek. Max dose: 40mg/day. Dosed QD–TID.	Onset: 20–60min Peak action: 2hr Duration: 4–6hr	See comments for methylphenidate.

From *Physicians' desk reference*[15] and Riddle[16].

MAOIs, monoamine oxidase inhibitors.

NOTE: Additional information for many of these drugs can be found in ch.29 (formulary).

NOTE: Most of these drugs have not been FDA approved for pediatric use. They are listed here based on material presented in *The Pediatric Clinics of North America*[18], October 1998 edition on Child and Adolescent Psychopharmacology, as a reference guide. It should be noted that most have not undergone rigorous extensive safety or efficacy testing in the pediatric age group.

26

PSYCHIATRY

Continued

TABLE 26.1

PSYCHIATRY DRUG FORMULARY—cont'd

Agent	Suggested dose	Kinetics	Side effects/comments
STIMULANTS (ADHD TREATMENT)—cont'd			
Dextroamphetamine extended release (Dexedrine Spansule) 5mg, 10mg, 15mg capsules	Starting dose: 5mg QD (or 0.3mg/kg/dose). Max dose: 40mg/day.	Onset: 60–90min Peak action: 8–10hr	See comments for methylphenidate.
Mixed Amphetamine Salts (Adderall) 5mg, 10mg, 20mg, 30mg	Starting dose: 2.5–5mg Qam. Increase by 2.5–5mg Qweek. Dosed QD–BID.	Onset: Estimated at 30min Duration: Estimated at 5–7hr	Limited information available.
Pemoline (Cyclert)	Starting dose: 37.5mg Qam. Increase by 18.75mg Qweek. Max dose: 112.5mg.	Onset: 2hr Duration: 12–24hr	Not first line for ADHD because of association with life-threatening liver failure. Follow LFTs. May also cause choreoathetoid movements. See comments for methylphenidate.
ANTIPSYCHOTICS			
Haloperidol (Haldol)	See ch. 29 (formulary).		Baseline HR, BP, LFTs. Check Q3mo, with dose changes. In general, anticholinergic effects: Orthostatic hypotension, sedation, weight gain, dystonic reactions.
Thioridazine (Mellaril)	See ch. 29 (formulary).		See comments for haloperidol.
Olanzapine (Zyprex)	Prepubescent: 2.5mg QD. Adol: 5mg QD Increase Q3–4 days to max: 20mg/day.		See comments for haloperidol.

Risperidone (Risperdal)	Prepubescent: 0.25mg/day. Adol: 0.5mg/day QD/ BID. Adult: 1mg BID. Increase Q week 1mg BID. Max: 3mg BID.	Renal/hepatic dosing. See comments for haloperidol.
ANXIOLYTICS		
Buspirone (Buspar)	Prepubescent: 2.5–5mg/day. Increase by 2.5mg/day Q3–4 days. Max: 20mg/day ÷ Q12hr. Adolescent: 5–10mg/day. Increase by 5mg/day Q3–4 days. Max: 60mg/day ÷ Q12hr.	Tachycardia, CNS effects (headache, insomnia, confusion, dizziness). GI effects.
Lorazepam (Ativan)	See ch. 29 (formulary).	
MOOD STABILIZERS		
Lithium	See ch. 29 (formulary). *Therapeutic level:* 0.6–1.5mEq/L.	Obtain levels Qweek until stable. Check renal, hepatic, thyroid panels; calcium CBC, ECG before therapy. Check renal fctn Q2–3 mo, thyroid Q6mo.
Divalproex sodium (Depakote)	15mg/kg/day ÷ BID–TID. Max: 60mg/kg. Therapeutic level: 50–60mEq/L.	β-HCG, CBC, LFTs before therapy. LFT, CBC Q6mo.

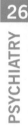

26

PSYCHIATRY

Continued

From *Physicians' desk reference*[15] and Riddle[16].

NOTE: Additional information for many of these drugs can be found in ch.29 (formulary).

NOTE: Most of these drugs have not been FDA approved for pediatric use. They are listed here based on material presented in *The Pediatric Clinics of North America*[18], October 1998 edition on Child and Adolescent Psychopharmacology, as a reference guide. It should be noted that most have not undergone rigorous extensive safety or efficacy testing in the pediatric age group.

TABLE 26.1

PSYCHIATRY DRUG FORMULARY—cont'd

Drug type/name	Dosage	Side effects/monitoring
MOOD STABILIZERS—cont'd		
Carbamezapine (Tegretol)	See ch. 29 (formulary).	CBC, LFTs, β-HCG before therapy.
ANTIDEPRESSANTS/ANXIOLYTICS		
Selective serotonin reuptake inhibitors (SSRIs)		
Fluoxetine (Prozac)	5–18 yr: 5–10mg/day. Max: 60mg/day.	Do not use if MAOIs used in previous 14 days. Can cause GI upset, CNS side effects (including headache, nervousness, sedation).
Fluvoxamine (Luvox)	8–17yr: 25mg initially QHS. Adjust by 25mg increments Q4–7 days. Max: 250mg/day ÷ BID.	Contraindications: MAOIs, cisapride, terfenadine aztemizole. Smoking increases levels.
Paroxetine (Paxil)	Child: initially 5–10mg/day. Max: 40mg/day.	Purpura, hyponatremia, cytochrome p450 system (multiple drug interactions). See comments for fluoxetine.
Sertraline (Zoloft)	OCD: 6–12yr: 25mg/day. Increase by 1-week intervals. 13–17 yr: 50mg/day. Max: 200mg/day.	See comments for fluoxetine.

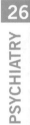

Tricyclics (TCAS)

Nortryptyline (Pamelor)	See ch. 29 (formulary).	Check CBC, LFTs, BP before therapy. ECG before therapy, with every dose increase, and Q1mo × 6mo then Q6mo. Check TCA level with each ECG. Side effects include anticholinergic effects (dry mouth, weight gain, sedation). Recommend slow taper.
Imipramine (Tofranil)	See ch. 29 (formulary).	See comments for nortryptyline.
Desipiramine (Norpramin)	6–12yr: 1–3mg/kg/day QHS or BID. Adol: 25–50mg/day.	Blood dyscrasia, GI side effects, photosensitivity, arrhythmias. See comments for nortryptyline. Does not cause weight gain. Level: 150–250mcg/ml.
Anafranil (Clomipramine)	>10yr: With food, 25mg/day. Increase over 2wk to 100mg/day or 3mg/kg/day in divided doses.	Seizures, anticholinergic effect, nausea, anorexia, weight gain.

From Physicians' desk reference[15] and Riddle[16].

NOTE: Additional information for many of these drugs can be found in ch.29 (formulary).

NOTE: Most of these drugs have not been FDA approved for pediatric use. They are listed here based on material presented in The Pediatric Clinics of North America[18], October 1998 edition on Child and Adolescent Psychopharmacology, as a reference guide. It should be noted that most have not undergone rigorous extensive safety or efficacy testing in the pediatric age group.

Continued

TABLE 26.1

PSYCHIATRY DRUG FORMULARY—cont'd

Drug type/name		Dosage	Side effects/monitoring
ANTIDEPRESSANTS/ANXIOLYTICS—cont'd			
Serotonin norepinephrine reuptake inhibitor			
Venlafaxine (Effexor)	8–12yr	Initially: 12.5mg/day × 3 days. Increase by 12.5mg BID × 3 days. Can increase to 12.5mg TID.	Nausea, dizziness, somnolence constipation, xerostomia.
	13–17yr	25mg/day × 3 days, then 25mg BID × 3 days, and 25mg TID.	
5-HT blockers			
Nefazodone (Serzone)		Begin 50mg BID. Titrate to effectiveness by 50mg Q3 days. Child: Max: 300mg/day. >12yr: 600mg/day.	Nausea, dizziness, priapism agitation, dry mouth, vision changes. Contraindications: MAOIs, aztemizole, cisapride, terfenadine.
Trazadone (Desyrel)		6–18 yr: initially 1.5–2mg/kg/day. Increase Q3-4 days prn. Max 6mg/kg/day + TID. Adol: initially 25–50mg/day. Increase to 100–150mg/day.	Priapism, fewer anticholinergic effects drowsiness, blurred vision. Monitor BP, mental status, LFTs.
Other			
Wellbutrin		>18 yr: 100mg BID × 3 days. Increase by 100mg TID (min: Q6hr). Max: 450mg/day, 150mg/dose/4hr.	CNS stimulation, weight change dry mouth, headache, GI effects. Contraindications: seizures, eating disorders, MAOIs.

From *Physicians' desk reference*[15] and Riddle[16].

MAOIs, monoamine oxidase inhibitors.

NOTE: Additional information for many of these drugs can be found in ch.29 (formulary).

NOTE: Most of these drugs have not been FDA approved for pediatric use. They are listed here based on material presented in *The Pediatric Clinics of North America*[18], October 1998 edition on Child and Adolescent Psychopharmacology, as a reference guide. It should be noted that most have not undergone rigorous extensive safety or efficacy testing in the pediatric age group.

26

PSYCHIATRY

VI. REFERENCES

1. American Psychiatric Association. *Diagnostic and statistical manual for mental disorders (DSM-IV),* 4th edn. Washington, DC: The Association; 1994.

2. American Academy of Pediatrics. *Classification of child and adolescent mental diagnoses in primary care: diagnostic and statistical manual for primary care (DSM-PC).* Elk Grove Village, IL: The Academy; 1996.

3. Conners CK. *Conners' rating scales.* Toronto: Multi-Health Systems; 1995.

4. Folstein MF, Folstein SE, McHugh PR. Mini-Mental State: a practical method for grading the cognitive state of patients for the clinician. *J Psychiatr Res* 1975; **12:**196–198.

5. Cockrell JR, Folstein MF. Mini-Mental State Examination (MMSE). *Psychopharmacol Bull* 1988; **24:**685–692.

6. Kovac M. The Children's Depression Inventory (CDI). *Psychopharmacol Bull* 1985; **21:**995–998.

7. Beck AT et al. Beck's Depression Inventory (BDI). *Arch Gen Psychiatry* 1961; **4:**561–571.

8. March JS, Parker JD, Sullivan K, Stallings P, Conners CK. The Multidimensional Anxiety Scale for Children (MASC): factor, structure, reliability, and validity. *J Am Acad Child Adolesc Psychiatry* **36(4):**554–565, 1997.

9. Lewis M, ed. *Child and adolescent psychiatry: a comprehensive textbook.* Baltimore: Williams & Wilkins; 1991.

10. Reviews in Child and Adolescent Psychiatry. Reprinted from *J Am Acad Child Adolesc Psychiatry.* Edited by Mina Dulcan.

11. American Academy of Child and Adolescent Psychiatry. AACAP official action: practice parameters for the assessment and treatment of children and adolescents with anxiety disorders. *J Am Acad Child Adolesc Psychiatry* 1997-1998; **36-37:**suppl.

12. Miller G. *The Substance Abuse Subtle Screening Inventory (SASSI): adolescent version.* Bloomington, IN: SASSI Institute; 1990.

13. Rahder E. *The adolescent assessment and referral manual (POSIT).* Rockville, MD: National Institute on Drug Abuse; 1991.

14. Weinberg NZ, Rahdert E, Colliver JD, Glantz MD. Adolescent substance abuse: a review of the past 10 years. *J Am Acad Child Adolesc Psychiatry* **37(3):**252–261, 1998.

15. *Physicians' desk reference, 53rd edn.* Montvale, NJ: Medical Economics; 1999.

16. Riddle MA, Subramaniam G, Walkup J. Efficacy of psychiatric medications in children and adolescents: a review of controlled trials. *Psychiatric Clinics of North America: annual drug therapy,* 1998.

17. Barkley RA, Edelbrach CS. Assessing situational variation in children's behavior problems: the home and school situations questionnaires. In Prinz R, ed. *Advances in behavioral assessment of children and families.* Greenwich, CT: JAI Press; 1987.
18. *Pediatr Clin North Am* 1998; **45(5)**.

I. PLAIN FILMS

A. CHEST

1. **Pneumonia:** Lobar or segmental consolidation and atelectasis are more typical of bacterial infections, whereas hyperinflation, bilateral patchy or streaky densities, and peribronchial thickening are more typical of nonbacterial disease.

2. **Atelectasis vs infiltrate**

   a. Atelectasis: When air is removed from the lung, the tissue collapses. Air may still remain in the larger bronchi, making air bronchograms on the radiograph. Collapse and reexpansion can happen very quickly.

   b. Infiltrate: A fluid (blood, pus, edema) that invades one of the compartments of the lung (bronchoalveolar air space or peribronchial interstitial space) shows as a density on a radiograph. Where alveolar air is displaced by fluid, but air remains in the bronchi, the classic pneumonic infiltrate with air bronchogram is seen. Where the infiltrate is interstitial, its borders are more vague, and bronchial walls may be thickened. Typically, infiltrates resolve in 2–6 weeks.

3. **Central line placement:** Central venous catheters ideally placed with the catheter tip at the junction of the superior vena cava and right atrium. Some extension into the right atrium is acceptable, but if the catheter is noted to curve to the patient's left on the posteroanterior (PA) film, the catheter may be positioned in the right ventricle (Fig. 27.1).

4. **Endotracheal tube (ETT) placement:** The end of the ETT should rest approximately 2–3cm above the carina, at the level of T3–T4. (This may vary somewhat depending on the size of the patient.) The lung fields should show symmetric aeration.

5. **Anatomy** (Fig. 27.2)

B. ABDOMEN:
Plain films of the abdomen are useful in evaluating for obstruction, pneumoperitoneum, and mass effect. In the radiologic evaluation of the acute abdomen, at least two films should be obtained.

1. **Supine:** Useful for evaluating bowel distention.

2. **Either a left lateral decubitus of the abdomen or a supine cross-table lateral film:** For free air, necrotizing enterocolitis, or intussusception.

3. **Chest radiologic examination:** Should always be considered so that pulmonary pathology, which can mimic an abdominal process, can be excluded.

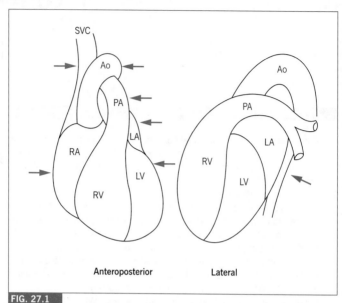

FIG. 27.1

Diagram of the heart. Arrows indicate contours seen on anteroposterior and lateral chest x-ray films. Ao, aorta; LA, left atrium; LV, left ventricle; PA, pulmonary artery; RA, right atrium; RV, right ventricle; SVC, superior vena cava. (From Kirks[1].)

C. **CERVICAL SPINE:** After immobilization in a collar, lateral/anteroposterior (lateral/AP) radiologic examinations of the cervical spine should be performed in all children who have sustained significant head trauma or deceleration injury or who have undergone unwitnessed trauma for which no history can be obtained. The seventh cervical vertebrae must be visualized. Flexion/extension films may be helpful, especially in patients with Down syndrome who are at risk for atlantoaxial subluxation. Odontoid views may be helpful in older children with suspected occipitocervical injury (e.g., whiplash). Cervical spine injuries are most common from the occiput to C3 in children and in the lower cervical spine in adults.

D. **AIRWAY FILMS:** The lateral view of the upper airway is the single most useful film for evaluating a child with stridor. If possible, this view should be obtained on inspiration. A radiologic workup should always include AP and lateral views of the chest, with inclusion of the upper airway on the AP chest film.

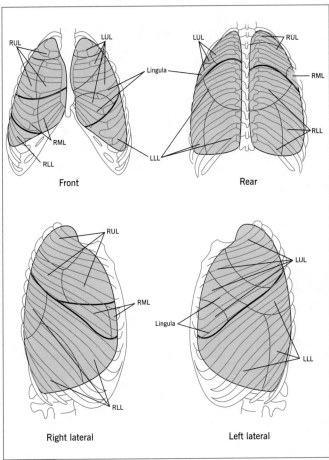

FIG. 27.2

Lung anatomy. LLL, left lower lobe; LUL, left upper lobe; RLL, right lower lobe; RML, right middle lobe; RUL, right upper lobe. Divisions within lobes indicate segments.

1. **Diagnosis of diseases based on airway radiologic examination** (Table 27.1 and Fig. 27.3).
2. **Foreign bodies**
a. Lower airway foreign bodies: In the absence of a radiopaque foreign body, radiologic findings include air trapping, hyperinflation, atelectasis, consolidation, pneumothorax, and pneumomediastinum. If suspected clinically or on the basis of an initially abnormal chest radiograph,

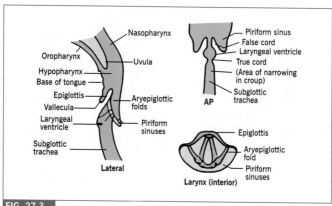

FIG. 27.3
Normal upper airway anatomy.

TABLE 27.1

DIAGNOSIS OF DISEASES BASED ON AIRWAY RADIOLOGIC EXAMINATION

Diagnosis	Findings on airway films
Croup	AP and lateral films with subglottic narrowing ('steeple sign')
Epiglottitis	Enlarged, indistinct epiglottis on lateral film ('thumb sign')
Vascular ring	AP and lateral films with narrowing; double or right aortic arch
Retropharyngeal abscess or pharyngeal mass	Soft tissue air or persistent enlargement of prevertebral soft tissues; more than half of a vertebral body above C3 and one vertebral body below C3
Immunodeficiency	Absence of adenoidal and tonsillar tissue after age 6mo

further evaluative studies should include expiratory films (cooperative patient), bilateral decubitus chest films (uncooperative patient), or airway fluoroscopy.

b. Esophageal foreign bodies: Esophageal foreign bodies usually lodge at one of three locations: At the thoracic inlet, at the level of the aortic arch–left mainstem bronchus, or at the gastroesophageal junction. Evaluation should include the following:

1) Lateral airway film.

2) AP film of the chest and abdomen (including the supraclavicular region).

3. **If these films are normal and an esophageal foreign body is still suspected:** A contrast study of the esophagus may reveal it. If perforation is suspected, use a nonionic, water-soluble contrast.

E. **EXTREMITY X-RAY STUDIES:** In suspected trauma, an adequate evaluation requires at least two views, usually an AP and a lateral. Restricting the film to include only the area of interest improves the resolution (e.g., for a thumb injury, ask for an image of the thumb, not the hand). In general, comparison films of the uninvolved extremity are not necessary, but they may be helpful in several instances, such as the evaluation of joint effusions (particularly the hip), suspected osteomyelitis, or pyarthrosis and/or the evaluation of subtle fractures, especially in areas of multiple ossification centers such as the elbow. **Bone age** determinations traditionally use a PA view of the left hand and wrist.

F. **SKELETAL SURVEY:** The skeletal survey is the appropriate radiologic series to order in cases of suspected child abuse or metastatic disease. This survey should include a lateral skull film with a cervical spine film, an AP chest film (bone technique), an oblique view of the ribs, AP view of the pelvis, an abdominal film (bone technique) with the lateral thoracic and lumbar spine, and AP long bone films. Classic findings are multiple epiphyseal and metaphyseal injuries of various ages. In addition, suspicion should be raised by fracture at unusual sites or solitary spiral and transverse fractures of the long bones, with a history of inconsistent trauma.

G. **SPINE FILMS:** Scoliosis is evaluated by an erect AP spine radiograph. PA views can be used in postpubertal girls to decrease breast radiation dose. For evaluation and management, see pp. 116–117. For spondylolysis and spondylolisthesis, oblique films should also be obtained.

II. CONVENTIONAL GRAY SCALE ULTRASONOGRAPHY

A. **APPLICATIONS**
1. Pyloric stenosis
2. Abdominal masses in young children
3. Intussusception
4. Tuboovarian abscess
5. Acute intracranial hemorrhage in newborns
6. Definition of renal pathology
7. Congenital hip dislocation in children <4 months of age
8. Fluid collections (e.g., hip effusions, pleural effusions, ascites)
9. Biliary tree and gallbladder evaluation.

B. **ADVANTAGES:** No radiation exposure, painless, no sedation required, portable.

C. **DISADVANTAGES:** Gas and fat may degrade image; operator dependent.

27

RADIOLOGY

D. **PREPARATION:** Obtain this test before barium studies. Patient must be well hydrated for pelvic and lower abdomen studies; no voiding for 1–3 hours.

III. COLOR DOPPLER FLOW IMAGING

Moving blood is detected by ultrasonographic frequency shifts. Can be used to evaluate deep vein thrombosis, vascular patency, intracranial blood flow, cardiac shunt flow, transplant vascularity, and testicular perfusion. Power Doppler, available in some centers, is particularly sensitive in detecting slow flow in small vessels (e.g., infant testes).

IV. COMPUTED TOMOGRAPHY (CT)

A. **APPLICATIONS**
1. **Modality of choice:** For the evaluation of acute intracranial trauma, hydrocephalus, pulmonary parenchymal disease, calcifying processes, abdominal and chest trauma, and complicated inflammatory bowel disease. In children with blunt abdominal trauma, a CT scan of the abdomen, including the lower portion of the chest, should be obtained.
2. **Three-dimensional CT reconstruction:** Useful for evaluating complex craniofacial injuries and other complex skeletal deformities.
B. **ADVANTAGES:** Less costly than magnetic resonance imaging (MRI), sensitive to calcium, operator-independent interpretation, wide field of view. Spiral scanning also decreases the need for sedation.
C. **DISADVANTAGES:** Ionizing radiation exposure, not sensitive to diffuse white matter or cutaneous abnormalities, limited scanning planes, and IV contrast exposure.
D. **INDICATIONS FOR ORAL AND IV CONTRAST:** For abdominal study, use both oral and IV contrast. For a chest study, use only IV contrast. Avoid oral contrast in the child with intractable vomiting. Avoid IV contrast if there is renal compromise or allergy to IV contrast.
E. **PREPARATION:** No solid foods 3 hours before study. No liquids 30 minutes before. Sedation protocols require longer periods without liquids.

V. SPECIAL CT SCANS

A. **ULTRAFAST CT:** This technique permits cine imaging of a dynamic process such as trachea shape with breathing, uses reduced radiation dosing, and takes only 50–100msec to complete. A disadvantage is a somewhat decreased image quality compared with conventional CT.
B. **HIGH-RESOLUTION CT:** This permits edge enhancement and is good for imaging lung parenchyma.

VI. MAGNETIC RESONANCE IMAGING (Table 27.2)

A. APPLICATIONS

1. **CNS:** Better than CT for evaluating the posterior fossa, brainstem, and spinal cord, including defects such as meningomyelocele. Excellent for evaluating demyelination disorders because it differentiates between areas of normal and abnormal myelin content. Useful in the workup of focal seizures in which a structural lesion may be involved. However, MRI may not reveal calcifications that characterize some neoplastic lesions. Useful in the evaluation of suspected intentional injury by detecting diffuse axonal injury and determining ages of multiple extraaxial hemorrhages.

2. **Mediastinal lymphadenopathy**

3. **Cardiac:** MRI provides excellent contrast between flowing blood and myocardium without the use of IV agents. Also used for detecting vascular anomalous vessels (e.g., vascular ring).

4. **Abdomen:** More sensitive than CT for evaluating the extent of hepatic tumors before surgical resection.

5. **Skeletal:** Useful in detecting early signs of osteomyelitis and avascular necrosis of the femoral head. Can detect the extension of bone tumors and marrow replacement by leukemic infiltrates.

B. **ADVANTAGES:** No ionizing radiation, multiple imaging planes, sensitive to the presence of abnormal tissues.

C. **DISADVANTAGES:** Difficult to accommodate critical care equipment. Patients with implanted ferromagnetic devices (e.g., pacemakers, implanted heart valves, osteotomy hardware) cannot be scanned. Sensitive to motion degradation. Frequently requires sedation. Poor signal from calcium and gas.

D. **INDICATIONS FOR CONTRAST:** Contrast is not used routinely; consult a radiologist.

E. **PREPARATION:** Depends on sedation protocol considerations; consider a mild anxiolytic for older children.

27

RADIOLOGY

TABLE 27.2

T1- AND T2-WEIGHTED IMAGING

	T1-weighted images	T2-weighted images
Fat	Increased	Intermediate
Flowing blood	No signal	No signal
Acute hematoma	Intermediate	Decreased
Subacute hematoma	Increased	Increased
Chronic blood (hemosiderin)	Decreased	Decreased
Muscle	Intermediate	Intermediate

Courtesy Laureen Sena, MD.
Increased means 'brighter'; *decreased* means 'darker'.

VII. SPECIAL TESTS

A. **GASTROINTESTINAL:** Barium usually contrast of choice. Water-soluble contrast medium should be used if perforation or leak is suspected. Gas-producing agents may be used for providing double contrast.

1. **Upper gastrointestinal study:** Contrast is ingested; esophagus, stomach, and duodenum are visualized by fluoroscopy and plain films. Test can be expanded to include small intestine if small bowel follow-through is requested.

a. Indications: Esophageal webs and rings, masses, gastric volvulus, gastroesophageal reflux evaluation (to exclude other causes of reflux symptoms); motility problems, ulcerations, strictures/obstruction, hiatal hernias, varices, and gastric outlet obstruction (e.g., pyloric stenosis). Limited sensitivity in detecting mucosal disease.

b. Preparation: <18 months: Nothing by mouth (NPO) for 3 hours before study. >18 months: NPO for 4 hours before. Clear liquids only after midnight. Consider bisacodyl pills/suppositories and magnesium citrate for older children.

2. **Barium enema**

a. Indications: Polyps, strictures/Hirschsprung's disease, colitis, volvulus, meconium ileus, intussusception.

b. Preparation: <18 months: Liquid diet starting evening before. >18 months: Liquid diet for 24 hours before. Consider bisacodyl/suppositories and enemas, and magnesium citrate for older children.

B. **GENITOURINARY**

1. **Voiding cystourethrogram:** Water-soluble contrast fills the bladder through a urinary catheter; the catheter is then removed. Plain films taken during filling and voiding.

a. Indications: Vesicoureteral reflux, abnormalities of bladder function and anatomy.

b. Preparation: No urination just before examination. (Some urine needs to be in the bladder.) Can be uncomfortable and requires urinary catheterization.

2. **Intravenous urogram:** Contrast given IV and timed plain films taken as contrast is excreted in the kidneys.

a. Indications: Collecting system abnormalities, duplex kidneys. Rarely first examination for urinary tract.

b. Preparation: No food or fluid 2–3 hours before. Invasive, requires IV contrast, which may aggravate renal failure.

VIII. COMMONLY USED NUCLEAR MEDICINE PROCEDURES
(Table 27.3)

TABLE 27.3
COMMONLY USED NUCLEAR MEDICINE PROCEDURES

Study/agent\	Indication	Patient preparation/technique	Physiology/mechanism
Musculoskeletal			
Bone scan ^{99m}Tc-MDP	Benign or metastatic bone disorders	No preparation	Localizes at sites of osteoblastic or osteoclastic activity
	Unexplained bone pain	IV injection	
	Child abuse	Delayed imaging at 3–4 hours	
Three-phase bone scan (^{99}Tc-MDP)	Infection or inflammation (osteomyelitis, septic arthritis), AVN, fracture	No preparation	Blood flow and extracellular information helpful in infection or inflammation
		Immediate blood flow, extracellular phases	
		Delayed imaging at 3–4hr	
Gallium scan (^{67}Ga citrate)	Infections	Bowel preparation	Ga^{2+} is an Fe^{2+} analog; binds to serum proteins
	Some tumors (Hodgkin's lymphoma)	Imaging times dependent on indication or interference from bowel activity (24, 48, 72, 96hr)	Partial excretion in colon
			Sometimes better for chronic infection
White blood cell scan (^{111}In-labeled WBCs)	Infections	Blood withdrawal	Localizes active inflammation or infection
		WBC labeling, reinjection	No bowel excretion
		Imaging at 24 and/or 48hr	
Neurologic			
Brain blood flow scan (^{99}Tc-DTPA)	Adjunct in assessment of brain death	No preparation	Absent perfusion is compatible with brain death

AVN, avascular necrosis; DTPA, diethylenetriaminepentaacetic acid.

Continued

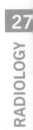

27

RADIOLOGY

TABLE 27.3

COMMONLY USED NUCLEAR MEDICINE PROCEDURES—cont'd

Study/agent	Indication	Patient preparation/technique	Physiology/mechanism
Neurologic—cont'd			
Brain scan (^{99m}Tc-ECD or ^{99m}Tc-HMPAO)	Localization of epileptic foci Cerebral vascular disease	No preparation	Ictal foci show increased flow Tracer follows blood flow
Cisternography (^{111}In-DTPA)	Hydrocephalus CSF leak	No preparation Tracer injected into subarachnoid space	Tracer follows CSF flow
CSF shunt patency (^{111}In-DTPA)	Assess patency of VP, LP, VA shunts	No preparation Injection into reservoir/shunt	Tracer follows CSF flow
Respiratory			
V/Q scan (^{99m}Tc-MAA perfusion, ^{133}Xe ventilation)	Assess congenital pulmonary or vascular anomalies Pulmonary embolus	No preparation	IV-injected MAA trapped in the pulmonary capillary bed ^{133}Xe gas inhaled
Gastrointestinal			
Gastric emptying or reflux study (^{99m}Tc-sulfur colloid)	Quantitative assessment of solid or liquid emptying Gastric reflux	NPO the evening before study	Tracer is not absorbed in the gastrointestinal tract Assess for GER or pulmonary aspiration
Hepatobiliary (^{99m}Tc-mebrofenin)	Neonatal hepatitis vs biliary atresia Biliary leak after trauma or transplant	Phenobarbital 2.5mg/kg Q12hr 3–5 days before imaging No preparation	Phenobarbital increases bile secretion; in hepatitis, helps in tracer transit In leaks, tracer extravasates into peritoneal cavity

Procedure	Indications	Preparation	Comments
Liver-spleen scan (^{99m}Tc-sulfur colloid)	Defining organs in congenital anomalies (splenosis, asplenia); Assess splenic function	No preparation	Tracer taken up by RES in liver (Kupffer's cells), spleen, bone marrow
Meckel's scan (^{99m}Tc-pertechnetate)	Gastrointestinal bleeding	(Optional) pentagastrin, cimetidine, glucagon	Tracer localizes to mucinous cells in Meckel's diverticula
Genitourinary			
Radionuclide cystogram (^{99m}Tc-pertechnetate)	Vesicoureteral reflux; Functional bladder capacity	Bladder catheterization; Direct infusion of tracer via bladder catheter	Dynamic imaging of bladder filling and voiding; Sensitive in detection of VUR
Renal scan ^{99m}Tc-DTPA or ^{99m}Tc-MAG$_3$	Renal function; Renovascular hypertension (RAS); Ureteral obstruction	Bladder catheterization (optional if no obstruction); Initial 30min imaging; Lasix washout 30min (optional)	^{99m}Tc-DTPA is excreted by filtration (GFR); Captopril challenge for RAS; Lasix washout slower in obstruction
^{99m}Tc-DMSA or ^{99m}Tc-glucoheptonate	Renal cortical scarring; Pyelonephritis	^{99m}Tc-DMSA: Imaging at 4hr; Glucoheptonate: Initial 2hr delayed imaging	Tracers localize in the renal tubules, providing an indicator of function
Testicular scan (^{99m}Tc-pertechnetate)	Suspected testicular torsion vs epididymitis	No preparation	Absent flow in torsion; increased in epididymitis

CSF, cerebrospinal fluid; LP, lumbar puncture; VA, ventriculoatrial; V/Q, ventilation/perfusion; MAA, macroaggregated albumin; PE, pulmonary embolism; VP, ventriculoperitoneal; GER, gastroesophageal reflux; GFR, glomerular filtration rate; RES, reticuloendothelial system; VUR, vesicoureteral reflux; RAS, renal artery stenosis. NPO, nothing by mouth;

27

RADIOLOGY

IX. REFERENCE

1. Kirks DR et al. *Practical pediatric imaging: diagnostic radiology of infants and children.* Boston: Little, Brown; 1991.

SURGERY

Karen E. Lantz, MD

I. GENERAL SURGERY

A. GASTROSCHISIS/OMPHALOCELE[1]

1. **Definitions**
   a. Gastroschisis: Abdominal wall defect separate from and usually to the right of the umbilicus; usually intestine/stomach/bladder/liver are outside the peritoneal cavity. May be complicated by bowel atresia (from ischemic insult) and malrotation.
   b. Omphalocele: Rotational anomaly associated with embryologic failure of intestines +/− viscera to return to the abdominal cavity; presents as intestines/organs (usually liver and stomach) covered by peritoneum and/or amniotic membrane at the umbilical orifice. Usually associated with other congenital anomalies (cardiac, genitourinary, nervous system); can be a part of pentalogy of Cantrell (omphalocele, ectopia cordis, intracardiac malformation, sternal cleft, diaphragmatic hernia).
2. **Studies:** Echocardiogram, renal ultrasonography for associated defects.
3. **Management**
   a. Immediate: NPO, nasogastric decompression, IV hydration; maintain moisture, limit contamination (bowel bag); surgical consultation.
   b. Definitive: Operative correction, either primary or staged; outcome depends on associated anomalies.

B. CONGENITAL DIAPHRAGMATIC HERNIA

1. **Definition:** Persistence of the posterolateral foramen of Bochdalek (most common on the left side), allowing abdominal cavity contents to penetrate the thoracic cavity.
2. **Clinical presentation:** Respiratory distress and cyanosis (secondary to pulmonary hypoplasia/hypertension), decreased breath sounds, displaced cardiac sounds, bowel sounds in chest, scaphoid abdomen, asymmetric chest wall movement.
3. **Studies:** Chest or abdominal radiograph with air-filled loops in affected hemithorax and mediastinal shift; often diagnosed on prenatal ultrasonography.
4. **Management**
   a. Immediate: Endotracheal intubation in delivery room (avoid mask ventilation secondary to resulting bowel distention and further respiratory compromise), NPO, nasogastric decompression, medical management of pulmonary hypertension.
   b. Definitive: Operative correction when pulmonary hypertension resolved (usually within 3–5 days).

28

C. **ESOPHAGEAL ATRESIA/TRACHEOESOPHAGEAL FISTULA**[2]
1. **Definition:** Atresia or partial absence of esophagus and/or communication (fistula) between the trachea and esophagus (Fig. 28.1).
2. **Clinical presentation:** Inability to pass nasogastric tube or swallow food, respiratory distress (cough, cyanosis, aspiration, pneumonia of the right upper lobe after feeding), excessive salivation. H-type fistulas (Fig. 28.1, *E*) usually present with cough and/or choking.
3. **Studies:** Chest and abdominal radiographs (distended stomach, coiled nasogastric tube); may need bronchoscopy and/or upper GI or swallow study (risk of aspiration). Echocardiogram to determine aortic arch position for surgical approach.
4. **Management**
a. Immediate: NPO, minimize gastroesophageal reflux (upright position, H_2-receptor blocker, prokinetic agent) and aspiration (sump tube in proximal esophageal stump, reverse Trendelenburg position); treatment of pneumonia if present.
b. Definitive: Operative esophageal anastomosis and/or ligation of fistula.
D. **PYLORIC STENOSIS**[4]
1. **Definition:** Hypertrophy of the pyloric sphincter, causing functional gastric outlet obstruction. Age usually 3–6 weeks, hereditary component, more common in firstborn boys.

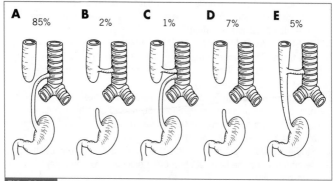

FIG. 28.1

Relative incidence of various types of esophageal atresia/tracheoesophageal fistula. **A,** Esophageal atresia with fistula to the distal pouch. **B,** Esophageal atresia with tracheoesophageal fistula to the proximal pouch of the esophagus. **C,** Esophageal atresia with two fistulas, one to each esophageal pouch. **D,** Esophageal atresia without fistula. **E,** Tracheoesophageal fistula without atresia, the so called H type. (Modified from Myers[3].)

2. **Clinical presentation:** Persistent, Progressive, Projectile <u>nonbilious</u> emesis; Poor weight gain; Peristaltic waves; Palpable Pyloric 'olive' (70–90%)[5]; Prominent metabolic alkalosis; and Paradoxic aciduria (late sign).

3. **Studies (after surgical consultation):** Ultrasonography (operator dependent, 90% sensitive, considered positive if muscle thickness >4mm and length >16mm)[6]; barium or gastrografin swallow ('string' sign); electrolytes (hypokalemic hypochloremic metabolic alkalosis).

4. **Management**

a. Immediate
   1) NPO, nasogastric decompression, surgical consultation, correction of dehydration and metabolic alkalosis with normal saline boluses, H_2-blocker for possible gastritis.
   2) If olive palpable, proceed to surgery without further imaging studies. If olive not palpable, contrast swallow to evaluate for other differential diagnoses (gastroesophageal reflux, antral web, malrotation). If unsure, ultrasonography to confirm presence or absence of olive.

b. Definitive: Operative pyloromyotomy.

E. **HIRSCHSPRUNG DISEASE**[7]

1. **Definition:** Congenital absence of intramural colonic ganglion cells, most commonly in the rectosigmoid colon but can extend proximally. Resulting inability of sphincter complex/bowel wall to relax causes a functional bowel obstruction.

2. **Clinical presentation:** Usually presents in first 24–48 hours of life with failure to pass meconium, abdominal distention, and vomiting. May present with chronic constipation, failure to thrive, acute enterocolitis.

3. **Studies:** Suction rectal biopsy (gold standard, necessary to confirm diagnosis), abdominal radiograph (gas-filled loops); barium enema (if obtained) may demonstrate distended bowel and narrowed aganglionic segment, transition zone. Avoid prior rectal examination/enema/bowel preparation before barium enema because they may obscure findings. Anorectal manometry may be useful in the diagnosis in older children[4].

4. **Management**

a. Immediate: NPO, nasogastric decompression.

b. Definitive: Leveling colostomy with resection of aganglionic segment at transition zone, followed by surgical pull-through in 3–6 months.

F. **INTUSSUSCEPTION**

1. **Definition:** Intestinal invagination (Fig. 28.2); usually idiopathic and around the ileocecal valve (ages 3–36 months, thought secondary to hypertrophic Peyer's patches). Lead points in older children may include polyps, Meckel's diverticulum, lymphoma, meconium ileus (cystic fibrosis), and hemorrhagic foci (Henoch–Schönlein purpura, inflammatory bowel disease)[5].

28

SURGERY

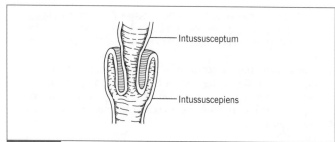

FIG. 28.2

Telescoping segment of proximal bowel (intussusceptum) into intussuscipiens. (From Silen[9].)

2. **Clinical presentation:** Intermittent colicky abdominal pain with legs drawn up, initially relieved by passage of stool; emesis becoming bilious; bloody 'currant jelly' stools (late finding); Dance sign (scaphoid right iliac fossa); palpation of mass (classically right upper quadrant 'sausage') on abdominal or rectal examination.

3. **Studies**

a. Plain radiograph: Small bowel obstruction, right upper quadrant soft tissue density and empty right lower quadrant.

b. Barium or air enema: May be performed in consultation with surgeon without initial radiograph if high clinical suspicion; must extend to small bowel to ensure no additional intussusception.

c. Abdominal sonography.

d. Upper GI with small bowel follow-through (in consultation with surgeon): If concerned about small-bowel obstruction. Especially important in patients with HSP.

4. **Management**

a. Immediate: NPO, nasogastric decompression; surgical consultation. In absence of peritonitis, reduction with air or barium enema (50–90% successful)[8], and postprocedure hospitalization (observe for 5–10% recurrence in first 24 hours).

b. Definitive: Laparotomy if failed reduction. Need to search for lead point if older child or small bowel involvement.

G. **INGUINAL HERNIA**[10]

1. **Definition:** Patency of the processus vaginalis with intraabdominal contents protruding into processus (Fig. 28.3). More common in boys (6:15). May be located on right side (60%) or left side (25%) or may be bilateral (15%).[6]

2. **Clinical presentation:** Prominent inguinal/periscrotal mass, accentuated by Valsalva maneuver. Transillumination reveals bowel (vs fluid in

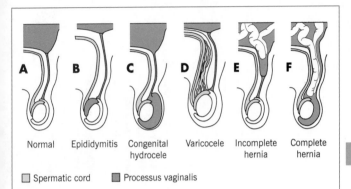

FIG. 28.3
Abnormalities of processus vaginalis or spermatic cord. **A,** Normal. **B,** Epididymitis. **C,** Congenital hydrocele. **D,** Varicocele. **E,** Incomplete hernia. **F,** Complete hernia. (From Zitelli[3].)

hydrocele), although this may be difficult to ascertain. Incarcerated hernias may present with pain, edema, erythema, and/or hematochezia.

3. **Studies:** If concerned about possible torsion, ultrasonography warranted.

4. **Management:** Prompt operative correction necessary secondary to high incidence of incarceration (30% in infants <1 year old[5]). Suspected incarcerated hernias require immediate surgical consultation and attempted reduction (sedation, nasogastric decompression, Trendelenburg position).

H. **ABDOMINAL MASSES**

1. **Differential (by age group):** See Table 28.1.

2. **Diagnosis**

a. History: Duration, growth pattern of mass; trauma, review of systems (fever, pain, emesis, diarrhea, urinary symptoms, bowel patterns).

b. Examination: Hypertension/hypotension, dysmorphisms, abdominal tenderness, mass (contour, consistency, location, continuity with other structures, mobility), transillumination (in infants), digital rectal examination, and/or pelvic examination (as indicated), neurologic examination.

3. **Studies and laboratory evaluation (by age group):** See Table 28.1.

4. **Management**

a. Immediate: Appropriate stabilization, including rehydration, correction of electrolyte abnormalities, tumor lysis management (see p. 524).

b. Definitive: Consultation (general surgery, urology, gynecology, oncology); possible biopsy, surgical excision, radiation, chemotherapy.

TABLE 28.1

ABDOMINAL MASSES

	Neonates	Early childhood	Adolescents
Differential	Hydronephrosis and/or enlarged bladder (PKD, PUV, UPJ obstruction)	Tumors (Wilms', neuroblastoma, rhabdomyosarcoma, non-Hodgkin's lymphoma, hepatic, ovarian)	Fecal material
	Renal vein thrombosis	Pyloric stenosis (3–6wk)	IBD
	Hepatoma/hemangioma	Intussusception (3–36mo)	Abscess
	Storage disease	Duplication cysts	Tumors (see Early childhood)
	Choledochal cyst	Mesenteric cysts	Pregnancy (intrauterine or ectopic)
	Duplication	Hydronephrosis	Ovarian cyst/torsion
	Ovarian cyst	Renal malformation	Pancreatic pseudocyst
	Teratomas	Fecal material	Choledochal cyst
	Hydrocolpos/hematocolpos	Choledochal cyst	Parasitic infections
	Adrenal hemorrhage	Bladder distention	PID/tuboovarian abscess
	Mesenteric/omental cyst	Pancreatic pseudocyst	Endometriosis
	Mesoblastic nephroma	Other congenital lesions	Bladder distention
	Volvulus		Hydrometrocolpos
	Other congenital lesions		

Studies to consider (in consultation with surgeon)	Sonography (renal) VCUG Scintigraphy MIBG scan	Sonography (abdomen) Abdominal CT with IV/PO contrast MRI Bone scan/chest CT/chest radiograph (if malignancy suspected) IV pyelography MIBG scan	Abdominal CT with IV/PO contrast Upper GI Sonography (pelvic, RUQ) Plain radiograph (obstruction, calcification) Bone scan/chest CT/chest radiograph Quantitative β-hCG ESR
Laboratory tests	Chromosomal studies (PKD) Urinalysis	Tumor markers (HVA, VMA, AFP, β-hCG, ferritin) Urinalysis	
All ages: Complete blood count with differential, electrolytes, chemistries, and liver and kidney function tests.			

PKD, polycystic kidney disease; PUV, pelvic urethral valve; UPJ, ureteropelvic junction; IBD, inflammatory bowel disease; PID, pelvic inflammatory disease; VCUG, voiding cystourethrography; RUQ, right upper quadrant; MIBG, ^{131}I-*meta*-iodobenzylguanidine; HVA, homovanillic acid; VMA, vanillyl mandelic acid; AFP, α-fetoprotein; β-hCG, β-human chorionic gonadotropin; ESR, erythrocyte sedimentation rate.

I. RECTAL PROLAPSE

1. **Definition:** Extension of full-thickness bowel (most common) or rectal mucosa through anus; can be associated with spina bifida (decreased perineal innervation and muscular atrophy), cystic fibrosis (large stools, weakened abdominal musculature, malnutrition), and hookworm or pinworm infestation; exacerbated by diarrheal illness/constipation.
2. **Clinical presentation:** Friable erythematous bowel extruding from anus.
3. **Studies:** Stool examination (ova/parasites), sweat test, sigmoidoscopy/lower GI (refractory cases).
4. **Management**
   a. Immediate: Manual reduction by parents or health care provider, sitz baths, stool softeners and bulking agents frequently sufficient.
   b. Definitive: Presacral sclerosing (with hypertonic saline or sodium maurate), resection of redundant bowel and sacrococcygeopexy, biofeedback.

J. GASTROINTESTINAL BLEEDING

See pp. 251–252.

K. ACUTE ABDOMEN[11]

1. **Differential:** Appendicitis, pancreatitis, intussusception, malrotation with volvulus, IBD, HSP, gastritis, bowel obstruction, mesenteric lymphadenitis, ectopic pregnancy, ovarian cyst/torsion, pelvic inflammatory disease, irritable bowel syndrome, urinary tract infection (UTI)/pyelonephritis, abscess, tumor (e.g., Wilms' tumor/neuroblastoma), nephrolithiasis, pneumonia, hepatitis, perforated ulcer (gastric/duodenal), sickle cell anemia, Meckel's diverticulitis, diabetes, cholecystitis, choledocholithiasis, JRA.
2. **Diagnosis**
   a. History: Course and characterization of pain, diarrhea, emesis +/− blood, fever, hematochezia, last oral intake, menstrual history, vaginal discharge/bleeding, urinary symptoms.
   b. Physical examination
      1) General: Vital signs, toxicity, rashes, arthritis, jaundice.
      2) Abdominal: Moderate to severe abdominal tenderness on palpation, rebound/guarding, rigidity, masses, change in bowel sounds.
      3) Rectal: Include testing for occult blood.
      4) Pelvic: Discharge, masses, adnexal/cervical motion tenderness.
3. **Studies**
   a. Radiology: Plain abdominal (obstruction, gallstones or kidney stones) and chest (pneumonia) radiographs, abdominal/pelvic ultrasonography, abdominal CT, contrast studies, endoscopy.
   b. Laboratory: Electrolytes, chemistry panel, CBC, liver and kidney function tests, coagulation studies, type and screen/crossmatch, urinalysis, amylase, lipase, GGT, gonorrhea/chlamydia cultures (or probes), quantitative β-hCG, antinuclear antibody, rheumatoid factor, ESR/CRP.

4. **Management**
a. Immediate: NPO, nasogastric decompression, rehydration, serial abdominal examinations, surgical/gynecologic/GI evaluation as indicated, pain control (may confound examination), antibiotics as indicated.
b. Definitive: Appropriate intervention, surgical or endoscopic exploration as warranted.

II. ORTHOPEDICS

A. DEVELOPMENTAL DYSPLASIA OF THE HIP[12]

1. **Definition**
a. A spectrum of subluxation to dislocation of one or both hip joints, often congenital and usually isolated (idiopathic); more severe variety involves femoral head/acetabular malformation.
b. Can be associated with additional anomalies, including clubfoot, metatarsus adductus, infantile scoliosis, and other contractures.
c. Often results from positioning (e.g., breech) exacerbated by intrauterine restriction, hormonal effects; 5–10% with positive family history; more common in firstborn girls.

2. **Clinical presentation:**
a. Limited abduction, leg held in adduction.
b. Asymmetric femoral length with knees and hips flexed 90° in supine position (Galeazzi sign).
c. Palpable 'clunk' with dislocation by posterior pressure (Barlow maneuver) and relocation by abduction/internal rotation (Ortolani maneuver); these two findings usually disappear by 3–4 months of age.

3. **Studies:** Anteroposterior/frog-leg radiograph (femoral head located laterally/superiorly, shallow acetabulum, delayed ossification, hypoplasia if teratogenic). Ultrasonography preferred in first 3–4 months if done by experienced sonographer.

4. **Management**
a. Referral to orthopedic surgeon: Pavlik harness (up to 6 months of age), closed or open reduction and serial spica casting (6–18 months), femoral osteotomy and open reduction (>18 months).[5]
b. Palpable 'clicks' usually associated with knee or tendon movements as contrasted with pathologic 'clunks' or sliding movement of the hip joint; if in doubt, early referral to an orthopedic surgeon or experienced sonographer is warranted.

B. COMPARTMENT SYNDROME[13]

1. **Definition:** Elevated muscle compartment/venous pressure (enclosed by surrounding fascia), which impairs blood flow/oxygenation/metabolism, resulting in nerve and muscle damage.

2. **Clinical presentation**
a. Can be seen in open and closed fractures, crush injuries, burns, and necrotizing fasciitis; most common with tibial fractures but also occurs

28

SURGERY

with displaced forearm and supracondylar humerus fractures. Chronic compartment syndrome occasionally seen in athletes.[14]

b. Severe unrelievable pain exacerbated by passive motion of the fingers or toes; swollen extremity that is tense to palpation.

c. **P**ain (earliest symptom), **P**allor, **P**aresthesias, **P**aralysis, **P**oikilothermia, **P**ulselessness (late finding).

3. **Studies:** Reading of intracompartmental pressure (<10mmHg normal; 20–30mmHg usually produces clinical symptoms).

4. **Management:** Emergent (within 6 hours of symptom onset) surgical fasciotomy (absolutely indicated if pressure >30mmHg).

C. **SPORTS-RELATED INJURIES**

1. **Shoulder**[15]

a. Clavicular fracture: Must obtain chest radiograph to rule out pneumothorax; treatment with sling for 6–8 weeks; consider figure-8 bandage for optimal alignment.

b. Separation: Laxity of the acromioclavicular joint; usually occurs secondary to fall and directly landing on shoulder or on outstretched hand; examination may reveal a positive crossover test (pain when patient reaches across chest to touch contralateral shoulder) and localized pain, crepitus, and/or swelling; conservative management with sling adequate in lower-grade (most) injuries.

c. Dislocation: Displacement of humeral head from glenoid socket, usually anteriorly; patient often holding injured arm in abduction and external rotation (if posterior dislocation, arm usually held across chest); usually with obvious asymmetry and deformity; limited range of motion; neurovascular status (usually axillary nerve; impaired sensation over lateral aspect of shoulder) may be compromised; with first-time dislocation, anteroposterior, lateral, and axillary/scapular radiographs necessary to rule out fracture; immediate reduction indicated to reduce neurovascular injury; referral to orthopedist or sports medicine physician indicated for further evaluation.

d. Subluxation: Repetitive partial dislocation, indicating unidirectional or multidirectional instability; may involve anterior (apprehension with abduction and external rotation), posterior (excessive movement with posteromedial force on elbow while shoulder/elbow flexed at 90 degrees), and/or inferior (sulcus sign [dimple over deltoid with humeral distraction]) instability; physical therapy indicated (strengthening only, not flexibility); some instability may require surgical correction.

e. 'Little League Shoulder'[16]: Stress fracture through the proximal humeral physis; patient usually 10–14 years old with insidious onset of shoulder pain with motion; examination may reveal generalized weakness and limited AROM in abduction, external and internal rotation; radiographs can show widening of the proximal humeral physis with fragmentation and sclerosis.

2. **Knee (must also evaluate for hip pathology)**
a. Instability
   1) Anterior cruciate ligament: Likely history of falling on hyperextended leg or twisting knee with planted foot. Usually large effusion +/− blood within initial few hours, limited or exaggerated range of motion; Lachman test (usually helpful only in acute setting before compensation by hamstrings; patient supine, knee flexed 20–30 degrees; evaluate excursion and endpoint when displacing tibia anteriorly with one hand on tibia, other on distal femur), pivot shift (more helpful with older injuries; patient supine with knee extended and in slight vagus, foot/tibia internally rotated; positive test equals pain with progressive knee flexion).
   2) Posterior cruciate ligament (less common): Posterior drawer test (one hand on femur, other on tibia; laxity when pushing tibia posteriorly), step-off, posterior/tibial sag sign (backward subluxation of tibia on femur with patient supine and muscles relaxed, knee flexed 90 degrees, and hip flexed 45 degrees).
   3) Medial/lateral collateral ligaments: Usually history of direct contact at lateral knee; pain and tenderness with palpation, varus/valgus stress* at 0 and 30 degrees.
   4) Medial/lateral menisci: Usually history of twisting motion. May have effusion, tenderness to palpation at joint line with knee flexed 90 degrees, positive McMurray test (knee fully flexed, rotate externally/internally, apply varus/valgus stress* to knee and extend to 90 degrees; pain and palpable click indicate positive test). If limited extension, refer to orthopedist for likely 'bucket-handle' tear.
   5) Management for instability: Rest, ice, and immobilization; referral to orthopedist indicated if severe injury, persistent pain or instability.
b. Osgood-Schlatter apophysitis: Knee pain and tenderness over tibial tuberosities (>50% bilateral)[16] with occasional avulsion; most common with open tibial physes (usually between 6 and 16 years); radiographs necessary only if clinical presentation unclear—usually normal with soft tissue swelling but may reveal an avulsion or occult pathology; conservative management with NSAIDs and relative rest.
c. Osteochondritis dissecans (OCD): Partial or complete separation of hyaline cartilage from supporting bone, most common in distal femur/medial femoral condyle; most occur in teenage years, male > female. Increasing pain with activity, positive Wilson test (flex knee 90 degrees and rotate tibia internally; anterior knee pain just before full extension, relieved by external rotation of tibia): Radiographs (including notch or tunnel view for femoral condyles) may show sclerosis or fragmentation; nonoperative treatment often successful with open physes, otherwise fragment removal/fixation necessary.

Varus stress: with femur stabilized, push or pull ankle medially. *Valgus stress:* with femur stabilized, push or pull ankle laterally.

d. Patellar instability: Dislocation of patella out of trochlear groove, usually from direct contact or pivoting maneuver. Accompanied by pain, swelling, and occasionally crepitus; often recurrent with disruption of the medial retinaculum; patient usually apprehensive with attempted patellar distraction; pain over medial adductor tubercle. Radiographs should include a 'sunrise' view; management includes symptomatic treatment and rehabilitation with flexibility and strength training; surgery if persistent hypermobility.

e. Patellofemoral dysfunction: Includes malalignment, lateral patellar compression syndrome (LPCS), chondromalacia. Gradual onset of pain, possible history of overuse or distant trauma; pain usually with squatting maneuvers, going up and down stairs, and prolonged knee flexion ('theater sign'); examination may reveal muscle tightness or crepitus. Radiographs may be helpful, may show patellar variants (bipartite patella, Sinding-Larsen-Johansson disease). Management should focus on physical therapy with strengthening and flexibility exercises.

3. Foot/Ankle

a. Sprains
   1) Classified as grade I (stretching, minor ligamentous injury), grade II partial tear of anterior talofibular ligament), and grade III (complete ligamentous disruption with inability to bear weight).
   2) Examination includes anterior drawer test (integrity of ATF ligament) and talar tilt (inversion stress to heel and ankle, integrity of calcaneofibular ligament); palpation must include first and fifth metatarsophalangeal joints and metatarsal heads, navicular and peroneal tubercles, head and dome of talus, bilateral malleoli, calcaneus, sinus tarsi (anterior to lateral malleolus), ligaments (anterior/posterior talofibular, calcaneofibular, deltoid), tendons, and proximal tibia/fibula.
   3) Look for hidden injuries (high sprain, disruption of syndesmosis [squeeze distal fibular shaft toward tibia, palpate interosseus membrane], Maisonneuve fracture with diastasis of mortise and fibular fracture, subtalar sprain).
   4) Radiographs (anteroposterior, lateral and oblique) recommended only if pain near malleoli, inability to bear weight, and point tenderness at posterior edge or tip of either malleolus.
   5) Conservative management, including early stress-controlled rehabilitation (maintain proprioception, strength); infrequent indication for weight-bearing cast with grade III injuries; persistent pain may indicate anterolateral soft tissue impingement, occult fracture; repetitive injury may result from peroneal weakness, loss of subtalar motion.

b. Sever (calcaneal) apophysitis: Inflammation of the open calcaneal growth plate. Evaluate older adolescents for stress fracture. Heel pain with direct pressure, medial-lateral compression. Conservative management with heel cup, orthotics, Achilles stretching.

c. Iselin apophysitis: Traction apophysitis/overuse osteochondritis and inflammation of fifth metatarsal tuberosity. Conservative management; healing can be complicated by nonunion, intermittent pain.

d. Accessory navicular: Normal variant (5–10% incidence)[17]; can cause medial ankle pain, usually chronic and insidious, that worsens with activity. Evaluation can include tenderness and palpation of ossicle, visualization of ossicle on radiographs. Conservative management indicated initially with orthotics, NSAIDs; walking cast if acute fracture or surgery if failed treatment.

e. Fractures: Radiographic indications include point tenderness and inability to bear weight; management includes non-weight-bearing immobilization; referral to orthopedist for casting, definitive management.

28

SURGERY

III. DENTAL SURGERY

A. DENTAL TRAUMA[8]

1. Definitions

a. Concussion: injury to supporting structures; can result in pulp hemorrhage/vasodilatation (tooth discoloration).

b. Luxation: Loosening/displacement of tooth disruption of anchoring periodontal ligament.

c. Fracture: Injury to enamel dentin and/or pulp (pulpitis can lead to necrosis and abscess formation).

d. Avulsion: Tooth separated from alveolar socket.

2. Diagnosis: Examine for pulp/dentin exposure, and dental fragments embedded in soft tissue, concurrent soft tissue injuries and skeletal injury.

3. Studies: Radiographs may show mandibular/maxillary fracture or loose fragments.

4. Management

a. Concussion, enamel fractures: Long-term observation, restoration with bonded filling, root canal (depends on severity).

b. Displacement injuries

　1) Primary teeth: Urgent referral to dentist, extraction likely.

　2) Secondary teeth: Surgical repositioning/splinting.

c. Fractures exposing dentin/pulp and root fractures: Urgent referral to dentist for pulp capping, pulpotomy, or splinting +/− root canal.

d. Avulsion

　1) Primary teeth: Observation; exclude tooth aspiration.

　2) Secondary teeth: Reimplantation requires short time interval, ideally 30 minutes. Storage of tooth in socket, saliva, or milk. Irrigation of avulsed site; splinting; probable root canal.

IV. OTOLARYNGOLOGY

A. PERITONSILLAR ABSCESS

1. Definition: Intraoral abscess surrounding one or both tonsils and extending across the soft palate; most caused by group A β-hemolytic streptococci and/or *S. aureus.* Usually affects school-age children.

2. **Clinical presentation:** Initial pharyngitis progressing to severe (usually unilateral) throat pain associated with high fever and dysphagia, trismus, torticollis, radiating ear pain. Examination reveals contralateral uvular deviation and erythematous mass, tender ipsilateral lymphadenopathy.

3. **Studies:** CBC, blood cultures, preoperative coagulation studies.

4. **Management:** Urgent ENT consultation, IV antibiotics; surgical drainage indicated if fluctuance or airway compromise. Consider diagnosis of tonsillar lymphoma.

B. **RETROPHARYNGEAL/PARAPHARYNGEAL ABSCESS**

1. **Definition:** Abscess involving one or more retropharyngeal lymph nodes (retropharyngeal abscess) or the lateral neck space (parapharyngeal abscess); occurs in children <4 years of age[5] (sporadic) and older children (posttraumatic). Group A β-hemolytic streptococci most common, can also involve *S. aureus* (as well as oral flora if traumatic).

2. **Clinical presentation:** Acutely worsening pharyngitis in toxic child with high fever, stridor, drooling, and respiratory distress; head held in hyperextension (retropharyngeal) or torticollis positioning (parapharyngeal).

a. Retropharyngeal: Erythematous mass with forward displacement of uvula and ipsilateral tonsil.

b. Parapharyngeal: Exquisitely tender anterolateral neck swelling with medial displacement of tonsil or lateral pharyngeal wall.

3. **Studies:** If patient stable, lateral neck radiograph (widening of prevertebral tissues [see p. 570]) and/or neck CT with IV contrast (abscess vs cellulitis).

4. **Management:** Urgent ENT consultation, IV antibiotics, probable surgical drainage (particularly with parapharyngeal involvement to prevent mediastinal extension). Risk of airway compromise, especially with sedation.

C. **CLEFT LIP/PALATE**

1. **Definition:** Failure of lip and palatal fusion during first trimester, causing unilateral or bilateral clefts of soft and/or hard palate. Can result in poor feeding, reflux, chronic middle ear effusions with hearing loss, speech difficulties, and dental/orthodontic problems.

2. **Clinical presentation:** Varied tissue involvement from exclusively lip and soft palate to bilateral involvement of the hard palate; usually isolated, but cleft palate may be associated with teratogens, positive family history, syndromes (trisomies 13 and 18, Pierre–Robin, and others). Submucosal cleft involves thinning of soft palate with a midline notch and can cause eustachian tube/middle ear problems.

3. **Management**

a. Education of feeding techniques and occupational therapy.

b. Surgical correction during first year of life; usually lip repair at 3 months, palate repair at 8 months.

c. Myringotomy tubes.

d. Psychologic support.

D. FOREIGN BODY ASPIRATION

1. **Definition:** Aspiration of small object into larynx, trachea, or bronchus, causing respiratory difficulty.

2. **Clinical presentation:** History of aspiration; acute or delayed development of cough, stridor, or wheezing (may be unilateral).

3. **Studies:** Radiographs including lateral neck and chest (radiopaque objects) and inspiratory/expiratory chest films (bilateral decubitus films if young, uncooperative patient; evaluate for asymmetric hyperinflation secondary to ball-valve effect of foreign body); fluoroscopy (mediastinal shift); bronchoscopy.

4. **Management**

a. Immediate: If complete airway obstruction, perform abdominal thrusts (>1 year) or back blows/chest thrusts (infants); if ineffective, may require emergent needle cricothyrotomy (see p. 10).

b. Definitive: Rigid bronchoscopy for object removal (ENT or general surgery).

V. UROLOGY

A. BLADDER/CLOACAL EXSTROPHY

1. **Definition:** Premature rupture of the cloacal membrane resulting in inadequate midline formation/closure of anterior bony pelvis, bladder, and genitalia ± intestinal involvement.

2. **Clinical presentation**

a. Bladder exstrophy: Anomalies include epispadias; exposure of inner bladder mucosa, trigone, and ureteral orifices; widespread pubic symphysis; hypoplastic or bifid genital structures.

b. Cloacal exstrophy: Above abnormalities plus omphalocele, myelomeningocele/hydrocephalus (>50% of patients), exposed bowel mucosa, and imperforate anus.

3. **Studies:** Upper urinary tract evaluation; chromosomal analysis if ambiguous genitalia.

4. **Management**

a. Immediate: Maintain moistened bladder surface with cellophane, urgent urologic consultation. Cloacal exstrophy may cause difficulties in gender assignment.

b. Definitive: Staged surgical correction ± pelvic osteotomy.

B. HYPOSPADIAS[18]

1. **Definition:** Abnormal location of the urethral meatus on the ventral penile surface.

2. **Clinical presentation:** Presence of dorsal hood/prepuce; description of meatus location (glandular, coronal, subcoronal, distal/mid/proximal

shaft, penoscrotal, scrotal, or perineal). More severe with presence of chordee (shortening of the ventral skin, causing curvature of the penis).

3. **Studies:** Voiding cystourethrography (VCUG) indicated only with severe anomaly or with history of UTIs. Consider evaluation for possible virilization if suggested by examination.
4. **Management:** Avoid circumcision; urology referral/surgical correction.

C. POSTERIOR URETHRAL VALVES

1. **Definition:** Abnormal tissue folds along the male membranous urethra, causing bladder outflow obstruction and subsequent dilatation of the upper urinary tract.
2. **Clinical presentation:** Unilateral or bilateral hydronephrosis/megaureter (on prenatal or postnatal sonography), oliguria, renal failure, flank mass/pain, voiding difficulties, UTI.
3. **Studies:** Sonography, VCUG, urinalysis, measurement of electrolytes, kidney function tests.
4. **Management**
   a. Immediate: Catheterization and bladder drainage, correction of electrolyte disturbances, dialysis (if needed for renal failure).
   b. Definitive: Transurethral ablation of abnormal tissue or urinary diversion (vesicostomy).

D. OBSTRUCTION OF THE URETEROPELVIC JUNCTION

1. **Definition:** Blockage of the normal ureteropelvic junction leading to hydronephrosis.
2. **Clinical presentation:** Hydronephrosis on prenatal ultrasonography; flank mass in infant; UTI, abdominal/flank pain in older child.
3. **Studies:** Electrolytes, kidney function tests, VCUG (vesicoureteral reflux [see p. 448]), sonography (hydronephrosis), diuretic nuclear renography.
4. **Management**
   a. Immediate: Antibiotic prophylaxis, urology consultation.
   b. Definitive: Surgical pyeloplasty if indicated.

E. HYDROCELE[10]

1. **Definition:** Collection of fluid inside the processus or tunica vaginalis (Fig. 28.3, C, p. 583).
2. **Clinical presentation:** Usually painless, swollen scrotum; transilluminates on examination.
3. **Studies:** Ultrasonography (determine whether testes have descended if not palpable on examination).
4. **Management:** Usual spontaneous resolution by 1 year of age; surgical correction warranted beyond the first year for communicating hydrocele (represents inguinal hernia). Cord hydroceles may require early urologic evaluation to rule out benign or possibly malignant growths.

F. TESTICULAR TORSION

1. **Definition:** Twisting of the spermatic cord resulting in decreased perfusion and ischemia of the testis.

2. **Clinical presentation**

a. Prenatal onset: Firm, nontender mass high in scrotum; present at birth.

b. Postnatal onset (usually adolescence): Acute (rarely chronic) scrotal pain and swelling, lower abdominal pain, nausea, emesis. Examination may reveal red/swollen/tender testis, elevation of testis (secondary to shortening of the spermatic cord), hydrocele, abnormal orientation of testis, absent cremasteric reflex, negative Prehn sign (see section on epididymitis, below).

3. **Studies:** Urinalysis (usually normal), nuclear medicine blood flow scan (evaluate for asymmetry), Doppler imaging/sonography (look for arterial flow; heterogeneity may indicate infarctions).

4. **Management:** Urgent surgical intervention (90% testicular survival if surgery within 8 hours of onset of symptoms); gentle manual detorsion (perform facing patient as if "opening a book"; less optimal and controversial, may be indicated if delay in surgical consultation).

G. EPIDIDYMITIS

1. **Definition:** Inflammation of the epididymis secondary to infection or anomalous collection of urine in vas deferens (Fig. 28.3).

2. **Clinical presentation:** Fever, tenderness, swollen epididymis (early) or inflammatory mass (late), present cremasteric reflex, positive Prehn's sign (pain relief with elevation of scrotum to level of pubic symphysis with patient in the supine position).

3. **Studies:** Urinalysis (pyuria), nuclear medicine flow study (increased flow to epididymis), Doppler ultrasonography, urine culture (if prepubertal), urethral swab for *N. gonorrhoeae* and *C. trachomatis* (if sexually active). Urinary tract imaging (if prepubertal) after resolution of acute symptoms.

4. **Management**

a. Immediate: Rule out torsion by sonography or nuclear medicine scan (or surgical exploration).

b. Definitive

    1) Prepubertal: Antibiotics to cover urinary pathogens (i.e., trimethoprim-sulfamethoxazole).

    2) Sexually active: Antibiotics to cover gonorrhea and chlamydia; treat partner.

H. VARICOCELE

1. **Definition:** Venous dilatation of spermatic cord vessels (Fig. 28.3, p. 583) with potential testicular damage.

2. **Clinical presentation:** Usually asymptomatic, rare before puberty; spontaneously decompresses in supine position.

3. **Studies:** None indicated in children (semen analysis in adults).

4. **Management:** Varicocelectomy if testicular size discrepancy; relative indications include large or painful varicoceles.

VI. REFERENCES

1. Dillon PW, Cilley RE. Newborn surgical emergencies: gastrointestinal anomalies, abdominal wall defects. *Pediatr Clin North Am* 1993; **40(6):**1289–1314.
2. Spitz L. Esophageal atresia and tracheoesophageal fistula in children. *Curr Opin Pediatr* 1993; **5(3):**347–352.
3. Myers MA, Aberdeen E. The esophagus. In: Ravitch MM, Welch KJ, Genson CD, et al, eds. *Pediatric surgery,* vol. 1. St Louis: Mosby; 1979.
4. Oldham KT, Columbani PM, Foglia RP. *Surgery of infants and children.* Philadelphia: Lippincott-Raven; 1996.
5. Zitelli BJ, Davis HW. *Atlas of pediatric physical diagnosis,* 3rd edn. St Louis: Mosby; 1997.
6. Way LW, ed. *Current surgical diagnosis and treatment,* 10th edn. Norwalk, CT: Appleton-Lange; 1994.
7. Skinner MA. Hirschsprung's disease. *Curr Prob Surg* 1996; **33(5):**389–460.
8. Barkin RM, ed. *Pediatric emergency medicine,* 2nd edn. St Louis: Mosby; 1997.
9. Silen W. *Cope's early diagnosis of the acute abdomen,* 18th edn. Oxford, England: Oxford University Press, 1991.
10. Skoog SJ, Conlin MU. Pediatric hernias and hydroceles: the urologist's perspective. *Urol Clin North Am* 1995; **22(1):**119–130.
11. Moir CR. Abdominal pain in infants and children. *Mayo Clin Proc* 1996; **71(10):**984–989.
12. Mooney JF III, Emans JB. Development dislocation of the hip: a clinical overview. *Pediatr Rev* 1995; **16(8):**299–303.
13. Mabee JR, Bostwick TL. Pathophysiology and mechanisms of compartment syndrome. *Orthopaed Rev* 1993; **22(2):**175–181.
14. Barnes M. Diagnosis and management of chronic compartment syndromes: a review of the literature. *Br J Sports Med* 1997; **31(1):**21–27.
15. Glockner SM. Shoulder pain: a diagnostic dilemma. *Am Fam Physician* 1995; **51(7):**1677–1687, 1690–1692.
16. Gomez JE. *Injuries unique to young athletes.* Paper presented at the 22nd Annual Sports Medicine Symposium, The University of Wisconsin-Madison, May 7, 1999.
17. Reider B. *Sports medicine: the school-age athlete,* 2nd edn. Philadelphia: WB Saunders; 1996.
18. Belman AB. Hypospadias update. *Urology* 1997; 49(2):166–172.

PART III

Formulary

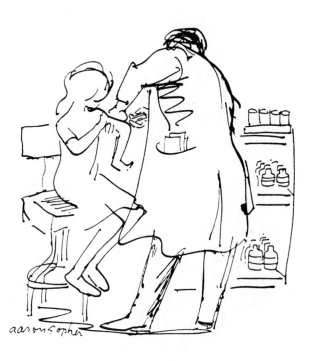

DRUG DOSES

Amy B. Hirshfeld, MD;
Aklil Getachew, MD;
and Jessica Sessions, MD

I. NOTE TO THE READER

The authors have made every attempt to check dosages and medical content for accuracy. Because of the incomplete data on pediatric dosing, many drug dosages will be modified after the publication of this text. We recommend that the reader check product information and published literature for changes in dosing, especially for newer medicines.

29

II. SAMPLE ENTRY

Pregnancy: Refer to explanation of pregnancy categories (on facing page).

Breast: Refer to explanation of breast-feeding categories (on facing page).

Kidney: Indicates need for caution or need for dose adjustment in renal failure. (See also ch. 32.)

How supplied

ACETAZOLAMIDE ← Generic name

Diamox ← Trade name and other names

Carbonic anhydrase inhibitor, diuretic ← Drug category

Tabs: 125, 250 mg

Suspension: 25, 30, 50 mg/ml ← Mortar and pestle: Indicates need for extemporaneous compounding by a pharmacist.

Capsules (sustained release): 500 mg

Injection (sodium): 500 mg/5 ml

Contains 2.05 mEq Na/500 mg drug

Yes   1   C

Diuretic (PO, IV)

Child: 5 mg/kg/dose QD-QOD

Adult: 250–375 mg/dose QD-QOD

Glaucoma

Child: 20–40 mg/kg/24 hr ÷ Q6 hr IM/IV; 8–30 mg/kg/24 hr ÷ Q6–8 hr PO

Adult: 1000 mg/24 hr ÷ Q6 hr PO; for rapid decrease in intraocular pressure, administer 500 mg/dose IV

Seizures: 8–30 mg/kg/24 hr ÷ Q6–12 hr PO

Max dose: 1 g/24 hr

Urine alkalinization: 5 mg/kg/dose PO repeated BID-TID

Management of hydrocephalus: see Chapter 22

Drug dosing

Contraindicated in hepatic failure, severe renal failure (GFR < 10 ml/min), and hypersensitivity to sulfonamides.

$T_{1/2}$: 2–6 hr; **do not use** sustained release capsules in seizures; IM injection may be painful; bicarbonate replacement therapy may be required during long-term use (see Citrate or Sodium Bicarbonate).

Possible side effects (more likely with long-term therapy) include GI irritation, paresthesias, sedation, hypokalemia, acidosis, reduced urate excretion, aplastic anemia, polyuria, and development of renal calculi.

Brief remarks about side effects, drug interactions, precautions, therapeutic monitoring, and other relevant information

III. EXPLANATION OF BREAST-FEEDING CATEGORIES

See Sample entry.

1 Compatible
2 Use with caution
3 Unknown with concerns
X Contraindicated
? Safety not established

IV. EXPLANATION OF PREGNANCY CATEGORIES

A Adequate studies in pregnant women have not demonstrated a risk to the fetus in the first trimester of pregnancy, and there is no evidence of risk in later trimesters.

B Animal studies have not demonstrated a risk to the fetus, but there are no adequate studies in pregnant women; OR animal studies have shown an adverse effect, but adequate studies in pregnant women have not demonstrated a risk to the fetus during the first trimester of pregnancy, and there is no evidence of risk in later trimesters.

C Animal studies have shown an adverse effect on the fetus, but there are no adequate studies in humans; or there are no animal reproduction studies and no adequate studies in humans.

D There is evidence of human fetal risk, but the potential benefits from the use of the drug in pregnant women may be acceptable despite its potential risks.

X Studies in animals or humans demonstrate fetal abnormalities or adverse reaction; reports indicate evidence of fetal risk. The risk of use in a pregnant woman clearly outweighs any possible benefit.

V. DRUG INDEX

Trade name	Generic name
2-PAM*	Pralidoxime chloride
3TC*	Lamivudine
5-FC*	Flucytosine
A-200 Pyrinate	Pyrethrins
Abbokinase	Urokinase
Abbokinase Open Cath	Urokinase
Abelcet	Amphotericin B lipid complex
Accolate	Zafirlukast
Accutane	Isotretinoin
Acular (ophth)	Ketorolac (ophth)
Acthar	ACTH
Actigall	Ursodiol
Adalat	Nifedipine
Adalat CC	Nifedipine
Adenine arabinoside	Vidarabine
Adenocard	Adenosine
Adrenalin	Epinephrine HCl
Advil	Ibuprofen
Aerobid	Flunisolide
Aerobid-M	Flunisolide
Afrin	Oxymetazoline
Aftate	Tolnaftate
Ak-poly-BAC	Polymyxin B sulfate and bacitracin
Akarpine	Pilocarpine HCl
Albuminar	Albumin, human
Albutein	Albumin, human
Aldactone	Spironolactone
Aldomet	Methyldopa
Aleve [OTC]	Naproxen sodium
Allegra	Fexofenadine
Allerest 12 Hour Nasal	Oxymetazoline
Alprostadil	Prostaglandin E_1
Alu-Tab	Aluminum hydroxide
Alupent	Metaproterenol
AmBisome	Amphotericin B, liposomal
Amicar	Aminocaproic acid
Amikin	Amikacin sulfate
Aminophyllin	Aminophylline
Amoxil	Amoxicillin
Amphocin	Amphotericin B
Amphojel	Aluminum hydroxide
Amphotec	Amphotericin B cholesteryl sulfate
Anacin	Aspirin
Anacin-3	Acetaminophen
Anaprox	Naproxen sodium
Ancef	Cefazolin
Ancobon	Flucytosine (5-FC)
Anectine	Succinylcholine
Antilirium	Physostigmine salicylate
Anitminth	Pyrantel pamoate
Apresoline	Hydralazine hydrochloride
Aqua-Mephyton	Vitamin K_1/phytonadione

*Common abbreviation or other name.

Trade name	Generic name
Aquachloral Supprettes	Chloral hydrate
Aquasol A	Vitamin A
Aquasol E	Vitamin E/alpha-tocopherol
Ara-A*	Vidarabine
Aralen	Chloroquine HCl/phosphate
Aristocort	Triamcinolone
ASA*	Aspirin
Astelin	Azelastine
Asthmanefrin	Epinephrine, racemic
Atarax	Hydroxyzine
Ativan	Lorazepam
Atretol	Carbamazepine
Atrovent	Ipratropium bromide
Augmentin	Amoxicillin-clavulanic acid
Auralgan	Antipyrine and benzocaine
Aventyl	Nortriptyline hydrochloride
Avita	Tretinoin
Avlosulfon	Dapsone
Azactam	Aztreonam
Azmacort	Triamcinolone
AZT*	Zidovudine
Azulfidine	Sulfasalazine
Bactocill	Oxacillin
Bactrim	Co-trimoxazole
Bactroban	Mupirocin
BAL	Dimercaprol
Beclovent	Beclomethasone dipropionate
Beconase	Beclomethasone dipropionate
Beconase AQ	Beclomethasone dipropionate
Benadryl	Diphenhydramine
Benemid	Probenecid
Benzac 10	Benzoyl peroxide
Benzac 5	Benzoyl peroxide
Betalin S	Thiamine (vitamin B_1)
Biaxin	Clarithromycin
Bicillin L-A	Penicillin G benzathine
Bicillin C-R	Penicillin G: benzathine and procaine
Bicillin C-R 900/300	Penicillin G: benzathine and procaine
Biltricide	Praziquantel
Brethine	Terbutaline
Bretylol	Bretylium tosylate
Brevibloc	Esmolol HCl
Bricanyl	Terbutaline
British anti-Lewisite*	Dimercaprol
Bromphen elixir	Brompheniramine
Bufferin	Aspirin
Bumex	Bumetanide
Buminate	Albumin, human
C-Lexin	Cephalexin
Cafergot	Ergotamine tartrate
Caffeine base	Caffeine
Caffeine citrate	Caffeine
Calan	Verapamil
Calciferol	Ergocalciferol
Calcijex	Calcitriol
Calcimar	Calcitonin
Calcium disodium versenate	EDTA calcium disodium

Trade name	Generic name
Camphorated opium tincture*	Paregoric
Capoten	Captopril
Carafate	Sucralfate
Carbatrol	Carbamazepine
Cardene	Nicardipine
Cardene SR	Nicardipine
Cardizem	Diltiazem
Cardizem CD	Diltiazem
Cardizem SR	Diltiazem
Carnitor	Carnitine
Catapres	Clonidine
Catapres TTS	Clonidine
Ceclor	Cefaclor
Cedax	Ceftibuten
Cefanex	Cephalexin
Cefizox	Ceftizoxime
Cefobid	Cefoperazone
Cefotan	Cefotetan
Ceftin	Cefuroxime axetil (PO)
Cefzil	Cefprozil
CellCept	Mycophenolate mofetil
Celontin Kapseals	Methsuximide
Cephulac	Lactulose
Ceptaz [arginine salt]	Ceftazidime
Cerebyx	Fosphenytoin
Cerumenex	Triethanolamine polypeptide oleate
Chemet	Succimer
Chibroxin	Norfloxacin
Childen's Advil	Ibuprofen
Children's Kapopectate	Attapulgite
Children's Motrin	Ibuprofen
Chlor-Trimeton	Chlorpheniramine maleate
Chloromycetin	Chloramphenicol
Cibacalcin	Calcitonin
Cibalith-S	Lithium
Ciloxan ophthalmic	Ciprofloxacin
Cipro	Ciprofloxacin
Cipro HC Otic	Ciprofloxacin
Claforan	Cefotaxime
Claritin	Loratadine
Claritin RediTabs	Loratadine
Claritin-D 12 Hour	Loratadine + pseudophrine
Claritin-D-24 Hour	Loratadine + pseudophrine
Cleocin	Clindamycin
Cleocin-T	Clindamycin
Clopra	Metoclopramide
Cloxapen	Cloxacillin
Co-Lav	Polyethylene glycol–electrolyte
Colace	Docusate sodium
Colovage	Polyethylene glycol–electrolyte
CoLyte	Polyethylene glycol–electrolyte
Compazine	Prochlorperazine
Cordarone	Amiodarone HCl
Cortef	Hydrocortisone
Corticotropin	ACTH

*Common abbreviation or other name.

Trade name	Generic name
Cortisporin	Polymyxin B sulfate, neomycin sulfate
Cortone acetate	Cortisone acetate
Coumadin	Warfarin
Crixivan	Indinavir
Crolom	Cromolyn
Cuprimine	Penicillamine
Cutivate	Fluticasone propionate
Cyclogyl	Cyclopentolate
Cyclomydril	Cyclopentolate/phenylephrine
Cylert	Pemoline
Cysticillin A.S.	Penicillin G preparations–procaine
Cytovene	Ganciclovir
d4T*	Stavudine
Dantrium	Dantrolene
Daraprim	Pyrimethamine
DDAVP	Desmopressin acetate
ddC*	Zalcitabine
ddI*	Didanosine
Decadron	Dexamethasone
Delta-Cortef	Prednisolone
Demerol	Meperidine HCl
Deodorized tincture of opium	Opium tincture
Depacon	Valproic acid
Depakene	Valproic acid
Depakote	Divalproex sodium
Depen	Penicillamine
Depo-Medrol	Methylprednisolone
Desferal Mesylate	Deferoxamine mesylate
Desquam-E 10	Benzoyl peroxide
Desquam-E 5	Benzoyl peroxide
Desyrel	Trazodone
Dexedrine	Dextroamphetamine
DHT	Dihydrotachysterol
DHT Intensol	Dihydrotachysterol
Dialume	Aluminum hydroxide
Diamox	Acetazolamide
Diapid	Lypressin
Diasorb	Attapulgite
Dideoxyinosine	Didanosine
Diflucan	Fluconazole
Digibind	Digoxin immune FAB (ovine)
Dilacor XR	Diltiazem
Dilantin	Phenytoin
Dilaudid	Hydromorphone HCl
Dimetane Extentabs	Brompheniramine
Dimetapp	Brompheniramine + phenylpropanolamine
Ditropan	Oxybutynin chloride
Diulo	Metolazone
Diurigen	Chlorothiazide
Diuril	Chlorothiazide
DMP-266*	Efavirenz
DMSA* [dimercaptosuccinic acid]	Succimer
Dobutrex	Dobutamine
Dolophine	Methadone HCl
Donnagel	Attapulgite
Dopastat	Dopamine
Dopram	Doxapram HCl

29

DRUG DOSES

Trade name	Generic name
Dramamine	Dimenhydrinate
Dridase	Oxybutynin chloride
Drisdol	Ergocalciferol
Dulcolax	Bisacodyl
Duragesic	Fentanyl
Duricef	Cefadroxil
Dynapen	Dicloxacillin sodium
Dyrenium	Triamterene
E-Mycin	Erythromycin
Elavil	Amitriptylline
Elimite	Permethrin
Emitrip	Amitriptylline
EMLA	Eutectic mixture of local anesthetic
Endep	Amitriptylline
Enovil	Amitriptylline
Epitol	Carbamazepine
Epivir	Lamivudine
Epivir-HBV	Lamivudine
Epoetin Alfa	Erythrpoietin
Epogen	Erythrpoietin
Epsom salts	Magnesium sulfate
Ery-Ped	Erythromycin
Erythrocin	Erythromycin
Esidrix	Hydrochlorothiazide
Eskalith	Lithium
Evac-Q-Mag	Magnesium citrate
Exosurf Neonatal	Pulmonary surfactant
Exsel (Rx)	Selenium sulfide
Famvir	Famiciclovir
Felbatol	Felbamate
Fentanyl Oralet	Fentanyl
Feosol	Iron preparations
Fer-In-Sol	Iron preparations
Fergon	Iron preparations
Ferralet	Iron preparations
Feverall	Acetominophen
Fiberall	Psyllium
FK506*	Tacrolimus
Flagyl	Metronidazole
Fleet	Sodium phosphate
Fleet Babylax	Glycerin
Fleet Phospho-soda	Sodium phosphate
Flonase	Fluticasone propionate
Florinef acetate	Fludrocortisone acetate
Flovent	Fluticasone propionate
Flovent Rotadisk	Fluticasone propionate
Floxin	Ofloxacin
Floxin Otic	Ofloxacin
Flumadine	Rimantadine
Fluohydrisone	Fludrocortisone acetate
Fluoritab	Fluoride
Folvite	Folic acid
Fortaz	Ceftazidime
Fortovase	Saquinavir
Foscavir	Foscarnet

*Common abbreviation or other name.

Trade name	Generic name
Fulvicin	Griseofulvin microcrystalline
Fungizone	Amphotericin B
Furadantin	Nitrofurantoin
Furomide	Furosemide
G-CSF*	Filgrastim
G-well	Lindane
Gabitril Filmtab	Tiagabine
Gamastan IV	Immune globulin (IM)
Gamimune-N	Immune globulin (IV)
Gamma benzene hexachloride*	Lindane
Gammagard	Immune globulin (IV)
Gammar	Immune globulin (IM)
Gammar–PIV	Immune globulin (IV)
Gantrisin	Sulfisoxazole
Garamycin	Gentamicin
Gas-X	Simethicone
Gastrocrom	Cromolyn
Geocillin	Carbenicillin
Geopen	Carbenicillin
Glucagon	Glucagon HCl
GoEvac	Polyethylene glycol–electrolyte
GoLYTELY	Polyethylene glycol–electrolyte
Grifulvin V	Griseofulvin microcrystalline
Grisactin	Griseofulvin microcrystalline
Haldol	Haloperidol
Hismanal	Astemizole
Hivid	Zalcitabine
Human Albumin	Albumin, human
Humatin	Paromycin sulfate
Hydro-T	Hydrochlorothiazide
Hyrocortone	Hydrocortisone
Hydrodiuril	Hydrochlorothiazide
Hyoscine	Scopolamine hydrobromide
Hyperstat	Diazoxide
Hytakerol	Dihydrotachysterol
IDV*	Indinavir
Imitrex	Sumatriptan succinate
Imodium	Loperamide
Imodium AD	Loperamide
Imuran	Azathioprine
Inapsine	Droperidol
Inderal	Propranolol
Indocin	Indomethacin
InfeD	Iron dextran
INH*	Isoniazid
Inocor	Amrinone lactate
Intal	Cromolyn
Intropin	Dopamine
Invirase (mesylate salt)	Saquinavir
Iosat	Potassium Iodide
Isoptin	Verapamil
Isopto	Scopolamine hydrobromide
Isopto Carpine	Pilocarpine HCl
Isuprel	Isoproterenol
Iveegam	Immune globulin
Janimine	Imipramine

29

DRUG DOSES

Trade name	Generic name
K-PHOS Neutral	Phosphorous supplements
Kabikinase	Streptokinase
Kantrex	Kanamycin
Kaopectate Advanced Formula	Attapulgite
Kaopectate Maximum Strength	Attapulgite
Kaopectate Tab Formula	Attapulgite
Kayexalate	Sodium polystyrene sulfonate
Keflex	Cephalexin
Keflin	Cephalothin
Kefurox	Cefuroxime (IV, IM)
Kefzol	Cefazolin
Kenalog	Triamcinolone
Ketalar	Ketamine
Klonopin	Clonazepam
Kondremul	Mineral oil
Konsyl	Psyllium
Kwell	Lindane
Kytril	Granisetron
Lamictal	Lamotrigine
Laniazid	Isoniazid
Lanoxin	Digoxin
Lariam	Mefloquine HCl
Lasix	Furosemide
Levocarnitine	Carnitine
Levophed	Norepinephrine bitartrate
Levothroid	Levothyroxine T_4
Lioresal	Baclofen
Liqui-E	Vitamin E/α-tocopherol
Lithane	Lithium
Lithobid	Lithium
Lithonate	Lithium
Lithotabs	Lithium
Loniten	Minoxidil
Lorabid	Loracarbef
Lotrimin	Clotrimazole
Lovenox	Enoxaparin
Luminal	Phenobarbitol
Luride	Fluoride
Luvox	Fluvoxamine
Maalox	Aluminum hydroxide with magnesium
Macrobid	Nitrofurantoin
Macrodantin	Nitrofurantoin
Mandol	Cefamandole
Maox	Magnesium oxide
Marcaine	Bupivicaine
Marinol	Dronabinol
Maxair	Pirbuterol acetate
Maxipime	Cefepime
Maxolon	Metoclopramide
Medipren	Ibuprofen
Medrol	Methylprednisolone
Mefoxin	Cefoxitin
Mellaril	Thioridazine
Mephyton	Vitamin K_1 phytonadione
Merrem	Meropenem

*Common abbreviation or other name.

Trade name	Generic name
Mestinon	Pyridostigmine bromide
Metamucil	Psyllium
Metaprel	Metaproterenol
Metro	Metronidazole
Mezlin	Mezlocillin
Miacalcin	Calcitonin
Miacalcin Nasal Spray	Calcitonin
Micronefrin	Epinephrine, racemic
Milk of magnesia	Magnesium hydroxide
Minipress	Prazosin HCl
Minocin	Minocycline
Mintezol	Thiabendazole
Mithracin	Plicamycin
Monistat	Miconazole
Motrin	Ibuprofen
Mucomyst	Acetylcysteine
Mucosil-10	Acetylcysteine
Mucosil-20	Acetylcysteine
Myambutol	Ethambutol HCl
Mycelex	Clotrimazole
Mycelex G	Clotrimazole
Mycifradin	Neomycin sulfate
Mycobutin	Rifabutin
Mycostatin	Nystatin
Mykrox	Metolazone
Mylanta	Aluminum hydroxide with magnesium
Mylanta Gas	Simethicone
Mylicon	Simethicone
Mysoline	Primidone
Nafcil	Nafcillin
Nallpen	Nafcillin
Naprosyn	Naproxen/naproxen sodium
Narcan	Naloxone
Nasacort	Triamcinolone
Nasacort AQ	Triamcinolone
Nasalcrom	Cromolyn
Nasalide	Flunisolide
Nasarel	Flunisolide
Nebcin	Tobramycin
NebuPent	Pentamidine isethionate
Nembutal	Pentobarbital
Neo-Calglucon	Calcium glubionate
Neo-Synephrine	Phenylephrine HCl
Neoral	Cyclosporin microemulsion
Neosporin	Neomycin/polymyxin B/±Bacitracin
Neosporin GU Irrigant	Neomycin/polymyxin B/±Bacitracin
Nephrox	Aluminum hydroxide
Neupogen	Filgrastim
Neurontin	Gabapentin
NeutraPhos	Phosphorous supplements
NeutraPhos-K	Phosphorous supplements with potassium
NFV*	Nelfinavir
Niferex	Iron preparations
Nilstat	Nystatin
Nipride	Nitroprusside
Nitro-bid	Nitroglycerin

Trade name	Generic name
Nitrostat	Nitroglycerin
Nix	Permethrin
Nizoral	Ketoconazole
Noctec	Chloral hydrate
Norcuron	Vecuronium bromide
Normodyne	Labetalol
Noroxin	Norfloxacin
Norpace	Disopyramide phosphate
Norvasc	Amlodipine
Norvir	Ritonavir
Nostrilla	Oxymetazoline
Novafed	Pseudoephedrine
NuLYTELY	Polyethylene glycol–electrolyte
Nuprin	Ibuprofen
NVP	Nevirapine
Nydrazid	Isoniazid
OCL	Polyethylene glycol–electrolyte
OcuClear	Oxymetazoline
Ocuflox	Ofloxacin
Ocusert Pilo	Pilocarpine HCl
Omnipen	Ampicillin
Os-Cal	Calcium carbonate
Osmitrol	Mannitol
Otocort	Polymyxin B sulfate, neomycin sulfate
Oxy-10	Benzoyl peroxide
Oxy-5	Benzoyl peroxide
Oxycontin	Oxycodone (slow release)
Pamelor	Nortriptyline hydrochloride
Panadol	Acetaminophen
Panmycin	Tetracycline HCl
Pavulon	Pancuronium bromide
Paxil	Paroxetine
Pediamycin	Erythromycin preparations
Pediapred	Prednisolone
Pediazole	Erythromycin ethylsuccinate + sulfamethizole
Pen Vee K	Penicillin V potassium
Pentacarinat	Pentamidine isethionate
Pentam 300	Pentamidine isethionate
Pentothal	Thiopental sodium
Pepcid	Famotidine
Pepcid AC [OTC]	Famotidine
Pepcid RPD	Famotidine
Pepto-Bismol	Bismuth subsalicylate
Percocet	Oxycodone and acetaminophen
Percodan	Oxycodone and aspirin
Percodan-Demi	Oxycodone and aspirin
Periactin	Cyproheptadine
Permapen	Penicillin G preparations–benzathine
Pfizerpen-AS	Penicillin G preparations–procaine
PGE$_1$*	Prostaglandin E$_1$
Phazyme	Simethicone
Phenergan	Promethazine
Phyllocontin	Aminophylline
Piligan	Pilocarpine HCl
Pima	Potassium Iodide

*Common abbreviation or other name.

Trade name	Generic name
Pin-Rid	Pyrantel pamoate
Pin-X	Pyrantel pamoate
Pipracil	Piperacillin
Pitressin	Vasopressin
Plasbumin-5	Albumin, human
Polycillin	Ampicillin
Polygam	Immune globulin
Polymox	Amoxicillin
Polysporin	Polymyxin B sulfate and bacitracin
Potassium Iodide Enseals	Potassium iodide
Potassium Phos	Phosphorous supplements with potassium
Prelone	Prednisolone
Prevalite	Cholestyramine
Prilosec	Omeprazole
Primacor	Milrinone
Primaxin	Imipenem-cilastatin
Principen	Ampicillin
Priscoline	Tolazoline
Procan SR	Procainamide
Procardia	Nifedipine
Procardia XL	Nifedipine
Procrit	Erythropoietin
Proglycem	Diazoxide
Prograf	Tacrolimus
Pronestyl	Procainamide
Pronto Plus	Pyrethrins
Propulsid	Cisapride
Prostaphlin	Oxacillin
Prostigmin	Neostigmine
Prostin VR	Prostaglandin E_1
Protopam	Pralidoxime chloride
Protostat	Metronidazole
Proventil	Albuterol
Provigan	Promethazine
Prozac	Fluoxetine hydrochloride
PTU*	Propylthiouracil
Pulmicort Turbuhaler	Budesonide
Pulmozyme	Dornase alfa/DNase
Pyopen	Carbenicillin
Pyrazinoic acid amide	Pyrazinamide
Pyridium	Phenazopyridine HCl
Pyrinyl	Pyrethrins
Quelicin	Succinylcholine
Questran	Cholestyramine
Questran Light	Cholestyramine
Rebetol	Ribavirin
Reese's Pinworm medicine	Pyrantel pamoate
Regitine	Phentolamine mesylate
Reglan	Metoclopramide
Regonol	Pyridostigmine bromide
Resectisol	Mannitol
Respigam	Respiratory syncytial virus immune
Retin-A	Trettinoin
Retin-A Micro	Trettinoin
Retrovir	Zidovudine
Rheaban Maximum Strength	Attapulgite
Rhinocort	Budesonide

29

DRUG DOSES

Trade name	Generic name
RID	Pyrethrins
Rifadin	Rifampin
Rimactane	Rifampin
Riobin	Riboflavin
Ritalin	Methylphenidate HCl
Ritalin SR	Methylphenidate HCl
Robinul	Glycopyrrolate
Rocaltrol	Calcitriol
Rocephin	Ceftriaxone
Rogaine	Minoxidil
Romazicon	Flumazenil
Roxicet 5/500	Oxycodone and acetaminophen
Roxicodone	Oxycodone
Roxilox	Oxycodone and acetaminophen
Roxiprin	Oxycodone and aspirin
Salicylazo-sulfapyridine	Sulfasalazine
Sandimmune	Cyclosporine
Sandostatin	Octreotide acetate
Sani-Supp	Glycerin
SAS*	Sulfasalazine
Scabene	Lindane
Selsun	Selenium sulfide
Senna-Gen	Senna
Senokot	Senna
Sensorcaine	Bupivicaine
Sensorcaine-MPF	Bupivicaine
Septra	Co-trimoxazole
Seraton	Psyllium
Serevent	Salmeterol
Serevent Diskus	Salmeterol
Silvadene	Silver sulfadiazine
Singulair	Montelukast
Slo-bid Gyrocaps	Theophylline
Slo-Phyllin Gyrocaps	Theophylline
Sodium Phos	Phosphorous supplements
Sofarin	Warfarin
Solfoton	Phenobarbitol
Solu-cortef	Hydrocortisone
Solu-Medrol	Methylprednisolone
Sporanox	Itraconazole
SPS	Sodium polystyrene sulfonate
SSD AF Cream	Silver sulfadiazine
SSD Cream	Silver sulfadiazine
SSKI	Potassium iodide
Staphcillin	Methicillin
Stimate	Desmopressin acetate
Streptase	Streptokinase
Stromectol	Ivermectin
Sublimaze	Fentanyl
Sulamyd	Sulfacetamide sodium
Sulfatrim	Co-trimoxazole
Sumycin	Tetracycline HCl
Suprax	Cefixime
Survanta	Beractant, pulmonary surfactant
Sustiva	Efavirenz

*Common abbreviation or other name.

Trade name	Generic name
Symadine	Amantadine hydrochloride
Symmetrel	Amantadine hydrochloride
Synagis	Palivizumab
Synthroid	Levothyroxine (T₄)
Tagamet	Cimetidine
Tagamet HB [OTC]	Cimetidine
Tambocor	Flecainide acetate
Tapazole	Methimazole
Tavist	Clemastine
Tazicef	Ceftazidime
Tazidime	Ceftazidime
Tegopen	Cloxacillin
Tegretol	Carbamazepine
Tegretol-XR	Carbamazepine
Tempra	Acetaminophen
Tenormin	Atenolol
Tensilon	Edrophonium chloride
Terramycin	Tetracycline HCl
Tetrahydrocannabinol*	Dronabinol
THC*	Dronabinol
TheoDur	Theophylline
Thermazene	Silver sulfadiazine
Thiuretic	Hydrochlorothiazide
Thorazine	Chlorpromazine
Thyro Block	Potassium iodide
Tiazac	Diltiazem
Ticar	Ticarcillin
Tigan	Trimethobenzamide HCl
Tilade	Nedocromil sodium
Timentin	Ticarcillin/clavulanate
Tinactin	Tolnaftate
TMP-SMX*	Co-trimoxazole
TOBI	Tobramycin
Tobrex	Tobramycin
Tofranil	Imipramine
Tolectin	Tolmetin sodium
Toradol	Ketorolac
Totacillin	Ampicillin
Trandate	Labetalol
Transderm Scop	Scopolamine hydrobromide
Tridil	Nitroglycerin
Trilisate	Choline magnesium trisalicylate
Trimox	Amoxicillin
Trobicin	Spectinomycin
Tums	Calcium carbonate
Tylenol	Acetaminophen
Tylox	Oxycodone and acetaminophen
Ultracef	Cefadroxil
Unasyn	Ampicillin/sulbactam
Unipen	Nafcillin
Urecholine	Bethanechol chloride
Uro-KP-Neutral	Phosphorous supplements
Urolene Blue	Methylene blue
V-Cillin K	Pencillin V potassium
Valium	Diazepam
Valtrex	Valacyclovir
Vancenase	Beclomethasone dipropionate

Trade name	Generic name
Vancenase AQ	Beclomethasone dipropionate
Vanceril	Beclomethasone dipropionate
Vanceril Double Strength	Beclomethasone dipropionate
Vancocin	Vancomycin
Vantin	Cefpodoxime proxetil
Vaponefrin	Epinephrine, racemic
Vasotec	Enalapril maleate
Vasotec IV	Enalaprilat
Velosef	Cephradine
Venoglobulin	Immune globulin
Ventolin	Albuterol
Vermizine	Piperazine
Vermox	Mebendazole
Versed	Midazolam
Vibramycin	Doxycycline
Videx	Didanosine
Vira-A	Vidarabine
Viracept	Nelfinavir
Viramine	Nevirapine
Virazole	Ribavirin
Visine LR	Oxymetazoline
Vistaril	Hydroxyzine
VitaCarn	Carnitine
Vitamin B_6*	Pyridoxine
Vitamin C	Ascorbic acid
VZIG*	Varicella-zoster immuneglobulin
WinRho-SD	Rh_o (D) immune globulin intravenous
Wycillin	Penicillin G preparations–procaine
Wydase	Hyaluronidase
Wymox	Amoxicillin
Xylocaine	Lidocaine
Zantac	Ranitidine HCl
Zantac 75 [OTC]	Ranitidine HCl
Zarontin	Ethosuximide
Zaroxolyn	Metalazone
Zemuron	Rocuronium
Zerit	Stavudine
Ziagen	Abacavir sulfate
Zinacef	Cefuroxime (IV, IM)/Cefuroxime axetil (PO)
Zithromax	Azithromycin
Zofran	Ondansetron
Zolicef	Cefazolin
Zoloft	Sertraline HCl
Zosyn	Piperacillin/tazobactam
Zovirax	Acyclovir
Zyflo	Zileuton
Zyloprim	Allopurinol
Zyrtec	Cetirizine

*Common abbreviation or other name.

FORMULARY

VI. DRUG DOSES

ABACAVIR SULFATE
Ziagen, 1592
Antiviral agent, nucleoside analogue reverse transcriptase inhibitor

No 3 C

Tabs: 300 mg
Oral Solution: 20 mg/ml (240 ml)

3 months to 16 years: 8 mg/kg/dose PO BID; **max dose:** 300 mg BID
Adults: 300 mg/dose PO BID

Fatal hypersensitivity reactions (5%) have been associated with signs or symptoms of fever, skin rash, fatigue, and gastrointestinal symptoms (nausea, vomiting, diarrhea, or abdominal pain). If signs or symptoms are present, discontinue drug immediately and monitor closely. **Do not** restart medication following hypersensitivity reaction because more severe life-threatening symptoms will recur. Adverse reactions not related to hypersensitivity include nausea, vomiting, diarrhea, decreased appetite, and insomnia. Lactic acidosis and severe hepatomegaly with steatosis have also been reported.

Use in combination with other anti-retrovirals. Drug is primarily metabolized by alcohol dehydrogenase and glucuronyl transferase. Ethanol decreases the elimination of abacavir. Pharmacokinetic properties in renal or hepatic impairment are incomplete. Doses may be administered with food or on an empty stomach.

ACETAMINOPHEN
Tylenol, Tempra, Panadol, Feverall, Anacin-3, and others
Analgesic, antipyretic

Yes 1 B

Tabs: 160, 325, 500, 650 mg
Chewable tabs: 80, 160 mg
Infant drops, solution/suspension: 80 mg/0.8 ml
Child solution/suspension: 160 mg/5 ml
Elixir: 80, 120, 160, 325 mg/5 ml

Caplet: 160, 325, 500, 650 mg
Gelcap: 500 mg
Sprinkle Capsules: 80, 160 mg
Suppositories: 80, 120, 125, 325, 650 mg
(Combination product with Codeine, see Codeine)

For explanation of icons, see p. 600.

Pediatric: 10–15 mg/kg/dose PO/PR Q4–6 hr
Dosing by age:
0–3 mo: 40 mg/dose
4–11 mo: 80 mg/dose
12–24 mo: 120 mg/dose
2–3 yr: 160 mg/dose
4–5 yr: 240 mg/dose
6–8 yr: 320 mg/dose
9–10 yr: 400 mg/dose
11–12 yr: 480 mg/dose
Adult: 325–650 mg/dose
Max dose: 4 g/24 hr, 5 doses/24 hr

Does not possess anti-inflammatory activity. May cause hemolysis at large doses in type A G6PD deficiency.

$T_{1/2}$: 1–3 hr, 2–5 hr in neonates; metabolized in the liver; see p. 22 for management of overdosage.

Some preparations contain alcohol (7%–10%) and/or phenylalanine; all suspensions should be shaken before use.

Adjust dose in renal failure (see p. 937).

ACETAZOLAMIDE

Diamox

Carbonic anhydrase inhibitor, diuretic
Tabs: 125, 250 mg
Suspension: 25, 30, 50 mg/ml
Capsules (sustained release): 500 mg
Injection (sodium): 500 mg/5 ml
Contains 2.05 mEq Na/500 mg drug

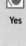 **Yes 1 C**

Diuretic (PO, IV)
Child: 5 mg/kg/dose QD-QOD
Adult: 250–375 mg/dose QD-QOD
Glaucoma
Child: 20–40 mg/kg/24 hr ÷ Q6 hr IM/IV; 8–30 mg/kg/24 hr ÷ Q6–8 hr PO
Adult: 1000 mg/24 hr ÷ Q6 hr PO; for rapid decrease in intraocular pressure, administer 500 mg/dose IV
Seizures: 8–30 mg/kg/24 hr ÷ Q6–12 hr PO
Max dose: 1 g/24 hr
Urine alkalinization: 5 mg/kg/dose PO repeated BID-TID
Management of hydrocephalus: see Chapter 22

Contraindicated in hepatic failure, severe renal failure (GFR <10 ml/min), and hypersensitivity to sulfonamides.

$T_{1/2}$: 2–6 hr; **do not use** sustained release capsules in seizures; IM injection may be painful; bicarbonate replacement therapy may be required during long-term use (see Citrate or Sodium Bicarbonate).

Possible side effects (more likely with long-term therapy) include GI irritation, paresthesias, excretion, hypokalemia, acidosis, reduced urate secretion, aplastic anemia, polyuria, and development of renal calculi.

ACETYLCYSTEINE

Mucomyst, Mucosil-10, Mucosil-20
Mucolytic, antidote for acetaminophen toxicity
Solution: 100 mg/ml (10%) or 200 mg/ml (20%) (4, 10, 30 ml)

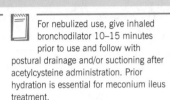

No   ?   B

For acetaminophen poisoning, see p. 22

Meconium Ileus: 5–10 ml/kg of 10% solution PR by soft rubber catheter. This may be given up to Q6 hr.
Nebulizer:
Children: 3–5 ml of 20% solution (diluted with equal volume of H_2O, or sterile saline to equal 10%), or 6–10 ml of 10% solution; administer TID-QID.
Adolescents: 5–10 ml of 10% or 20% solution; administer TID-QID.

For nebulized use, give inhaled bronchodilator 10–15 minutes prior to use and follow with postural drainage and/or suctioning after acetylcysteine administration. Prior hydration is essential for meconium ileus treatment.

May induce bronchospasm, stomatitis, drowsiness, rhinorrhea, nausea, vomiting, and hemoptysis.

ACTH

Corticotropin, Acthar
Polypeptide
Aqueous (inj): 25, 40 U/vial
Gel: 40, 80 U/ml (1, 5 ml)
1 unit = 1 mg

No   ?   C

Antiinflammatory:
Aqueous: 1.6 U/kg/24 hr IV, IM, or SC ÷ Q6–8 hr
Gel: 0.8 U/kg/24 hr ÷ Q12–24 hr IM
Infantile spasms: many regimens exist
Gel: 20–40 U/24 hr IM QD × 6 weeks or 150 U/m^2/24 hr IM ÷ BID for 2 weeks; followed by a gradual taper.

Contraindicated in acute psychoses, CHF, Cushing's disease, TB, peptic ulcer, ocular herpes, fungal infections, recent surgery, sensitivity to porcine products. IV administration for diagnostic purposes only. **Gel dosage form is only for the IM route.**

Can have hypersensitivity reaction. Similar adverse effects as corticosteroids.

ACYCLOVIR

Zovirax
Antiviral   Yes 1 C
Capsules: 200 mg
Tabs: 400, 800 mg
Suspension: 200 mg/5 ml
Ointment: 5% (15 g)
Inj (with sodium): 500 mg/10 ml, 1000 mg/20 ml
Contains 4.2 mEq Na/1 g drug

IMMUNOCOMPETENT:
*Neonatal HSV and HSV
encephalitis: All ages:* 30 mg/kg/
24 hr or 1500 mg/m²/24 hr ÷ Q8 hr IV ×
14–21 days. Higher doses of 45–60 mg/
kg/24 hr ÷ Q8 hr IV can be used in term
infants.
Mucocutaneous HSV (including genital):
Initial infection:
    IV: 15 mg/kg/24 hr or 750 mg/m²/
    24 hr ÷ Q8 hr × 5–7 days
    PO: 1200 mg/24 hr ÷ Q8 hr × 7–
    10 days
Recurrence:
    PO: 1200 mg/24 hr ÷ Q8 hr or
    1600 mg/24 hr ÷ Q12 hr × 5 days
Chronic suppressive therapy:
    PO: 800–1000 mg/24 hr ÷ 2–5 ×
    day for up to 1 year
Zoster:
    IV: 30 mg/kg/24 hr or 1500 mg/m²/
    24 hr ÷ Q8 hr × 7–10 days
    PO: 4000 mg/24 hr ÷ 5 × 24 hr × 5–
    7 days for patients ≥ 12 yr
Varicella:
    IV: 30 mg/kg/24 hr or 1500 mg/m²/
    24 hr ÷ Q8 hr × 7–10 days
    PO: 80 mg/kg/24 hr ÷ QID × 5 days
    (begin treatment at earliest
    signs/symptoms; **max dose:** 3200 mg/
    24 hr
Max dose of oral acyclovir in children =
80 mg/kg/24 hr
IMMUNOCOMPROMISED:
HSV:
    IV: 750–1500 mg/m²/24 hr ÷ Q8 hr ×
    7–14 days

PO: 1000 mg/24 hr ÷ 3–5 times/
24 hr × 7–14 days
HSV Prophylaxis:
    IV: 750 mg/m²/24 hr ÷ Q8 hr during
    risk period
    PO: 600–1000 mg/24 hr ÷ 3–5
    times/24 hr during risk period
Varicella or Zoster:
    IV: Same as immunocompetent dosing
    × 7–10 days
    PO: 250–600 mg/m²/dose 4–5 times/
    24 hr
CMV Prophylaxis:
    IV: 1500 mg/m²/24 hr ÷ Q8 hr during
    risk period
    PO: 800–3200 mg/24 hr ÷ Q6–24 hr
    during risk period
Max dose of oral acyclovir in children =
80 mg/kg/24 hr.
TOPICAL:
    Apply 0.5 inch ribbon of 5% ointment
    for 4 inch square surface area 6 times a
    day × 7 days.

See most recent edition of the AAP
Red Book for further details. Oral
absorption is unpredictable
(15–30%). Use ideal body weight for
obese patients when calculating dosages.
    Adequate hydration and slow (1 hr) IV
administration are essential to prevent
crystallization in renal tubules; dose
alteration necessary in patients with
impaired renal function (see p. 928).
    Can cause renal impairment; has been
infrequently associated with headache,
vertigo, insomnia, encephalopathy, GI
tract irritation, rash, urticaria, arthralgia,
fever, and adverse hematologic effects.

For explanation of icons, see p. 600.

ADENOSINE
Adenocard
Antiarrhythmic
Inj: 3 mg/ml (2 ml)

No ? C

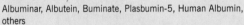

Supraventricular tachycardia:
Children: 0.1–0.2 mg/kg rapid IV push over 1–2 seconds; may increase dose by 0.05 mg/kg increments every 2 min to **max** of 0.25 mg/kg (up to 12 mg), or until termination of SVT
Max single dose: 12 mg

Contraindicated in 2nd and 3rd degree AV block or sick-sinus syndrome unless pacemaker placed.
Follow each dose with NS flush. $T_{1/2}$: <10 seconds.
May precipitate bronchoconstriction. Side effects include facial flushing, headache, shortness of breath, dyspnea, nausea, chest pain, lightheadedness.

ALBUMIN, HUMAN
Albuminar, Albutein, Buminate, Plasbumin-5, Human Albumin, others
Blood product derivative, plasma volume expander
Inj: 5% (50 mg/ml); 25% (250 mg/ml); each contains 130–160 mEq Na/L

No ? C

Hypoproteinemia:
Children: 0.5–1 g/kg/dose IV over 30–120 min
Adult: 25 g/dose IV over 30–120 min; repeat Q1–2 days PRN
Hypovolemia:
Children: 0.5–1 g/kg/dose IV rapid infusion
Adult: 25 g/dose IV rapid infusion; may repeat PRN
Max dose: 6 g/kg/24 hr or 250 g/48 hr

Contraindicated in cases of CHF or severe anemia; rapid infusion may cause fluid overload; hypersensitivity reactions may occur; may cause rapid increase in serum sodium levels.
Caution: 25% concentration contraindicated in preterm infants due to risk of IVH. For infusion, use 5 micron filter or larger. Both 5% and 25% products are isotonic but differ in oncotic effects. Dilutions of the 25% product should be made with D5W or NS.

ALBUTEROL

Proventil, Ventolin

Beta-2-adrenergic agonist

No 2 C

Tabs: 2, 4 mg
Sustained release tabs: 4, 8 mg
Oral solution: 2 mg/5 ml (473 ml)
Aerosol inhaler: 90 mcg/actuation (200 actuations/inhaler) (17 g)
Rotacaps for inhalation: 200 mcg/capsule
Nebulization solution: 0.5% (5 mg/ml) (20 ml)
Prediluted nebulized solution: 2.5 mg in 3 ml NS (0.083%)

 Oral:
Children <6 yr: 0.3 mg/kg/24 hr
PO ÷ TID; **max dose:** 12 mg/24 hr
6–11 yr: 6 mg/24 hr PO ÷ TID; **max dose:** 24 mg/24 hr
12 yr and adults: 2–4 mg/dose PO TID-QID; **max dose:** 32 mg/24 hr
Inhalations:
Aerosol (MDI): 1–2 puffs (90–180 mcg) Q4–6 hr PRN
Rotacaps: 200–400 mcg Q4–6 hr
Nebulization:
<1 yr: 0.05–0.15 mg/kg/dose Q4–6 hr
1–5 yr: 1.25–2.5 mg/dose Q4–6 hr
5–12 yr: 2.5 mg/dose Q4–6 hr
>12 yr: 2.5–5 mg/dose Q6 hr
For use in acute exacerbations more aggressive dosing may be employed.

Nebulization may be given more frequently than indicated. In such cases, consider cardiac monitoring and monitoring of serum potassium for hypokalemia. Systemic effects are dose related. Please verify the concentration of the nebulization solution used.

Possible side effects include tachycardia, palpitations, tremor, insomnia, nervousness, nausea, and headache.

The use of tube spacers or chambers may enhance efficacy of the metered dose inhalers.

For systemic use, use with caution in breastfeeding; inhaled route is likely to be compatible.

ALLOPURINOL

Zyloprim and others
Uric acid lowering agent, xanthine oxidase inhibitor   **Yes   1   C**
Tabs: 100, 300 mg
Suspension: 10, 20 mg/ml

 Child: 10 mg/kg/24 hr PO ÷ BID-QID; **Max dose:** 800 mg/24 hr
Adult: 200–300 mg/24 hr PO ÷ BID-TID

Adjust dose in renal insufficiency (see p. 937). Must maintain adequate urine output and alkaline urine.

Drug interactions: increases serum theophylline level; may increase the incidence of rash with ampicillin and amoxicillin; and increase risk of hypersensitivity reactions with ACE inhibitors and thiazide diuretics.

Side effects include rash, neuritis, hepatotoxicity, GI disturbance, bone marrow suppression, and drowsiness.

ALPROSTADIL
See Prostaglandin E₁

ALUMINUM HYDROXIDE

Amphojel, Dialume, Nephrox, Alu-Tab, and others
Antacid   **Yes   ?   C**
Tabs: 300, 500, 600 mg
Caps: 400, 475, 500 mg
Suspension: 320 mg/5 ml, 450 mg/5 ml, 600 mg/5 ml, 675 mg/5 ml (150, 360 ml)
Each 15 ml contains <0.3 mEq Na.

Doses in ml are based on the 320 mg/5 ml suspension concentration):

Peptic ulcer:
  Child: 5–15 ml PO Q3–6 hr or 1–3 hr PC and HS
  Adult: 15–45 ml PO Q3–6 hr or 1–3 hr PC and HS
Prophylaxis against GI bleeding:
  Neonates: 1 ml/kg/dose Q4 hr PRN
  Infant: 2–5 ml PO Q1–2 hr
  Child: 5–15 ml PO Q1–2 hr
  Adults: 30–60 ml PO Q1–2 hr
Hyperphosphatemia:
  Child: 50–150 mg/kg/24 hr ÷ Q4–6 hr PO
  Adult: 30–40 ml TID-QID PO between meals and QHS

 Use with **caution** in patients with renal failure and upper GI hemorrhage.

Interferes with the absorption of several orally administered medications, including digoxin, indomethicin, isoniazid, tetracyclines, and iron.

May cause constipation, decreased bowel motility, encephalopathy, and phosphorus depletion.

ALUMINUM HYDROXIDE WITH MAGNESIUM HYDROXIDE

Maalox, Mylanta, and others   **Yes   ?   C**
Antacid

Tabs: [Al (OH)$_3$:Mg (OH)$_2$]
  200 mg: 200 mg + Simethicone 20 mg
  400 mg: 400 mg + Simethicone 40 mg
Chewable tabs:
  200 mg: 200 mg (Maalox, Mylanta)

Suspension:
Mylanta: each 5 ml contains 200 mg ALOH, 200 mg MgOH, and 20 mg Simethicone
Maalox: each 5 ml contains 225 mg ALOH, 200 mg MgOH
Many other combinations exist
Contains 0.03–0.1 mEq Na/5 ml

 Same as for aluminum hydroxide preparations. **Do not use** combination product for hyperphosphatemia.

 May have laxative effect. May cause hypokalemia. Use with **caution** in patients with renal insufficiency (magnesium), gastric outlet obstruction.

Interferes with the absorption of the benzodiazepines, chloroquine, digoxin, phenytoin, tetracyclines, and iron.

AMANTADINE HYDROCHLORIDE

Symadine, Symmetrel, and others
Antiviral agent   **Yes   2   C**
Capsule: 100 mg
Syrup: 50 mg/5 ml (480 ml)

 Influenza A prophylaxis and treatment:
  1–9 yr: 5 mg/kg/24 hr PO ÷ QD-BID; **max dose:** 150 mg/24 hr
  >9 yr:
  < 40 kg: 5 mg/kg/24 hr PO ÷ QD-BID; **max dose** 200 mg/24 hr
  ≥ 40 kg: 200 mg 24 hr ÷ QD-BID
Prophylaxis (Duration of Therapy):
  Single exposure: at least 10 days
  Repeated/uncontrolled exposure: up to 90 days
  Use with influenza A vaccine when possible
Symptomatic treatment (Duration of Therapy):
  Continue for 24–48 hr after disappearance of symptoms

 Use with **caution** in patients with liver disease, seizures, renal disease, and in those receiving CNS stimulants. **Dose must be adjusted in patients with renal insufficiency (see p. 937).**

May cause dizziness, anxiety, depression, mental status change, rash (livedo reticularis), nausea, orthostatic hypotension, edema, CHF, and urinary retention.

For treatment of influenza A, it is best to initiate therapy immediately after the onset of symptoms (within 2 days).

AMIKACIN SULFATE

Amikin
Antibiotic, aminoglycoside   **Yes   ?   C**
Injection: 50, 250 mg/ml
Pre-Mixed IV Infusion: 500 mg in 100 ml normal saline

Neonates: See table below.
Infants and Children:
15–22.5 mg/kg/24 hr ÷ Q8 hr IV/IM
Adults:
15 mg/kg/24 hr ÷ Q8–12 hr IV/IM
Initial max dose: 1.5 g/24 hr, then monitor levels

Adjust dose in renal failure (see p. 928). Rapidly eliminated in patients with cystic fibrosis, burns, and in febrile neutropenic patients. CNS penetration is poor beyond early infancy.

Therapeutic levels: peak, 20–30 mg/L; trough 5–10 mg/L. Recommended serum sampling time at steady-state: trough within 30 minutes prior to the 3rd consecutive dose and peak 30–60 minutes after the administration of the 3rd consecutive dose. Peak levels of 25–30 mg/L have been recommended for pulmonary, bone, life-threatening infections and in febrile neutropenic patients.

May cause ototoxicity, nephrotoxicity, neuromuscular blockade, and rash. Loop diuretics may potentiate the ototoxicity of all aminoglycoside antibiotics.

NEONATES: IV/IM

Postconceptional age (wk)	Postnatal age (days)	Dose (mg/kg/dose)	Interval (hr)
≤29*	0–28	7.5	24
	>28	10	24
30–36	0–14	10	24
	>14	7.5	12
≥37	0–7	7.5	12
	>7	7.5	8

*Or significant asphyxia.

AMINOCAPROIC ACID
Amicar and others
Hemostatic agent
Tabs: 500 mg
Syrup: 250 mg/ml (480 ml) (contains potassium sorbate)
Injection: 250 mg/ml (contains 0.9% benzyl alcohol)

Yes ? C

For explanation of icons, see p. 600.

Antidepressant:

Children (PO): Start with 1 mg/kg/24 hr ÷ TID for 3 days; then increase to 1.5 mg/kg/24 hr. Dose may be gradually increased to a maximum of 5 mg/kg/24 hr if needed. Monitor ECG, BP, and heart rate for doses >3 mg/kg/24 hr.

Adolescents (PO): 10 mg TID with 20 mg QHS; dose may be gradually increased up to a maximum of 200 mg/24 hr if needed.

Adults:

PO: 40–100 mg/24 hr ÷ QHS-BID; dose may be gradually increased up to 300 mg/24 hr if needed; gradually decrease dose to lowest effective dose when symptoms are controlled.

IM: 20–30 mg QID (convert to oral therapy as soon as possible)

Augment analgesia for chronic pain:

Initial: 0.1 mg/kg/dose QHS PO; increase as needed and tolerated over 2–3 weeks to 0.5–2 mg/kg/dose QHS

Contraindicated in narrow angle glaucoma, seizures, severe cardiac disorders and patients who received MAO inhibitors within 14 days. See p. 39 for management of toxic ingestion.

$T_{1/2}$ = 12–18 hr (children) and 24–48 hr (adult). Maximum antidepressant effects may not occur for 2 or more weeks after initiation of therapy. **Do not abruptly discontinue therapy in patients receiving high doses for prolonged periods.**

Therapeutic Levels (sum of amitriptyline and nortriptyline): 100–250 ng/ml. Recommended serum sampling time: obtain a single level 8 or more hours after an oral dose (following 4–5 days of continuous dosing).

Side effects include sedation, urinary retention, constipation, dry mouth, dizziness, drowsiness, and arrhythmia. QHS dosing during first weeks of therapy will reduce sedation. Monitor ECG, BP, CBC at start of therapy and with dose changes. Decrease dose if PR interval reaches 0.22 sec, QRS reaches 130% baseline, HR rises above 140/min, or if BP is more than 140/90. Tricyclics may cause mania.

Children:

Loading dose: 100–200 mg/kg IV/PO

Maintenance: 100 mg/kg/dose Q4–6 hr; **max dose:** 30 g/24 hr

Contraindications: DIC, hematuria. Dose should be reduced by 75% in oliguria or end stage renal disease. Hypercoagulation may be produced when given in conjunction with oral contraceptives.

May cause nausea, diarrhea, malaise, weakness, headache, decreased platelet function, and hypotension. Elevation of serum potassium may occur, especially in patients with renal impairment.

AMINOPHYLLINE

Aminophyllin, Phyllocontin, and others
Bronchodilator, methylxanthine   **No   1   C**
Tabs: 100, 200 mg (79% theophylline)
Liquid (oral): 105 mg/5 ml (240 ml) (86% theophylline)
Injection: 25 mg/ml (79% theophylline)
Suppository: 250, 500 mg (79% theophylline)
Tablet (sustained release): 225 mg (79% theophylline)
Note: Pharmacy may dilute IV and oral dosage forms to enhance accuracy of neonatal dosing.

AMLODIPINE

Norvasc
Calcium channel blocker, antihypertensive   **No   ?**
Tabs: 2.5, 5, 10 mg

IV loading: 6 mg/kg IV over 20 min (each 1.2 mg/kg dose raises the serum theophylline concentration 2 mg/L)

IV maintenance: Continuous IV drip:
  Neonates: 0.2 mg/kg/hr
  6 wk–6 mo: 0.5 mg/kg/hr
  6 mo–1 yr: 0.6–0.7 mg/kg/hr
  1–9 yr: 1–1.2 mg/kg/hr
  9–12 yr and young adult smokers: 0.9 mg/kg/hr
  12 yr healthy nonsmokers: 0.7 mg/kg/hr

The above total daily doses may also be administered IV ÷ Q4–6 hr.

PO:
  Infants: (see Theophylline and convert to mg of Aminophylline)
  1–9 yr: 27 mg/kg/24 hr ÷ Q4–6 hr
  9–12 yr: 20 mg/kg/24 hr ÷ Q6 hr
  >12–16 yr: 16 mg/kg/24 hr ÷ Q6 hr
  Adults: 12.5 mg/kg/24 hr ÷ Q6 hr
Neonatal apnea:
  Loading dose: 5–6 mg/kg IV or PO
  Maintenance dose: 1–2 mg/kg/dose Q6–8 hr, IV or PO

Consider mg of theophylline available when dosing aminophylline.

Monitoring serum levels is essential especially in infants and young children. Intermittent dosing for infants and children 1–5 yr may require Q4 hr dosing regimen due to enhanced metabolism. Side effects: restlessness, GI upset, headache, tachycardia, seizures (may occur in absence of other side effects with toxic levels).

Therapeutic level (theophylline): for asthma, 10–20 mg/L; for neonatal apnea, 6–13 mg/L.

Recommended Guidelines for obtaining levels:
IV bolus: 30 min after infusion
IV continuous; 12–24 hr after initiation of infusion
PO liquid, immediate-release tab:
  Peak: 1 hr post dose
  Trough: just before dose
PO sustained-release:
  Peak: 4 hr post dose
  Trough: just before dose
Ideally, obtain levels after steady state has been achieved (after at least one day of therapy). See Theophylline for drug interactions.

Use in breastfeeding may cause irritability in infant.

Children PO:
  <1 yr: 600–800 mg/1.73 m²/24 hr ÷ Q12–24 hr then reduce to 200–400 mg/1.73 m²/24 hr
  ≥ 1 yr: 10–15 mg/kg/24 hr ÷ Q12–24 hr × 4–14 days and/or until adequate control achieved then reduce to 5 mg/kg/24 hr ÷ Q12–24 hr if effective
Children IV (limited data):
  5 mg/kg over 30 minutes followed by a continuous infusion starting at 5 micrograms (mcg)/kg/min; infusion may be increased up to a maximum of 10 mcg/kg/min or 20 mg/kg/24 hr.
Adults PO:
  Loading dose: 800–1600 mg QD for 1–3 wk
  Maintenance: 600–800 mg QD × 1 mo, then 200–400 mg QD
Use lowest effective dose to minimize adverse reactions.
Adults IV:
  Loading dose: 150 mg over 10 minutes (15 mg/min) followed by 360 mg over 6 hrs (1 mg/min); followed by a maintenance dose of 0.5 mg/min. Supplemental boluses of 150 mg over 10 minutes may be given for breakthrough VF or hemodynamically unstable VT and the maintenance infusion may be increased to suppress the arrhythmia.

Contraindicated i
node dysfunction, bradycardia, 2nd ar
AV block.

Long elimination half-life (
Major metabolite is active.

Increases cyclosporin, digoxi
phenytoin, tacrolimus, warfarin,
channel blockers, theophylline, a
quinidine levels.

Proposed therapeutic level with c
oral use: 1–2.5 mg/L.

Asymptomatic corneal microdeposi
should appear in all patients. Alters liv
enzymes, thyroid function. Pulmonary
fibrosis reported in adults. May cause
worsening of preexisting arrhythmias with
bradycardia and AV block. May also cause
anorexia, nausea, vomiting, dizziness,
paresthesias, ataxia, tremor, and hypo- and
hyper-thyroidism.

Intravenous continuous infusion
concentration for peripheral administration
should not exceed 2 mg/ml and **must be**
diluted with D5W. The preservative-free
intravenous product is available as an
orphan drug from Academic
Pharmaceuticals, Inc. at (847) 735-1170.

AMIODARONE HCI
Cordarone
Antiarrhythmic, Class III
Tabs: 200 mg
Suspension: 5 mg/ml
Inj: 50 mg/ml (3 ml) (contains 20.2 mg/ml benzyl alcohol and 100 mg/ml polysorbate 80 or Tween 80)
Inj (without benzyl alcohol and polysorbate 80): 15 mg/ml (10 ml)
Contains 37% iodine by weight.

No 3 D

AMITRIPTYLINE
Elavil, Emitrip, Endep, Enovil
Antidepressant, tricyclic
Tabs: 10, 25, 50, 75, 100, 150 mg
Inj: 10 mg/ml (10 ml)

No 3

Children:
Hypertension (data limited to retrospective analysis in Pediatric BMT patients): 0.1–0.2 mg/kg/dose QD PO; dosage may be increased to 0.3 mg/kg/dose QD.

Adult:

Hypertension: 5–10 mg/dose QD PO; use 2.5 mg/dose QD PO in small, fragile, geriatric patients or those with hepatic insufficiency.

Max. dose: 10 mg/24 hr

Use with caution in combination with other antihypertensive agents.

Reduce dose in hepatic insufficiency. Allow 3–5 days of continuous initial dose therapy before making dosage adjustments because of the drug's gradual onset of action and lengthy elimination half-life.

Dose-related side effects include edema, dizziness, flushing, and palpitations. Other side effects include headache, fatigue, nausea, abdominal pain, and somnolence.

AMMONIUM CHLORIDE

Diuretic, urinary acidifying agent

Tabs: 500 mg
Enteric coated tabs: 500 mg
Injection: 5 mEq/ml (26.75%);
1 mEq = 53 mg

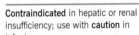

Yes   ?   B

 Urinary acidification:
Child: 75 mg/kg/24 hr ÷ Q6 hr PO or IV

Max dose: 6 g/24 hr

Adult: 1.5 g/dose IV Q6 hr. Max dose: 6 g/24 hr IV or 8–12 g/24 hr PO ÷ Q6 hr

Injection: Dilute to concentration not >0.4 mEq/ml.

Infusion **not to exceed** 50 mg/kg/hr or 1 mEq/kg/hr.

Contraindicated in hepatic or renal insufficiency; use with **caution** in infants.

May produce acidosis, hyper-ammonemia, and GI irritation. Monitor serum chloride level, acid/base status, and ammonia.

Administer oral doses after meals.

AMOXICILLIN

Amoxil, Trimox, Wymox, Polymox, and others
Antibiotic, aminopenicillin   **Yes   1   B**
Drops: 50 mg/ml (15, 30 ml)
Suspension: 125, 250 mg/5 ml (80, 100, 150, 200 ml)
Caps: 250, 500 mg
Chewable tabs: 125, 250 mg

 Child: 20–50 mg/kg/24 hr ÷ TID
PO
Adult: 250–500 mg/dose TID PO
Max dose: 2–3 g/24 hr
Recurrent otitis media prophylaxis: 20 mg/
kg/dose QHS PO
SBE prophylaxis: See pp. 162–163

Renal elimination. Adjust dose in
renal failure (see p. 928). Serum
levels about twice those achieved
with equal dose of ampicillin. Fewer GI
effects, but otherwise similar to ampicillin.
Side effects: rash and diarrhea.

Higher doses of 75–90 mg/kg/24 hr ÷
TID PO have been recommended for
resistant strains of *S. pneumoniae* in
acute otitis media.

AMOXICILLIN-CLAVULANIC ACID

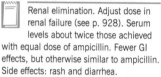

Augmentin
Antibiotic, aminopenicillin with beta-lactmase inhibitor   **Yes   1   B**
Tabs:
For TID dosing: 250, 500 (with
125 mg clavulanate)
For BID dosing: 875 mg amoxicillin
(with 125 mg clavulanate)
Chewable tabs:
For TID dosing: 125, 250 mg
amoxicillin (31.25 and 62.5 mg
clavulanate, respectively)
For BID dosing: 200, 400 mg
amoxicillin (28.5 and 57 mg
clavulanate)

Suspension:
For TID dosing: 125, 250 mg
amoxicillin 5 ml (31.25 and 62.5 mg
clavulanate/5 ml) (75, 100, 150 ml)
For BID dosing: 200, 400 mg
amoxicillin/5 ml (28.5 and 57 mg
clavulanate/5 ml) (50, 75, 100 ml)
Contains 0.63 mEq K^+ 125 mg
clavulanate

Dosage based on amoxicillin component.
Children <3 months: 30 mg/kg/ 24 hr ÷BID PO (recommended dosage form is 125 mg/5 ml suspension)
Children 3 months and older:
  TID dosing (see remarks):
    20–40 mg/kg/24 hr ÷ TID PO
  BID dosing (see remarks):
    25–45 mg/kg/24 hr ÷ BID PO
Adult: 250–500 mg/dose TID PO or 750 mg/dose BID PO for more severe and respiratory infections
Max dose: 2 g/24 hr

Clavulanic acid extends the activity of amoxicillin to include beta-lactamase producing strains of *H. influenzae, M. catarrhalis, N. gonorrhoeae,* some *S. aureus.* **Adjust dose in renal failure (see p. 928).**

The BID dosing schedule is associated with less diarrhea. For BID dosing, the 875 mg tablet, the 200 mg, 400 mg chewable tablets or the 200mg/5ml, 400mg/5ml suspensions should be used. These BID dosage forms contain phenylalanine and should not be used by phenyketonurics. For TID dosing, the 250 mg, 500 mg tablets, the 125 mg, 250 mg chewable tablets or the 125mg/5ml, 250mg/5ml suspensions should be used.

AMPHOTERICIN B
Fungizone, Amphocin
Antifungal
Injection: 50 mg vials
Oral Suspension: 100 mg/ml (24 ml)
Cream: 3% (20 g)
Lotion: 3% (30 ml)
Ointment, topical: 3% (20 g)

Yes   ?   B

Topical: Apply BID-QID
IV: mix with D$_5$W to concentration 0.1 mg/ml (peripheral administration) or 0.2 mg/ml (central line only). pH >4.2. Infuse over 2–6 hr.
Test dose: 0.1 mg/kg/dose IV **up to max** 1 mg (followed by remaining initial dose)
Initial dose: 0.25–0.5 mg/kg/24 hr
Increment: Increase as tolerated by 0.25–0.5 mg/kg/24 hr QD or QOD
Maintenance: 0.25–1 mg/kg/24 hr -or- QOD: 1.5 mg/kg/dose QOD
Max dose: 1.5 mg/kg/24 hr
Intrathecal: 25–100 mcg Q48–72 hr Increase to 500 mcg as tolerated.
Oral candidiasis: 100 mg QID PO

Monitor renal, hepatic, electrolyte, and hematologic status closely.
Hypercalciuria, hypokalemia, hypomagnesemia, RTA, renal failure, acute hepatic failure, hypotension, and phlebitis may occur. **For dosing information in renal failure (see p. 928).**

Common infusion-related reactions include fever, chills, headache, hypotension, nausea, vomiting; may premedicate with acetaminophen and diphenhydramine 30 min before and 4 hr after infusion. Meperidine useful for chills. Hydrocortisone, 1 mg/mg ampho (max 25 mg) added to bottle may help prevent immediate adverse reactions.

Salt loading with 10–15 ml/kg of NS infused prior to each dose may minimize the risk of nephrotoxicity.

AMPHOTERICIN B CHOLESTERYL SULFATE

No ? B

Amphotec
Antifungal
Inj: 50, 100 mg (vials)
(formulated as a 1:1 molar ratio of amphotericin B complexed to cholesteryl sulfate)

IV: Start at 3–4 mg/kg/24 hr QD, dose may be increased to 6 mg/kg/24 hr if necessary.

Mix with D$_5$W to concentration of 0.16–0.83 mg/ml.

Test dose: 10 ml of the diluted solution administered over 15–30 minutes has been recommended.

Infusion Rate: Give first dose at 1 mg/kg/hr, if well tolerated, infusion time can be gradually shortened to a minimum of 2 hr.

Monitor renal, hepatic, electrolyte, and hematologic status closely.

Thrombocytopenia, tachycardia, hypokalemia, hypomagnesemia, hypocalcemia, hyperglycemia, diarrhea, dyspnea, back pain, and increases in aminotransferases and bilirubin may occur.

Common infusion-related reactions include fever, chills, rigors, nausea, vomiting, hypotension, and headache; may premedicate with acetaminophen, diphenhydramine and meperidine (see Amphotericin B remarks).

Doses as high as 7.5 mg/kg/24 hr have been used to treat invasive fungal infections in BMT patients.

AMPHOTERICIN B LIPID COMPLEX

No ? B

Abelcet
Antifungal
Inj: 5 mg/ml (20 ml)
(formulated as a 1:1 molar ratio of amphotericin B to lipid complex comprised of dimyristoylphosphatidylcholine and dimyristoylphosphatidylglycerol)

For explanation of icons, see p. 600.

IV: 2.5–5 mg/kg/24 hr QD
Mix with D_5W to concentration
1 mg/ml or 2 mg/ml for fluid
restricted patients.
Infusion Rate: 2.5 mg/kg/hr; shake the
infusion bag every 2 hours if total infusion
time exceeds 2 hours.

Monitor renal, hepatic, electrolyte,
and hematologic status closely.
Thrombocytopenia, anemia,
leukopenia, hypokalemia, hypomagnesemia diarrhea, respiratory failure,
skin rash, and increases in liver enzymes
and bilirubin may occur.

Common infusion-related reactions
include fever, chills, rigors, nausea,
vomiting, hypotension, and headache;
may premedicate with acetaminophen,
diphenhydramine and meperidine (see
Amphotericin B remarks).

AMPHOTERICIN B, LIPOSOMAL

AmBisome
Antifungal

No   ?   B

Inj: 50 mg (vials)
(formulated in liposomes composed of hydrogenated soy phosphatidylcholine,
cholesterol, distearoylphosphatidylglycerol, and alpha-tocopherol)

IV: 3–5 mg/kg/24 hr QD
Mix with D_5W to concentration 1–
2 mg/ml (0.2–0.5 mg/ml may be
used for infants and small children).
Infusion Rate: Administer dose over 2
hours; infusion may be reduced to 1 hour
if well tolerated.

Monitor renal, hepatic, electrolyte,
and hematologic status closely.
Thrombocytopenia, tachycardia,
hypokalemia, hypomagnesemia,
hypocalcemia, hyperglycemia, diarrhea,
dyspnea, skin rash, low back pain, and
increases in liver enzymes and bilirubin
may occur.

Common infusion-related reactions
include fever, chills, rigors, nausea,
vomiting, hypotension, and headache;
may premedicate with acetaminophen,
diphenhydramine and meperidine (see
Amphotericin B remarks).

AMPICILLIN

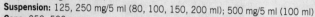

Omnipen, Polycillin, Principen, Totacillin
Antibiotic, aminopenicillin

Yes   2   B

Drops: 100 mg/ml (20 ml)
Suspension: 125, 250 mg/5 ml (80, 100, 150, 200 ml); 500 mg/5 ml (100 ml)
Caps: 250, 500 mg
Injection: 125, 250, 500 mg; 1, 2, 10 g
Contains 3 mEq Na/1 g IV drug

Neonate IM/IV:
<7 days:
<2 kg: 50–100 mg/kg/24 hr IM/
IV ÷ Q12 hr
≥ 2 kg: 75–150 mg/kg/24 hr IM/IV ÷
Q8 hr
≥ 7 days:
<1.2 kg: 50–100 mg/kg/24 hr ÷
Q12 hr IM/IV
1.2–2 kg: 75–150 mg/kg/24 hr ÷
Q8 hr IM/IV
>2 kg: 100–200 mg/kg/24 hr ÷ Q6 hr
IM/IV
Child:
Mild-moderate infections: 100–200
mg/kg/24 hr ÷ Q6 hr IM/IV
50–100 mg/kg/24 hr ÷ Q6 hr PO
Max PO dose: 2–3 g/24 hr

Severe infections: 200–400 mg/kg/
24 hr ÷ Q4–6 hr IM/IV
Adult:
500–3000 mg Q4–6 hr IM/IV
250–500 mg Q6 hr PO
Max IV/IM dose: 12 g/24 hr

Use higher doses to treat CNS
disease. CSF penetration occurs
only with inflammed meninges.
Adjust dose in renal failure (see p. 929).
Produces the same side effects as
penicillin, with cross-reactivity. Rash
commonly seen at 5–10 days. May cause
interstitial nephritis, diarrhea, and
pseudomembranous enterocolitis.
**Breastfeeding adverse effects are rare,
but three potential problems exist for the
nursing infant: bowel flora modification,
allergic response, and interference of
culture results for fever work-up.**

AMPICILLIN/SULBACTAM

Unasyn
Antibiotic, aminopenicillin with beta-lactamase inhibitor

Yes   ?   B

Injection:
1.5 g = ampicillin 1 g + sulbactam 0.5 g
3 g = ampicillin 2 g + sulbactam 1 g
Contains 5 mEq Na per 1.5 g drug combination

For explanation of icons, see p. 600.

Dosage based on ampicillin component
Child: 100–200 mg/kg/24 hr ÷ Q6 hr IM/IV
Severe Infections: 200–400 mg/kg/24 hr ÷ Q4–6 hr IM/IV
Adult: 1–2 g Q6–8 hr IM/IV
Max dose: 8 g ampicillin/24 hr

Similar spectrum of antibacterial activity to that of ampicillin with the added coverage of beta-lactamase–producing organisms.
Adjust dose in renal failure (see p. 929). Similar CSF distribution and side effects to ampicillin.

AMRINONE LACTATE
Inocor
Adrenergic agonist
Injection: 5 mg/ml (20 ml)

No ? C

Neonate: 0.75 mg/kg IV bolus over 2–3 min, followed by maintenance infusion of 3–5 mcg/kg/min
Children and Adults: 0.75 mg/kg IV bolus over 2–3 min, followed by maintenance infusion of 5–10 mcg/kg/min.
(IV bolus may need to be repeated in 30 min in neonates and children)
Max dose: 10 mg/kg/24 hr

Onset of action: 2–5 minutes with peak effects in 10 minutes.
Monitor for hypotension (which can be controlled with NS fluid boluses), arrhythmias, thrombocytopenia, hepatotoxicity, and GI effects; monitor fluid and electrolytes. Diuresis may result from improvement in cardiac output and may require dosage reduction of diuretics.

ANTIPYRINE AND BENZOCAINE
Auralgan and others
Otic analgesic, cerumenolytic
Otic solution: Antipyrine 5.4%, Benzocaine 1.4% (10, 15 ml)

No ? C

Otic Analgesia: Fill external ear canal (2–4 drops) Q1–2 hr PRN.
After instillation of the solution, a cotton pledget should be moistened with the solution and inserted into the meatus.
Cerumenolytic: Fill external ear canal (2–4 drops) TID–QID for 2–3 days

Benzocaine sensitivity may develop. **Contraindicated** if tympanic membrane perforated or PE tubes in place.

ASCORBIC ACID
vitamin C, others
Water soluble vitamin

No   1   A/C

Tabs: 25, 50, 100, 250, 500 mg, 1 g
Chewable tabs: 60, 100, 250, 500, 1000 mg
Tabs (timed release): 0.5, 1, 1.5 g
Caplet: 500 mg
Caps (timed release): 500 mg
Injection: 250, 500 mg/ml

Liquid: 35 mg/0.6 ml (50 ml)
Solution: 100 mg/ml (50 ml)
Syrup: 500 mg/ml (120, 480 ml)
Lozenges: 60 mg
Contains approximately 5 mEq Na/1 g drug

Scurvy PO/IM/IV/SC
Children: 100–300 mg/24 hr ÷ QD-BID for at least 2 weeks
Adults: 100–250 mg QD-BID for at least 2 weeks
See pp. 485–486 for U.S. RDA

Adverse reactions: nausea, vomiting, heartburn, flushing, headache, faintness, dizziness, hyperoxaluria. Oral dosing is preferred, but can give parenterally (IM preferred).
Pregancy Category changes to "C" if used in doses above the RDA.

ASPIRIN
ASA, Anacin, Bufferin, and various trade names
Nonsteroidal antiinflammatory agent, antiplatelet agent, analgesic

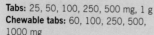

Yes   2   C/D

Tabs: 325, 500 mg
Tabs, enteric-coated: 81, 165, 325, 500, 650, 975 mg
Tabs, time-release: 81, 650, 800 mg
Tabs, buffered: 325, 500 mg
Tabs, caffeinated: 400 mg ASA + 32 mg caffeine
Tabs, chewable: 81 mg
Suppository: 60, 120, 125, 130, 195, 200, 300, 325, 600, 650 mg, and 1.2 g

Analgesic/antipyretic: 10–15 mg/kg/dose PO Q4–6 hr up to total 60–80 mg/kg/24 hr **Max dose:** 4 g/24 hr
Anti-inflammatory: 60–100 mg/kg/24 hr PO ÷ Q6–8 hr
Kawasaki disease: 80–100 mg/kg/24 hr PO ÷ QID during febrile phase until defervesces then decrease to 3–5 mg/kg/24 hr PO QAM. Continue for at least 8 weeks or until both platelet count and ESR normal.

 Do not use in children <16 yr for treatment of chicken pox or flu-like symptoms (risk of Reye's syndrome), in combination with other non-steroidal anti-inflammatory drugs, or in severe renal failure. Use with **caution** in bleeding disorders, renal dysfunction, gastritis, and gout. May cause GI upset, allergic reactions, liver toxicity, and

decreased platelet aggregation. See p. 37 for management of overdose.

Drug Interactions: may increase effects of methotrexate, valproic acid, and warfarin which may lead to toxicity (protein displacement). Buffered dosage forms may decrease absorption of ketoconazole, tetracycline.

Therapeutic levels: antipyretic/analgesic: 30–50 mg/L, antiinflammatory: 150–300 mg/L, Tinnitus may occur at levels of 200–400 mg/L. Recommended serum sampling time at steady state: obtain trough level just prior to dose following 1–2 days of continuous dosing. Peak levels obtained 2 hours (for non-sustained release dosage forms) after a dose may be useful for monitoring toxicity.

Pregnancy category changes to "D" if full-dose aspirin is used during the 3rd trimester. **Adjust dose in renal failure (see p. 927).**

ASTEMIZOLE
Hismanal
Antihistamine, less sedating
Tabs: 10 mg

No ? C

 <6 yr: 0.2 mg/kg/24 hr PO QD
6–12 yr: 5 mg/24 hr PO QD
>12 yr: 10 mg/24 hr PO QD
Max dose: 10 mg/24 hr

 Long elimination half-life. Less sedating than traditional antihistamines. High doses may cause cardiovascular complications. Avoid use in hepatic disease. Can result in severe life-threatening cardiac arrhythmias if given with drugs that reduce hepatic metabolism; e.g., erythromycin, itraconazole, ketoconazole, cimetidine, ciprofloxacin. This drug is a substrate of CYP450 3A4 (see p. 924).

ATENOLOL
Tenormin
Beta-1 selective adrenergic blocker
Injection: 0.5 mg/ml (10 ml)
Tab: 25, 50, 100 mg
Suspension: 2 mg/ml

Yes   2   C

Children: 1–1.2 mg/kg/dose PO QD
Max dose: 2 mg/kg/24 hr
Adults: 25–100 mg/dose PO QD
Max dose: 200 mg/24 hr

Contraindicated in pulmonary edema, cardiogenic shock. May cause bradycardia, hypotension, second or third degree AV block, dizziness, fatigue, lethargy, headache. Wheezing and dyspnea have occurred when daily dosage exceeds 100 mg/24 hr. **Avoid** abrupt withdrawal of the drug. Does not cross the blood-brain barrier; lower incidence of CNS side effects compared to propranolol. **Adjust dose in renal impairment (see p. 937).** IV administration rate **not to exceed** 1 mg/min.

ATROPINE SULFATE
Anticholinergic agent
Tabs: 0.4, 0.6 mg
Injection: 0.05, 0.1, 0.3, 0.4, 0.5, 0.8, 1 mg/ml
Ointment (ophthalmic): 0.5%, 1% (3.5 g)
Solution (ophthalmic): 0.5%, 1%, 2% (1, 2, 5, 15 ml)

No   1   C

Pre-anesthesia dose:
Child: 0.01 mg/kg/dose SC/IV/IM,
max dose: 0.4 mg/dose; min dose:
0.1 mg/dose; may repeat Q4–6 hr
Adult: 0.5 mg/dose SC/IV/IM
Cardiopulmonary Resuscitation:
Child: 0.02 mg/kg/dose IV Q5 min ×
2–3 doses PRN; min dose: 0.1 mg;
max single dose: 0.5 mg in children,
1 mg in adolescents; max total dose:
1 mg children, 2 mg adolescents
Adult: 0.5–1 mg/dose IV Q5 min; max
dose: 2 mg
Bronchospasm: 0.05 mg/kg/dose in
2.5 ml NS; min dose 0.25 mg; max dose:
1 mg Q6–8 hr via nebulizer
Ophthalmic:
Child: (0.5% solution) 1–2 drops in
each eye QD-TID
Adult: (1% solution) 1–2 drops in each
eye QD-TID

Contraindicated in glaucoma,
obstructive uropathy, tachycardia,
thyrotoxicosis. **Caution** in patients
sensitive to sulfites.

Doses <0.1 mg have been associated
with paradoxical bradycardia. Side effects
include: dry mouth, blurred vision, fever,
tachycardia, constipation, urinary
retention, CNS signs (dizziness,
hallucinations, restlessness, fatigue,
headache).

In case of bradycardia, may give via
endotracheal tube (dilute with NS to
volume of 1–2 ml). Use injectable
solution for nebulized use; can be mixed
with albuterol for simultaneous
administration.

ATTAPULGITE

Children's Kapopectate, Diasorb, Donnagel, Kaopectate Advanced
Formula, Kaopectate Maximum Strength, Kaopectate Tab Formula, **No ? B**
Rheaban Maximum Strength
Antidiarrheal
Liquid: 600 mg/15 ml (180, 240, 360, 480 ml); 750 mg/15 ml (120, 354 ml)
Chewable Tabs: 300, 600 mg
Tabs: 750 mg
Caplets: 750 mg

*PO (Administer dose after each
loose stool).*
3–6 yrs: 300–750 mg/dose PRN
up to a maximum of 7 doses/24 hr or
2250 mg/24 hr
6–12 yrs: 600–1500 mg/dose PRN up
to a maximum of 7 doses/24 hr or
4500 mg/24 hr
>12 yrs and Adults: 1200–3000 mg/
dose PRN up to a maximum of 8 doses/
24 hr or 9000 mg/24 hr

Plain Kaopectate's active
ingredients are kaolin and pectin.
Different versions of Kaopectate
may contain different active ingredients.
Do not use in children <3 years old,
diarrhea caused by *C. difficile* or other
toxigenic bacterias. Allow a 2–3 hour
interval between the administration of
attapulgite and other medications
(concurrent administration may lead to
reduced absorption). Prolonged use or
excessive doses may cause constipation.

AZATHIOPRINE
Imuran
Immunosuppressant
Suspension: 2, 50 mg/ml
Tabs: 50 mg
Injection: 100 mg (20 ml)

Yes   ?   D

Immunosuppression:
Initial: 3–5 mg/kg/24 hr IV/PO QD
Maintenance: 1–3 mg/kg/24 hr
IV/PO QD

Toxicity: bone marrow suppression, rash, stomatitis, hepatotoxicity, alopecia, arthralgias, and GI disturbances. Use ¼–⅓ dose when given with allopurinol. Monitor CBC, platelets, total bilirubin, alkaline phosphatase, BUN, creatinine. **Adjust dose in renal failure (see p. 937).**

AZELASTINE
Astelin
Nasal Antihistamine
Nasal Spray: 1% (137 mcg/spray), 100 actuations (17 ml)

Yes   ?   C

≥12 yrs and adults: 2 sprays each nostril BID

Use with **caution** in asthmatics. Reduced dosages have been recommended in patients with renal and hepatic dysfunction.

Drowsiness may occur despite the nasal route of administration (avoid concurrent use of alcohol or CNS depressants). Bitter taste, nasal burning, epistaxis may also occur.

AZITHROMYCIN

No ? B

Zithromax
Antibiotic, macrolide
Tablets: 250, 600 mg
Capsules: 250 mg
Suspension: 100 mg/5 ml (15 ml), 200 mg/5 ml (15, 22.5, 30 ml)
Oral Powder (Sachet): 1 g
Inj: 500 mg

Children:
Otitis Media or Community Acquired Pneumonia (≥6 months old): 10 mg/kg PO day 1 (**not to exceed** 500 mg), followed by 5 mg/kg/24 hr PO QD (**not to exceed** 250 mg/24 hr) on days 2–5
Pharyngitis/Tonsillitis (≥2 yrs old): 12 mg/kg/24 hr PO QD × 5 days (**not to exceed** 500 mg/24 hr)
M. avium complex prophylaxis: 20 mg/kg/dose PO Q 7 days (**not to exceed** 1,200 mg/dose)
Adolescents and Adults:
Respiratory tract, skin, and soft tissue infection: 500 mg PO day 1, then 250 mg/24 hr PO on days 2–5
Uncomplicated chlamydial urethritis or cervicitis: single 1 g dose PO
M. avium complex prophylaxis: 1,200 mg PO Q 7 days
Acute PID (Chlamydia): 500 mg IV QD × 1–2 days followed by 250 mg PO QD to complete a 7–10 day regimen.

Contraindicated in hypersensitivity to macrolides. Can cause increase in hepatic enzymes, cholestatic jaundice, GI discomfort, pain at injection site (IV use). Compared to other macrolides, less risk for drug interactions. CNS penetration is poor.

Aluminum- and magnesium-containing antacids decrease absorption. Capsules and oral suspension should be administered on an empty stomach, at least 1 hour before or two hours after meals. Tablets and oral powder (sachet) may be administered with food. Intravenous administration is over 1–3 hours; do not give as a bolus or IM injection.

Single 2 g oral dose may be adequate treatment for *N. gonorrhoeae* urethritis or cervicitis.

AZTREONAM

Yes 1 B

Azactam
Antibiotic, monobactam
Injection: 0.5, 1, 2 g
Each 1 g drug contains approximately 780 mg L-Arginine

Neonate:
30 mg/kg/dose:
<1.2 kg and 0–4 wk age: Q12 hr IV/IM
1.2–2 kg and 0–7 days: Q12 hr IV/IM
1.2–2 kg and >7 days: Q8 hr IV/IM
>2 kg and 0–7 days: Q8 hr IV/IM
>2 kg and >7 days: Q6 hr IV/IM
Children:
90–120 mg/kg/24 hr ÷ Q6–8 hr IV/IM
Cystic fibrosis:
150–200 mg/kg/24 hr ÷ Q6–8 hr IV/IM
Maximum Dose: 8 g/24 hr

Well-absorbed IM. Low cross-allergenicity between aztreonam and other beta-lactams. Adverse reactions: thrombophlebitis, eosinophilia, leukopenia, neutropenia, thrombocytopenia, elevation of liver enzymes, hypotension, seizures, confusion. Good CNS penetration. **Adjust dose in renal failure (see p. 929).**

BACLOFEN

Lioresal
Centrally acting skeletal muscle relaxant
Tabs: 10, 20 mg
Suspension: 5, 10 mg/ml
Intrathecal Inj: 0.5, 2 mg/ml

Yes   1   C

Dosage increments are made at 3 day intervals until desired effect or maximum dose is achieved.
Children; PO:
≥ *2 yr:* 10–15 mg/24 hr ÷ Q8 hr
  Max dose, <8 yr: 40 mg/24 hr
  Max dose, ≥ 8 yr: 60 mg/24 hr
Adults; PO:
5 mg TID; **max dose:** 80 mg/24 hr

Avoid abrupt withdrawal of drug. Use with **caution** in patients with seizure disorder, impaired renal function. Approximately 70-80% of the drug is excreted in the urine unchanged. Administer oral doses with food or milk.
  Adverse effects: drowsiness, fatigue, nausea, vertigo, psychiatric disturbances, rash, urinary frequency, hypotonia. Intrathecal dosing in children is not well established.

BECLOMETHASONE DIPROPIONATE

Beclovent, Beconase, Beconase AQ, Vanceril, Vanceril Double
Strength, Vancenase, Vancenase AQ

No ? C

Corticosteroid

Inhalation, oral: 42 mcg/inhalation (80 inhalations, 6.7 g; 200 inhalations, 16.8 g)

Inhalation, oral (double strength): 84 mcg/inhalation (40 inhalations, 5.4 g; 120 inhalations, 12.2 g)

Inhalation, nasal: 42 mcg/inhalation (80 inhalations, 6.7 g; 200 inhalations, 16.8 g)

Spray, aqueous nasal: 42 mcg/inhalation (200 metered doses, 25 g); 84 mcg/inhalation (120 metered doses, 19 g)

Oral Inhalation (1 inhalation = 42 mcg):
  6–12 yr: 1–2 inhalations TID-QID or 2–4 inhalations BID; **max** 10 inhalations/24 hr
  >12 yr: 2 inhalations TID-QID; **max** 20 inhalations/24 hr

Oral Inhalation, Double Strength (1 inhalation = 84 mcg):
  6–12 yr: 2 inhalations BID; **max** 5 inhalations/24 hr
  >12 yr: 2 inhalations BID; **max** 10 inhalations/24 hr

Oral Inhalation (NIH-National Heart Lung and Blood Institute recommendations): see pp. 911–912.

Nasal Inhalation:
  6–12 yr: 1 spray each nostril TID
  >12 yr: 1 spray each nostril BID-QID or 2 sprays each nostril BID

Aqueous nasal spray:
  >6 yr and adults: 1–2 sprays each nostril BID

Not recommended for children <6 yr. Dose should be titrated to lowest effective dose. **Avoid** using higher than recommended doses, since hypothalamic, pituitary, or adrenal suppression may occur.

Rinse mouth and gargle with water after oral inhalation; may cause thrush. Consider using with spacers for oral inhalation.

BENZOYL PEROXIDE

Benzac 5, Benzac 10, Benzamycin, Desquam-E 5,
Desquam-E 10, Oxy-5, Oxy-10 and various other names

No ? C

Topical Acne Product

Liquid Wash: 2.5% (240 ml), 5% (120, 150, 240 ml), 10% (120, 150, 240 ml)

Bar: 5% (113 g), 10% (106, 113 g)

Lotion: 5% (25, 30, 50, 60 ml), 5.5% (25 ml), 10% (12, 30, 60)

Cream: 5% (18, 113.4 g), 10% (18, 28, 113.4 g)

Gel: 2.5% (30, 45, 60, 90, 113 g), 4% (42.5, 90 g), 5% (45, 60, 90, 113.4 g), 6% (42.5%), 10% (45, 60, 90, 113.4 g), 20% (30, 60 g)

Cleanser: 10% (85.1 g)

Combination product with erythromycin:
Gel: 30 mg erythromycin and 50 mg benzoyl peroxide per g (23.3 g)

Children and Adults:
Cleanser, Liquid Wash, or Bar: Wet affected area prior to application. Apply and wash QD–BID; rinse thoroughly and pat dry. Modify dose frequency or concentration to control the amount of drying or peeling.
Lotion, Cream, or Gel: Cleanse skin and apply small amounts over affected areas QD initially; increase frequency to BID–TID if needed. Modify dose frequency or concentration to control drying or peeling.

Avoid contact with mucous membranes, eyes. May cause skin irritation, stinging, dryness, peeling, erythema, edema, and contact dermatitis. Concurrent use with tretinoin (Retin-A) will increase risk of skin irritation. Any single application resulting in excessive stinging or burning may be removed with mild soap and water.

BERACTANT
See Surfactant, pulmonary

BETHANECHOL CHLORIDE
Urecholine and other brand names
Cholinergic agent
Tabs: 5, 10, 25, 50 mg
Suspension: 1 mg/ml
Injection: 5 mg/ml

No   ?   C

Children:
Abdominal distention/urinary retention
PO: 0.6 mg/kg/24 hr ÷ Q6–8 hr
SC: 0.12–0.2 mg/kg/24 hr ÷ Q6–8 hr
Gastroesophageal reflux:
0.1–0.2 mg/kg/dose 30 min.–1 hr AC and HS; **max:** 4 doses/24 hr
Adults:
PO: 10–50 mg Q6–12 hr
SC: 2.5–5 mg TID-QID, up to 7.5–10 mg Q4 hr for neurogenic bladder

Contraindicated in asthma, mechanical GI or GU obstruction, peptic ulcer disease, hyperthyroidism, cardiac disease, seizure disorder. May cause hypotension, nausea, bronchospasm, salivation, flushing, abdominal cramps. **Warning: severe hypotension may occur when given with ganglionic blockers (trimethaphan). Do not give IV or IM.** Atropine is the antidote.

BISACODYL

Dulcolax and various other names
Laxative, stimulant

No ? B

Tabs (enteric-coated): 5 mg
Suppository: 5, 10 mg
Enema: 10 mg/30 ml (37.5 ml)
Powder: 1.5 mg with tannic acid, 2.5 g/packet (25s, 50s)

Oral:
Child: 0.3 mg/kg/24 hr or 5–10 mg to be given 6 hr before desired effect
Adult (>12 yr): 5–15 mg QD
Rectal:
<2 yr: 5 mg
2–11 yr: 5–10 mg
>11 yr: 10 mg

Do not chew or crush tablets; do not give within 1 hr of antacids or milk. **Do not use** in newborn period. May cause abdominal cramps, nausea, vomiting, rectal irritation. Oral usually effective within 6–10 hr; rectal usually effective within 15–60 min.

BISMUTH SUBSALICYLATE

Pepto-Bismol
Antidiarrheal, gastrointestinal ulcer agent

Yes 2 C/D

Liquid: 262 mg/15 ml (120, 240, 360, 480 ml), 524 mg/15ml
(120, 240, 360 ml)
Caplet: 262 mg
Chewable Tabs: 262 mg
Contains 102 mg salicylate per 262 mg tablet; or 129 mg salicylate per 15 ml of the 262 mg/15 ml suspension.

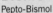

Diarrhea:
Children: 100 mg/kg/24 hr ÷ 5 equal doses for 5 days

Dosage by age; give following dose Q 30 min to 1 hr PRN **up to a maximum 8 doses/24 hrs:**

  3–6 yrs: 87.3 mg (⅓ tablet or 5 ml of 262 mg/15 ml)

  6–9 yrs: 174.7 mg (⅔ tablet or 10 ml of 262 mg/15 ml)

  9–12 yrs: 262 mg (1 tablet or 15 ml of 262 mg/15 ml)

  Adults: 524 mg (2 tablets or 30 ml of 262 mg/15 ml)

H. pylori *gastric infection (in combination with ampicillin and metronidazole or with tetracycline and metronidazole for adults; doses not well established for children):*

  <10 yr: 262 mg PO QID × 6 weeks

  ≥10 yr–adults: 524 mg PO QID × 6 weeks

Generally not recommended in children <16 yr with chicken pox or flu-like symptoms (risk of Reye's Syndrome), in combination with other non-steroidal anti-inflammatory drugs, or in severe renal failure. Use with **caution** in bleeding disorders, renal dysfunction, gastritis, and gout. May cause darkening of tongue and/or black stools, GI upset, impaction, and decreased platelet aggregation.

Drug combination appears to have antisecretory and antimicrobial effects with some anti-inflammatory effects. Absorption of bismuth is negligible, whereas approximately 80% of the salicylate is absorbed.

Pregnancy category changes to "D"during the third trimester. **Adjust dose in renal failure (see p. 937).**

BRETYLIUM TOSYLATE
Bretylol
Antiarrhythmic, class III
Injection: 50 mg/ml (10, 20 ml)
Pre-mixed injection: 2, 4 mg/ml in D5W (250 ml)

Yes   ?   C

IV: 5–10 mg/kg/dose; may repeat Q10–20 min for **total dose** of 30 mg/kg.

IM: 2–5 mg/kg × 1

Maintenance dose (IM, IV): 5 mg/kg/dose Q6–8 hr

Contraindicated in arrhythmias induced by digoxin toxicity. May cause initial hypertension followed by hypotension. May cause PVCs and increased sensitivity to digitalis and catecholamines. **Reduce dose in renal failure, see p. 938).**

BROMPHENIRAMINE ± PHENYLPROPANOLAMINE

Bromphen Elixir, Dimetane Extentabs and various other names; in combination with phenylpropanolamine - Bromanate, Dimetapp, and various other names

Yes 1/? C

Antihistamine ± decongestant
Elixir: 2 mg/5 ml (120, 480 ml) (contains 3% alcohol)
Tablets: 4, 8, 12 mg
Extended release Tabs: 8, 12 mg
Inj: 10 mg/ml (10 ml)
In combination with phenylpropanolamine:
Elixir: Brompheniramine 2 mg + Phenylpropanolamine 12.5 mg/5 ml

(120, 240, 480 ml) (some preparations contain 2.3% alcohol)
Tablets or Capsules (liquid filled):
Brompheniramine 4 mg + Phenylpropanolamine 25 mg
Extended Release Tablets:
Brompheniramine 12 mg + Phenylpropanolamine 75 mg

BROMPHENIRAMINE:
Oral:
<6 yr: 0.5 mg/kg/24 hr ÷ Q6–8 hr; **maximum dose:** 6–8 mg/24 hr
6–12 yr: 2–4 mg/dose Q6–8 hr; **maximum dose:** 12–16 mg/24 hr
>12 yr: 4–8 mg/dose Q6–8 hr or 8–12 mg of the sustained release dosage form Q8–12 hr; **maximum dose:** 24 mg/24 hr
IV/IM/SC:
<12 yr: 0.5 mg/kg/24 hr ÷ Q6–8 hr
≥12 yr: 5–20 mg Q6–12 hr; **maximum dose:** 40 mg/24 hr
BROMPHENIRAMINE + PHENYLPROPANOLAMINE:
Oral, Elixir:
7–24 mon: 2.5 ml TID–QID
2–4 yr: 3.75 ml TID–QID
4–12 yr: 5 ml TID-QID
Adult: 5–10 ml TID–QID
Oral, Immediate Release Tab or Cap:
Adult: 1 tab or cap TID–QID
Oral, Sustained Release Tab:
Adult: 1 tab BID

Contraindicated in narrow-angle glaucoma, bladder neck obstruction, asthma, and with concurrent use of MAO inhibitors. In addition, phenylpropanolamine containing product is **contraindicated** in severe hypertension, coronary artery disease, diabetes mellitus, and thyroid disease. Discontinue use 48 hours prior to allergy skin testing. Generally not recommended for treating URIs for infants. No proven benefit for infants/toddlers with URIs.

Both products may cause drowsiness, fatigue, CNS excitation, xerostomia, blurred vision, wheezing. Excessive doses or chronic usage of the phenypropanolamine containing product may cause hypertension, myocardial injury, or atrioventricular conduction block.

Dosage adjustment may be necessary in renal failure for patients receiving the combination product since phenylpropanolamine is significantly excreted in the urine (86%).

Brompheniramine is compatible with breastfeeding, but the safety is not established for phenylpropanolamine.

BUDESONIDE
Pulmicort Turbuhaler, Rhinocort
Corticosteroid

No **?** **C**

Nasal aerosol: 32 mcg/actuation (7 g, delivers approx 200 sprays)
Oral Inhaler: 200 mcg/metered dose (1 inhaler delivers approx 200 doses)

 Oral Inhalation:
Children ≥6 yr: Start at 1 inhalation (200 mcg) BID and increase, as needed, up to a **maximum** of 4 inhalations/24 hr
Adult:
No prior steroid use: 1–2 inhalations BID; **Max dose:** 4 inhalations/24 hr
Prior inhaled steriod use: Start at 1–2 inhalations BID and increase, as needed, up to a **maximum** of 8 inhalations/24 hr
Prior oral steroid use: Start at 2–4 inhalations BID; **max dose:** 8 inhalations/24 hr
Oral Inhalation (NIH-National Heart Lung and Blood Institute recommendations): see pp. 911–912.

Nasal Inhalation:
>6 yr: Initial: 2 sprays in each nostril QAM and QHS or, 4 sprays in each nostril QAM. Reduce dose gradually to the lowest effective dose after resolution of symptoms.
Max total dose: 250 mcg/24 hr (8 sprays)

Reduce maintenance dose to as low as possible to control symptoms. May cause pharyngitis, cough, epistaxis, and nasal irritation. Rinse mouth after each use via the oral inhalation route. Although not yet approved in the United States, nebulized budesonide has been shown effective in mild to moderate croup at doses of 2 mg × 1. Ref: *N Engl J Med* 331(5):285.

BUMETANIDE
Bumex
Loop diuretic

No **?** **C**

Tabs: 0.5, 1, 2 mg
Injection: 0.25 mg/ml (some preparations may contain 1% benzyl alcohol)

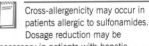

Children: PO, IM, IV
≥6 *mo:* 0.015–0.1 mg/kg/dose QD-QOD
Adults:
    PO: 0.5–2 mg/dose QD-BID
    IM/IV: 0.5–1 mg over 1–2 min. May give additional doses Q2–3 hr PRN
Usual max dose (PO/IM/IV): 10 mg/24 hr

Cross-allergenicity may occur in patients allergic to sulfonamides. Dosage reduction may be necessary in patients with hepatic dysfunction. Administer oral doses with food.

Side effects include cramps, dizziness, hypotension, headache, electrolyte losses (hypokalemia, hypocalcemia, hyponatremia, hypochloremia), and encephalopathy. May also lead to metabolic alkalosis.

BUPIVICAINE

Marcaine, Sensorcaine, Sensorcaine-MPF, Bupivicaine Spinal, and others

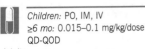

No   ?   C

Local Anesthetic
Inj (preservative-free): 0.25%, 0.5%, 0.75% (2.5, 5, 7.5 mg/ml, respectively)
Inj: 0.25%, 5% (some preparations may contain 1 mg/ml methylparabens)
Injection with 1:200,000 epi (preservative-free): 0.25%, 0.5%, 0.75%
Injection with 1:200,000 epi: 0.25%, 0.5%
Spinal Injection (preservative-free): 0.75% in dextrose 8.25%

Caudal block: 1–3.7 mg/kg; with or without epinephrine
Epidural block: 1.25 mg/kg

Contraindicated in patients allergic to other amide-type anesthetics, regional intravenous anesthesia (Bier Block), obstetrical paracervical block. May cause hypotension, asystole,

seizures, and respiratory arrest. Prolonged use, particularly in neonates and infants, may lead to toxicity. Use with **caution** in severe liver disease.

Solutions containing epinephrine contain metabisulfate, which can induce allergic reactions including anaphylaxis. See Chapter 30 for additional information.

CAFFEINE

Caffeine base, caffeine citrate
Methylxanthine, respiratory stimulant

No   1   B

Injectable and oral liquid: 20 mg/ml (citrate salt) = 10 mg/ml (caffeine base) (also available as powder for compounding)

Doses expressed in mg of caffeine citrate. To convert to mg of caffeine base divide citrate dose by 2.

Neonatal apnea:
  Loading dose: 10–20 mg/kg IV/PO × 1
  Maintenance dose: 5–10 mg/kg/dose PO/IV QD, to begin 24 hr after loading dose

Avoid use in symptomatic cardiac arrhythmias. Caffeine benzoate formulation has been associated with causation of kernicterus in neonates.

Therapeutic levels: 5–25 mg/L. Cardiovascular, neurologic, or GI toxicity reported at serum levels >50 mg/L. Recommended serum sampling time: obtain trough level within 30 minutes prior to an oral dose. Steady-state is typically achieved 3 weeks following the initiation of therapy. Levels obtained prior to steady-state are useful for preventing toxicity.

CALCITONIN

Calcimar, Cibacalcin, Miacalcin, Miacalcin Nasal Spray
Hypercalcemia antidote, antiosteoporotic   No   ?   B
Injection:
  Salmon: 200 U/ml (2 ml); contains phenol
  Human (Cibacalcin): 0.5 mg (1 ml)
Nasal Spray:
  Salmon: 200 U/metered dose (2 ml, provides 14 doses)

Ostegenesis Imperfecta:
  6 mon.–15 yrs: (Salmon calcitonin) 2 U/kg/dose IM/SC 3 times per week with oral calcium supplements.
Hypercalcemia (adult doses):
  Salmon calcitonin: Start with 4 U/kg/dose IM/SC Q12 hr; if response is unsatisfactory after 1 or 2 days, increase dose to 8 U/kg/dose Q12 hr. If response remains unsatisfactory after 2 more days, increase to a **maximum** of 8 U/kg/dose Q6 hr.
Paget's Disease (adult doses):
  Salmon calcitonin:
    IM/SC: Start with 100 U QD initially, followed by a usual maintenance dose of 50 U QD OR 50–100 U Q 1–3 days
    Intranasal: 1–2 sprays (200–400 U) QD

Human calcitonin: Start with 0.5 mg SC QD initially, followed by a usual maintenance dose of 0.5 mg SC 2–3 times per week OR 0.25 mg SC QD

Contraindicated in patients sensitive to salmon protein or gelatin. If using salmon calcitonin product, prepare a 10 U/ml dilution with normal saline and administer 0.1 ml intradermally as a skin test (observe for 15 minutes). Nausea, abdominal pain, flushing, and inflamation at the injection site has been reported with IM/SC route of administration. Nasal irritation, rhinitis, epistaxis may occur with use of the nasal spray. If the injection volume exceeds 2 ml, use IM route and multiple sites of injection.

For explanation of icons, see p. 600.

CALCITRIOL

1,25-dihydroxycholecalciferol, Rocaltrol, Calcijex
Active form Vitamin D, fat soluble   No   2   A/D
Caps: 0.25, 0.5 mcg
Inj: (Calcijex) 1, 2 mcg/ml (1 ml)

Renal failure:
Children:
  Oral: Suggested dose range
0.01–0.05 mcg/kg/24 hr. Titrate in
0.005–0.01 mcg/kg/24 hr increments
Q4–8 wk based on clinical response.
  IV: 0.01–0.05 mcg/kg/dose given
  3 ×/week
Adults:
  Initial: 0.25 mcg/dose PO QD–QOD
  Increment: 0.25 mcg/dose PO Q4–
  8 wk. Usual dose is 0.5–1 mcg/
  24 hr.
Adult: IV: 0.5 mcg/24 hr given 3
×/week. Usual dose is 0.5–3 mcg/24 hr
given 3 ×/week

Most potent vitamin D metabolite
available. Monitor serum calcium
and phosphorus. **Avoid**
concomitant use of Mg^{++}-containing
antacids. IV dosing applies if patient
undergoing hemodialysis.

Contraindicated in patients with
hypercalcemia, vitamin D toxicity. Side
effects include: weakness, headache,
vomiting, constipation, hypotonia,
polydipsia, polyuria, myalgia, metastatic
calcification, etc.

Pregnancy category changes to "D" if
used in doses above the recommended
daily allowance.

CALCIUM CARBONATE

Tums, Os-Cal, and others; 40% Elemental Ca
Calcium supplement, antacid   No   ?   C
Tab, chewable: 350, 420, 500, 550, 750, 850, 1000, 1250 mg
Tab: 500, 650, 1000, 1250, 1500 mg
Lozenge: 600 mg
Susp: 400 mg/5 ml, 1000 mg/5 ml, 1250 mg/5 ml
Caps: 1250, 1500 mg
Powder: 6500 mg/packet
Each 1000 mg of salt contains 20 mEq elemental Ca (400 mg elemental Ca)

Doses expressed in mg of
elemental Calcium. To convert to
mg of salt, divide elemental dose
by 0.4.
Hypocalcemia:
  Neonates: 50–150 mg/kg/24 hr ÷
  Q4–6 hr PO; max dose: 1 g/24 hr
  Children: 45–65 mg/kg/24 hr PO ÷ QID
  Adults: 1–2 g/24 hr PO ÷ TID-QID

Side effects: constipation,
hypercalcemia, hypophosphatemia,
hypomagnesemia, nausea,
vomiting, headache, confusion. May
reduce absorption of tetracycline, iron,
and effectiveness of polystrene sulfonate.
May potentiate effects of digoxin. Some
products may contain trace amounts of
Na. Administer each dose with meals or
with lots of fluid.

CALCIUM CHLORIDE

27% Elemental Ca
Calcium supplement   **No   ?   C**
Injection: 100 mg/ml (10%) (1.36 mEq Ca/ml); each gram of salt contains 13.6 mEq (270 mg) elemental Ca

 Doses expressed in mg of CaCl
Cardiac arrest:
Infant/Child: 20 mg/kg/dose IV (0.2 ml/kg/dose) Q10 min
Adults: 250–500 mg/dose IV (2.5–5 ml/dose) Q10 min or 2–4 mg/kg/dose Q10 min
MAXIMUM IV ADMINISTRATION RATES:
IV push: **Do not exceed** 100 mg/min
IV infusion: **Do not exceed** 45–90 mg/kg/hr with a **maximum concentration** of 20 mg/ml.

Use IV with extreme caution. Extravasation may lead to necrosis. Hyaluronidase may be helpful for extravasation. Central-line administration is preferred IV route of administration. **Do not administer IM or SC route.**
Rapid IV infusion associated with bradycardia, hypotension, and peripheral vasodilation. May cause hyperchloremic acidosis.

CALCIUM GLUBIONATE

Neo-Calglucon; 6.4% Elemental Ca
Calcium supplement   **No   ?   C**
Syrup: 1.8 g/5 ml (480 ml) (1.2 mEq Ca/ml); each gram of salt contains 3.2 mEq (64 mg) elemental Ca.

 Doses expressed in mg Calcium glubionate
Neonatal hypocalcemia: 1200 mg/kg/24 hr PO ÷ Q4–6 hr
Maintenance:
Infant/Child: 600–2000 mg/kg/24 hr PO ÷ QID; **max dose:** 9 g/24 hr
Adult: 6–18 g/24 hr PO ÷ QID

Side effects include GI irritation, dizziness, and headache. Best absorbed when given before meals. Absorption inhibited by high phosphate load. High osmotic load of syrup (20% sucrose) may cause diarrhea.

CALCIUM GLUCEPTATE

(8.2% Ca)
8.2% Elemental Ca

No ? C

Calcium Supplement

Injection: 220 mg/ml (22%) (0.9 mEq Ca/ml); each gram of salt contains 4.1 mEq (82 mg) elemental Ca.

Doses expressed in mg of Calcium gluceptate

Hypocalcemia:

Children: 200–500 mg/kg/24 hr IV ÷ Q6 hr

Adult: 500–1100 mg/dose IV as needed

Cardiac arrest:

Children: 110 mg/kg/dose IV Q10 min

MAXIMUM IV ADMINISTRATION RATES:

IV push: **Do not exceed** 100 mg/min

IV infusion: **Do not exceed** 150–300 mg/kg/hr with a **maximum concentration** of 55 mg/ml.

See calcium gluconate.

CALCIUM GLUCONATE

9% Elemental Ca

Calcium supplement

No ? C

Tabs: 500, 650, 975, 1000 mg

Injection: 100 mg/ml (10%) (0.45 mEq Ca^{++}/ml); each gram of salt contains 4.8 mEq (90 mg) elemental Ca

Doses expressed in mg Calcium gluconate

Maintenance/hypocalcemia:

Neonates: IV: 200–800 mg/kg/24 hr ÷ Q6 hr

Infants:

IV: 200–500 mg/kg/24 hr ÷ Q6 hr

PO: 400–800 mg/kg/24 hr ÷ Q6 hr

Child: 200–500 mg/kg/24 hr IV or PO ÷ Q6 hr

Adult: 5–15 g/24 hr IV or PO ÷ Q6 hr

For cardiac arrest:

Infants and children: 100 mg/kg/dose (1 ml/kg/dose) IV Q10 min

Adults: 500–800 mg/dose (5–8 ml/dose) IV Q10 min

Max dose: 3 g/dose

MAXIMUM IV ADMINISTRATION RATES:

IV push: **Do not exceed** 100 mg/min

IV infusion: **Do not exceed** 120–240 mg/kg/hr with a **maximum concentration** of 50 mg/ml

Avoid peripheral infusion as extravasation may cause tissue necrosis. IV infusion associated with hypotension and bradycardia. Also associated with arrythmias in digitalized patients. May precipitate when used with bicarbonate. **Do not use scalp veins! Do not administer IM or SC.**

CALCIUM LACTATE
13% Elemental Ca
Calcium supplement
Tabs: 325, 650 mg; each gram of salt contains 6.5 mEq (130 mg) elemental Ca

No ? C

 Doses expressed in mg of Calcium lactate.
Infants: 400–500 mg/kg/24 hr PO ÷ Q4–6 hr
Children: 500 mg/kg/24 hr PO ÷ Q6–8 hr
Adult: 1.5–3 g PO Q8 hr
Max dose: 9 g/24 hr

Give with meals. Do not dissolve tablets in milk.

CAPTOPRIL
Capoten
Angiotensin converting enzyme inhibitor, anti-hypertensive
Tabs: 12.5, 25, 50, 100 mg
Suspension: 1 mg/ml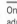

 Yes 1 C/D

 Neonates: 0.1–0.4 mg/kg/24 hr PO ÷ Q6–8 hr
Infants: Initially 0.15–0.3 mg/kg/dose; titrate upward if needed; **max dose:** 6 mg/kg/24 hr ÷ QD-QID
Children: Initially 0.3–0.5 mg/kg/dose Q8 hr; titrate upward if needed; **max dose:** 6 mg/kg/24 hr ÷ BID-QID
Adolescents and adults: Initially 12.5–25 mg/dose PO BID–TID; increase weekly if necessary by 25 mg/dose to **max dose:** 450 mg/24 hr

Onset within 15–30 min of administration. Peak effect within 1–2 hr. **Adjust dose with renal failure, see p. 938.** Should be administered on an empty stomach 1 hr before or 2 hr after meals. Titrate to minimal effective dose.

Use with **caution** in collagen vascular disease. May cause rash, proteinuria, neutropenia, cough, angioedema, hyperkalemia, hypotension, or diminution of taste perception (with long-term use). Known to decrease aldosterone and increase renin production.

Pregnancy category is a "C" during the first trimester but changes to a "D" for the second and third trimester.

CARBAMAZEPINE
Atretol, Epitol, Tegretol, Tegretol-XR, Carbatrol
Anticonvulsant   **Yes   1   C**

Tabs: 200 mg
Chewable tabs: 100 mg
Extended release tabs: 100, 200, 400 mg
Extended release caps: 200, 300 mg
Suspension: 100 mg/5 ml (450 ml)

<6 yr:
Initial: 10–20 mg/kg/24 hr PO ÷
BID-TID (QID for suspension)
Increment: q5–7 days up to 35
mg/kg/24 hr PO
6–12 yr:
Initial: 10 mg/kg/24 hr PO ÷ BID up to
max dose: 100 mg/dose BID
Increment: 100 mg/24 hr at 1 wk
intervals (÷ TID-QID) until desired
response is obtained
Maintenance: 20–30 mg/kg/24 hr PO ÷
BID-QID; usual maintenance dose is
400–800 mg/24 hr; **max dose:**
1000 mg/24 hr
>12 yr:
Initial: 200 mg PO BID
Increment: 200 mg/24 hr at 1 wk
intervals (÷ BID-QID) until desired
response is obtained
Maintenance: 800–1200 mg/24 hr
PO ÷ BID-QID
Max dose:
12–15 yr: 1000 mg/24 hr
Adult: 1.6–2.4 g/24 hr

Contraindicated for patients taking
MAO inhibitors or who are sensitive
to tricyclic antidepressants.
Erythromycin, verapamil, cimetidine, and
INH may increase serum levels.
Carbamazepine may decrease activity of
warfarin, doxycycline, oral contraceptives,
cyclosporin, theophylline, phenytoin,
benzodiazepines, ethosuximide, and
valproic acid. Carbamazepine is a
substrate and inducer of CYP 450 3A3-4
(see p. 924).

Suggested dosing intervals for specific
dosage forms:
extended release tabs or caps (BID);
chewable and immediate release tablets
(BID–TID); suspension (QID). Doses may
be administered with food. Do not crush
or chew extended release dosage forms.
Do not administer the oral suspension
simultaneously with other liquid
medicines or diluents.

Drug metabolism typically increases
after the first month of therapy due to
hepatic autoinduction. $T_{1/2}$ = 25–65 hrs,
initially. $T_{1/2}$ for children = 8–14 hrs. $T_{1/2}$
for adults = 12–17 hrs.

Therapeutic blood levels: 4–12 mg/L.
Recommended serum sampling time:
obtain trough level within 30 minutes
prior to an oral dose. Steady-state is
typically achieved one month following
the initiation of therapy (following
enzymatic autoinduction). Levels obtained
prior to steady-state are useful for
preventing toxicity.

Side effects include sedation, dizziness,
diplopia, aplastic anemia, neutropenia,
urinary retention, nausea, SIADH, and
Stevens-Johnson syndrome. Pretreatment
CBCs and LFTs is suggested. Patient
should be monitored for hematologic and
hepatic toxicity. **Adjust dose in renal
impairment, see p. 938).**

See p. 27 for management of
ingestions.

CARBENICILLIN

Geocillin, Geopen, Pyopen
Antibiotic, penicillin (extended spectrum)
Yes   ?   B
Tabs (as Indanyl sodium): 382 mg; each 382 mg tab contains 1 mEq Na

Mild infection:
Children: 30–50 mg/kg/24 hr PO
÷ Q6 hr; **max dose:** 2–3 g/24 hr
Adults (UTI): 382–764 mg PO Q6 hr

Use with **caution** in penicillin allergic patients. Most frequent side effects are nausea, vomiting, diarrhea, abdominal cramps, and flatulence. May cause hepatotoxicity. Furry tongue is a reported side effect. **Adjust dose in renal failure, see p. 929).**

CARNITINE

Levocarnitine, Carnitor, VitaCarn
L-Carnitine
No   ?   B
Tabs: 330 mg
Caps: 250 mg
Solution: 100 mg/ml (118 ml)
Injection: 200 mg/ml (5ml) (preservative free)

Oral:
Children: 50–100 mg/kg/24 hr
PO ÷ Q8–12 hr; increase slowly as needed and tolerated to **max dose** of 3 g/
24 hr
Adults: 330 mg to 1 g/dose BID-TID PO
IV:
Children and Adults: 50 mg/kg as loading dose; may follow with 50 mg/
kg/24 hr IV infusion; maintenance:
50 mg/kg/24 hr ÷ Q4–6 hr; increase to **maximum** of 300 mg/kg/24 hr if needed.

May cause nausea, vomiting, abdominal cramps, diarrhea, body odor. Give bolus IV infusion over 2–3 minutes.

CEFACLOR
Ceclor
Antibiotic, cephalosporin (2nd generation) Yes 1 B
Caps: 250, 500 mg
Extended release tabs: 375, 500 mg
Suspension: 125, 187, 250, 375 mg/5 ml (75, 150 ml)

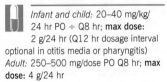 *Infant and child:* 20–40 mg/kg/
24 hr PO ÷ Q8 hr; **max dose:**
2 g/24 hr (Q12 hr dosage interval
optional in otitis media or pharyngitis)
Adult: 250–500 mg/dose PO Q8 hr; **max
dose:** 4 g/24 hr

Use with **caution** in patients with
penicillin allergy or renal
impairment. May cause positive
Coomb's test or false-positive test for
urinary glucose. Serum sickness reactions
have been reported in patients receiving
multiple courses of cefaclor. **Adjust dose
in renal failure (see p. 929).**

CEFADROXIL
Duricef, Ultracef
Antibiotic, cephalosporin (1st generation) Yes 1 B
Suspension: 125, 250, 500 mg/5 ml (50, 100 ml)
Tabs: 1 g
Caps: 500 mg

Infant and child: 30 mg/kg/24 hr
PO ÷ Q12 hr
Adult: 1–2 g/24 hr PO ÷ Q12 hr;
max dose: 2 g/24 hr

See cephalexin. Side effects include
nausea, vomiting,
pseudomembranous colitis,
pruritus, neutropenia, vaginitis, and
candidiasis. **Adjust dose in renal failure
(see p. 929).**

CEFAMANDOLE
Mandol
Antibiotic, cephalosporin (2nd generation) Yes 1 B
Injection: 0.5, 1, 2, 10 g (3.3 mEq Na/g)

Child: 50–150 mg/kg/24 hr IM/IV
÷ Q4–6 hr
Adult: 4–12 g/24 hr IM/IV ÷ Q4–
8 hr; **max dose:** 12 g/24 hr, 2 g/dose

See cefaclor. May cause elevated
liver enzymes, coagulopathy,
transient neutropenia, and
disulfiram-like reaction with ethanol. Does
not penetrate well into cerebrospinal fluid.
Adjust dose in renal failure (see p. 929).

CEFAZOLIN

Ancef, Kefzol, Zolicef, others
Antibiotic, cephalosporin (1st generation)
Injection: 0.25, 0.5, 1, 5, 10, 20 g (2.1 mEq Na/g)

Yes   1   B

Neonate IM, IV:
Postnatal age ≤7 days: 40 mg/kg/24 hr ÷ Q12 hr
Postnatal age >7 days:
  ≤2000 g: 40 mg/kg/24 hr ÷ Q12 hr
  >2000 g: 60 mg/kg/24 hr ÷ Q8 hr
Infant >1 mo/children: 50–100 mg/kg/24 hr ÷ Q8 hr IV/IM; **max dose:** 6 g/24 hr
Adult: 2–6 g/24 hr ÷ Q6–8 hr IV/IM; **max dose:** 12 g/24 hr

See cephalexin. Use with **caution** in renal impairment or in penicillin-allergic patients. Does not penetrate well into cerebrospinal fluid. May cause phlebitis, leukopenia, thrombocytopenia, transient liver enzyme elevation, false-positive urine reducing substance. **Adjust dose in renal failure (see p. 929).**

CEFEPIME

Maxipime
Antibiotic, cephalosporin (4th generation)
Injection: 0.5, 1, 2 gm
Each 1 g drug contains 725 mg L-Arginine

Yes   1   B

Children ≥2 months: 100 mg/kg/24 hr ÷ Q12 hr IV/IM
  Meningitis or serious infections: 150 mg/kg/24 hr ÷ Q8 hr IV/IM
  Max dose: 6 gm/24 hr
Cystic Fibrosis: 150 mg/kg/24 hr ÷ Q8 hr IV/IM, up to a **maximum** of 6 g/24 hr.
Adult: 1–4 g/24 hr ÷ Q12 hr IV/IM
  Severe Infections: 6 g/24 hr ÷ Q8 hr IV/IM
  Max dose: 6 g/24 hr

Use with **caution** in patients with penicillin allergy or renal impairment. Good activity against *P. aeruginosa* and other gram-negative bacterias plus most gram positives *(S. aureus)*. May cause thrombophlebitis, gastrointestinal discomfort, transient increases in liver enzymes. **Adjust dose in renal failure (see p. 930).**

CEFIXIME
Suprax
Antibiotic, cephalosporin (3rd generation)
Tabs: 200, 400 mg
Suspension: 100 mg/5 ml (50, 100 ml)

Yes   1   B

 Infant and child: 8 mg/kg/24 hr ÷ Q12–24 hr PO; **max dose:** 400 mg/ 24 hr
Adolescent/Adult: 400 mg/24 hr ÷ Q12–24 hr PO
Uncomplicated cervical, urethral, or rectal infections due to N. gonorrhoeae: 400 mg × 1 PO

 Use with **caution** in patients with penicillin allergy or renal failure. Adverse reactions include diarrhea, abdominal pain, nausea, headaches. Do not use tablets for the treatment of otitis media due to reduced bioavailability. **Adjust dose in renal failure (see p. 930).**

CEFOPERAZONE
Cefobid
Antibiotic, cephalosporin (3rd generation)
Injection: 1, 2, 10 g (1.5 mEq Na/g)

No   1   B

 Infant and child: 100–200 mg/kg/24 hr ÷ Q8–12 hr IV/IM
Adult: 2–4 g/24 hr ÷ Q12 hr IV/IM; **max dose:** 12 g/24 hr

 Use with **caution** in penicillin-allergic patients or in patients with hepatic failure, or biliary obstruction. Drug is extensively excreted in bile. May cause disulfiram-like reaction with ethanol. Bleeding and brusing may occur especially in patients with vitamin K deficiency. Does not penetrate well into cerebrospinal fluid.

CEFOTAXIME
Claforan
Antibiotic, cephalosporin (3rd generation)
Injection: 0.5, 1, 2, 10 g (2.2 mEq Na/g)

Yes   1   B

Neonates: IV/IM:
Postnatal age ≤7 days:
<2000 g: 100 mg/kg/24 hr ÷ Q12 hr
≥2000 g: 100–150 mg/kg/24 hr ÷ Q8–12 hr
Postnatal age >7 days:
<1200 g: 100 mg/kg/24 hr ÷ Q12 hr
≥1200 g: 150 mg/kg/24 hr ÷ Q8 hr
Infant and child: (<50 kg): 100–200 mg/kg/24 hr ÷ Q6–8 hr IV/IM (see remarks)
Meningitis: 200 mg/kg/24 hr ÷ Q6 hr IV/IM (see remarks)
Max dose: 12 g/24 hr
Adult: (≥50 kg): 1–2 g/dose Q6–8 hr IV/IM
Severe Infection: 2 g/dose Q4–6 hr IV/IM
Max dose: 12 g/24 hr

Use with **caution** in penicillin-allergic patients or in presence of renal impairment (reduce dosage). Toxicities similar to other cephalosporins: allergy, neutropenia, thrombocytopenia, eosinophilia, positive Coomb's test, elevated BUN, creatinine, and liver enzymes.

Good CNS penetration. 225–300 mg/kg/24 hr ÷ Q6–8 hr, in combination with vancomycin (60 mg/kg/24 hr), has been recommended for meningitis due to penicillin-resistant pneumococci. 150–225 mg/kg/24 hr ÷ Q6–8 hr has been recommended for infections outside the CSF due to penicillin-resistant pneumococci. *Pediatrics* 99(2);1997:293.
Adjust dose in renal failure (see p. 930).

CEFOTETAN
Cefotan
Antibiotic, cephalosporin (2nd generation)
Injection: 1, 2, 10 g (3.5 mEq Na/g)

Yes   **1**   **B**

Infant and child: 40–80 mg/kg/24 hr ÷ Q12 hr IV/IM
Adult: 2–6 g/24 hr ÷ Q12 hr IV/IM
Max dose: 6 g/24 hr

Use with **caution** in penicillin-allergic patients or in presence of renal impairment. Has good anaerobic activity. May cause disulfiram-like reaction with ethanol. CSF penetration is poor. **Adjust dose in renal failure (see p. 930).**

CEFOXITIN

Mefoxin

Antibiotic, cephalosporin (2nd generation)

Injection: 1, 2, 10 g (2.3 mEq Na/g)

Yes 1 B

 Infant and child: 80–160 mg/kg/24 hr ÷ Q4–8 hr IM/IV
Adult: 4–12 g/24 hr ÷ Q6–8 hr IM/IV
Max dose: 12 g/24 hr

Use with **caution** in penicillin-allergic patients or in presence of renal impairment. Has good anaerobic activity. CSF penetration is poor.

Adjust dose in renal failure (see p. 931).

CEFPODOXIME PROXETIL

Vantin

Antibiotic, cephalosporin (2nd generation)

Tabs: 100, 200 mg

Suspension: 50, 100 mg/5 ml (100 ml)

Yes 1 B

 5 mo–12 yr: 10 mg/kg/24 hr PO ÷ Q12–24 hr; **max dose:** 400 mg/24 hr
≥13 yr–adult: 200–800 mg/24 hr PO ÷ Q12 hr
Uncomplicated gonorrhea: 200 mg PO × 1

Use with **caution** in penicillin-allergic patients or in presence of renal impairment. May cause diarrhea, nausea, vomiting, vaginal candidiasis.

Tablets should be administered with food to enhance absorption. Suspension may be administered without regard to food. High doses of antacids or H_2 blockers may reduce absorption.

Adjust dose in renal failure (see p. 931).

CEFPROZIL
Cefzil
Antibiotic, cephalosporin (2nd generation)
Tabs: 250, 500 mg
Suspension: 125 mg/5 ml, 250 mg/5 ml (50, 75, 100 ml)

Yes   1   B

 Otitis Media:
   6 mo–12 yr: 30 mg/kg/24 hr PO ÷ Q12 hr
Pharyngitis/Tonsillitis:
   2–12 yrs: 15 mg/kg/24 hr PO ÷ Q12 hr
Other:
   ≥12 yr: 500–1000 mg/24 hr PO ÷ Q12–24 hr
Max dose: 1 g/24 hr

Use with **caution** in penicillin-allergic patients or in presence of renal impairment. Absorption is not affected by food. **Adjust dose in renal failure (see p. 931).**

CEFTAZIDIME
Fortaz, Tazidime, Tazicef, Ceptaz [arginine salt]
Antibiotic, cephalosporin (3rd generation)
Injection: 0.5, 1, 2, 6, 10 g
(Fortaz, Tazicef, Tazidime contains 2.3 mEq Na/g drug)
(Ceptaz contains 349 mg L-arginine/g drug)

Yes   1   B

 Neonates: IV/IM:
   Postnatal age ≤7 days: 100 mg/kg/24 hr ÷ Q12 hr
Postnatal age >7 days:
   <1200 g: 100 mg/kg/24 hr ÷ Q12 hr
   ≥1200 g: 150 mg/kg/24 hr ÷ Q8 hr
Infant and child: 90–150 mg/kg/24 hr ÷ Q8 hr IV/IM
Meningitis: 150 mg/kg/24 hr ÷ Q8 hr IV/IM

Cystic fibrosis: 150 mg/kg/24 hr ÷ Q8 hr IV/IM
Adult: 2–6 g/24 hr ÷ Q8–12 hr IV/IM
Max dose: 6 g/24 hr

Use with **caution** in penicillin-allergic patients or in presence of renal impairment. Good Pseudomonas coverage and CSF penetration. **Adjust dose in renal failure (see p. 931).**

CEFTIBUTEN

Cedax
Antibiotic, cephalosporin (3rd generation)   **Yes**   **1**   **B**
Suspension: 90 mg/5 ml (30, 60, 90, 120 ml); 180 mg/5 ml (30, 60, 120 ml)
Tabs: 400 mg

Children: 9 mg/kg/24 hr PO QD
≥12 yr: 400 mg PO QD
Max dose: 400 mg/24 hr

Use with **caution** in penicillin-allergic patients or in presence of renal impairment. Suspension should be administered 2 hours before or 1 hour after a meal. **Adjust dose in renal failure (see p. 931).**

CEFTIZOXIME
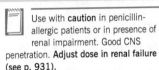

Cefizox
Antibiotic, cephalosporin (3rd generation)   **Yes**   **1**   **B**
Injection: 0.5, 1, 2, 10 g (2.6 mEq Na/g)

Infant and child: 150–200 mg/kg/24 hr ÷ Q6–8 hr IV/IM
Adult: 2–12 g/24 hr ÷ Q8–12 hr IV/IM
Uncomplicated gonorrhea: 1 g IM × 1
Max dose: 12 g/24 hr

Use with **caution** in penicillin-allergic patients or in presence of renal impairment. Good CNS penetration. **Adjust dose in renal failure (see p. 931).**

CEFTRIAXONE
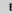

Rocephin
Antibiotic, cephalosporin (3rd generation)   **No**   **1**   **B**
Injection: 0.25, 0.5, 1, 2, 10 g (3.6 mEq Na/g)

Neonate:
*Gonococcal ophthalmia or
prophylaxis:* 25–50 mg/kg/dose
IM/IV × 1; **max dose:** 125 mg/dose
Infant and child: 50–75 mg/kg/24 hr ÷
Q12–24 hr IM/IV (see remarks)
  *Meningitis (including penicillin resistant
  pneumococci):* 100 mg/kg/24 hr IM/IV
  ÷ Q12 hr; **max dose:** 4 g/24 hr
  Acute otitis media: 50 mg/kg IM × 1;
  max dose: 1g
Adult: 1–4 g/24 hr ÷ Q12–24 hr IV/IM;
max dose: 4 g/24 hr
  Uncomplicated gonorrhea: 125 mg
  IM × 1
  Chancroid: 250 mg IM × 1

Use with **caution** in penicillin-
allergic patients or in presence of
renal impairment. May cause
reversible cholelithiasis, sludging in
gallbladder, and jaundice.

Use with **caution in neonates** and
continuous dosing because of risk for
hyperbilirubinemia. Consider using an
alternative 3rd generation cephalosporin
with similar activity.

80–100 mg/kg/24 hr ÷ Q12–24 hr has
been recommended for infections outside
the CSF due to penicillin-resistant pneumococci. Pediatrics 99(2);1997:293.

CEFUROXIME (IV, IM)/CEFUROXIME AXETIL (PO)
CEFUROXIME AXETIL (PO)

Yes 1 B

IV: Zinacef, Kefurox; PO: Ceftin
Antibiotic, cephalosporin (2nd generation)
Injection: 0.75, 1.5, 7.5 g (2.4 mEq Na/g)
Tabs: 125, 250, 500 mg
Suspension: 125, 250 mg/5 ml (50, 100 ml)

IM/IV:
  Neonates: 20–60 mg/kg/24 hr ÷
  Q12 hr
Infant/Child: 75–150 mg/kg/24 hr ÷
Q8 hr;
Max dose: 6 g/24 hr
Adults: 750–1500 mg/dose Q8 hr;
Max dose: 9 g/24 hr
PO:
Children:
  Pharyngitis:
    Suspension: 20 mg/kg/24 hr ÷
    Q12 hr; **max dose:** 500 mg/24 hr
    Tab: 125 mg Q12 hr
  Otitis Media/Impetigo:
    Suspension: 30 mg/kg/24 hr ÷
    Q12 hr; **max dose:** 1 g/24 hr

  Tab: 250 mg Q12 hr
  Adults: 250–500 mg BID
  Max dose: 1 g/24 hr

Use with **caution** in penicillin-
allergic patients or in presence of
renal impairment. May cause
thrombophlebitis at the infusion site. Not
recommended for meningitis.

Tablets and suspension are NOT
bioequivalent and are NOT substitutable
on a mg/mg basis. Administer suspension
with food. **Adjust dose in renal failure
(see p. 931).**

CEPHALEXIN
Keflex, Cefanex, C-Lexin, and others
Antibiotic, cephalosporin (1st generation)

Yes   1   B

Tabs: 250, 500 mg, 1 g
Caps: 250, 500 mg
Suspension: 125 mg/5 ml, 250 mg/5 ml (60, 100, 200 ml)
Drops: 100 mg/ml (10 ml)

 Infant and Child: 25–100 mg/kg/24 hr PO ÷ Q6 hr
Adult: 1–4 g/24 hr PO ÷ Q6 hr
Max dose: 4 g/24 hr

Some cross-reactivity with penicillins. Use with **caution** in renal insufficiency. Administer doses on an empty stomach; 2 hours before and 1 hour after meals. Less frequent dosing (Q8-12 hr) can be used for uncomplicated infections. **Adjust dose in renal failure (see p. 931).**

CEPHALOTHIN
Keflin
Antibiotic, cephalosporin (1st generation)

Yes   1   B

Injection: 1, 2 g (2.8 mEq Na/g)

 Neonates:
IV: <2 kg:
  0–7 days: 40 mg/kg/24 hr ÷ Q12 hr
  >7 days: 40–60 mg/kg/24 hr ÷ Q8–12 hr
≥2 kg:
  0–7 days: 60 mg/kg/24 hr ÷ Q8 hr
  >7 days: 80 mg/kg/24 hr ÷ Q6 hr
Infant and child: 80–160 mg/kg/24 hr ÷ Q4–6 hr IV or deep IM
Adults: 2–12 g/24 hr ÷ Q4–6 hr IV/IM
Max dose: 12 g/24 hr

Some cross-reactivity with penicillins. Use with **caution** in renal insufficiency. May cause phlebitis. Similar spectrum to cefazolin but with a longer $T_{1/2}$. CSF penetration is poor. **Adjust dose in renal failure (see p. 931).**

CEPHRADINE
Velosef, and others
Antibiotic, cephalosporin (1st generation)
Suspension: 125 mg/5 ml, 250 mg/5 ml (100, 200 ml)
Caps: 250, 500 mg
Injection: 0.25, 0.5, 1, 2 gm (6 mEq Na/1g)

     Yes   1   B

    Child: PO: 25–50 mg/kg/24 hr ÷ Q6–12 hr
Adult: PO: 1–4 g/24 hr ÷ Q6–12 hr
Max dose: 4 g/24 hr

Some cross-reactivity with penicillins. Use with **caution** in renal insufficiency. Does not penetrate well into cerebrospinal fluid.
Adjust dose in renal failure (see p. 931).

CETIRIZINE
Zyrtec
Antihistamine, less-sedating
Syrup: 5 mg/5 ml (120 ml)
Tabs: 5, 10 mg

    Yes   ?   B

    Children 2–5 yr: Initial dose: 2.5 mg PO QD; if needed, may increase dose to a **maximum** of 5 mg/24hr.
≥6 yr–Adult: 5–10 mg PO QD

May cause headache, pharyngitis, GI symptoms, dry mouth, sedation.
Has NOT been implicated in causing cardiac arrhythmias when used with other drugs that are metabolized by hepatic microsomal enzymes (e.g., ketoconazole, erythromycin).
Dosage adjustment is recommended in renal or hepatic impairment (see p. 938).

CHARCOAL, ACTIVATED
See Chapter 2

CHLORAL HYDRATE
Noctec, Aquachloral Supprettes
Sedative, hypnotic
Caps: 250, 500 mg
Syrup: 250, 500 mg/5 ml
Suppository: 324, 500, 648 mg

Yes 1 C

 Children:
Sedative: 25–50 mg/kg/24 hr
PO/PR ÷ Q6–8 hr; **max dose:**
500 mg/dose
Sedation for procedures: 25–100
mg/kg/dose PO/PR;
max dose: 1 g/dose (infants); 2 g/dose
(children)
Adult:
Sedative: 250 mg/dose TID PO/PR
Hypnotic: 500–1000 mg/dose PO/PR;
max dose: 2 g/24 hr

Contraindicated in patients with
hepatic or renal disease. May
cause GI irritation, paradoxical
excitement, hypotension, and
myocardial/respiratory depression. Chronic
administration in neonates can lead to
accumulation of active metabolites.
Requires same monitoring as other
sedatives.
   Not analgesic. Peak effects occur within
30-60 minutes. Do not exceed 2 weeks of
chronic use. **Avoid** use in severe renal
failure. Sudden withdrawal may cause
delirium tremens.

CHLORAMPHENICOL
Chloromycetin and others
Antibiotic
Caps: 250 mg
Injection: 1 g (2.25 mEq Na/1g)
Otic solution: 0.5% (15 ml)
Ophthalmic solution: 0.5% (2.5, 7.5, 15 ml)
Ophthalmic ointment: 1% (3.5 g)
Powder for ophthalmic solution: 25 mg (preservative-free)
Topical cream: 1% (30 g)

Yes 3 C

Neonates IV:
Loading dose: 20 mg/kg
Maintenance dose:

≤7 days: 25 mg/kg/24 hr QD
>7 days:

≤2 kg: 25 mg/kg/24 hr QD
>2 kg: 50 mg/kg/24 hr ÷ Q12 hr
The first maintenance dose should be
given 12 hours after the loading dose
Infants/children/adults: 50–75 mg/kg/
24 hr IV/PO ÷ Q6 hr
Meningitis: 75–100 mg/kg/24 hr IV ÷
Q6 hr
Max dose: 4 g/24 hr
Ophthalmic: 1–2 drops or ribbon of
ointment in each eye Q3–6 hr
Topical: apply to affected area TID-QID

Dose recommendations are just
guidelines for therapy; monitoring
of blood levels is essential in
neonates and infants. Follow hematologic
status for dose related or idiosyncratic
marrow suppression. "Gray baby"
syndrome may be seen with levels >50
mg/L. Use with **caution** in G6PD
deficiency, renal or hepatic dysfunction,
and neonates.

Concomitant use of phenobarbital and
rifampin may lower chloramphenicol
serum levels. Phenytoin may increase
chloramphenicol serum levels.
Chloramphenicol may increase phenytoin
levels, reduce metabolism of oral
anticoagulants, and decrease absorption
of vitamin B_{12}. Chloramphenicol in an
inhibitor of CYP 450 2B6 (see p. 924).

Therapeutic levels: 15–25 mg/L for
meningitis; 10–20 mg/L for other
infections. Trough: 5–15 mg/L for
meningitis; 5–10 mg/L for other infections.
Recommended serum sampling time:
trough (IV/PO) within 30 minutes prior to
next dose; peak (IV) 30 minutes after the
end of infusion; peak (PO) 2 hours after
oral administration. Time to achieve
steady-state: 2-3 days for newborns;
12–24 hrs for children and adults. **Note:**
higher serum levels may be achieved using
the oral, rather than the IV route.

CHLOROQUINE HCl/PHOSPHATE
Aralen
Amebicide, antimalarial
Tabs: 250, 500 mg as phosphate (150, 300 mg base, respectively)
Suspension: 16.67 mg/ml as phosphate (10 mg/ml base)
Injection: 50 mg/ml as HCl (40 mg/ml base) (5 ml)

Yes   1   C

Doses expressed in mg of Chloroquine base:

Malaria Prophylaxis (start 1 week prior to exposure and continue for 4 weeks after leaving edemic area):
Children: 5 mg/kg/dose PO Q week; **max dose:** 300 mg/dose
Adult: 300 mg/dose PO Q week
Malaria Treatment:
Children: 10 mg/kg/dose (**max dose:** 600 mg/dose) PO × 1; followed by 5 mg/kg/ dose (**max dose:** 300 mg/dose) 6 hours later and then once daily for 2 days
Adult: 600 mg/dose PO × 1; followed by 300 mg/dose 6 hours later and then once daily for 2 days

 For treatment of malaria, consult with ID specialist or see the latest edition of the AAP Red Book.
Use with **caution** in liver disease, G6PD deficiency, or concomitant hepatotoxic drugs. May cause nausea, vomiting, blurred vision, retinal and corneal changes, headaches, confusion, and hair depigmentation.
Adjust dose in renal failure (see p. **938**).

CHLOROTHIAZIDE
Diuril, Diurigen
Thiazide diuretic
Tabs: 250, 500 mg
Suspension: 250 mg/5 ml (237 ml)
Injection: 500 mg (5 mEq Na/1g)

Yes 1 D

 <6 mo: 20–40 mg/kg/24 hr ÷ Q12 hr PO/IV
≥6 mo: 20 mg/kg/24 hr ÷ Q12 hr PO/IV
Adults: 250–1000 mg/dose QD-QID PO/IV
Max dose: 2 g/24 hr

Use with **caution** in liver and severe renal disease. May increase serum calcium, bilirubin, glucose, uric acid. May cause alkalosis, pancreatitis, dizziness, hypokalemia, and hypomagnesemia.
Avoid IM or subcutaneous administration.

CHLORPHENIRAMINE MALEATE
Chlor-Trimeton and others
Antihistamine
Tabs: 4 mg
Sustained release caps and tabs: 8, 12 mg
Chewable tab: 2 mg
Syrup: 2 mg/5 ml (120, 473 ml)
Injection: 10 mg/ml

No ? B

Children: 0.35 mg/kg/24 hr PO ÷ Q4–6 hr or dose based on age below

2–6 yr: 1 mg/dose PO Q4–6 hr; **max dose:** 6 mg/24 hr
6–12 yr: 2 mg/dose PO Q4–6 hr; **max dose:** 12 mg/24 hr
Sustained release (6–12 yr): 8 mg/dose PO PRN

≥12 yrs/adults: 4 mg/dose Q4–6 hr PO; **max dose:** 24 mg/24 hr
Sustained release: 8–12 mg PO BID
IV/SC/IM: 5–20 mg × 1; **max dose:** 40 mg/24 hr

Use with **caution** in asthma. May cause sedation, dry mouth, blurred vision, urinary retention, polyuria, and disturbed coordination. Young children may be paradoxically excited.
Administer oral doses with food. Sustained release forms are not recommended in children less than 6 years old.

CHLORPROMAZINE
Thorazine
Antiemetic, antipsychotic, phenothiazine derivative
Tabs: 10, 25, 50, 100, 200 mg
Extended-release caps: 30, 75, 150, 200, 300 mg
Syrup: 10 mg/5 ml (120 ml)
Suppository: 25, 100 mg
Oral concentrate: 30 mg/ml (120 ml), 100 mg/ml (60, 240 ml)
Injection: 25 mg/ml

No   3   C

Children >6 mo:
IM or IV: 2.5–4 mg/kg/24 hr ÷ Q6–8 hr
PO: 2.5–6 mg/kg/24 hr ÷ Q4–6 hr
PR: 1 mg/kg/dose Q6–8 hr
Max IM/IV dose:
<5 yr: 40 mg/24 hr
5–12 yr: 75 mg/24 hr
Adult:
IM/IV: Initial: 25 mg; repeat with 25–50 mg/dose, if needed, Q1–4 hr **up to max** of 400 mg/dose Q4–6 hr
PO: 10–25 mg/dose Q4–6 hr; **max dose:** 2 g/24 hr
PR: 50–100 mg/dose Q6–8 hr

Adverse effects include drowsiness, jaundice, lowered seizure threshold, extrapyramidal/ anticholinergic symptoms, hypotension (more with IV), arrhythmias, agranulocytosis, neuroleptic malignant syndrome. May potentiate effect of narcotics, sedatives, other drugs. Monitor BP closely. ECG changes include prolonged PR interval, flattened T waves and ST depression.

For explanation of icons, see p. 600.

CHOLESTYRAMINE

Questran, Questran Light, Prevalite
Antilipemic, binding resin

No ? B

Powder: 4 g anhydrous resin per 9 g packet (9, 378 g); Questran Light: 4 g anhydrous resin per 5 g packet with aspartame (5, 210 g); Prevalite: 4 g anhydrous resin per 5.5 g packet with aspartame (5.5 g)

All doses based in terms of anhydrous resin.
Children: 240 mg/kg/24 hr ÷ TID. Give PO as slurry in water, juice, or milk before meals.
Adult: 3–4 g of cholestyramine BID-QID
Max dose: 32 g/24 hr

May cause constipation, abdominal distention, vomiting, vitamin deficiencies (A, D, E, K), and rash. Hyperchloremic acidosis may occur with prolonged use.
Give other oral medications 4–6 hr after cholestyramine or 1 hr before dose to avoid decreased absorption.

CHOLINE MAGNESIUM TRISALICYLATE

Trilisate
Nonsteroidal antiinflammatory agent

Yes ? C

Combination of choline salicylate and magnesium salicylate (1:1.24 ratio, respectively); strengths expressed in terms of mg salicylate:
Tabs: 500, 750, 1000 mg
Liquid: 500 mg/5 ml

Dose based on total salicylate content.
Children: 30–60 mg/kg/24 hr ÷ TID-QID
Adults: 500 mg–1.5 g QD-TID

Avoid use in patients with suspected varicella or influenza due to concerns of Reye's syndrome. Use with **caution** in severe renal failure because of risk for hypermagnesemia, or in peptic ulcer disease. Less GI irritation than aspirin and other NSAIDs. No antiplatelet effects.
Therapeutic salicylate levels, see aspirin. 500 mg choline magnesium trisalicylate is equivalent to 650 mg aspirin.

CIMETIDINE

Tagamet, Tagamet HB [OTC]
Histamine-2-antagonist
Tabs: 100 (OTC), 200, 300, 400, 800 mg
Injection: 150 mg/ml
Syrup: 300 mg/5 ml (240, 470 ml) (contains 2.8% alcohol)

Yes   1   B

Neonates: 5–20 mg/kg/24 hr IM/PO/IV Q6–12 hr
Infants: 10–20 mg/kg/24 hr IM/PO/IV ÷ Q6–12 hr
Children: 20–40 mg/kg/24 hr IM/PO/IV ÷ Q6 hr
Adults (PO/IM/IV): 300 mg/dose QID or 400 mg/dose BID or 800 mg/dose QHS
Ulcer prophylaxis: 400–800 mg PO QHS
Max dose: 2400 mg/24 hr

Diarrhea, rash, myalgia, confusion, neutropenia, gynecomastia, elevated liver function tests, or dizziness may occur.

Inhibits cytochrome P-450 oxidase system, therefore increases levels of hepatically metabolized drugs (i.e. theophylline, phenytoin, lidocaine, diazepam, warfarin). See p. 924. Cimetidine may decrease the absorption of iron, ketoconazole, and tetracyclines.
Adjust dose in renal failure (see p. 938).

CIPROFLOXACIN

Cipro, Ciloxan ophthalmic, Cipro HC Otic
Antibiotic, quinolone
Tabs: 100, 250, 500, 750 mg
Oral Suspension: 250 mg/5 ml, 500 mg/5 ml (100 ml)
Injection: 10 mg/ml
Ophthalmic solution: 3.5 mg/ml (2.5, 5 ml)
Otitic Suspension (Cipro HC Otic): 2 mg/ml Ciprofloxacin + 10 mg/ml Hydrocortisone (10 ml)

Yes   3   C

Children:
PO: 20–30 mg/kg/24 hr ÷ Q12 hr;
max dose: 1.5 g/24 hr
IV: 10–20 mg/kg/24 hr ÷ Q12 hr; **max dose:** 800 mg/24 hr
Cystic Fibrosis:
PO: 40 mg/kg/24 hr ÷ Q12 hr; **max dose:** 2 g/24 hr
IV: 30 mg/kg/24 hr ÷ Q8 hr; **max dose:** 1.2 g/24 hr
Adults:
PO: 250–750 mg/dose Q12 hr
IV: 200–400 mg/dose Q12 hr
Ophthalmic: 1–2 drops Q2 hr while awake × 2 days, then 1–2 gtts Q4 hr while awake × 5 days
Otitic:
>1 yr and Adults: 3 drops to affected ear(s) BID × 7 days

Can cause GI upset, renal failure, seizures. GI symptoms, headache, restlessness, rash are common side effects. Like other quinolones, ciprofloxacin has caused arthropathy in immature animals; use **with caution in children less than 18 years old.**

Inhibits CYP 450 1A2. Ciprofloxacin can increase effects and/or toxicity of theophylline, warfarin, cyclosporine.

Do not administer antacids or other divalent salts with or within 2–4 hours of oral ciprofloxacin dose. **Adjust dose in renal failure (see p. 931).**

CISAPRIDE
Propulsid
GI stimulant, prokinetic agent
Suspension: 1 mg/ml (450 ml)
Tabs: 10, 20 mg

No   1   C

Neonates: 0.1–0.2 mg/kg/dose Q6–12 hr PO
Infants and Children: 0.2–0.3 mg/kg/dose TID-QID PO; **max dose:** 10 mg/dose
Adults: 10 mg QID, administer 15 min AC and QHS PO; **max dose:** 20 mg/dose

Contraindicated in patients taking medications that inhibit cytochrome P-450 3A4 to increase serum cisapride serum levels (substrate); potentially resulting in fatal cardiac arrhythmias. These medications include: ketoconazole, itraconazole, miconazole, fluconazole, erythromycin, clarithromycin, troleandomycin, nefazodone, indinavir,

and ritonavir. Do not use in patients with cardiac disease (especially, torsades de pointes, long QT syndrome, sinus node dysfunction, and 2nd or 3rd degree AV block). **Avoid concomitant use of drugs known to prolong the QT interval (i.e. quinidine, procainamide, sotalol, tricyclic antidepressants, maprotiline, phenothiazines, astemizole, and sparfloxacin).**

Use in premature infants is controversial due to concerns of immature drug metabolism.

Frequent adverse reactions are headaches and GI disturbance. Cisapride can decrease the absorption of digoxin.

CITRATE MIXTURES
Alkalinizing agent, electrolyte supplement

| | | | No   ?   C |

Each ml contains (mEq):

	Na	K	Citrate or HCO$_3^-$
Polycitra or Cytra-3	1	1	2
Polycitra-LC or Cytra-LC	1	1	2
Polycitra-K or Cytra-K	0	2	2
Bicitra or Cytra-2	1	0	1
Oracit	1	0	1

LC, low calorie (contains no sucrose, sorbitol, glycerin).

Dilute in water or juice and administer doses after meals and at bedtime.

All mEq doses based on citrate
Children: 5–15 ml/dose Q6–8 hr PO or 2–3 mEq/kg/24 hr PO ÷ Q6–8 hr
Adult: 15–30 ml/dose Q6–8 hr PO or 100–200 mEq/24 hr ÷ Q6–8 hr

Contraindicated in severe renal impairment and acute dehydration.
Use with **caution** in patients already receiving potassium supplements or who are sodium restricted. May have laxative effect and cause hypocalemia and metabolic alkalosis.

Adjust dose to maintain desired pH. 1 mEq of citrate is equivalent to 1 mEq HCO$_3$ in patients with normal hepatic function.

CLARITHROMYCIN
Biaxin
Antibiotic, macrolide
Film tabs: 250, 500 mg
Granules for suspension: 125, 250 mg/5 ml (50, 100 ml)

Yes   2   C

For explanation of icons, see p. 600.

Children:
Acute Otitis Media,
Pharyngitis/Tonsillitis, Pneumonia,
Acute Maxillary Sinusitis, or
Uncomplicated Skin Infections: 15 mg/
kg/24 hr PO ÷ Q12 hr
M. avium *complex prophylaxis:* 15
mg/kg/24 hr PO ÷ Q12 hr
Max dose: 1 g/24 hr
Adult:
Pharyngitis/Tonsillitis, Acute Maxillary
Sinusitis, Bronchitis, Pneumonia, or
Uncomplicated Skin Infections:
250–500 mg/dose Q12 hr PO
M. avium *complex prophylaxis:* 500 mg/
dose Q12 hr PO

Contraindicated in patients allergic
to erythromycin. May cause cardiac
arrhythmias in patients also
receiving terfenadine, astemizole, and
cisapride. Side effects: diarrhea, nausea,
abnormal taste, dyspepsia, abdominal
discomfort (< erythromycin but >
azithromycin), headache. May increase
carbamazepine, theophylline, cyclosporin,
tacrolimus levels. Inhibits CYP 450 3A4
(see p. 924).
 **Adjust dose in renal failure (see p.
932).** Doses, regardless of dosage form,
may be administered with food.

CLEMASTINE

Tavist
Antihistamine   No   2   B
Available as clemastine fumarate salt:
Tabs: 1.34 mg (1 mg base) [OTC], 2.68 mg (2 mg base)
Syrup: 0.67 mg/5 ml (0.5 mg/5 ml base) (120 ml) (contains 5.5% alcohol)

Doses expressed as Clemastine
base
Infants and Children <6 yr:
0.05 mg/kg/24 hr ÷ BID–TID PO; **max
dose:** 1 mg/24 hr
6–12 yr: 0.5 mg BID PO; **max dose:**
3 mg/24 hr
>12 yr: 1 mg BID PO dose, if needed,
may increase dose **up to a maximum of**
6 mg/24 hr

Contraindicated in narrow-angle
glaucoma, bladder neck
obstruction, stenosing peptic ulcer.
May cause dizziness, drowsiness, dry
mouth, and constipation.

CLINDAMYCIN

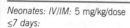

Cleocin-T, Cleocin, and others
Antibiotic

No   1   B

Caps: 75, 150, 300 mg
Oral liquid: 75 mg/5 ml (100 ml)
Injection: 150 mg/ml (contains 9.45 mg/ml benzyl alcohol)
Solution, topical: 1% (30, 60, 480 ml)
Gel: 1% (7.5, 30 g)
Lotion: 1% (60 ml)
Vaginal cream: 2% (40 g)

Neonates: IV/IM: 5 mg/kg/dose
≤7 days:
  ≤2 kg: Q12 hr
  >2 kg: Q8 hr
>7 days:
  <1.2 kg: Q12 hr
  1.2–2 kg: Q8 hr
  >2 kg: Q6 hr
Children:
  PO: 10–30 mg/kg/24 hr ÷ Q6–8 hr
  IM/IV: 25–40 mg/kg/24 hr ÷ Q6–8 hr
Adults:
  PO: 150–450 mg/dose Q6–8 hr; **max dose: 1.8 g/24 hr**
  IM/IV: 1200–1800 mg/24 hr IM/IV ÷ Q6–12 hr; **max dose: 4.8 g/24 hr**
Topical: apply to affected area BID

Not indicated in meningitis; CSF penetration is poor.

Pseudomembranous colitis may occur up to several weeks after cessation of therapy. May cause diarrhea, rash, Stevens-Johnson syndrome, granulocytopenia, thrombocytopenia, or sterile abscess at injection site.

Clindamycin may increase the neuromuscular blocking effects of tubocurarine, pancuronium. **Do not exceed IV infusion rate of 30 mg/min** because hypotension, cardiac arrest has been reported with rapid infusions.

CLONAZEPAM

Klonopin
Benzodiazepine

No   3   C

Tabs: 0.5, 1, 2 mg
Suspension: 100 mcg/ml

For explanation of icons, see p. 600.

Children: <10 yr or <30 kg:
Initial: 0.01–0.03 mg/kg/24 hr ÷ Q8 hr PO
Increment: 0.25–0.5 mg/24 hr Q3 days, up to **max maintenance dose** of 0.1–0.2 mg/kg/24 hr ÷ Q8 hr
Children ≥10 yr or ≥30 kg and Adults:
Initial: 1.5 mg/24 hr PO ÷ TID
Increment: 0.5–1 mg/24 hr Q3 days; **max dose:** 20 mg/24 hr

Contraindicated in severe liver disease and acute narrow angle glaucoma. Drowsiness, behavior changes, increased bronchial secretions, GI, CV, GU, and hematopoietic toxicity (thrombocytopenia, leukopenia) may occur. Use with **caution** in patients with renal impairment. Do not discontinue abruptly. $T_{1/2}$ = 24–36 hr.

Therapeutic levels: 20–80 ng/ml. Recommended serum sampling time: obtain trough level within 30 minutes prior to an oral dose. Steady-state is typically achieved 5–8 days of continuous therapy using the same dose.

CLONIDINE
Catapres, Catapres TTS
Central alpha-adrenergic agonist, antihypertensive
Tabs: 0.1, 0.2, 0.3 mg
Transdermal patch: 0.1, 0.2, 0.3 mg/24 hr (7 day)
Injection, epidural: 100 mcg/ml (preservative free, 10 ml)

No   ?   C

Children (PO): 5–7 mcg/kg/24 hr ÷ Q6–12 hr; if needed, increase at 5–7 day intervals to 5–25 mcg/kg/24 hr ÷ Q6 hr; **max dose:** 0.9 mg/24 hr
Adult (PO): 0.1 mg BID initially; increase in 0.1 mg/24 hr increments at weekly intervals until desired response is achieved, **max dose:** 2.4 mg/24 hr
Transdermal patch, adults: Initial 0.1 mg/24 hr patch for first week. May increase dose of patch to 0.3 mg/24 hr PRN. Patches last for 7 days.

Side effects: dry mouth, dizziness, drowsiness, fatigue, constipation, anorexia, arrhythmias, local skin reactions with patch. **Do not abruptly discontinue; signs of sympathetic overactivity may occur; taper gradually over >1 wk.**

$T_{1/2}$: 44–72 hr (neonates), 6–20 hr (adults). Onset of action: 0.5–1 hr for oral route, 2–3 days for transdermal route. Applying >2 of the 0.3 mg/24 hr patches does not provide additional benefit.

CLOTRIMAZOLE

Lotrimin, Mycelex, Mycelex G
Antifungal

No   ?   B

Cream: 1% (15, 30, 45, 90 g)
Solution: 1% (10, 30 ml)
Vaginal tabs: 100, 500 mg
Vaginal cream: 1% (45, 90 g)
Oral troche: 10 mg
Lotion: 1% (30 ml)
Twin Pack: Tab 500 mg (1) and vaginal cream 1% (7 g)

Topical: apply to skin BID × 4–8 wks
Vaginal Candidiasis: (vaginal tabs)
100 mg/dose QHS × 7 days, or
200 mg/dose QHS × 3 days, or
500 mg/dose QHS × 1, or
1 applicator dose (5 g) of 1% vaginal cream QHS × 7–14 days
>3 yr - adult:
Thrush: Dissolve slowly (15–30 minutes) one troche in the mouth 5 times/24 hr × 14 days

May cause erythema, blistering, or urticaria with topical use. Liver enzyme elevation, nausea and vomiting may occur with troches.

CLOXACILLIN

Tegopen, Cloxapen
Antibiotic, penicillin (penicillinase resistant)

No   ?   B

Caps: 250, 500 mg
Oral solution: 125 mg/5 ml (100, 200 ml)
Sodium content:
    250 mg tab = 0.6 mEq
    125 mg suspension = 0.48 mEq

Infant/child: 50–100 mg/kg/24 hr PO ÷ Q6 hr
Adults: 250–500 mg/dose PO Q6 hr
Max dose: 4 g/24 hr

Contraindicated in patients with a history of penicillin allergy. Use with **caution** in cephalosporin hypersensitivity. May cause nausea, vomiting, and diarrhea. Administer doses on an empty stomach.

For explanation of icons, see p. 600.

CO-TRIMOXAZOLE

Trimethoprim-Sulfamethoxazole, TMP-SMX;
Bactrim, Septra, Sulfatrim, others

Yes   1   C

Antibiotic, sulfonamide derivative

Tabs (reg strength): 80 mg TMP/400 mg SMX
Tabs (double strength): 160 mg TMP/800 mg SMX
Suspension: 40 mg TMP/200 mg SMX per 5 ml (20, 100, 150, 200, 480 ml)
Injection: 16 mg TMP/ml and 80 mg SMX/ml

Doses based on TMP component.
Minor infections (PO or IV):
  Child: 8–10 mg/kg/24 hr ÷ BID
  Adult (>40 kg): 160 mg/dose BID
UTI prophylaxis: 2–4 mg/kg/24 hr PO QD
Severe infections and Pneumocystis carinii pneumonitis (PO or IV): 20 mg/kg/24 hr ÷ Q6–8 hr
Pneumocystis prophylaxis (PO or IV): 5–10 mg/kg/24 hr ÷ BID or 150 mg/m²/24 hr ÷ BID for 3 consecutive days/wk; **max dose:** 320 mg/24 hr

Not recommended for use with infants <2 mo. May cause kernicterus in newborns; may cause blood dyscrasias, crystalluria, glossitis, renal or hepatic injury, GI irritation, rash, Stevens-Johnson syndrome, hemolysis in patients with G6PD deficiency. **Do not use drug at term during pregnancy.**

Reduce dose in renal impairment (see p. 932). See p. 367 for PCP prophylaxis guidelines.

CODEINE

Various brands
Narcotic, analgesic, antitussive

Yes   1   C/D

Tabs: 15, 30, 60 mg
Injection: 30, 60 mg/ml
Syrup: 60 mg/5 ml
Oral solution: 15 mg/5 ml
In combination with acetaminophen
Elixir (7% alcohol), Suspension,
Solution: Acetaminophen 120 mg and
codeine 12 mg/5 ml
Caps: Acetaminophen 325 + 15 mg
codeine
  Acetaminophen 325 + 30 mg
  codeine

Acetaminophen 325 + 60 mg
codeine
Tabs: (all contain 300 mg
acetaminophen per tab)
  Tylenol #1: 7.5 mg codeine
  Tylenol #2: 15 mg codeine
  Tylenol #3: 30 mg codeine
  Tylenol #4: 60 mg codeine
Tabs:
  Acetaminophen 650 mg + codeine
  30 mg
  Acetaminophen 500 mg + codeine
  30 mg

Analgesic:
Children: 0.5–1 mg/kg/dose Q4–6 hr IM, SC, or PO; **max dose:** 60 mg/dose
Adults: 15–60 mg/dose Q4–6 hr IM, SC, or PO
Antitussive (all doses PRN): 1–1.5 mg/kg/24 hr ÷ Q4–6 hr; alternatively dose by age
Children (2–6 yr): 2.5–5 mg/dose Q4–6 hr; **max** 30 mg/24 hr
Children (6–12 yr): 5–10 mg/dose Q4–6 hr; **max** 60 mg/24 hr
Adults: 10–20 mg/dose Q4–6 hr; **max** 120 mg/24 hr

Do not use in children <2 yr old as antitussive. Not intended for IV use, due to large histamine release and cardiovascular effects. Side effects: CNS and respiratory depression, constipation, cramping, hypotension, pruritis. May be habit forming.

For analgesia, use with acetaminophen orally. See p. 896 for equianalgesic dosing. **Adjust dose in renal failure (see p. 938).**

Pregnancy risk factor changes to a "D" if used for prolonged periods or in high doses at term.

COLFOSCERIL PALMITATE
See Surfactant, pulmonary

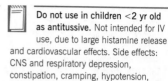

CORTISONE ACETATE
Cortone acetate
Corticosteroid
Tabs: 5, 10, 25 mg
Injection: 50 mg/ml (IM only)

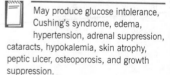

No ? D

Anti-inflammatory/ immunosuppressive:
PO: 2.5–10 mg/kg/24 hr ÷ Q6–8 hr
IM: 1–5 mg/kg/24 hr ÷ Q12–24 hr
Physiologic replacement:
PO: 0.5–0.75 mg/kg/24 hr ÷ Q8 hr
IM: 0.25–0.35 mg/kg/dose QD

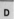
May produce glucose intolerance, Cushing's syndrome, edema, hypertension, adrenal suppression, cataracts, hypokalemia, skin atrophy, peptic ulcer, osteoporosis, and growth suppression.

See p. 907 for doses based on body surface area and other uses. IM form slowly absorbed over several days.

CROMOLYN
Intal, Nasalcrom, Crolom, Gastrocrom
Anti-allergic agent

 No ? B

Caps: 20 mg (for inhalation via "spinhaler")
Nebulized solution: 10 mg/ml (2 ml)
Aerosol inhaler: 800 mcg/spray (112 inhalations, 8.1g; 200 inhalations, 14.2 g)
Capsule: 100 mg
Oral Concentrate: 100 mg/5 ml
Ophthalmic: 4% (2.5, 10 ml)
Nasal spray (OTC): 4% (5.2 mg/spray) (100 sprays, 13 ml; 200 sprays, 26 ml)

Spin Inhalant: 20 mg Q6–8 hr
Nebulization: 20 mg Q6–8 hr
Nasal: 1 spray each nostril TID-QID
Aerosol inhaler:
  Children: 1–2 puffs TID-QID
  Adult: 2–4 puffs TID-QID
Ophthalmic: 1–2 gtts 4–6 ×/24 hr
Food Allergy/Inflammatory Bowel disease:
  Children >2 yr: 100 mg PO QID; give 15–20 min AC and QHS; **max dose:** 40 mg/kg/24 hr
  Adults: 200–400 mg PO QID; give 15–20 min AC and QHS
Systemic mastocytosis:
  <2 yr: 20 mg/kg/24 hr ÷ QID PO; **max dose:** 30 mg/kg/24 hr
  2–12 yr: 100 mg PO QID; **max dose:** 40 mg/kg/24 hr
  Adults: 200 mg PO QID

May cause rash, cough, bronchospasm, nasal congestion. May cause headache, diarrhea with oral use. Use with **caution** in patients with renal or hepatic dysfunction. Bronchospasm and pharyngeal irritation may occur when using spinhaler product.

Therapeutic response often occurs within 2 weeks, however, a 4–6 week trial may be needed to determine maximum benefit. For exercise induced asthma, give no longer than 1 hour before activity. Oral concentrate and contents of capsule can only be diluted in water. Nebulized solution can be mixed with albuterol nebs.

CYCLOPENTOLATE
Cyclogyl, and others
Anticholinergic, mydriatic agent

 No ? C

Solution: 0.5%, 1%, 2% (2, 5, 15 ml)

Infant: 1 drop of 0.5% OU 5–10 min before exam

Children: 1 drop of 0.5–1% OU, followed by repeat drop, if necessary, in 5 minutes

Adult: 1 drop of 1% OU followed by another drop OU in 5 min; use 2% solution for heavily pigmented iris

 Do not use in narrow-angle glaucoma. May cause a burning sensation, behavioral disturbance, tachycardia, loss of visual accommodation. To minimize absorption, apply pressure over nasolacrimal sac for at least 2 min. CNS and cardiovascular side effects are common with the 2% solution in children.

Onset of action: 15–60 minutes. Observe patient closely for at least 30 min after dose.

CYCLOPENTOLATE/PHENYLEPHRINE
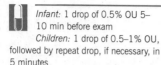

Cyclomydril

Anticholinergic/sympathomimetic, mydriatic agent

No   ?   C

Solution: 0.2% cyclopentolate/1% phenylephrine (2, 5 ml)

 1 drop OU Q5–10 min; **max dose:** 3 drops per eye

 Used to induce mydriasis. See cyclopentolate for comments.

CYCLOSPORINE, CYCLOSPORINE MICROEMULSION

Sandimmune, Neoral

Immunosuppressant

No   X   C

Injection: 50 mg/ml; contains 32.9% alcohol and 650 mg/ml polyoxyethylated castor oil

Oral solution: 100 mg/ml (50 ml); contains 12.5% alcohol

Cap: 25, 50, 100 mg; contains 12.7% alcohol

Neoral Cap: 25, 100 mg

Neoral Solution: 100 mg/ml (50 ml)

Neoral products contain 9.5% alcohol

Neoral manufacturer recommends a 1:1 conversion ratio with Sandimmune. Due to its better absorption, however, lower doses of Neoral may be required.

Oral: 15 mg/kg as a single dose given 4–12 hr pre-transplant; give same daily dose for 1–2 wk post-transplant, then reduce by 5% per wk to 5–10 mg/kg/24 hr ÷ Q12–24 hr

IV: 5–6 mg/kg as a single dose given 4–12 hr pretransplant; administer over 2–6 hr; give same daily dose post-transplant until patient able to tolerate oral form

May cause nephrotoxicity, hepatotoxicity, hypomagnesemia, hyperkalemia, hyperuricemia, hypertension, hirsutism, acne, GI symptoms, tremor, leukopenia, sinusitis, gingival hyperplasia, headache. Use **caution** with concomitant use of other nephrotoxic drugs such as amphotericin b and aminioglycosides.

Plasma concentrations increased with the use of fluconazole, ketoconazole, erythromycin, verapamil, and corticosteroids. Plasma concentrations decreased with the use of carbamazepine, rifampin, phenobarbital, and phenytoin. Cyclosporine is a substrate for CYP450 3A4 (see p. 924).

Children may require dosages 2–3 times higher than adults. T-tube clamping may increase absorption. Plasma half-life 6–24 hrs.

Monitor trough levels (just prior to a dose at steady-state). Steady-state is generally achieved after 3–5 days of continuous dosing. Interpretation will vary based on treatment protocol and assay methodology (RIA monoclonal vs. RIA polyclonal vs. HPLC) as well as whole blood vs. serum sample.

CYPROHEPTADINE

Periactin
Antihistamine
Tabs: 4 mg
Syrup: 2 mg/5 ml (473 ml); contains 5% alcohol

No   ?   B

Children: 0.25–0.5 mg/kg/24 hr ÷ Q8–12 hr PO

Adult: Start with 12 mg/24 hr ÷ TID PO; dosage range: 12–32 mg/24 hr ÷ TID PO

Max dose:
2–6 yr: 12 mg/24 hr
7–14 yr: 16 mg/24 hr
Adults: 0.5 mg/kg/24 hr

Contraindicated in neonates, patients currently on MAO inhibitors, and patients suffering from asthma, glaucoma, or GI/GU obstruction. May produce anti-cholinergic side effects including appetite stimulation.

DANTROLENE

Dantrium
Skeletal muscle relaxant   No   ?   C
Cap: 25, 50, 100 mg
Injection: 20 mg (3 gm mannitol/20 mg drug)
Suspension: 5 mg/ml

Chronic spasticity:
Children: (<5 yr)
Initial: 0.5 mg/kg/dose PO BID
Increment: Increase frequency to TID-QID at 4–7 day intervals, then increase doses by 0.5 mg/kg/dose
Max dose: 3 mg/kg/dose PO BID-QID, up to 400 mg/24 hr
Malignant Hyperthermia:
Prevention:
PO: 4–8 mg/kg/24 hr ÷ Q6 hr × 1–3 days before surgery
IV: 2.5 mg/kg over 1 hr beginning 1.25 hr before anesthesia, additional doses PRN
Treatment: 1 mg/kg IV, repeat PRN to **max cumulative dose** of 10 mg/kg, then continue 4–8 mg/kg/24 hr PO ÷ Q6 hr for 1–3 days

Contraindicated in active hepatic disease. Monitor transaminases for hepatotoxicity. Use with **caution** in children with cardiac or pulmonary impairment. May cause change in sensorium, weakness, diarrhea, constipation, incontinence, and enuresis. **Avoid unnecessary exposure to sunlight. Avoid extravasation into tissues.** A decrease in spasticity sufficient to allow daily function should be therapeutic goal. Discontinue if benefits are not evident in 45 days.

DAPSONE

Avlosulfon
Antibiotic, sulfone derivative   Yes   1   C
Tabs: 25, 100 mg
Suspension: 2 mg/ml ; also see remarks

For explanation of icons, see p. 600.

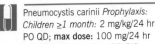

Pneumocystis carinii *Prophylaxis:*
Children ≥1 month: 2 mg/kg/24 hr
PO QD; **max dose:** 100 mg/24 hr
Adult: 100 mg/24 hr PO ÷ QD-BID;
other combination regimens with
pyrimethamine and leucovorin can be
used (See *MMWR* June 27, 1997; Vol.
46, No. RR-12)
Leprosy:
Children: 1–2 mg/kg/24 hr PO QD for a
minimum of 3 years; **max dose:** 100
mg/ 24 hr
Adult: 50–100 mg PO QD for 3–10
years (in combination with rifampin
600 mg PO QD × first 6 months is
recommended)

May cause hemolysis in G6PD
deficiency, or methemoglobin
reductase deficiency (primarily
results in methemoglobinemia), or
hemoglobin M. Side effects include:
hemolytic anemia (dose related),
agranulocytosis, aplastic anemia, nausea,
vomiting, hyperbilirubinemia, headache,
nephrotic syndrome, and hypersensitivity
reaction (sulfone syndrome).
   Suspension may not be absorbed as
well as tablets.
2 mg/ml suspension product is also
available via an IND for PCP prophylaxis
from Jacobus Pharmaceutical Company
(609) 921-7447.

DEFEROXAMINE MESYLATE
Desferal Mesylate
Chelating agent
Injection: 500 mg

No   ?   C

Acute iron poisoning:
Children:
IV: 15 mg/kg/hr or
IM: 50 mg/kg/dose Q6 hr
Max dose: 6 g/24 hr
Adult:
IV: 15 mg/kg/hr
IM: 1 g × 1, then 0.5 g Q4 hr × 2;
may repeat 0.5 g Q4–12 hr
Max dose: 6 g/24 hr
Chronic iron overload:
Children:
IV: 15 mg/kg/hr
SC: 20–40 mg/kg/dose QD as
infusion over 8–12 hr
Adult:
IM: 0.5–1 g/dose QD
SC: 1–2 g/dose QD as infusion over
8–24 hr

Contraindicated in anuria. Not
approved for use in primary
hemochromatosis. May cause
flushing, erythema, urticaria, hypotension,
tachycardia, diarrhea, leg cramps, fever,
cataracts, hearing loss. Iron mobilization
may be poor in children <3 yr.
   Maximum IV infusion rate: 15
mg/kg/hr. SC route is via a portable
controlled-infusion device and is not
recommended in acute iron poisoning.

DESMOPRESSIN ACETATE
DDAVP, Stimate

Vasopressin analog, synthetic; hemostatic agent

No 2 B

Tabs: 0.1, 0.2 mg

Nasal Solution: DDAVP, 100 mcg/ml (2.5 ml); Stimate, 1500 mcg/ml (2.5 ml); both preparations contain 9 mg NaCl/ml

Injection: 4 mcg/ml (1, 10 ml); 15 mcg/ml (1, 2 ml)

Nasal Spray: 100 mcg/ml, 10 mcg/spray (50 sprays, 5 ml); contains 7.5 mg NaCl/ml

Conversion: 100 mcg = 400 IU arginine vasopressin

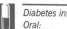

Diabetes insipidus:
Oral:
  Children: Start with 0.05 mg BID; titrate to effect
  Adult: Start with 0.05 mg BID; titrate dose to effect; usual dose range: 0.1–0.2 mg/24 hr ÷ BID-TID
Intranasal:
  3 mo–12 yr: 5–30 mcg/24 hr ÷ QD-BID
  Adults: 10–40 mcg/24 hr ÷ QD-TID; titrate dose to achieve control of excessive thirst and urination; **max intranasal dose:** 40 mcg/24 hr
IV/SC: 2–4 mcg/24 hr ÷ BID
Hemophilia A and von Willebrand's disease:
  Intranasal: 2–4 mcg/kg/dose
  IV: 0.2–0.4 mcg/kg/dose over 15–30 min
Nocturnal enuresis (>6 yr):
  Oral: 0.2 mg at bedtime, titrated to 0.6 mg to achieve desired effect

Intranasal: 20 mcg at bedtime, range 10–40 mcg; divide dose by 2 and administer each one-half dose per nostril.

Use with **caution** in hypertension and coronary artery disease. May cause headache, nausea, hyponatremia, nasal congestion, abdominal cramps, and hypertension.

Injection may be used SC or IV at approximately 10% of intranasal dose. Adjust fluid intake to decrease risk of water intoxication. Peak effects: 1–5 hr with intranasal route; 1.5–3 hr with IV route; and 2–7 hr with PO route.

For hemophilia A and von Willebrand's disease administer dose intranasally, 2 hours before procedure; IV, 30 minutes before procedure.

DEXAMETHASONE

No ? C

Decadron and other brand names
Corticosteroid

Tabs: 0.25, 0.5, 0.75, 1, 1.5, 2, 4, 6 mg
Injection: 4, 10, 20, 24 mg/ml (sodium phosphate; some preparations contain benzyl alcohol)
IM Injection: 8, 16 mg/ml (acetate)
Elixir: 0.5 mg/5 ml (some preparations contain 5% alcohol)
Oral Solution: 0.1, 1 mg/ml (some preparations contain 30% alcohol)
Oral Inhalation: 84 mcg/metered dose (12.6 g)
Nasal Spray: 84 mcg/metered dose (170 sprays; 12.6 g)
Opthalmic Ointment: 0.05% (3.5 g)
Opthalmic Solution: 0.1% (5 ml)

Cerebral Edema:
  Loading dose: 1–2 mg/kg/dose PO, IV, IM × 1
  Maintenance: 1–1.5 mg/kg/24 hr ÷ Q4–6 hr; **max dose:** 16 mg/24 hr
Airway Edema: 0.5–2 mg/kg/24 hr PO, IV, IM ÷ Q6 hr (begin 24 hr before extubation and continue for 4–6 doses after extubation)
Croup: 0.6 mg/kg/dose IV, IM × 1 (use sodium phosphate injection)
Antiemetic:
  Initial: 10 mg/m²/dose IV; max: 20 mg
  Subsequent: 5 mg/m²/dose Q6 hr IV
Anti-inflammatory:
  Children: 0.08–0.3 mg/kg/24 hr PO, IV, IM ÷ Q6–12 hr
  Adults: 0.75–9 mg/24 hr PO, IV, IM ÷ Q6–12 hr

Meningitis:
  >6 weeks old: 0.6 mg/kg/24 hr IV ÷ Q6 hr × 2 days; initiate prior to or with the first dose of antibiotic

Toxicity: same as for prednisone. Use in meningitis (other than Haemophilus influenzae type b) remains controversial. Consult ID specialist or latest edition of Red Book.
  Oral peak serum levels occur 1–2 hr and within 8 hr following IM administration. For other uses, doses based on body surface area, and dose equivalence to other steroids, see p. 913.

DEXTROAMPHETAMINE

Dexedrine and many other brand names
CNS stimulant
Tabs: 5, 10 mg
Sustained-release caps: 5, 10, 15 mg

No   X   C

 Attention Deficit Hyperactivity Disorder:

3–5 yr: 2.5 mg/24 hr QAM; increase by 2.5 mg/24 hr at weekly intervals to a **max dose** of 40 mg/24 hr
≥6 yr: 5 mg/24 hr QAM; increase by 5 mg/24 hr at weekly intervals to a **max dose** of 40 mg/24 hr

Narcolepsy:

6–12 yr: 5 mg/24 hr ÷ QD-TID; increase by 5 mg/24 hr at weekly intervals to a **max dose** of 60 mg/24 hr
>12 yr: 10 mg/24 hr ÷ QD-TID; increase by 10 mg/24 hr at weekly intervals to a **max dose** of 60 mg/24 hr

Use with **caution** in presence of hypertension or cardiovascular disease. Not recommended for <3 yr olds. Medication should generally not be used in children <5 yr old as diagnosis of ADHD in this age group is extremely difficult and should be only done in consultation with a specialist. Interrupt administration occasionally to determine need for continued therapy. Many side effects, including insomnia, restlessness, anorexia, psychosis, headache, vomiting, abdominal cramps, dry mouth, growth failure. Tolerance develops. (Same guidelines as for methylphenidate apply.) Do not give with MAO inhibitors, general anesthetics.

DIAZEPAM

Valium, and others
Benzodiazepine; anxiolytic, anticonvulsant
Tabs: 2, 5, 10 mg
Oral solution: 1 mg/ml, 5 mg/ml (contains 19% alcohol)
Injection: 5 mg/ml (contains 40% propylene glycol, 10% alcohol, and 1.5% benzyl alcohol)
Emulsified Injection (Dizac, Diazemuls): 5 mg/ml

No   3   D

Sustained-release cap: 15 mg
Pediatric Rectal Gel (Diastat): 2.5, 5, 10 mg (5 mg/ml concentration with 4.4 cm rectal tip delivery system)
Adult Rectal Gel (Diastat): 10, 15, 20 mg (5 mg/ml concentration with 6 cm rectal tip delivery system)

For explanation of icons, see p. 600.

Sedative/muscle relaxant:
Children:
 IM or IV: 0.04–0.2 mg/kg/dose
 Q2–4 hr; **max dose:** 0.6 mg/kg within
 an 8-hr period
 PO: 0.12–0.8 mg/kg/24 hr ÷ Q6–
 8 hr
Adults:
 IM or IV: 2–10 mg/dose Q3–4 hr PRN
 PO: 2–10 mg/dose Q6–12 hr PRN
Status epilepticus:
 Neonate: 0.3–0.75 mg/kg/dose IV
 Q15–30 min × 2–3 doses
 >1 mo: 0.2–0.5 mg/kg/dose IV
 Q15–30 min; **max total dose:** <5 yr: 5
 mg; ≥5 yr: 10 mg
 Adults: 5–10 mg/dose IV Q10–15 min;
 max total dose: 30 mg
 Rectal dose (using IV dosage form):
 0.5 mg/kg/dose followed by 0.25
 mg/kg/dose in 10 minutes PRN
 Rectal Gel: all doses rounded to the
 nearest available dosage strength;
 repeat dose in 4–12 hrs PRN
 2–5 yr: 0.5 mg/kg/dose
 6–11 yr: 0.3 mg/kg/dose
 ≥12 yr: 0.2 mg/kg/dose
Diazepam IV Emulsion:
 Status Epilepticus & Severe Recurrent
 Seizures:
 >30 days old –5 yr: 0.2–0.5 mg
 slow IV Q2–5 min PRN **up to a total
 max** of 5 mg
 Children ≥5 yr: 1 mg slow IV Q2–
 5 min PRN **up to a total max** of
 10 mg
 Adult: 5–10 mg slow IV × 1; if

needed repeat in 10–15 min intervals
up to a total max of 30 mg (therapy
may be repeated in 2–4 hr with
caution)
*Tetanus Spasms (Respiratory assistance
should be available):*
 Infants >30 days old: 1–2 mg slow
 IV Q3–4 hr PRN
 ≥5 yr: 5–10 mg slow IV Q3–4 hr PRN

Hypotension and respiratory
depression may occur. Use with
caution in glaucoma, shock, and
depression. Do not use in combination
with protease inhibitors. Concurrent use
with CNS depressants, cimetidine, erythromycin, and valproic acid may enhance the
effects of diazepam.

Administer the conventional IV product
undiluted no faster than 2 mg/min. Do not
mix with IV fluids.

The injectable emulsion product must
always be handled with strict aspectic
technique because it is an excellent
growth media for microorganisms. Doses
of this product must be injected slowly (no
faster than 5 mg/min) and must not be
administered through filters with pore
sizes <5 microns or via polyvinyl chloride
infusion sets.

In status epilepticus, diazepam must be
followed by long-acting anticonvulsants.
Onset of anticonvulsant effect: 1–3 min
with IV route; 2–10 min with rectal route.
For management of status epilepticus, see
p. 15). For management of neonatal
seizures, see p. 474).

DIAZOXIDE

Hyperstat, Proglycem
Antihypertensive agent, antihypoglycemic agent   No   ?   C
Injection: 15 mg/ml
Caps: 50 mg
Suspension: 50 mg/ml (30 ml); contains 7.25% alcohol

Hypertensive crisis: 1–3 mg/kg IV up to a maximum of 150 mg/dose; repeat Q5–15 min PRN, then Q4–24 hr

Hyperinsulinemic hypoglycemia (due to insulin-producing tumors):
   Newborns and infants: 8–15 mg/kg/24 hr ÷ Q8–12 hr PO
   Children and adults: 3–8 mg/kg/24 hr ÷ Q8–12 hr PO (start at lowest dose)

May cause hyponatremia, salt and water retention, GI disturbances, ketoacidosis, rash, hyperuricemia, weakness, hypertrichosis, and arrhythmias. Monitor BP closely for hypotension. Hyperglycemia occurs in majority of patients. Hypoglycemia should be treated initially with IV glucose; diazoxide should be introduced only if refractory to glucose infusion.

Peak antihypertensive effect with IV administration occurs within 5 minutes with a duration of 3–12 hours. Hyperglycemic effect with PO administration occurs within 1 hour with a duration of 8 hours.

DICLOXACILLIN SODIUM

Dynapen, and others
Antibiotic, penicillin (penicillinase-resistant)   No   ?   B
Caps: 125, 250, 500 mg; contains 0.6 mEq Na/250 mg
Oral suspension: 62.5 mg/5 ml (80, 100, 200 ml; contains 2.9 mEq Na/62.5 mg)

Children (<40 kg):
   Mild/moderate infections: 12.5–25 mg/kg/24 hr PO ÷ Q6 hr
   Severe infections: 50–100 mg/kg/24 hr PO ÷ Q6 hr
Adults (≥40 kg): 125–500 mg/dose PO Q6 hr; **max dose:** 4 g/24 hr

Toxicity and side effects similar to cloxacillin. Limited experience in neonates and very young infants. Higher doses (50–100 mg/kg/24 hr) are indicated following IV therapy for osteomyelitis.

Administer 1–2 hr before meals or 2 hr after meals. Use of the oral suspension dosage form may be limited by the resultant dose volume of the 62.5 mg/5 ml concentration.

For explanation of icons, see p. 600.

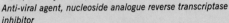

DIDANOSINE
Videx, Dideoxyinosine, ddI
Anti-viral agent, nucleoside analogue reverse transcriptase inhibitor

No   3   B

Tabs (buffered, chewable/dispersable): 25, 50, 100, 150 mg
Oral powder, buffered (single-dose packets for solution): 100, 167, 250, 375 mg
Oral pediatric powder (for 10 mg/ml solution): 2, 4 g

Neonates and Infants <3 months:
100 mg/m²/24 hr ÷ Q12 hr PO
Children <13 yr:
Usual dose (in combination with other antiretrovirals): 180 mg/m²/24 hr ÷ Q12 hr PO
Dose range: 180–300 mg/m²/24 hr ÷ Q12 hr; higher dose may be required for CNS disease
Alternative Pediatric dosing based on 200 mg/m²/24 hr, see the table below.
Adolescent/Adult:
<60 kg: 125 mg Q12hr PO (using tablets) or 167 mg Q12 hr PO (using buffered oral solution); see remarks for additional adolescent dosing information
≥60 kg: 200 mg Q12hr PO (using tablets) or 250 mg Q12 hr PO (using buffered oral solution)

Side effects include: headaches, diarrhea, abdominal pain, nausea, vomiting, peripheral neuropathy (dose related), electrolyte abnormalities, hyperuricemia, increased liver enzymes, retinal depigmentation, CNS depression, rash/pruritis, myalgia, and pancreatitis

(dose related, more in adults). Use with caution in patients on sodium restriction (264.5 mg Na/buffered tablet, 1380 mg Na/single dose packet).

Adolescent Dosing: patients in early puberty (Tanner I-II) should be dosed with pediatric regimens and those in late puberty (Tanner V) should be dosed with adult regimens. Adolescents at Tanner III-IV can be dosed by either pediatric or adult regimen with close monitoring of efficacy and toxicity.

Administer all doses on empty stomach. Impairs absorption of drugs requiring an acidic environment and drugs that have impaired absorption impaired in the presence of divalent ions. (e.g., ketoconazole and fluoroquinolones, respectively). Separate dosing when used in combination with the following drugs: 1 hr before or after ddI (indinavir); 2 hr before or after ddI (delavirdine, ritonavir, fluoroquinolones, ketoconazole, itraconazole, tetracyclines, and dapsone). Consult package insert for additional details.

ALTERNATIVE PEDIATRIC DOSING

BSA	*Chewable tablets	Peds powder dose
<0.4	25mg Q12hr	31mg Q12hr
0.5–0.7	50mg Q12hr	62mg Q12hr
0.8–1	75mg Q12hr	94mg Q12hr
1.1–1.4	100mg Q12hr	125mg Q12hr

*Use at least two tablets to ensure adequate buffering capacity (e.g., give two 25mg tablets for 50mg dose).

DIGOXIN
Lanoxin
Antiarrhythmic agent, inotrope
Yes **1** **C**
Caps: 50, 100, 200 mcg
Tabs: 125, 250, 500 mcg
Elixir: 50 mcg/ml (60 ml); may contain 10% alcohol
Injection: 100, 250 mcg/ml; may contain propylene glycol and alcohol

Digitalizing: Total digitalizing dose (TDD) and maintenance doses in mcg/kg/24 hr (see table below).
Initial: 1/2 TDD, then 1/4 TDD Q8–18 hr × 2 doses; obtain ECG 6 hr after dose to assess for toxicity
Maintenance (see table below):
  <10 yr: Give maintenance dose ÷ BID
  ≥10 yr: Give maintenance dose QD

Contraindicated in patients with ventricular dysrhythmias. Use with caution in renal failure. May cause AV block or dysrhythmias. In the patient treated with digoxin, cardioversion or calcium infusion may lead to ventricular fibrillation (pretreatment with lidocaine may prevent this). For signs and symptoms of toxicity, see p. 29).

Excreted via the kidney; **adjust dose in renal failure (see p. 938).** Therapeutic concentration: 0.8–2 ng/ml. Higher doses may be required for supraventricular tachycardia. Neonates, pregnant women, and patients with renal, hepatic, or heart failure may have falsely elevated digoxin levels, due to the presence of digoxin-like substances.

$T_{1/2}$: premature infants, 61–170 hr; full-term neonates, 35–45 hr; infants, 18–25 hr; and children, 35 hr.

Recommended serum sampling at steady-state: obtain a single level from 6 hours post dose to just before the next scheduled dose following 5–8 days of continuous dosing. Levels obtained prior to steady-state may be useful in preventing toxicity.

DIGOXIN DIGITALIZING AND MAINTENANCE DOSES

Age	TDD		Maintenance	
	PO	IV/IM	PO	IV/IM
Premature	20	15	5	3–4
Full term	30	20	8–10	6–8
<2yr	40–50	30–40	10–12	7.5–9
2–10yr	30–40	20–30	8–10	6–8
>10yr and <100kg	10–15	8–12	2.5–5	2–3

TTD, total digitalizing dose.

For explanation of icons, see p. 600.

DIGOXIN IMMUNE FAB (OVINE)
Digibind
Antidigoxin antibody
Injection: 38 mg

No ? C

First, determine total body digoxin load (TBL):
TBL (mg) = serum digoxin level (ng/ml) × 5.6 × wt (kg) ÷ 1000, OR TBL (mg) = mg digoxin ingested × 0.8
Then, calculate digoxin immune Fab dose:
Dose in number of digoxin immune Fab vials: # vials = TBL ÷ 0.5
Infuse IV over 15–30 min (through 0.22 micron filter).

Contraindicated if hypersensitivity to sheep products, or if renal or cardiac failure. May cause rapidly developing severe hypokalemia, decreased cardiac output, rash, edema. Digoxin therapy may be reinstituted in 3–7 days, when toxicity has been corrected. See p. 29 for additional information.

DIHYDROTACHYSTEROL
DHT, Hytakerol, DHT Intensol
Fat-soluble vitamin D analog
Solution: 0.2 mg/ml (20% alcohol)
Solution (in oil): 0.25 mg/ml (15 ml)
Caps: 0.125 mg
Tabs: 0.125, 0.2, 0.4 mg
1 mg = 120,000 IU vitamin D_2

No ? A/D

Hypoparathyroidism:
Neonates: 0.05–0.1 mg/24 hr PO
Infants/young children: Initial, 1–5 mg/24 hr PO × 4 days, then 0.5–1.5 mg/24 hr PO
Older children/adults: Initial, 0.75–2.5 mg/24 hr PO × 4 days, then 0.2–1.5 mg/24 hr PO
Nutritional Rickets: 0.5 mg × 1 PO, or 13–50 mcg/24 hr PO QD until healing
Renal Osteodystrophy:
Children/Adolescents: 0.1–0.5 mg/24 hr PO
Adults: 0.1–0.6 mg/24 hr PO

Use with **caution** in patients with renal stones, renal failure, and heart disease. Monitor serum Ca^{++} and PO_4. Toxicities include hypercalcemia or hypervitaminosis D. May cause nausea, vomiting, anorexia, and renal damage.

Activated by 25-hydroxylation in liver; does not require 1-hydroxylation in kidney. More potent than vitamin D_2 but more rapidly inactivated (half-life is hours vs. weeks). Titrate dose with patient response. Oral Ca^{++} supplementation may be required.

Pregnancy category changes to "D" if used in doses above RDA.

DILTIAZEM

Cardizem, Cardizem SR, Cardizem CD, Dilacor XR, Tiazac
Calcium channel blocker, antihypertensive

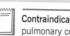

No   1   C

Tabs: 30, 60, 90, 120 mg
Extended Release Tabs: 120, 180, 240 mg
Extended Release Caps:
Cardizem SR: 60, 90, 120 mg
Cardizem CD: 120, 180, 240, 300 mg
Dilacor XR: 180, 240 mg
Tiazac: 120, 180, 240, 300, 360 mg
Inj: 5 mg/ml

Children: 1.5–2 mg/kg/24 hr PO ÷ TID-QID; **max dose:** 3.5 mg/kg/ 24 hr
Adolescents:
Immediate Release: 30–120 mg/dose PO TID-QID; usual range 180–360 mg/24 hr.
Extended Release: 120–300 mg/24 hr PO ÷ QD-BID (BID dosing with Cardizem SR ; QD dosing with Cardizem CD, Dilacor XR, Tiazac)

Contraindicated in acute MI with pulmonary congestion, 2nd or 3rd degree heart block, and sick sinus syndrome. Dizziness, headache, edema, nausea, vomiting, heart block, and arrhythmias may occur.

May increase levels and/or effect of cyclosporin, carbamazepine, fentanyl, digoxin, benzodiazepines, and beta-blockers. Cimetidine may increase diltiazem serum levels.

Maximal antihypertensive effect seen within 2 weeks.

DIMENHYDRINATE

Dramamine and other brand names
Antiemetic, antihistamine

No   ?   B

Tabs/Caps: 50 mg
Tabs (chewable): 50 mg (aspartame)
Injection: 50 mg/ml (benzyl alcohol and propylene glycol)
Solution: 12.5 mg/4 ml, 15.62 mg/5 ml (some preparations may contain 5% alcohol)

For explanation of icons, see p. 600.

Children (<12 yr): 5 mg/kg/24 hr ÷ Q6 hr PO/IM/IV
Adult: 50–100 mg/dose Q4–6 hr PRN PO/IM/IV
Max PO doses:
  2–6 yr: 75 mg/24 hr
  6–12 yr: 150 mg/24 hr
  Adults: 400 mg/24 hr
Max IM dose: 300 mg/24 hr

 Causes drowsiness and anticholinergic side effects. May mask vestibular symptoms and cause CNS excitation in young children. **Caution** when taken with ototoxic agents or history of seizures. **Use should be limited to management of prolonged vomiting of known etiology.** Not recommended in children <2 yr. Toxicity resembles anti-cholinergic poisoning.

DIMERCAPROL
BAL, British anti-Lewisite
Heavy metal chelator (arsenic, gold, mercury, lead
Injection (in oil): 100 mg/ml (3 ml)

No ? D

 Give all injections deep IM.
Lead poisoning: Administer BAL with Ca-EDTA. See p. 34 for details.
Arsenic or gold poisoning:
  Days 1 and 2: 2.5–3 mg/kg/dose Q6 hr
  Day 3: 2.5–3 mg/kg/dose Q12 hr
  Days 4–14: 2.5–3 mg/kg/dose Q24 hr
Mercury poisoning: 5 mg/kg × 1, then 2.5 mg/kg/dose QD–BID × 10 days

 Contraindicated in hepatic or renal insufficiency. May cause hypertension, tachycardia, GI disturbance, headache, fever (30% of children), nephrotoxicity, transient neutropenia. Symptoms are usually relieved by antihistamines. Urine should be kept alkaline to protect the kidneys. Use cautiously in patients with G6PD deficiency. **Do** not use concomitantly with iron. See p. 35 for additional information.

DIPHENHYDRAMINE
Benadryl and other brand names
Antihistamine
Elixir (14% alcohol): 12.5 mg/5 ml
Syrup (some contain 5% alcohol): 12.5 mg/5 ml
Liquid: 6.25mg/5 ml
Caps/Tabs: 25, 50 mg
Chewable Tabs: 12.5 mg (aspartame)

Yes ? B

Injection: 10, 50 mg/ml
Cream: 1, 2%
Lotion: 1% (75 ml)
Topical Gel: 1, 2%
Topical Spray: 1%
Topical Stick: 2%

Children: 5 mg/kg/24 hr ÷ Q6 hr PO/IM/IV

Max dose: 300 mg/24 hr

Adult: 10–50 mg/dose Q4–8 hr PO/IM/IV

Max dose: 400 mg/24 hr

For anaphylaxis or phenothiazine overdose: 1–2 mg/kg IV slowly.

Contraindicated with concurrent MAO inhibitor use, acute attacks of asthma, GI or urinary obstruction. Use with **caution** in infants and young children, and do not use in neonates due to potential CNS effects. Side effects include sedation, nausea, vomiting, xerostoma, blurred vision and other reactions common to antihistamines. CNS side effects more common than GI disturbances. May cause paradoxical excitement in children. **Adjust dose in renal failure (see p. 938).**

DISOPYRAMIDE PHOSPHATE

Norpace and others

Antiarrhythmic agent, class Ia

Caps: 100, 150 mg

Extended-release caps (CR): 100, 150 mg

Suspension: 1 mg/ml, 10 mg/ml

Yes   1   C

<1 yr: 10–30 mg/kg/24 hr ÷ Q6 hr PO

1–4 yr: 10–20 mg/kg/24 hr ÷ Q6 hr PO

4–12 yr: 10–15 mg/kg/24 hr ÷ Q6 hr PO

12–18 yr: 6–15 mg/kg/24 hr ÷ Q6 hr PO

Adult:

<50 kg: 100 mg/dose Q6 hr PO or 200 mg (extended-release) Q12 hr PO

≥50 kg: 150 mg/dose Q6 hr PO or 300 mg (extended-release) Q12 hr PO

Max dose: 1.6 g/24 hr

Contraindicated in 2nd or 3rd degree heart block. May cause decreased cardiac output. Anticholinergic effects may occur. Causes dose-related AV block, wide QRS, increased QTc, ventricular dysrhythmias. **Modify dose in renal (see p. 938)** or hepatic failure.

Erythromycin may increase serum levels. Phenytoin, phenobarbital, and rifampin may decrease serum levels.

Therapeutic levels: 3–7 mg/L.

DIVALPROEX SODIUM

Depakote

Anticonvulsant

Enteric coated tabs: 125, 250, 500 mg

Sprinkle caps: 125 mg

No   1   D

Dose: see Valproic Acid

 Remarks: see Valproic Acid. Preferred over valproic acid for patients on ketogenic diet.

DOBUTAMINE

Dobutrex
Sympathomimetic agent
Injection: 12.5 mg/ml (contains sulfites)

No   ?   C

 Continuous IV infusion: 2.5– 15 mcg/kg/min;
Max recommended dose: 40 mcg/ kg/min
To prepare infusion: see inside front cover

 Contraindicated in IHSS. Tachycardia, arrhythmias (PVCs), and hypertension may occasionally occur (especially at higher infusion rates). Correct hypovolemic states before use. Increases AV conduction, may precipitate ventricular ectopic activity.

Monitor BP and vital signs. $T_{1/2}$: 2 min. Peak effects in 10–20 min.

DOCUSATE SODIUM

Colace and others
Stool softener, laxative
Caps: 50, 100, 240, 250 mg
Tabs: 100 mg
Syrup: 16.7 mg/5 ml, 20 mg/5 ml
Solution: 10 mg/ml, 50 mg/ml (5% alcohol)

No   ?   C

 PO: (take with liquids)
<3 yr: 10–40 mg/24 hr ÷ QD-QID
3–6 yr: 20–60 mg/24 hr ÷ QD-QID
6–12 yr: 40–150 mg/24 hr ÷ QD-QID
>12 yr: 50–500 mg/24 hr ÷ QD-QID
Rectal: Older children and adults: add 50–100 mg of oral solution to enema fluid.

Oral dosage effective only after 1–3 days of therapy. Incidence of side effects is exceedingly low. Oral solution is bitter; give with milk, fruit juice, or formula to mask taste.

A few drops of the 10 mg/ml solution may be used in the ear as a cerumenolyic. Effect is usually seen within 15 min.

DOPAMINE

Intropin, Dopastat, and others
Sympathomimetic agent
Injection: 40, 80, 160 mg/ml
Prediluted in D$_5$W: 0.8, 1.6, 3.2 mg/ml

No   ?   C

Low dose: 2–5 mcg/kg/min IV; increases renal blood flow; minimal effect on heart rate and cardiac output

Intermediate dose: 5–15 mcg/kg/min IV; increases heart rate, cardiac contractility, and cardiac output, and to a lesser extent, renal blood flow.

High dose: >20 mcg/kg/min IV; alpha adrenergic effects are prominent; decreases renal perfusion

Max dose recommended: 20–50 mcg/kg/ min IV

To prepare infusion: see inside front cover

Do not use in pheochromocytoma, tachyarrhythmias, or hypovolemia.
Monitor vital signs and blood pressure continuously. Correct hypovolemic states. Tachyarrhythmias, ectopic beats, hypertension, vasoconstriction, vomiting may occur. Use cautiously with phenytoin since hypotension and bradycardia may be exacerbated.

Should be administered through a central-line or large vein. Extravasation may cause tissue necrosis; treat with phentolamine. Do not administer into an umbilical arterial catheter.

DORNASE ALFA/DNASE

Pulmozyme
Inhaled mucolytic
Sol: 1 mg/ml (2.5 ml)

No   ?   B

Patients >5 yr: 2.5 mg via nebulizer QD. Some patients may benefit from 2.5 mg BID

Contraindicated in patients with hypersensitivity to epoetin alfa.
Voice alteration, pharyngitis, laryngitis may result. These are generally reversible without dose adjustment.

Should not mix with other nebulized drugs. A beta-agonist may be useful before administration to enhance drug distribution. Chest physiotherapy should be incorporated into treatment regimen.

For explanation of icons, see p. 600.

DOXAPRAM HCl
Dopram
CNS stimulant

No ? B

Injection: 20 mg/ml (20 ml)
Contains 0.9% benzyl alcohol

 Methylxanthine-refractory neonatal apnea: Load with 2.5–3 mg/kg over 15 min, followed by a continuous infusion of 1 mg/kg/hr titrated to the lowest responsive dose; **Max dose:** 2.5 mg/kg/hr

Hypertension occurs with higher doses (greater than 1.5 mg/kg/hr). May also cause tachycardia, arrhythmias, seizure, hyperreflexia, hyperpyrexia, and sweating. Avoid extravasation into tissues.

DOXYCYCLINE
Vibramycin and others
Antibiotic, tetracycline derivative

Yes 2 D

Caps: 50, 100 mg
Tabs: 50, 100 mg
Syrup: 50 mg/5 ml (30 ml)
Suspension: 25 mg/5 ml (60 ml)
Injection: 100, 200 mg

 Initial:
  ≤45 kg: 5 mg/kg/24 hr ÷ BID PO/IV × 1 day to max dose of 200 mg/24 hr
  >45 kg: 100 mg BID PO/IV × 1 day
Maintenance:
  ≤45 kg: 2.5–5 mg/kg/24 hr ÷ QD-BID PO/IV
  >45 kg: 100–200 mg/24 hr ÷ QD-BID PO/IV
Max adult dose: 300 mg/24 hr
PID: see p. 392.
Malaria Prophylaxis (start 1–2 days prior to exposure and continue for 4 weeks after leaving edemic area):
  >8 yr: 2 mg/kg/24 hr PO QD; **max dose:** 100 mg/24 hr
  Adult: 100 mg PO QD

Use with **caution** in hepatic and renal disease. May cause increased intracranial pressure. **Do not use** in children <8 yr; may result in tooth enamel hypoplasia and discoloration. May cause GI symptoms, photosensitivity, hemolytic anemia, hypersensitivity reactions.
  Infuse IV over 1–4 hr. Avoid prolonged exposure to direct sunlight. See Tetracycline.

DRONABINOL
Tetrahydrocannabinol, THC, Marinol
Antiemetic
Caps: 2.5, 5, 10 mg

No   ?   C

Antiemetic:
Children & Adult (PO): 5 mg/m²/
dose 1–3 hrs prior to chemotherapy,
then Q2–4 hr **up to a maximum** of
6 doses/24 hr; doses may be gradually
increased to a maximum of 15 mg/m²/
dose if needed and tolerated
Appetite Stimulant:
Adult (PO): 2.5 mg BID 1 hr before
lunch and dinner; if not tolerated,
reduce dose to 2.5 mg QHS.
Max dose: 20 mg/24 hr (Use caution
when increasing doses because of
increased risk of dose-related adverse
reactions at higher dosages).

Contraindicated in patients with
history of substance abuse and
mental illness, allergy to sesame
oil. Use with **caution** in heart disease,
seizures, hepatic disease (reduce dose if
severe). Side effects: euphoria, dizziness,
difficulty concentrating, anxiety, mood
change, sedation, hallucinations, hypotension, excessively increased appetite,
and habit forming potential.

Onset of action: 0.5–1 hr. Duration of
psychoactive effects 4–6 hr, appetite
stimulation 24 hr.

DROPERIDOL
Inapsine
Sedative, antiemetic
Injection: 2.5 mg/ml

No   ?   C

For explanation of icons, see p. 600.

Antiemetic/Sedation:
Children: 0.03–0.07 mg/kg/dose IM or IV over 2–5 min; if needed, may give 0.1–0.15 mg/kg/dose; **max dose:** 2.5 mg/dose
Dosage Interval:
Antiemetic: PRN Q4–6 hr
Sedation: repeat dose in 15–30 minutes if necessary
Adult: 2.5–5 mg IM or IV over 2–5 min
Dosage Interval:
Antiemetic: PRN Q3–4 hr
Sedation: repeat dose in 15–30 minutes if necessary

 Side effects include hypotension, tachycardia, extrapyramidal side effects such as dystonia, feeling of motor restlessness, laryngospasm, bronchospasm. May lower seizure threshold. QT interval prolongation has been associated with use.

Onset in 3–10 minutes. Peak effects within 10–30 minutes. Duration of 2–4 hr. Often given as adjunct to other agents.

EDROPHONIUM CHLORIDE

Tensilon
Anti-cholinesterase agent, antidote for neuromuscular blockade   **Yes**   **?**   **C**
Injection: 10 mg/ml (1, 10, 15 ml)

Test for Myasthenia Gravis (IV):
Neonates: 0.1 mg single dose
Infants and Children:
Initial: 0.04 mg/kg/dose × 1
Max: 1 mg for <34 kg, 2 mg for ≥34 kg
If no response after 1 min, may give 0.16 mg/kg/dose for a total of 0.2 mg/kg
Total max dose: 5 mg for <34 kg, 10 mg for ≥ 34 kg
Adult: 2 mg test dose IV; if no reaction, give 8 mg after 45 sec

May precipitate cholinergic crisis, arrhythmias, bronchospasm. Keep atropine available in syringe and have resuscitation equipment ready. Hypersensitivity to test dose (fasciculations or intestinal cramping) is indication to stop giving drug. **Contraindicated** in GI or GU obstruction, or arrhythmias. Dose may need to be reduced in chronic renal failure.

Short duration of action with IV route (5–10 minutes). Antidote: Atropine 0.01–0.04 mg/kg/dose.

EDTA CALCIUM DISODIUM
Calcium disodium versenate
Chelating agent, antidote for lead toxicity
Injection: 200 mg/ml (5 ml)

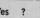

Yes ? C

 Lead Poisoning: see pp. 32–35 for classification, treatment and dosing.

 May cause renal tubular necrosis. **Do not use** if anuric. Follow urinalysis and renal function. Monitor ECG continuously for arrhythmia when giving IV. Rapid IV infusion may cause sudden increase in intracranial pressure in patients with cerebral edema. May cause zinc and copper deficiency. Monitor Ca^{++} and PO_4.

IM route preferred. Give IM with 0.5% procaine.

EFAVIRENZ
Sustiva, DMP-266
Antiviral agent, non-nucleoside reverse transcriptase inhibitor
Capsules: 50, 100, 200 mg

No 3 C

For explanation of icons, see p. 600.

Children ≥3 yrs and weighing ≥10 kg: daily PO dose administered QD (see table)

Body weight (kg)	Dose (mg)
10–<15	200
15–<20	250
20–<25	300
25–<32.5	350
32.5–<40	400
≤40	600

Adults: 600 mg/dose PO QD

Do not use as a single agent for HIV or added on as a sole agent to a failing regimen. Therapy should always be initiated in combination with at least one other antiretroviral agent to which the patient has not been previously exposed.

Dizziness, somnolence, insomnia, abnormal hallucinations, and euphoria are common side effects. Skin rashes (usually mild-moderate maculopapular eruptions) may occur within the first 2 weeks of initiating therapy and usually resolves (with continuing the drug) within 1 month.

Rash is more common in children and more often of greater severity. **Discontinue** therapy in patients developing severe rash associated with blistering, desquamation, mucosal involvement, or fever. Diarrhea, fever, cough, nausea, vomiting, pancreatitis, and elevations in liver enzymes and serum lipids have been reported.

Drug is a substrate and inducer of CYP 450 3A4; and may also inhibit other CYP 450 isoenzymes (2C9, 2C19, and 3A4). See p. 924. Monitor effect/serum levels of drugs metabolized by the aforementioned CYP 450 isoenzymes (eg. warfarin, rifampin). Increases serum levels of nelfinavir and ritonavir; and decreases levels of indinavir and saquinavir. Should **not** be administered with astemizole, cisapride, midazolam, triazolam, or ergot derivatives because competition for CYP 450 3A4 may result in inhibition of metabolism and toxicity of these drugs.

Pharmacokinetics in hepatic or renal impairment have not been adequately evaluated. Doses may be administered with or without food; however, high fat meals may increase absorption.

EMLA

Eutectic mixture of lidocaine and prilocaine
Topical Analgesic

No ? B

Cream: lidocaine 2.5% + prilocaine 2.5%; 5 g kit (with dressings); 30 g tube
Topical Anesthetic Disc: lidocaine 2.5% + prilocaine 2.5%; 1 g (box of 2's or 10's)

See p. 899 for maximum application area in cm².

Use with **caution** in patients with G6PD deficiency and in patients with renal and hepatic impairment. Prilocaine has been associated with methemoglobinemia.

Must apply 60–90 minutes in advance under an occlusive dressing. Wipe cream off before procedure.

ENALAPRIL MALEATE, ENALAPRILAT

Vasotec, Vasotec IV

Angiotensin converting enzyme inhibitor, antihypertensive   **Yes   1   D**

Tabs: 2.5, 5, 10, 20 mg (Enalapril)

Injection: 1.25 mg/ml (Enalaprilat); contains benzyl alcohol

Infants & Children:
PO: 0.1 mg/kg/24 hr ÷ QD–BID;
increase PRN over 2 wk
Max dose: 0.5 mg/kg/24 hr
IV: 0.005–0.01 mg/kg/dose Q8–24 hr
Adult:
PO: 2.5–5 mg/24 hr QD initially to **max
dose** of 40 mg/24 hr ÷ QD-BID
IV: 0.625–1.25 mg/dose IV Q6 hr

Use with **caution** in bilateral renal
artery stenosis. Side effects:
nausea, diarrhea, headache,
dizziness, hyperkalemia, hypoglycemia,
hypotension, and hypersensitivity. Cough
is a reported side effect of ACE inhibitors.

Enalapril (PO) is converted to its active
form (Enalapriat) by the liver. Administer
IV over 5 min. Reduce dose in renal
impairment. **Adjust dose in renal failure
(see p. 939).**

ENOXAPARIN

Lovenox

Anticoagulant, low molecular weight heparin   **No   ?   B**

Inj: 40 mg/0.4 ml, 30 mg/0.3 ml

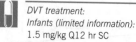

DVT treatment:
Infants (limited information):
1.5 mg/kg Q12 hr SC
Children and Adults: 1 mg/kg Q12 hr
SC
DVT prophylaxis:
Adults: 30 mg BID SC × 7–10 days;
initiate therapy 12–24 hrs after surgery
provided hemostasis is established. 40
mg QD SC has also been used.

Inhibits thrombosis by inactivating
factor Xa without significantly
affecting bleeding time, platelet
function, PT, or APTT at recommended
doses. Dosages of enoxaparin, heparin, or
other low molecular weight heparins
cannot be used interchangeably on a unit-

for-unit (or mg-for-mg) basis because of
differences in pharmacokinetics and
activity. Peak anti-factor Xa activity is
achieved after 4 hours of dose.

Contraindicated in major bleeding and
drug-induced thrombocytopenia. May
cause fever, confusion, edema, nausea,
hemorrhage, thrombocytopenia,
hypochromic anemia, and pain/erythema
at injection site.

Administer by deep SC injection by
having the patient lie down. Rotate
administration between the left and right
anterolateral and left and right posterolateral abdominal wall. See package insert
for detailed SC administration recommendations. To minimize bruising, do not rub
the injection site.

For explanation of icons, see p. 600.

EPINEPHRINE HCl
Adrenalin and others
Sympathomimetic agent

No ? C

1:1000 (Aqueous):
Injection: 1 mg/ml (1, 30 ml vials; 2 ml pre-filled syringe)
1:200 (Sus-phrine long-acting suspension):
Injection: 5 mg/ml (0.3, 5 ml)
1:10,000 (Aqueous):
Injection: 0.1 mg/ml (3, 10 ml prefilled syringe)
1:100,000 (Aqueous):
Injection: 0.01 mg/ml (5 ml)
Epi-pen: 0.3 mg autoinjection (2 ml of 1:1000 solution)

Epi-pen Jr: 0.15 mg autoinjection (2 ml of 1:2000 solution)
Aerosol: 0.16, 0.2, 0.25 mg epinephrine base/spray (15, 22.5 ml)
Oral Inhalation Solution: 1% (10 mg/ml or 1:100) (7.5 ml)
Ophthalmic Solution: 0.1% (1, 30 ml); 0.5% (15 ml); 1% (1, 10, 15 ml); 2% (10, 15 ml)
Nasal Solution: 0.1% (1 mg/ml or 1:1000) (30 ml)

Cardiac Uses:
Neonate:
   Asystole and bradycardia: 0.1–0.3 ml/kg of 1:10,000 solution (0.01–0.03 mg/kg) IV/ET Q3–5 min
Infants and Children:
   Bradycardia/Asystole and Pulseless arrest: **see inside front cover and inside back cover**
   Bradycardia, asystole, and pulseless arrest (first dose): 0.01 mg/kg of 1:10,000 solution (0.1 ml/kg) IO/IV; **max dose:** 1 mg (10 ml)
   Asystole and pulseless arrest (subsequent doses) and all ET doses: 0.1 mg/kg of 1:1000 solution (0.1 ml/kg) IO/IV/ET Q3–5 min. If doses are not effective, increase dose to 0.2 mg/kg of 1:1000 solution (0.2 mg/kg).
Adults:
   Asystole: 1–5 mg IV/ET Q3–5 min
IV drip (all ages): 0.1–1 mcg/kg/min; titrate to effect; to prepare infusion, see inside front cover.

Respiratory uses:
Bronchodilator:
1:1000 (Aqueous)
   Infants and Children: 0.01 ml/kg/dose SC (**max single dose** 0.5 ml); repeat Q15 min × 3–4 doses or Q4 hr PRN
   Adults: 0.3–0.5 ml/dose
1:200 (Susphrine suspension)
   Infants and Children: 0.005 ml/kg/dose SC (**max single dose** 0.15 ml); repeat Q8–12 hr PRN
   Adults: 0.1–0.3 ml/dose
Inhalation: 1–2 puffs Q4 hr PRN
Nebulization: (alternative to racemic epinephrine): 0.5 ml/kg of 1:1000 solution diluted in 3 ml NS; **max doses:** ≤ 4 yr: 2.5 ml/dose; >4 yr: 5 ml/dose

Hypersensitivity reactions: For asthma and certain allergic manifestations (e.g., angioedema, urticaria, serum sickness, anaphylactic shock) use epinephrine SC. The adult IV dose for hypersensitivity reactions or to relieve bronchospasm usually ranges from 0.1 to 0.25 mg injected slowly. Neonates may be given a dose of 0.01 mg/kg body weight; for the infant, 0.05 mg is an adequate initial dose and this may be repeated at 20 to 30 minute intervals in the management of asthma attacks.

May produce arrhythmias, tachycardia, hypertension, headaches, nervousness, nausea, vomiting. Necrosis may occur at site of repeated local injection.

Concomitent use of non-cardiac selective beta-blockers or tricyclic antidepressants may enhance epinephrine's pressor response. Chlorpromazine may reverse the pressor response.

ETT doses should be diluted with NS to a volume of 3–5 ml before administration. Follow with several positive pressure ventilations.

EPINEPHRINE, RACEMIC
Vaponefrin, Micronefrin, Asthmanefrin
Sympathomimetic agent
Solution: 2.25% (1.25% epinephrine base) (7.5, 15, 30 ml); 2% (1% epinephrine base) (15, 30 ml)

No   ?   C

Croup (using 2.25% solution): 0.05 ml/kg/dose diluted to 3 ml with NS. Given via nebulizer over 15 min PRN, but not more frequently than Q1–2 hr. **Max dose:** 0.5 ml

Tachyarrhythmias, headache, nausea, palpitations reported.
Rebound airway edema may occur. Cardio-respiratory monitoring should be considered if administered more frequently than Q1–2 hr.

ERGOCALCIFEROL

Drisdol, Calciferol
Vitamin D2

No ? A/D

Caps/Tabs: 50,000 IU (1.25 mg)
Injection: 500,000 IU/ml
Drops: 8000 IU/ml (200 mcg/ml) (60 ml)
1 mg = 40,000 IU vitamin D activity

Dietary supplementation:
  Preterm: 400–800 IU/24 hr PO
  Infants/Children: 400 IU/24 hr PO;
please refer to p. 485, for details.
Renal Failure:
  Children: 4000–40,000 IU/24 hr PO
  Adult: 20,000 IU/24 hr PO
Rickets: Vitamin D dependent:
  Children: 3000–5000 IU/24 hr PO;
  max dose: 60,000 IU/24 hr
  Adults: 10,000–60,000 IU/24 hr PO;
some may require 500,000 IU/24 hr
Nutritional Rickets:
  *Adults and Children with Normal GI
  absorption:* 2000–5000 IU/24 hr PO ×
  6–12 wk
  Malabsorption:
    Children: 10,000–25,000 IU/24 hr
    PO
    Adults: 10,000–300,000 IU/24 hr
    PO
*Vitamin D resistant rickets (with
phosphate supplementation):*
  Children: Initial dose 400,000–
  800,000 IU/24 hr PO; increase daily

dose by 10,000–20,000 IU PO Q3–
4 mo if needed.
  Adults: 10,000–60,000 IU/24 hr PO
*Hypoparathyroidism (with calcium
supplementation):*
  Children: 50,000–200,000 IU/24 hr
  PO
  Adults: 25,000–200,000 IU/24 hr PO

Monitor serum Ca, PO_4, and
alkaline phosphate. Serum Ca =
PO_4 product should be <70 mg/dl
to avoid ectopic calcification. Titrate
dosage to patient response. Watch for
symptoms of hypercalcemia: weakness,
diarrhea, polyuria, metastatic calcification,
nephrocalcinosis. Vitamin D_2 is activated
by 25-hydroxylation in liver and
1-hydroxylation in kidney.
  Oral route is preferred. May use IM
route in cases of fat malabsorption.
Injectable for IM administration only.
  Pregnancy category changes to "D" if
used in doses above the RDA.

ERGOTAMINE TARTRATE

Cafergot and others
Ergot alkaloid   Yes   X   X
Tabs: 1 mg and 100 mg caffeine
Sublingual tabs: 2 mg
Suppository: 2 mg and 100 mg caffeine
Drug also available in combinations with belladonna alkaloids and/or phenobarbital.

Older children and adolescents:
PO/SL: 1 mg at onset of migraine
attack, then 1 mg Q30 min PRN
up to **max** 3 mg.
Adults:
PO/SL: 2 mg at onset of migraine
attack, then 1–2 mg Q30 min up to
6 mg per attack.
Suppository: 2 mg at first sign of attack;
follow with second dose (2 mg) after
1 hr, **max dose** 4 mg per attack, **not** to
exceed 10 mg/week.

Caution in renal or hepatic disease.
May cause paresthesias, GI
disturbance, angina-like pain,
rebound headache with abrupt
withdrawal, or muscle cramps. Avoid use
during pregnancy. **Contraindicated** in
pregnancy and breastfeeding.

ERYTHROMYCIN ETHYLSUCCINATE AND ACETYLSULFISOXAZOLE

Pediazole   Yes   1   C
Antibiotic, macrolide + sulfonamide derivative
Suspension: 200 mg erythromycin and 600 mg sulfa/5 ml (100, 150, 200 ml)

Otitis media: 50 mg/kg/24 hr (as
erythromycin) and 150 mg/kg/
24 hr (as sulfa) ÷ Q6 hr PO, or
give 1.25 ml/kg/24 hr ÷ Q6 hr PO
Max dose: 2 g erythromycin, 6 g
sulfisoxasole/24 hr

See adverse effects of erythromycin
and sulfisoxazole. **Not** recommended in infants <2 month old.
Do **not** use in renal impairment because
dosage adjustments are inconsistent for
sulfisoxazole and erythromycin.

For explanation of icons, see p. 600.

ERYTHROMYCIN PREPARATIONS
Erythrocin, Pediamycin, E-Mycin, Ery-Ped, and others
Antibiotic, macrolide

Yes   1   B

Erythromycin base:
Tabs: 250, 333, 500 mg
Delayed release tabs: 250, 333, 500 mg
Delayed release caps: 250 mg
Topical Ointment: 2% (25 g)
Topical Gel: 2% (30, 60 g)
Topical Solution: 1.5%, 2% (60 ml)
Topical Swab: 2% (60s)
Ophthalmic ointment: 0.5% (3.5, 3.75 g)

Erythromycin Ethyl Succinate (EES):
Suspension: 200, 400 mg/5 ml (60, 100, 200 ml)
Oral Drops: 100 mg/2.5 ml (50 ml)

Chewable Tabs: 200 mg
Tabs: 400 mg

Erythromycin Estolate:
Suspension: 125, 250 mg/5 ml
Oral Drops: 100 mg/ml (10 ml)
Chewable Tabs: 125, 250 mg
Tabs: 500 mg
Caps: 125, 250 mg

Erythromycin Stearate:
Tabs: 250, 500 mg

Erythromycin gluceptate:
Injection: 1000 mg

Erythromycin lactobionate:
Injection: 500, 1000 mg

Oral:
Neonates:
  <1.2 kg: 20 mg/kg/24 hr ÷ Q12 hr PO
  ≥ 1.2 kg:
    0–7 days: 20 mg/kg/24 hr ÷ Q12 hr PO
    >7 days: 30 mg/kg/24 hr ÷ Q8 hr PO
  Chlamydial conjunctivitis and pneumonia: 50 mg/kg/24 hr ÷ Q6 hr PO × 14 days.
Children:
  30–50 mg/kg/24 hr ÷ Q6–8 hr; **max dose:** 2 g/24 hr
Adults: 1–4 g/24 hr ÷ Q6 hr; **max dose:** 4 g/24 hr

Parenteral:
  Children: 20–50 mg/kg/24 hr ÷ Q6 hr IV
  Adults: 15–20 mg/kg/24 hr ÷ Q6 hr IV
  Max dose: 4 g/24 hr
Rheumatic fever prophylaxis: 500 mg/24 hr ÷ Q12 hr PO
Endocarditis prophylaxis: See p. 162.
Ophthalmic: Apply 0.5 inch ribbon to affected eye BID-QID
Pertussis: Estolate salt: 50 mg/kg/24 hr ÷ Q6 hr PO × 14 days
Preoperative bowel prep: 20 mg/kg/dose PO erythromycin base × 3 doses, with neomycin, 1 day before surgery

Avoid IM route (pain, necrosis). GI side effects common (nausea, vomiting, abdominal cramps). Use with **caution** in liver disease. Estolate may cause cholestatic jaundice, although hepatotoxicity is uncommon (2% of reported cases). Inhibits CYP 450 1A2, 3A3/4 isoenzymes, see p. 924. May produce elevated digoxin, theophylline, carbamazepine, cyclosporine, methylprednisolone levels.

Contraindicated in combination with astemizole, cisapride, or terfenadine.

Oral therapy should replace IV as soon as possible. Give oral doses after meals. Because of different absorption characteristics, higher oral doses of EES are needed to achieve therapeutic effects. May produce false positive urinary catecholamines. Formulations of IV lactobionate dosage form may contain benzyl alcohol.

Adjust dose in renal failure (see p. 932).

ERYTHROPOIETIN
Epoetin Alfa, Epogen, Procrit
Recombinant human erythropoietin
Inj: 2000, 3000, 4000, 10,000, 20,000 U/ml
Multidose vials contain 1% benzyl alcohol.

No   ?   C

Renal failure: SC/IV
Initial: 50–100 U/kg 3x/wk; may increase dose if hematocrit does not rise by 5–6 points after 8 wk; maintenance doses are individualized
AZT treated HIV patients: SC/IV
100 U/kg/dose 3x/wk × 8 wk; the dose may be increased by 50–100 U/kg/dose given 3x/wk; **max dose** 300 U/kg/dose given 3x/wk
Anemia of prematurity:
25–100 U/kg/dose SC 3x/wk; alternatively, 200 U/kg/dose IV/SC QD to QOD for 2–6 wk may be used

Evaluate serum iron, ferritin, TIBC before therapy. Iron supplementation recommended during therapy unless iron stores are already in excess. Monitor Hct, BP, clotting times, platelets, BUN, serum creatinine. Peak effect in 2–3 wk. Reduce dose when target Hct is reached, or when Hct increases >4 points in any 2-wk period. May cause hypertension, seizure, hypersensitivity reactions, headache, edema, dizziness. SC route provides sustained serum levels compared to IV route.

ESMOLOL HCl
Brevibloc
Beta-1-selective adrenergic blocking agent, antihypertensive agent, class II antiarrhythmic

No   ?   C

Injection: 10, 250 mg/ml; contains 25% propylene glycol

Titrate to individual response.
Loading dose: 100–500 mcg/kg IV over 1 min
Maintenance dose: 25–100 mcg/kg/min as infusion
If inadequate response, may re-administer loading dose above, and/or increase maintenance dose by 25–50 mcg/kg/min in increments of Q5–10 min
Usual maintenance dose range: 50–500 mcg/kg/min

$T_{1/2}$ = 9 minutes. May cause bronchospasm, congestive heart failure, nausea, vomiting. May increase digoxin level by 10%–20%. Morphine may increase esmolol level by 46%. Administer **only** in monitored setting.

ETHAMBUTOL HCl
Myambutol
Antituberculosis drug

Yes   1   B

Tabs: 100, 400 mg

Tuberculosis:
Infants, children, adolescents, and adults: 15–25 mg/kg/dose PO QD or 50 mg/kg/dose PO twice weekly
Max dose: 2.5 g/24 hr
Nontuberculous mycobacterial infection:
Children, adolescents, and adults: 15–25 mg/kg/24 hr PO; **max dose:** 1 g/24 hr
M. avium *complex prophylaxis in AIDS* (use in combination with other medications):
Infants, children, adolescents, and adults: 15 mg/kg/dose PO QD; **max dose:** 900 mg/dose

May cause reversible optic neuritis, especially with larger doses. Obtain baseline ophthalmologic studies before beginning therapy and then monthly. Follow visual acuity, visual fields, and (red-green) color vision. Assessment of visual acuity may be difficult in young children. **Discontinue** if any visual deterioration occurs. Monitor uric acid, liver function, heme status, and renal function. May cause GI disturbances. Give with food. **Adjust dose in renal failure (see p. 932).**

ETHOSUXIMIDE
Zarontin
Anticonvulsant
Caps: 250 mg
Syrup: 250 mg/5 ml

Yes 1 C

 Children:
Oral:
  ≤ 6 yr: Initial: 15 mg/kg/24 hr ÷
BID; **max:** 500 mg/24 hr; increase as
needed Q4–7 days; usual maintenance
dose: 15–40 mg/kg/24 hr ÷ BID
>6 yr and Adults: 250 mg BID;
increase by 250 mg/24 hr as needed
Q4–7 days; usual maintenance dose:
20–40 mg/kg/24 hr ÷ BID
Max dose: 1500 mg/24 hr

 Use with **caution** in hepatic and
renal disease. Ataxia, anorexia,
drowsiness, sleep disturbances,
rashes, and blood dyscrasias are rare
idiosyncratic reactions. May cause lupus-
like syndrome; may increase frequency of
grand mal seizures in patients with mixed
type seizures. Drug of choice for absence
seizures.
  Therapeutic levels: 40–100 mg/L.
$T_{1/2}$ = 24–42 hr. Recommended serum
sampling time at steady-state: obtain
trough level within 30 minutes prior to the
next scheduled dose after 5-10 days of
continuous dosing.
  To minimize GI distress, may administer
with food or milk. Abrupt withdrawl of
drug may precipitate absence status.

FAMCICLOVIR
Famvir
Antiviral
Tabs: 125, 250, 500 mg

Yes ? B

 >18 yrs:
Herpes Zoster: 500 mg Q8hr PO ×
  7 days; initiate therapy promptly as
soon as diagnosis is made.
Genital Herpes Simplex: 125 mg Q12hr
PO × 5 days

Drug is converted to its active form
(penciclovir). Better absorption
than PO acyclovir. May cause
headache, diarrhea, nausea, and
abdominal pain. Concomitant use with
probenecid and other drugs eliminated by
active tubular secretion may result in
decreased penciclovir clearance. **Adjust
dose in renal failure (see p. 932).**

FORMULARY

FAMOTIDINE

Pepcid, Pepcid AC [OTC], Pepcid RPD
Histamine-2-receptor antagonist

  Yes 1 B

Injection: 10 mg/ml (multidose vials contain 0.9% benzyl alcohol)
Liquid: 40 mg/5 ml (contains parabens)
Tabs: 10 (OTC), 20, 40 mg
Disintegrating Oral Tabs: 20, 40 mg (contains aspartame)
Chewable Tabs: 10 mg (OTC)

Children:
  IV: Initial: 0.6–0.8 mg/kg/24 hr ÷ Q8–12 hr up to a **max** of 40 mg/24 hr
  PO: Initial: 1–1.2 mg/kg/24 hr ÷ Q8–12 hr up to a **max** of 40 mg/24 hr
Adult:
  Duodenal Ulcer:
    PO: 20 mg BID or 40 mg QHS × 4–8 weeks then maintenance therapy at 20 mg QHS
    IV: 20 mg BID

A 12 hr dosage interval is generally recommended; however, infants and young children may require an 8 hr interval because of enhanced elimination. Headaches, dizziness, constipation, diarrhea, and drowsiness have occurred. **Adjust dose in severe renal failure (see p. 939).**

FELBAMATE

Felbatol
Anticonvulsant

   No ? C

Tabs: 400, 600 mg
Suspension: 600 mg/5 ml

Lennox-Gastaut for Children 2–14 yr (adjunctive therapy):
Start at 15 mg/kg/24 hr PO ÷ TID-QID; increase dosage by 15 mg/kg/24 hr increments at weekly intervals up to a **maximum** of 45 mg/kg/24 hr or 3600 mg/24 hr. See remarks.

Children ≥ 14 yr - Adults:
Adjunctive therapy: Start at 1200 mg/24 hr PO ÷ TID-QID; increase dosage by 1200 mg/24 hr at weekly intervals up to a **maximum** of 3600 mg/day. See remarks.

Monotherapy (as initial therapy): Start at 1200 mg/24 hr PO ÷ TID-QID. Increase dose under close clinical supervision at 600 mg increments Q 2 weeks to 2400 mg/24 hr. **Max dose:** 3600 mg/24 hr.

Conversion to monotherapy: Start at 1200 mg/24 hr ÷ PO TID-QID for 2 weeks; then increase to 2400 mg/24 hr for 1 week. At week 3 increase to 3600 mg/24 hr. See remarks for dose reduction instructions of other antiepileptic drugs.

Drug should be prescribed under strict suppervision by a specialist.
Contraindicated in blood dyscrasias or hepatic dysfunction (prior or current); and hypersensitivity to meprobamate. Aplastic anemia and hepatic failure leading to death have been associated with drug. May cause headache, fatigue, anxiety, GI disturbances, gingival hyperplasia, increased liver enzymes, and bone marrow suppression. **Obtain serum levels of concurrent anticonvulsants.** Monitor liver enzymes, bilirubin, CBC with differential, platelets at baseline and every 1–2 weeks.

When initiating adjunctive therapy (all ages), reduce other antiepileptic drugs (AEDs) by 20% to control plasma levels of concurrent phenytoin, valproic acid, phenobarbital and carbamazepine. Further reductions of concomitant AEDs dosage may be necessary to minimize side effects caused by drug interactions.

When converting to monotherapy, reduce other AEDs by ⅓ at start of felbamate therapy. Then after 2 weeks and at the start of increasing the felbamate dosage, reduce other AEDs by an additional ⅓. At week 3, continue to reduce other AEDs as clinically indicated.

Carbamazepine levels may be decreased; whereas phenytoin and valproic acid levels may be increased. Phenytoin and carbamazepine may increase felbamate clearance; valproic acid may decrease its clearance.

FENTANYL
Sublimaze, Duragesic, Fentanyl Oralet
Narcotic; analgesic, sedative
Injection: 50 mcg/ml
SR patch (Duragesic): 25, 50, 75, 100 mcg/hr
Oralet lozenge: 200, 300, 400 mcg

Yes   1   B/D

For explanation of icons, see p. 600.

Titrate dose to effect.
IV/IM: 1–2 mcg/kg/dose Q30–60 min PRN
Continuous IV infusion: 1 mcg/kg/hr; titrate to effect; usual infusion range 1–3 mcg/kg/hr
PO (Oralet): Sedation: 10–15 mcg/kg/dose up to max of 400 mcg/dose
Transdermal: Safety and efficacy have not been established in pediatrics.
See p. 896 for equianalgesic dosing

Highly lipophilic and may deposit into fat tissue. IV onset of action 1–2 minutes with peak effects in 10 minutes. IV duration of action 30–60 minutes. Give IV dose over 3–5 minutes. Rapid infusion may cause respiratory depression and chest wall rigidity. Respiratory depression may persist beyond the period of analgesia. Transdermal onset of action 6–8 hours with a 72 hour duration of action. *See p. 896 for pharmacodynamic information with IM and PO routes.*

Pregancy category changes to "D" if drug is used for prolonged periods or in high doses at term.

FERROUS SULFATE
See Iron Preparations

FEXOFENADINE
Allegra
Antihistamine, less-sedating

 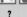 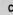

Yes   ?   C

Caps: 60 mg
Note: drug also available in combination with pseudoephedrine (Allegra-D extended-release tabs: 60 mg fexofenadine + 120 mg pseudoephedrine)

>12 yr - Adult: 60 mg PO BID
Reduce dose to 60 mg PO QD if CrCl <40 ml/min.

May cause drowsiness, fatigue, headache, dyspepsia, nausea, and dysmenorrhea. Has **not** been implicated in causing cardiac arrhythmias when used with other drugs that are metabolized by hepatic microsomal enzymes (e.g., ketoconazole, erythromycin).

FILGRASTIM
Neupogen, G-CSF
Colony stimulating factor
Injection: 300 mcg/ml

No   ?   C

IV/SC: 5–10 mcg/kg/dose QD × 14 days or until ANC of 10,000/mm³. Dosage may be increased by 5 mcg/kg/24 hr if desired effect is not achieved within 7 days.
Discontinue therapy when ANC >10,000/mm³.

Individual protocols may direct dosing. May cause bone pain, fever, rash. Monitor CBC, uric acid, and LFTs. Use with **caution** in patients with malignancies with myeloid characteristics. **Contraindicated** for patients sensitive to *E. coli*–derived proteins.

SC routes of administration are preferred because of prolonged serum levels over IV route. If used via IV route and GCSF final concentration <15 mcg/ml, add 2 mg albumin/ ml of IV fluid to prevent drug adsorption to the IV administration set.

FLECAINIDE ACETATE
Tambocor
Antiarrhythmic, class Ic
Tabs: 50, 100, 150 mg
Suspension: 5 mg/ml

Yes   1   C

Children: Initial: 1–3 mg/kg/24 hr ÷ Q8 hr PO; usual range: 3–6 mg/kg/24 hr ÷ Q8 hr PO, monitor serum levels to adjust dose if needed
Adults:
Sustained V tach: 100 mg PO Q12 hr; may increase by 50 mg Q12 hr every 4 days to **max dose** of 600 mg/24 hr
PSVT/PAF: 50 mg PO Q12 hr; may increase dose by 50 mg Q12 hr every 4 days to **max dose** of 300 mg/24 hr

May aggravate LV failure, sinus bradycardia, preexisting ventricular arrhythmias. May cause AV block, dizziness, blurred vision, dyspnea, nausea, headache, increased PR or QRS intervals. **Reserve for life-threatening cases.**

Therapeutic trough level: 0.2–1 mg/L. Recommended serum sampling time at steady-state: obtain trough level within 30 minutes prior to the next scheduled dose after 2–3 days of continuous dosing for children; after 3–5 days for adults.

Adjust dose in renal failure (see p. 939).

For explanation of icons, see p. 600.

FLUCONAZOLE

Diflucan

Antifungal agent

  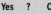

Yes   ?   C

Tabs: 50, 100, 150, 200 mg

Injection: 2 mg/ml; contains 9 mEq Na/2 mg drug

Oral Suspension: 10 mg/ml, 40 mg/ml

Neonates:
Loading dose: 6–12 mg/kg IV/PO, then maintenance (see table)

Children:
Loading dose: 10 mg/kg IV/PO, then
Maintenance: (begin 24 hr after loading dose) 3–6 mg/kg/24 hr IV/PO QD

Adults:
Oropharyngeal and esophageal candidiasis: Loading dose of 200 mg PO/IV followed by 100 mg QD 24 hr after; doses up to max dose of 400 mg/24 hr may be used for esophageal candidiasis

Systemic candidiasis: Loading dose of 400 mg PO/IV, followed by 200 mg QD 24 hr later

Cryptococcal meningitis: Loading dose of 400 mg PO/IV, followed by 200–400 mg QD 24 hr later

Bone Marrow Transplant Prophylaxis: 400 mg PO/IV Q24hr

Vaginal candidiasis: 150 mg PO × 1

Cardiac arrhythmias may occur when used with cisapride, terfenadine, astemizole. Concomitant administration of fluconazole with any of these drugs is **contraindicated.** May cause nausea, headache, rash, vomiting, abdominal pain, hepatitis, cholestasis, and diarrhea.

PO and IV doses are equivalent. Loading doses (mg/kg or mg amounts) are twice the maintenance dose amount.

Inhibits CYP 450 2C9/10 and CYP 450 3A3/4 (weak inhibitor), see p. 924. May increase effects or levels of cyclosporin, phenytoin, theophylline, warfarin, oral hypoglycemics, and AZT. Rifampin increases fluconazole metabolism.

Adjust dose in renal failure (see p. 932).

NEONATAL MAINTENANCE DOSING

Postconceptional age (wk)	Postnatal age (days)	Dose (mg/kg/dose)	Dosing interval (hr) & time (hr) to start 1st maint. dose after load
≤29	0–14	5–6	72
	>14	5–6	48
30–36	0–14	3–6	48
	>14	3–6	24
37–44	0–7	3–6	48
	>7	3–6	24
≥45	>0	3–6	24

FLUCYTOSINE
Ancobon, 5-FC, 5-Fluorocytosine
Antifungal agent
Caps: 250, 500 mg
Oral liquid: 10 mg/ml

Yes 3 C

 Neonates: 80–160 mg/kg/24 hr ÷ Q6 hr PO
Children and Adults: 50–150 mg/kg/24 hr ÷ Q6 hr PO

Monitor CBC, BUN, serum creatinine, alkaline phos, AST, ALT.
Common side effects: nausea, vomiting, diarrhea, rash, CNS disturbance, anemia, leukopenia, and thrombocytopenia.

Therapeutic levels: 25–100 mg/L. Recommended serum sampling time at steady-state: obtain peak level 2-4 hours after oral dose following 4 days of continuous dosing. Peak levels of 40-60 mg/L have been recommended for systemic candidiasis. Prolonged levels above 100 mg/L can increase risk of bone marrow suppression.
Adjust dose in renal failure (see p. 932).

FLUDROCORTISONE ACETATE
Florinef acetate, 9-Fluorohydrocortisone, Fluohydrisone
Corticosteroid
Tabs: 0.1 mg

No ? C

 Infants: 0.05–0.1 mg/24 hr QD PO
Children and Adults: 0.05–0.2 mg/24 hr QD PO

Contraindicated in CHF and systemic fungal infections. Has primarily mineralocorticoid activity. May cause hypertension, hypokalemia, acne, rash, bruising, headaches, GI ulcers and growth suppression.

Monitor BP and serum electrolytes. See pp. 908–909 for steroid potency comparison.

Drug Interactions: drug's hypokalemic effects may induce digoxin toxicity; phenytoin and rifampin may increase fludrocortisone metabolism.

FLUMAZENIL
Romazicon
Benzodiazepine antidote
Injection: 0.1 mg/ml (5, 10 ml)

No ? C

*Children, IV; Reversal of
benzodiazepine sedation:
Initial dose:* 0.01 mg/kg (**max
dose:** 0.2 mg), then 0.005–0.01 mg/kg
(**max dose:** 0.2 mg) given Q 1 minute
to a maximum total cumulative dose of
1 mg. Doses may be repeated in 20
minutes up to a **maximum** of 3 mg in
1 hour.

Does not reverse narcotics. Onset
of benzodiazepine reversal occurs
in 1–3 minutes. *Reversal effects of
flumazenil ($T_{1/2}$ approx 1 hr) may wear off
sooner than benzodiazepine effects.* If
patient does not respond after cumulative
1–3 mg dose, suspect agent other than
benzodiazepines.

May precipitate seizures, especially in
patients taking benzodiazepines for
seizure control or in patients with tricyclic
antidepressant overdose.

See p. 26 for complete management of
suspected ingestions.

FLUNISOLIDE
Nasalide, Nasarel, Aerobid, Aerobid-M
Corticosteroid
Nasal solution: 25 mcg/spray (200 sprays/bottle) (25 ml)
Oral aerosol inhaler: 250 mcg/dose (100 doses/inhaler) (7 g)

No ? C

For all dosage forms, reduce to lowest effective maintenance dose to control symptoms

Nasal Solution:
  Children (6–14 yr):
    Initial: 1 spray per nostril TID or 2 sprays per nostril BID; max dose: 4 sprays per nostril/24 hr
  Adults:
    Initial: 2 sprays per nostril BID; **max dose:** 8 sprays per nostril/24 hr
Inhaler:
  Children (6-15 yr): 2 puff BID
  Adults: 2 puffs BID up to **max** 8 puffs/24 hr
  NIH-National Heart Lung and Blood Institute recommendations: see pp. 911–912.

Stop gradually after 3 wk if no clinical improvement is seen.

Shake inhaler well before use. In children, spacer devices may enhance drug delivery of inhaled form. Rinse mouth after administering drug by inhaler to prevent thrush. Patients using nasal solution should clear nasal passages before use.

FLUORIDE
Luride, Fluoritab, and others
Mineral

No   ?   C

Concentrations and strengths based on fluoride ion:
Drops: 0.125 mg/drop, 0.25 mg/drop
Oral Solution: 0.2, 0.5, 2, 2.25, 5.5, 5.9 mg/ml
Chewable Tabs: 0.25, 0.5, 1 mg
Tabs: 1 mg
Lozenges: 1 mg   See p. 487 for fluoride-containing multivitamins.

All doses/24 hr **(see table):**
Recommendations from American Academy of Pediatrics and American Dental Association.

Acute overdose: GI distress, salivation, CNS irritability, tetany, seizures, hypocalcemia, hypoglycemia, cardiorespiratory failure. Chronic excess use may result in mottled teeth or bone changes.

Take with food, but **not** milk, to minimize GI upset. The doses have been decreased due to concerns over dental fluorosis.

| | Concentration of fluoride in drinking water (ppm) | | |
Age	<0.3	0.3–0.6	>0.6
Birth–6mo	0	0	0
6mo–3yr	0.25mg	0	0
3–6yr	0.5mg	0.25mg	0
6–16yr	1mg	0.5mg	0

For explanation of icons, see p. 600.

FORMULARY

FLUOXETINE HYDROCHLORIDE

Prozac
Antidepressant, selective serotonin reuptake inhibitor

No 3 B

Liquid: 20 mg/5 ml
Caps: 10, 20 mg

Depression:
Children >5 yr:
  5–10 mg QD PO.
Max dose: 20 mg/24 hr
Adults: Start at 20 mg QD PO. May increase after several weeks by 20 mg/24 hr increments to **max** of 80 mg/24 hr. Doses >20 mg/24 hr should be divided BID.

Contraindicated in patients taking MAO inhibitors due to possibility of seizures, hyperpyrexia, and coma. May increase the antidepressant effects of tricyclic antidepressants. May cause headache, insomnia, nervousness, drowsiness, GI disturbance, and weight loss. Increased bleeding diathesis with unaltered prothrombin time may occur with warfarin. May displace other highly protein bound drugs. Inhibits CYP 450 2C19, 2D6, and 3A3/4 drug metabolism isoenzymes (see p. 924).

FLUTICASONE PROPIONATE

Flonase, Cutivate, Flovent, Flovent Rotadisk
Corticosteroid

No ? C

Nasal Spray: 50 mcg/actuation (9, 16 g)
Topical Cream: 0.05% (15, 30, 60 g)
Topical Ointment: 0.005% (15, 60 g)
Aerosol Inhaler (MDI):
  44 mcg/actuation (7.9 g = 60 doses/inhaler, 13 g = 120 doses/inhaler)
  110 mcg/actuation (13 g = 120 doses/inhaler)
  220 mcg/actuation (13 g = 120 doses/inhaler)

Dry Powder Inhalation (DPI) (all strengths come in a package of 15 rotadisks where each rotadisk provides 4 doses for a total of 60 doses per package):
  50 mcg/dose (delivers approximately 44 mcg/dose)
  100 mcg/dose (delivers approximately 88 mcg/dose)
  250 mcg/dose (delivers approximately 220 mcg/dose)

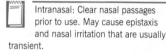

Intranasal (Allergic Rhinitis):
≥4 yr and Adolescents: 1 spray (50 mcg) per nostril QD. Dose can be increased to 2 sprays (100 mcg) per nostril QD if inadequate response or severe symptoms. Reduce to 1 spray per nostril QD once symptoms are controlled.

Max dose: 2 sprays (100 mcg) per nostril/24 hr

Adults: Initial 200 mcg/24 hr [2 sprays (100 mcg) per nostril QD; OR 1 spray (50 mcg) per nostril BID]. Reduce to 1 spray per nostril QD once symptoms are controlled

Max dose: 2 sprays (100 mcg) per nostril/24 hr

Oral Inhalation: **DIVIDE ALL 24hr DOSES BID.** Reduce to the lowest effective dose when asthma symptoms are controlled.

Converting from other asthma regimens (see table).
NIH-National Heart Lung and Blood Institute recommendations: see pp. 911–912.

Topical: Apply to affected areas BID

Intranasal: Clear nasal passages prior to use. May cause epistaxis and nasal irritation that are usually transient.

Oral Inhalation: Rinse mouth after each use. May cause dysphonia, oral thrush, and dermatitis.

Topical Use: Avoid application/contact to face, eyes, and open skin.

CONVERSION FROM OTHER ASTHMA REGIMENS TO FLUTICASONE

Age	Previous use of bronchodilators only (max dose)	Previous use of inhaled corticosteroid (max dose)	Previous use of oral corticosteroid (max dose)
Children (4–11yr)	MDI: 88mcg/24hr (176mcg/24hr) DPI: 100mcg/24hr (200mcg/24hr)	MDI: 88mcg/24hr (176mcg/24hr) DPI: 100mcg/24hr (200mcg/24hr	Dose not available
Age 12yr and Adults	MDI: 176mcg/24hr (800mcg/24hr) DPI: 200mcg/24hr (1000mcg/24hr)	MDI: 176–440mcg/ 24hr (800mcg/24hr) DPI: 200–500mcg/ 24hr (1000mcg/24hr)	MDI:1760mcg/24hr (1760mcg/24hr) DPI: 2000mcg/24hr (2000mcg/24hr)

FLUVOXAMINE
Luvox
Antidepressant, selective serotonin reuptake inhibitor
Tabs: 50, 100 mg

 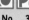

No   3   C

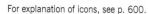

Obsessive Compulsive Disorder:
>8yr: Start at 25 mg PO QHS.
Dose may be increased by 25 mg/
24 hr Q 4–7 days up to a **maximum** of
200 mg/24 hr. Total daily doses
>50 mg/24 hr should be divided BID.
Adults: Start at 50 mg PO QHS. Dose
may be increased by 50 mg/24 hr Q4–
7 days up to a **maximum** of 300 mg/
24 hr. Total daily doses >100 mg/24 hr
should be divided BID.

Contraindicated with
coadministration of astemizole,
terfenadine, or MAO inhibitors.
Inhibits CYP 450 2C19, and 3A3/4, see
p. 924. When used with warfarin, may
increase warfarin plasma levels by 98%
and prolong PT. Side effects include:
headache, insomnia, somnolence,
nausea, diarrhea, dyspepsia, and dry
mouth.
Titrate dose to lowest effective dose.
May increase toxicity and/or levels of
theophylline, caffeine, and tricyclic
antidepressants.

FOLIC ACID
Folvite and others
Water-soluble vitamin
Tabs: 0.4, 0.8, 1 mg
Oral solution: 1 mg/ml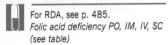
Injection: 5 mg/ml; contains 1.5% benzyl alcohol

No   1   A

For RDA, see p. 485.
Folic acid deficiency PO, IM, IV, SC
(see table)

Normal levels: serum >3 ng/ml,
RBC 153–605 ng/ml. May mask
hematologic effects of vitamin B_{12}
deficiency, but will not prevent progression
of neurologic abnormalities.
Women of child-bearing age considering
pregnancy should take at least 0.4 mg QD
before and during pregnancy to reduce
risk of neural tube defects in the fetus.

FOLIC ACID DEFICIENCY (PO, IM, IV, SC)		
Infants	Children (1–10yr)	Adults (>11yr)
Initial dose		
15mcg/kg/dose; max dose 50mcg/24 hr	1mg/dose	1–3mg/dose ÷ QD-TID
Maintenance		
30–45mcg/24hr QD	0.1–0.4mg/24hr QD	0.5mg/24hr QD; Pregnant/lactating women: 0.8mg/24hr QD

FOSCARNET
Foscavir
Antiviral agent
Injection: 24 mg/ml (250, 500 ml)

Yes   3   C

 Adolescents and Adults, IV:
CMV Retinitis:
  Induction: 180 mg/kg/24 hr ÷
  Q8 hr × 14–21 days
  Maintenance: 90–120 mg/kg/24 hr
  QD
Acyclovir-resistant herpes simplex:
40 mg/kg/dose Q8 hr or 40–60
mg/kg/dose Q12 hr for up to 3 weeks or
until lesions heal

Use with **caution** in patients with
renal insufficiency. **Discontinue** use
if Cr ≥2.9 mg/dl. **Adjust dose in
renal failure (see p. 932).**
  May cause peripheral neuropathy,
seizures, hallucinations, GI disturbance,
increased LFTs, hypertension, chest pain,
EKG abnormalities, coughing, dyspnea,
bronchospasm, and renal failure. Hypocalcemia (increased risk if given with
pentamidine), hypokalemia, hypomagnesemia may also occur.

FOSPHENYTOIN
Cerebyx
Anticonvulsant
Inj: 50 mg phenytoin equivalent (75 mg fosphenytoin)/1 ml
(2, 10 ml)

No   1   D

All doses are expressed as phenytoin sodium equivalents (PE):
Children: see phenytoin and use the conversion of 1 mg phenytoin = 1 mg PE
Adults:
Loading Dose:
Status Epilepticus: 15–20 mg PE/kg IV
Nonemergent loading: 10–20 mg PE/kg IV/IM
Initial Maintenance Dose: 4–6 mg PE/kg/24 hr IV/IM

All doses should be prescribed and dispensed in terms of mg phenytoin sodium equivalents (PE) to avoid medication errors. Safety in pediatrics has **not** been fully established.
Use with **caution** in patients with porphyria. Consider amount of phosphate delivered by fosphenytoin in patients with phosphate restrictions. Side effects: hypokalemia (with rapid IV administration), slurred speech, dizziness, ataxia, rash, exfoliative dermatitis, nystagmus, diplopia, tinnitus.

Abrupt withdrawal may cause status epilepticus. BP and EKG monitoring should be present during IV loading dose administration. Maximum IV infusion rate: 150 mg PE/min. IM administration may be administered via 1 or 2 injection sites and is not recommended in status epilepticus.

Therapeutic levels: 10–20 mg/L (free and bound phenytoin) OR 1–2 mg/L (free only). Recommended peak serum sampling times: 4 hours following an IM dose or 2 hours following an IV dose.

See phenytoin remarks for drug interactions.

FUROSEMIDE

Furomide, Lasix, and others
Loop diuretic
Tabs: 20, 40, 80 mg
Injection: 10 mg/ml
Oral liquid: 10 mg/ml (60, 120 ml), 40 mg/5 ml

No   ?   C

IM, IV, PO:
Neonates: 0.5–1 mg/kg/dose Q8–24 hr; **max PO dose:** 6 mg/kg/dose, **max IV dose:** 2 mg/kg/dose.
Infants and Children: 0.5–2 mg/kg/dose Q6–12 hr; **max dose:** 6 mg/kg/dose.
Adults: 20–80 mg/24 hr ÷ Q6–12 hr; **max dose:** 600 mg/24 hr.
Continuous IV infusion:
Children and Adults: 0.05 mg/kg/hr, titrate to effect.

Use with **caution** in hepatic disease. Ototoxicity may occur in presence of renal disease, especially when used with aminoglycosides. May cause hypokalemia, alkalosis, dehydration, hyperuricemia, and increased calcium excretion. Prolonged use in premature infants may result in nephrocalcinosis. **Max rate** of intermittent IV dose: 0.5 mg/kg/min.

GABAPENTIN
Neurontin
Anticonvulsant
Caps: 100, 300, 400 mg

Yes   ?   C

>12 yr and Adults (PO):
Day 1: 300 mg at bedtime
Day 2: 300 mg BID
Day 3: 300 mg TID
Usual effective doses: 900–1800 mg/
24 hr ÷ TID
Doses as high as 3.6 g/24 hr have been
tolerated.

Side effects include somnolence,
dizziness, ataxia, fatigue, and
nystagmus. Do **not** withdraw
medication abruptly. Drug is not
metabolized by the liver and is primarily
excreted in the urine unchanged.

May be taken with or without food. In
TID dosing schedule, interval between
doses should not exceed 12 hr. **Adjust
dose in renal impairment (see p. 939).**

GANCICLOVIR
Cytovene
Antiviral agent
Injection: 500 mg; contains 4 mEq Na per 1 gm drug
Caps: 250, 500 mg

Yes   ?   C

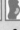
Cytomegalovirus (CMV) infections:
Children >3 mo and adults:
Induction therapy (duration 14–
21 days): 10 mg/kg/24 hr ÷ Q12 hr
IV
Maintenance therapy: 5 mg/kg/dose
QD IV or 6 mg/kg/dose QD IV for
5 days/wk
Oral maintenance therapy (adults):
1000 mg PO TID with food
Prevention of CMV in transplant
recipients:
Children and adults:
Induction therapy (duration 7–14
days): 10 mg/kg/24 hr ÷ Q12 hr IV
Maintenance therapy: same as above
Oral maintenance therapy (adults):
same as above
Prevention of CMV in HIV-Infected
individuals:
Infants and Children: 5 mg/kg/dose QD
IV

Adolescent and adults:
IV: 5–6 mg/kg/dose QD for 5–7 days/
wk
PO: 1000 mg PO TID with food

Limited experience with use in
children <12 yr old. Use with
extreme caution. **Reduce dose in
renal failure (see p. 933).** Oral absorption
is poor. Common side effects:
neutropenia, thrombocytopenia, retinal
detachment, confusion. Drug reactions
alleviated with dose reduction or
temporary interruption. Minimum dilution
is 10 mg/ml and should be infused IV
over ≥1 hr. IM and SC administration
are **contraindicated** because of high pH
(pH = 11).

GCSF
See Filgrastim

GENTAMICIN
Garamycin and others
Antibiotic, aminoglycoside
Injection: 10, 40 mg/ml
Ophthalmic ointment: 0.3% (3.5 g)
Ophthalmic drops: 0.3% (5 ml)
Topical ointment: 0.1% (15 g)
Topical cream: 0.1% (15 g)
Intrathecal injection: 2 mg/ml

Yes ? C

Parenteral (IM or IV):
Neonate/Infant (**see table**)
Children: 6–7.5 mg/kg/24 hr ÷ Q8 hr
Adults: 3–6 mg/kg/24 hr ÷ Q8 hr
Cystic Fibrosis: 7.5–10.5 mg/kg/24 hr ÷ Q8 hr
Intrathecal/intraventricular:
  >3 mo: 1–2 mg QD
  Adult: 4–8 mg QD
Ophthalmic ointment: apply Q6–8 hr
Ophthalmic drops: 1–2 drops Q4 hr

Use with **caution** in patients receiving anesthetics or neuromuscular blocking agents, and in patients with neuromuscular disorders. May cause nephrotoxicity and ototoxicity. Ototoxicity may be potentiated with the use of loop diuretics. Eliminated more quickly in patients with cystic fibrosis, neutropenia, and burns. **Adjust dose in renal failure (see p. 933).** Monitor peak and trough levels.
  Therapeutic peak levels:
    6–10 mg/L general
    8–10 mg/L in pulmonary infections, neutropenia, and severe sepsis
  Therapeutic trough levels: <2 mg/L. Recommended serum sampling time at steady-state: trough within 30 minutes prior to the 3rd consecutive dose and peak 30–60 minutes after the administration of the 3rd consecutive dose.

NEONATAL/INFANT GENTAMICIN DOSING (IM, IV)

Postconceptional age (wk)	Postnatal age (days)	Dose (mg/kg/dose)	Interval (hr)
≤29*	0–28	2.5	24
	>28	3	24
30–36	0–14	3	24
	>14	2.5	12
≥37	0–7	2.5	12
	>7	2.5	8

*Or significant asphyxia

GLUCAGON HCl
Glucagon
Antihypoglycemic agent
Injection: 1, 10 mg/vial (1 unit = 1 mg)

No   ?   B

Hypoglycemia, IM, IV, SC:
Neonates/Infants: 0.025–0.3 mg/kg/dose Q30 min PRN;
max dose: 1 mg/dose
Children: 0.03–0.1 mg/kg/dose Q20 min PRN; **max dose:** 1 mg/dose
Adults: 0.5–1 mg/dose Q20 min PRN

 High doses have cardiac stimulatory effect and have had some success in beta-blocker overdose. May cause nausea, vomiting, urticaria, and respiratory distress. Do **not** delay glucose infusion; dose for hypoglycemia is 2–4 ml/kg of Dextrose 25%.

GLYCERIN
Fleet Babylax, Sani-Supp, and others
Osmotic Laxative
Rectal solution: 4 ml per application (6 doses)
Suppository: infant, adult

No   ?   C

 Constipation:
Neonate: 0.5 ml/kg/dose rectal solution PR as an enema QD–BID PRN
Children <6 yr: 2–5 ml rectal solution PR as an enema or 1 infant suppository PR QD–BID PRN
>6 yr-adults: 5–15 ml rectal solution PR as an enema or 1 adult suppository PR QD–BID PRN

 Onset of action: 15-30 min. May cause rectal irritation, abdominal pain, bloating, and dizziness. Insert suppository high into rectum and retain for 15 minutes.

GLYCOPYRROLATE
Robinul
Anticholinergic agent
Tabs: 1, 2 mg
Injection: 0.2 mg/ml

Yes   ?   B

Respiratory antisecretory:
IM/IV:
Children: 0.004–0.01 mg/kg/dose Q4–8 hr
Adults: 0.1–0.2 mg/dose Q4–8 hr
Max dose: 0.2 mg/dose or 0.8 mg/24 hr
Oral:
Children: 0.04–0.1 mg/kg/dose Q4–8 hr
Adults: 1–2 mg/dose BID-TID
Reverse neuromuscular blockade:
Children and adults: 0.2 mg IV for every 1 mg neostigmine or 5 mg pyridostigmine

Use with **caution** in hepatic and renal disease, ulcerative colitis, asthma, glaucoma, ileus, or urinary retention. Atropine-like side effects: tachycardia, nausea, constipation, confusion, bronchospasm, blurred vision, and dry mouth. These may be potentiated if given with other drugs with anticholinergic properties. IV dosage form may be used orally.

GRANISETRON
Kytril
Antiemetic agent, 5-HT$_3$ antagonist
Inj: 1 mg/ml (1, 4 ml)
Tabs: 1 mg

No   ?   B

IV:
Children ≥2 yr and adults: 10–20 mcg/kg/dose 15–60 minutes before chemotherapy; the same dose may be repeated 2–3 times following chemotherapy (within 24 hrs after chemotherapy) as a treatment regimen. Alternatively, a single 40 mcg/kg/dose 15–60 minutes before chemotherapy has been used.
PO:
Adults: 2 mg/24 hr ÷ QD-BID; initiate first dose 1 hour prior to chemotherapy

Use with **caution** in liver disease. May cause hypertension, hypotension, arrythmias, agitation, and insomnia. Inducers or inhibitors of the CYP-450 drug metabolizing enzymes may increase or decrease, respectively, the drug's clearance (see p. 924).

Griseofulvin microcrystalline 731

FORMULARY

GRISEOFULVIN MICROCRYSTALLINE

No ? C

Grifulvin V, Grisactin, Fulvicin
Antifungal agent
Microsize:
Tabs: 250, 500 mg
Caps: 125, 250 mg
Suspension: 125 mg/5 ml (120 ml); contains 0.2% alcohol
Ultramicrosize tabs: 125, 165, 250, 330 mg
250 mg ultra is approx 500 mg micro

Microsize:
Children >2 yr: 10–20 mg/kg/24 hr PO ÷ QD-BID; give with milk, eggs, fatty foods
Adult: 500–1000 mg/24 hr PO ÷ QD-BID
Max dose: 1 g/24 hr
Ultramicrosize:
Children >2 yr: 5–10 mg/kg/24 hr PO ÷ QD-BID
Adults: 330–750 mg/24 hr PO ÷ QD-BID
Max dose: 750 mg/24 hr

Contraindicated in porphyria, hepatic disease. Monitor hematologic, renal, and hepatic function, especially for courses >4–6 weeks. May cause leukopenia. Possible cross-reactivity in penicillin-allergic patients. Usual treatment period is 4–6 wk for tinea capitis and 4–6 months for tinea unguium. Photosensitivity reactions may occur. May reduce effectiveness or decrease level of oral contraceptives, warfarin, and cyclosporin. Phenobarbital may enhance clearance of griseofulvin. Coadministration with fatty meals will increase the drug's absorption.

HALOPERIDOL

No 3 C

Haldol and others
Antipsychotic agent
Injection (IM use only):
  Lactate: 5 mg/ml
  Decanoate (long acting): 50, 100 mg/ml
Tabs: 0.5, 1, 2, 5, 10, 20 mg
Solution: 2 mg/ml

Children 3–12 yr:
PO: Initial dose at 0.025–0.05 mg/kg/24 hr ÷ BID-TID. If necessary, increase daily dosage by 0.25–0.5 mg/24 hr Q5–7 days PRN up to a **maximum** of 0.15 mg/kg/24 hr. Usual maintenance doses for specific indications include the following:

Agitation: 0.01–0.03 mg/kg/24 hr QD PO

Psychosis: 0.05–0.15 mg/kg/24 hr ÷ BID-TID PO

Tourette's syndrome: 0.05–0.075 mg/kg/24 hr ÷ BID-TID PO; may increase daily dose by 0.5 mg Q5–7 days.

IM, as lactate, for 6–12 yrs old: 1–3 mg/dose Q4–8 hr; **max dose:** 0.15 mg/kg/24 hr

>12 yr:
Acute agitation: 2–5 mg/dose IM as lactate or 1–15 mg/dose PO; repeat in 1 hr PRN

Psychosis: 2–5 mg/dose Q4–8 hr IM PRN or 1–15 mg/24 hr ÷ BID-TID PO

Tourette's: 0.5–2 mg/dose BID-TID PO

Use with **caution** in patients with cardiac disease because of the risk of hypotension and in patients with epilepsy since the drug lowers the seizure threshold. Extrapyramidal symptoms, drowsiness, headache, tachycardia, ECG changes, nausea, and vomiting can occur.

Acutely aggravated patients may require doses as often as Q60 min. Decanoate salt is given every 3–4 **weeks** in doses that are 10–15 times the individual patient's stabilized oral dose.

HEPARIN SODIUM
Various trade names
Anticoagulant

No   1   B

Injection: 10, 100, 1000, 2000, 2500, 5000, 7500, 10,000, 15000, 20,000, 40,000 U/ml
120 U = approx 1 mg
Product's origin is from either beef lung or porcine intestinal mucosa.

For explanation of icons, see p. 600.

Anticoagulation:
Infants and Children:
Initial: 50 U/kg IV bolus
Maintenance: 10–25 U/kg/hr as IV
infusion or 50–100 U/kg/dose Q4 hr
IV
Adults:
Initial: 50–100 U/kg IV bolus
Maintenance: 15–25 U/kg/hr as IV
infusion or 75–125 U/kg/dose Q4 hr
IV
See p. 315 for dosage adjustments.
DVT prophylaxis:
Adults: 5000 U/dose SC Q8–12 hr until
ambulatory
Heparin flush:
Peripheral IV: 1–2 ml of 10 U/ml
solution Q4 hr
Central lines: 2–3 ml of 100 U/ml
solution Q24 hr

TPN (central line) and arterial line: add
heparin to make final concentration of
0.5–1 U/ml
**Flush dose should be less than
heparinizing dose!**

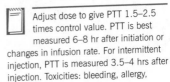

Adjust dose to give PTT 1.5–2.5
times control value. PTT is best
measured 6–8 hr after initiation or
changes in infusion rate. For intermittent
injection, PTT is measured 3.5–4 hrs after
injection. Toxicities: bleeding, allergy,
alopecia, thrombocytopenia.

Use preservative-free heparin in
neonates. **Note:** heparin flush doses may
alter PTT in small patients; consider using
more dilute heparin in these cases.

Antidote: Protamine sulfate (1 mg per
100 U heparin in previous 4 hr). For low
molecular weight heparin, see enoxaparin.

HYALURONIDASE
Wydase
Antidote, extravasation
Injection: 150 U/ml
Powder for injection: 150, 1500 U
🖉: Pharmacy can make a 15 U/ml dilution.

No ? C

Infants and Children: Dilute to 1
5 U/ml; give 1 ml (15U) by
injecting 5 separate injections of
0.2 ml (3U) at borders of extravasation
site SC or ID using a 25- or 26-gauge
needle

Contraindicated in dopamine and
alpha-agonist extravasation. May
cause urticaria. Administer as early
as possible (minutes to 1 hour) after IV
extravasation.

HYDRALAZINE HYDROCHLORIDE
Apresoline
Antihypertensive, vasodilator
Tabs: 10, 25, 50, 100 mg
Injection: 20 mg/ml
Oral liquid: 1.25, 2, 4 mg/ml

Yes   1   C

Hypertensive crisis:
Children: 0.1–0.2 mg/kg/dose IM or IV Q4–6 hr PRN; **max dose:** 20 mg/dose
Adults: 10–40 mg IM or IV Q4–6 hr PRN
Chronic hypertension:
Infants and children: Start at 0.75–1 mg/kg/24 hr PO ÷ Q6–12 hr (**max dose:** 25 mg/dose). If necessary, increase dose over 3–4 weeks up to a **maximum** of: 5 mg/kg/24 hr for infants and 7.5 mg/kg/24 hr for children; or 200 mg/24 hr
Adults: 10–50 mg/dose PO QID; **max dose:** 300 mg/24 hr

Use with caution in severe renal and cardiac disease. Slow acetylators, patients receiving high dose chronic therapy and those with renal insufficiency are at highest risk of lupus-like syndrome (generally reversible). May cause reflex tachycardia, palpatations, dizziness, headaches, and GI discomfort. Drug undergoes first pass metabolism. Onset of action: PO: 45-60 minutes; IV: 10–20 minutes; IM: 5–10 minutes.
Adjust dose in renal failure (see p. 939).

HYDROCHLOROTHIAZIDE
Esidrix, Hydro-T, Thiuretic, Hydrodiuril, and others
Diuretic, thiazide
Tabs: 25, 50, 100 mg
Caps: 12.5 mg
Solution: 10 mg/ml

Yes   1   D

Neonates and Infants <6 months: 2–4 mg/kg/24 hr ÷ BID PO
≥6 months and Children: 2 mg/kg/24 hr ÷ BID PO
Adults: 25–100 mg/24 hr ÷ QD-BID PO; **max dose:** 200 mg/24 hr

See chlorothiazide. May cause fluid and electrolyte imbalances, hyperuricemia. Drug may not be effective when creatinine clearance is less than 25–50 ml/min.

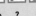

HYDROCORTISONE
Solu-cortef, Hydrocortone, Cortef, and others
Corticosteroid

No   ?   C

Hydrocortisone base
Tabs: 5, 10, 20 mg
Rectal cream: 1%, 2.5%
Cypionate
Suspension: 10 mg/5 ml (120 ml)
Na Phosphate
Injection: 50 mg/ml

Na Succinate (Solu-Cortef)
Injection: 100, 250, 500,
1000 mg/vial
Acetate (Hydrocortone)
Injection: 25, 50 mg/ml
Suppository: 25 mg
Rectal foam aerosol: 10%
(90 mg/dose) (20 g)

Status asthmaticus:
Children:
Load (optional): 4–8 mg/kg/dose
IV; **max dose: 250 mg**
Maintenance: 8 mg/kg/24 hr ÷ Q6 hr
IV
Adults: 100–500 mg/dose Q6 hr IV
Physiologic Replacement:
PO: 0.5–0.75 mg/kg/24 hr ÷ Q8 hr
IM: 0.25–0.35 mg/kg/dose QD
Anti-inflammatory/immunosuppressive:
Children:
PO: 2.5–10 mg/kg/24 hr ÷ Q6–8 hr
IM/IV: 1–5 mg/kg/24 hr ÷ Q12–24 hr
Adolescents and Adults:
PO/IM/IV: 15–240 mg/dose Q12 hr
Acute adrenal insufficiency (see p. 907
for additional information) (IM/IV)

Infants and Young Children:
Load: 1–2 mg/kg/dose IV bolus
Maintenance: 25–150 mg/24 hr ÷
Q6–8 hr
Older Children:
Load: 1–2 mg/kg/dose IV bolus
Maintenance: 150–250 mg/24 hr ÷
Q6–8 hr

For doses based on body surface
area and topical preparations, see
p. 907. Na succinate used for IV,
IM dosing. Na phosphate may be give IM,
SC, or IV. Acetate form recommended for
intraarticular, intralesional, soft tissue use,
but not for IV use.

HYDROMORPHONE HCl
Dilaudid and others
Narcotic, analgesic

Yes   ?   B/D

Tabs: 1, 2, 3, 4, 8 mg
Injection: 1, 2, 3, 4, 10 mg/ml (contains benzyl alcohol)
Suppository: 3 mg
Oral liquid: 1 mg/ml

Analgesia, titrate to effect:
Children:
  IV: 0.015 mg/kg/dose Q4–6 hr PRN
  PO: 0.03–0.08 mg/kg/dose Q4–6 hr PRN
Adolescents and Adults:
  IM, IV, SC: 1–2 mg/dose Q4–6 hr PRN
  PO: 1–4 mg/dose Q4–6 hr PRN

Refer to p. 897 for equianalgesic doses and patient-controlled analgesia dosing. Less pruritus than morphine. Similar profile of side effects to other narcotics. Use with **caution** in infants and young children, and **do not use** in neonates due to potential CNS effects. Dose reduction recommended in renal insufficiency or severe hepatic impairment. Pregnancy category changes to"D" if used for prolonged peroids or in high doses at term.

HYDROXYZINE

Atarax, Vistaril
Antihistamine, anxiolytic
Tabs (HCl): 10, 25, 50, 100 mg
Caps (pamoate): 25, 50, 100 mg
Syrup (HCl): 10 mg/5 ml
Suspension (pamoate): 25 mg/5 ml (120 ml)
Injection (HCl): 25, 50 mg/ml

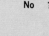

No   ?   C

Oral:
  Children: 2 mg/kg/24 hr ÷ Q6–8 hr
  Adult: 25–100 mg/dose Q4–6 hr PRN
IM:
  Children: 0.5–1 mg/kg/dose Q4–6 hr PRN
  Adult: 25–100 mg/dose Q4–6 hr PRN; **max dose:** 600 mg/24 hr

May potentiate barbiturates, meperidine, and other depressants. May cause dry mouth, drowsiness, tremor, convulsions, blurred vision, hypotension. May cause pain at injection site. IV administration is **not** recommended.

IBUPROFEN
Motrin, Advil, Nuprin, Medipren, Children's Advil, Children's Motrin, and others

Yes 1 B/D
Nonsteroidal anti-inflammatory agent
Suspension: 100 mg/5 ml (120, 480 ml)
Suspension: 100 mg/5 ml (60, 120 ml)
Oral Drops: 40 mg/ml (15 ml)
Chew Tabs: 50, 100 mg
Caplets: 100 mg
Tabs: 100, 200, 300, 400, 600, 800 mg

Children:
Analgesic/Antipyretic: 5–10 mg/kg/dose Q6–8 hr PO; **max dose:** 40 mg/kg/24 hr PO
JRA: 30–50 mg/kg/24 hr ÷ Q6 hr PO; **max dose:** 2400 mg/24 hr
Adults:
Inflammatory disease: 400–800 mg/dose Q6–8 hr PO
Pain/fever/dysmenorrhea: 200–400 mg/dose Q4–6 hr PO
Max dose: 3.2 g/24 hr

Contraindicated with active GI bleeding and ulcer disease. GI distress (lessened with milk), rashes, ocular problems, granulocytopenia, anemia may occur. Inhibits platelet aggregation. Use **caution** with aspirin hypersensitivity, or hepatic/renal insufficiency, dehydration, and patients receiving anticoagulants. May increase serum levels and effects of digoxin, methotrexate and lithium. May decrease the effects of antihypertensives, furosemide, and thiazide diuretics. Pregnancy category changes to "D" if used in 3rd trimester or near delivery.

IMIPENEM-CILASTATIN
Primaxin
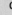
Yes ? C
Antibiotic
Injection: 250, 500, 750 mg. Each gram contains 3.2 mEq Na.

Neonates:
<1 wk: 40–50 mg/kg/24 hr ÷ Q12 hr IV
1–4 wks: 60–75 mg/kg/24 hr ÷ Q8 hr IV
Children (4 wks–3 months): 100 mg/kg/24hr ÷ Q6 hr IV
Children (>3 months): 60–100 mg/kg/24 hr ÷ Q6 hr IV; **max dose:** 4 g/24 hr
Adults: 250–1000 mg/dose Q6–8 hr IV; **max dose:** 4 g/24 hr or 50 mg/kg/24 hr, whichever is less

For IV use, give slowly over 30–60 minutes. Adverse effects: pruritus, urticaria, GI symptoms, seizures, dizziness, hypotension, elevated LFTs, blood dyscrasias, and penicillin allergy. CSF penetration is variable but best with inflamed meninges. Higher doses of 90 mg/kg/24 hr have been used in older children with cystic fibrosis. **Adjust dose in renal insufficiency (see p. 933).**

IMIPRAMINE

Tofranil, Janimine
Antidepressant, tricyclic
Tabs: 10, 25, 50 mg
Caps: 75, 100, 125, 150 mg
Injection: 12.5 mg/ml

No   3   D

Antidepressant:
Children:
   Initial: 1.5 mg/kg/24 hr ÷ TID PO;
Increase 1–1.5 mg/kg/24 hr Q3–
4 days to **max** of 5 mg/kg/24 hr
Adolescent:
   Initial: 25–50 mg/24 hr ÷ QD-TID
PO; dosages exceeding 100 mg/24 hr
are generally not necessary
Adult:
   Initial: 75–100 mg/24 hr ÷ TID
PO/IM; **max** initial IM dose: 100
mg/24 hr
   Maintenance: 50–300 mg/24 hr QHS
PO; **max** PO dose: 300 mg/24 hr
Enuresis (≥6 yrs):
   Initial: 10–25 mg QHS PO
   Increment: 10–25 mg/dose at 1–2 wk
intervals until **max dose** for age or
desired effect achieved. Continue for
2–3 mo, then taper slowly
   Max dose:
   6–12 yr: 50 mg/24 hr
   12–14 yr: 75 mg/24 hr
Augment analgesia for chronic pain:
   Initial: 0.2–0.4 mg/kg/dose QHS PO;
increase 50% every 2–3 days to **max** of
1–3 mg/kg/dose QHS PO

Contraindicated in narrow-angle
glaucoma and patients who used
MAO inhibitors within 14 days. See
p. 39 for management of toxic ingestion.
Side effects include sedation, urinary
retention, constipation, dry mouth,
dizziness, drowsiness, and arrhythmia.
QHS dosing during first weeks of therapy
will reduce sedation. Monitor ECG, BP,
CBC at start of therapy and with dose
changes. Tricyclics may cause mania.

   Therapeutic reference range (sum of
imipramine and desipramine) =
150–250 ng/ml. Levels >1000 ng/ml are
toxic; however, toxicity may occur at
>300 ng/ml.

   Recommended serum sampling times at
steady-state: obtain trough level within
30 minutes prior to the next scheduled
dose after 5–7 days of continuous
therapy. Carbamazepine may reduce
imipramine levels. Cimetidine, fluoxetine,
fluvoxamine, labetolol, quinidine may
increase imipramine levels.

   PO route preferred. May be given IM.
Do not discontinue abruptly in patients
receiving long-term high dose therapy.

For explanation of icons, see p. 600.

IMMUNE GLOBULIN
IM: Gammar-IM, Gamastan
IV: Sandoglobulin, Gammagard. Gamimune-N, Gammar-IV,
Iveegam, Polygam, Venoglobulin

 No ? C

IM preparations
Gammar-IM: 165 ± 15 mg/ml
Gamastan: 165 ± 5 mg/ml
IV preparations
Gamimune-N: 5%, 10%
Polygam S/D: 5%, 10%

Gammar-IV: 5%
Sandoglobulin: 6%, 12%
Venoglobulin I: 5%
Venoglobulin S: 5%
Gammagard S/D: 5%, 10%

See indications and doses on p. 333.

General Guidelines for administration (see package insert of specific products): Begin infusion at 0.01 ml/kg/min, double rate every 15–30 min, up to max of 0.08 ml/kg/min. If adverse reactions occur, stop infusion until side effects subside and may restart at rate that was previously tolerated.

May cause flushing, chills, fever, headache, hypotension.

Hypersensitivity reaction may occur when IV form is administered rapidly. Gamimune-N contains maltose and may cause an osmotic diuresis. May cause **anaphylaxis** in IgA-deficient patients due to varied amounts of IgA. Some products are IgA depleted. Consult a pharmacist.

Delay immunizations after IVIG administration (see p. 351).

INDINAVIR
Crixivan, IDV
Anti-viral agent, protease inhibitor
Caps: 200, 400 mg

 No 3 C

Children: 500 mg/m²/dose PO Q8 hr; **max dose:** 800 mg/dose *Adolescents and Adults:* 800 mg PO Q8 hr

Reduce dose in mild-moderate hepatic impairment. May cause GI discomfort, headache, metallic taste, hyperbilirubinemia, dizziness, nephrolithiasis, hyperglycemia, and body fat redistribution.

Like other protease inhibitors, indinavir inhibits the CYP-450-3A4 isoenzyme to increase the effects or toxicities of many drugs. Concomitant use with astemizole, terfenadine, cisapride, ergot alkaloid derivatives, triazolam, and/or midazolam is **contraindicated.** Rifampin and nevirapine can decrease indinavir levels; whereas ketoconazole and itraconazole can increase levels. **Carefully review the patients' medication profile for potential interactions!**

Administer doses on an empty stomach (1 hr before or 2 hrs after a meal) with adequate hydration (48 ounces/24 hr in adults). If didanosine is included in the regimen, space 1 hour apart on an empty stomach. Capsules are sensitive to moisture and should be stored with a desiccant. **Non-compliance can quickly promote resistant HIV strains.**

INDOMETHACIN
Indocin
Nonsteroidal antiinflammatory agent
Caps: 25, 50 mg
Sustained-release caps: 75 mg
Injection: 1 mg
Suppositories: 50 mg
Suspension: 25 mg/5 ml

Yes 1 B/D

Anti-inflammatory:
>14 yr old: 1–3 mg/kg/24 hr ÷ TID-QID PO; **max dose: 200 mg/24 hr**
Adults: 50–150 mg/24 hr ÷ BID-QID PO; **max dose: 200 mg/24 hr**
Closure of ductus arteriosus:
Infuse intravenously over 20–30 minutes:

Age	Dose (mg/kg/dose (Q12–24hr))		
	#1	#2	#3
<48hr	0.2	0.1	0.1
2–7 days	0.2	0.2	0.2
>7 days	0.2	0.25	0.25

In <1500 g infants, 0.1–0.2 mg/kg/dose IV Q24 hr may be given for an additional 3–5 days

Contraindicated in active bleeding, coagulation defects, necrotizing enterocolitis, and renal insufficiency. May cause (especially in neonates) decreased urine output, platelet dysfunction, decreased GI blood flow. Monitor renal and hepatic function before and during use. **Reduction in cerebral flow associated with rapid IV infusion.** Fatal hepatitis reported in treatment of JRA.

Pregnancy category changes to "D" if used for greater than 48 hours or after 34 weeks gestation or close to delivery.

INSULIN

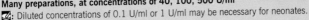

Pancreatic hormone   **Yes   1   B**
Many preparations, at concentrations of 40, 100, 500 U/ml
📋: Diluted concentrations of 0.1 U/ml or 1 U/ml may be necessary for neonates.

Insulin preparations: See pp. 914–915
Hyperkalemia: See p. 241
DKA: See p. 207

When using insulin drip with new IV tubing, fill the tubing with the insulin infusion solution and wait for 30 minutes (prior to connecting tubing to the patient). Then flush the line and connect the IV line to the patient to start the infusion. This will ensure proper drug delivery. **Adjust dose in renal failure (see p. 939).**

IPECAC

Emetic agent   **No   ?   C**
Syrup: 70 mg/ml (15, 30, 473, 4000 ml); contains 1.5–2% alcohol

See p. 20 for indications.
6–12 mos: 10 ml ipecac followed by 10–20 ml/kg water
1–5 yr: 15 ml ipecac followed by 120 ml water
≥5 yr and Adults: 30 ml followed by 200–300 ml of water

Do not administer if patient is unconscious, lacks a gag reflex, has seizures, or had ingested corrosives, strong acids or bases, volatile oils. May cause GI irritation, cardiotoxicity, myopathy. **Do not** use ipecac fluid extract as it is 14 times more potent. May repeat dose once if emesis does not occur within 20–30 minutes. Follow dose administration with water; **do not** adminster with milk or carbonated beverages.

IPRATROPIUM BROMIDE
Atrovent

Anticholinergic agent   **No   1   B**
Aerosol: 18 mcg/dose (200 actuations per canister)
Nebulized Solution: 500 mcg/2.5 ml
Nasal Spray: 0.03% (21 mcg per actuation, 30 ml); 0.06% (42 mcg per actuation, 15 ml)

Inhaler:
  <12 yr: 1–2 puffs TID-QID
  ≥12 yr: 2–3 puffs QID up to 12 puffs/24 hr
Nebulized treatments:
  Infants and Children: 250 mcg/dose TID-QID
  >12 yr and Adults: 250–500 mcg/dose TID-QID
Nasal Spray:
  >12 yr and Adults: 2 sprays per nostril BID-TID

Use with **caution** in narrow-angle glaucoma or bladder neck obstruction, though ipratropium has fewer anticholinergic systemic effects than atropine. May cause anxiety, dizziness, headache, GI discomfort, and cough with inhaler or nebulized use. Epistaxis, nasal congestion, and dry mouth/throat have been reported with the nasal spray.

Shake inhaler well prior to use. Nebulized solution may be mixed of albuterol. Safety and efficacy of use with the nasal spray beyond 4 days on patients with the common cold have not been established.

Breastfeeding safety **extrapolated** from safety of atropine.

For explanation of icons, see p. 600.

I

FORMULARY

IRON DEXTRAN

InfeD

Parenteral iron

No ? C

Injection: 50 mg/ml (50 mg elemental Fe/ml)

Products containing phenol 0.5% are only for IM administration; products containing sodium chloride 0.9% can be administered via the IM or IV route.

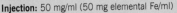

Inject test dose (see comments)
Iron deficiency anemia: Total replacement dose of iron dextran (ml) = $0.0476 \times$ wt(kg) $\times$ (desired Hgb [g/dl] – measured Hgb [g/dl]) + 1 ml/5 kg body weight (up to max of 14 ml).

Acute blood loss: Total replacement dose of iron dextran (ml) = $0.02 \times$ blood loss (ml) $\times$ hematocrit expressed as fraction. Assumes 1 ml of RBC = 1 mg elemental iron.

If no reaction to test dose, give remainder of replacement dose ÷ over 2–3 daily doses.

Max *daily (IM) dose:*
  <5 kg: 0.5 ml (25 mg)
  5–10 kg: 1 ml (50 mg)
  >10 kg: 2 ml (100 mg)

Oral therapy with iron salts is preferred. Numerous adverse effects including anaphylaxis, fever, hypotension, rash, myalgias, arthralgias. Use "Z-track" technique for IM administration. **Inject test dose:** 25 mg IM/IV (12.5 mg for infants).

May begin treatment dose after 1 hour. **Maximum** rate of IV infusion: 50 mg/min. For IV infusion, diluting in NS may lower the incidence of phlebitis. Direct IV push administration is **NOT** recommended. Not recommended in infants <4 months of age. Compatible with parenteral nutrition solutions.

IRON PREPARATIONS
Fergon, Fer-In-Sol, Ferralet, Feosol, Niferex, and others

Oral iron supplements

No   ?   A

Ferrous sulfate (20% elemental Fe):
Drops (Fer-In-Sol): 75 mg (15 mg Fe)/0.6 ml (50 ml); 125 mg (25 mg Fe)/1 ml (50 ml)
Syrup (Fer-In-Sol): 90 mg (18 mg Fe)/5 ml (5% alcohol)
Elixir (Feosol): 220 mg (44 mg Fe)/5 ml (5% alcohol)
Capsules: 250 mg (50 mg Fe)
Tabs: 195 mg (39 mg Fe), 300 mg (60 mg Fe), 324 mg (65 mg Fe)

Ferrous gluconate (12% elemental Fe):
Elixir: 300 mg (34 mg Fe)/5 ml (7% alcohol)
Tabs: 240 mg (27 mg Fe, as Fergon), 300 mg (34 mg Fe), 320 mg (37 mg Fe), 325 mg (38 mg Fe)

Sustained-release caps: 320 mg (37 mg Fe), 435 mg (50 mg Fe)
Caps: 86 mg (10 mg Fe), 325 mg (38 mg Fe), 435 mg (50 mg Fe)
Ferrous sulfate, exsiccated/dried (30% elemental Fe):
Tabs: 200 mg (65 mg Fe)
Extended release tabs: 160 mg (50 mg Fe)
Caps: 190 mg (60 mg Fe)
Extended release caps: 159 mg (50 mg Fe)

Polysaccharide-Iron Complex (Niferex) (expressed in mg elemental Fe):
Tabs: 50 mg
Caps: 150 mg
Elixir: 100 mg/5 ml (10% alcohol)

Iron deficiency anemia:
Premature Infants: 2–4 mg elemental Fe/kg/24 hr ÷ QD-BID PO; **max dose:** 15 mg elemental Fe/24 hr
Children: 3–6 mg elemental Fe/kg/24 hr ÷ QD-TID PO
Adults: 60 mg elemental Fe BID-QID
Prophylaxis:
Children: Give dose below PO ÷ QD-TID
    Premature: 2 mg elemental Fe/kg/24 hr
    Full-term: 1–2 mg elemental Fe/kg/24 hr
    Max dose: 15 mg elemental Fe/24 hr
Adults: 60 mg elemental Fe/24 hr PO ÷ QD-BID

Iron preparations are variably absorbed. Less GI irritation when given with or after meals. Vitamin C, 200 mg per 30 mg iron, may enhance absorption. Liquid iron preparations may stain teeth. Give with dropper or drink through straw. May produce constipation, dark stools (false positive guaiac is controversial), nausea, and epigastric pain. Iron and tetracycline inhibit each other's absorption. Antacids may decrease iron absorption.

For explanation of icons, see p. 600.

ISONIAZID

Yes   1   C

INH, Nydrazid, Laniazid
Antituberculous agent
Tabs: 50, 100, 300 mg
Syrup: 50 mg/5 ml (473 ml)
Injection: 100 mg/ml

See pp. 402–403 for details and
length of therapy.
Prophylaxis:
Infants and Children: 10–15 mg/kg (up
to 300 mg) PO QD. After 1 month of
daily therapy and in cases where daily
compliance cannot be ensured, may
change to 20–40 mg/kg (up to 900 mg)
per dose PO, given twice weekly.
Adults: 300 mg PO QD
Treatment:
Infants and Children:
10–15 mg/kg (up to 300 mg) PO QD or
20–30 mg/kg (up to 900 mg) per dose
twice weekly with rifampin for
uncomplicated pulmonary tuberculosis
in compliant patients
Adults:
5–10 mg/kg (up to 300 mg) PO QD or
15 mg/kg (up to 900 mg) per dose
twice weekly with rifampin
For INH-resistant TB: Discuss with Health
Dept., or consult ID specialist.

Should **not** be used alone for
treatment. Peripheral neuropathy,
optic neuritis, seizures,
encephalopathy, psychosis, hepatic side
effects may occur with higher doses,
especially in combination with rifampin.
Follow LFTs monthly. Supplemental
pyridoxine (1–2 mg/kg/24 hr) is
recommended. May cause false positive
urine glucose test. Inhibits hepatic
microsomal enzymes; decrease dose of
carbamazepine, diazepam, phenytoin,
and prednisone. May be given IM (same
as oral doses) when oral therapy is not
possible. **Adjust dose in renal failure (see
p. 933).**

ISOPROTERENOL

No   ?   C

Isuprel and others
Adrenergic agonist
Isoproterenol HCl:
  Tabs: 10, 15 mg (sublingual)
  Solutions for nebulization:
    0.25% (2.5 mg/ml) (0.5 ml, 15 ml)
    0.5% (5 mg/ml) (0.5, 10, 60 ml)
    1% (10 mg/ml) (10 ml)
  Aerosol: 131 mcg/dose (300 metered doses per 15 ml; 10, 15 ml)
  Injection: 0.2 mg/ml (1, 5 ml ampules)
Isoproterenol Sulfate:
  Aerosol 80 mcg/dose (300 metered doses per 15 ml; 15, 22.5 ml)

Aerosol: 1–2 puffs up to 6x/24 hr
Nebulized solution:
Children: 0.05 mg/kg/dose =
0.01 ml/kg/dose of 0.5% Sol (min dose: 0.5 mg; max dose: 1.25 mg) diluted with NS to 2 ml Q4 hr PRN
Adults: 2.5–5 mg/dose = 0.25–0.5 ml of 1% solution diluted with NS to 2 ml Q4 hr PRN
IV Infusion:
Children: 0.05–2 mcg/kg/min; start at minimum dose and increase every 5–10 min by 0.1 mcg/kg/min until desired effect or onset of toxicity; max dose: 2 mcg/kg/min
Adults: 2–20 mcg/kg/min
See inside front cover for preparation of infusion
Sublingual:
Children: 5–10 mg/dose Q3-4 hr; max dose: 30 mg/24 hr
Adults: 10–20 mg/dose Q3-4 hr; max dose: 60 mg/24 hr

Use with care in CHF, ischemia, or aortic stenosis. May cause flushing, ventricular arrhythmias, profound hypotension, anxiety, and myocardial ischemia. Patients with continuous IV infusion should have heart rate, respiratory rate, and blood pressure monitored. Not for treatment of asystole or for use in cardiac arrests, unless bradycardia is due to heartblock. Continuous infusion use for bronchodilatation must be gradually tapered over a 24–48 hr period to prevent rebound bronchospasm. Tolerance may occur with prolonged use.

ISOTRETINOIN
Accutane
Retinoic acid, vitamin A derivative
Caps: 10, 20, 40 mg

No   3   X

Cystic acne: 0.5–2 mg/kg/24 hr ÷ BID PO × 15–20 wk
Dosages as low as 0.05 mg/kg/24 hr have been reported to be beneficial.

Caution in females during childbearing years. **Contraindicated** during pregnancy; known teratogen. May cause conjunctivitis, xerosis, pruritus, epistaxis, anemia, hyperlipidemia, pseudotumor cerebri, cheilitis, bone pain, muscle aches, skeletal changes, lethargy, nausea, vomiting, elevated ESR. To avoid additive toxic effects, **do not** take vitamin A concomitantly. Monitor CBC, ESR, triglycerides, and LFTs.

ITRACONAZOLE

Sporanox
Antifungal Agent
Caps: 100 mg
Oral solution: 10 mg/ml (150 ml)

No   3   C

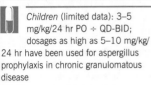

Children (limited data): 3–5 mg/kg/24 hr PO ÷ QD-BID; dosages as high as 5–10 mg/kg/24 hr have been used for aspergillus prophylaxis in chronic granulomatous disease

Adults:

Blastomycosis and nonmeningeal histoplasmosis: 200 mg PO QD up to a **maximum** of 400 mg/24 hr PO ÷ BID (**max dose:** 200 mg/dose)

Aspergillosis and severe infections: 600 mg/24 hr PO ÷ TID × 3–4 days, followed by 200–400 mg/24 hr PO ÷ BID; **max dose:** 600 mg/24 hr ÷ TID

Oral solution and capsule dosage form should **NOT** be used interchangeably. Only the oral solution has been demonstrated effective for oral and/or esophageal candidasis. Use with **caution** in hepatic impairment. May cause GI symptoms, headaches, rash, liver enzyme elevation, hepatitis, and hypokalemia.

Like ketoconazole, it inhibits the activity of the CYP-450 3A4 drug metabolizing isoenzyme (see p. 924). Thus the coadministration of terfenadine, astemizole, and cisapride is **contraindicated.** See remarks in ketoconazole for additional drug interaction information.

Administer oral solution on an empty stomach, but administer capsules with food. Achlorhydria reduces absorption of the drug.

IVERMECTIN
Stromectol
Anthelmintic
Tabs: 6 mg

No ? C

 Cutaneous larva migrans, scabies, or strongyloidiasis: 0.2 mg/kg PO × 1; dosing by body weight (see table)

CUTANEOUS LARVA MIGRANS, SCABIES, STRONGYLOIDIASIS

Weight (kg)	Single oral dose
15–24	3mg (½tablet)
25–35	6mg (1tablet)
36–50	9mg (1½tablets)
51–65	12mg (2tablets)
66–79	15mg (2½tablets)
≥80	0.2mg/kg

200 mcg/kg/dose QD PO × 2 days can also be used for strongyloidiasis.
Onchocerciasis: 0.15 mg/kg PO × 1; dosing by body weight (see table):

ONCHOCERCIASIS

Weight (kg)	Single oral dose
15–25	3mg (½tablet)
26–44	6mg (1tablet)
45–64	9mg (1½tablets)
65–84	12mg (2tablets)
≥85	0.15mg/kg

Dose may be repeated every 3–12 months.

Adverse reactions experienced in strongyloidiasis include: diarrhea, nausea, vomiting, pruritus, rash, dizziness, and drowsiness.

Adverse reactions experienced in onchocerciasis include cutaneous or systemic allergic/ inflammatory reactions of varying severity (Mazzotti reaction) and ophthalmological reactions. Specific reactions may include arthralgia/synovitis, lymph node enlargement and tenderness, pruritus, edema, fever, orthostatic hypotension, and tachycardia. Antihistamines and/or aspirin have been used for most mild to moderate cases. Therapy for postural hypotension may include oral hydration, recumbency, IV normal saline, and/or IV steroids.

For explanation of icons, see p. 600.

KANAMYCIN

Kantrex
Antibiotic, aminoglycoside
Caps: 500 mg
Injection: 37.5, 250, 333, 500 mg/ml

Yes   1   D

 Neonatal IV/IM administration: (see table)
Infants and Children: IM/IV: 15–30 mg/kg/24 hr ÷ Q8–12 hr
Adults: IV/IM: 15 mg/kg/24 hr ÷ Q8–12 hr
PO administration for GI bacterial overgrowth: 150–250 mg/kg/24 hr ÷ Q6 hr; **max dose:** 4 g/24 hr

Renal toxicity and ototoxicity may occur. Give over 30 min if IV.
Poorly absorbed orally, PO used to treat GI bacterial overgrowth.

Therapeutic levels: peak: 15–30 mg/L; trough: <5–10 mg/L. Recommended serum sampling time at steady-state: trough within 30 minutes prior to the 3rd consecutive dose and peak 30–60 minutes after the administration of the 3rd consecutive dose. **Adjust dose in renal failure (see p. 933).**

NEONATAL DOSING		
	<7days	≥7days
BW<2kg	15mg/kg/24hr ÷ Q12hr	22.5mg/kg/24hr ÷ Q8
BW≥2kg	20mg/kg/24hr ÷ Q12hr	30mg/kg/24hr ÷ Q8

KETAMINE

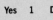

Ketalar
General anesthetic
Injection: 10, 50, 100 mg/ml

No   3   B

Children:
Sedation:
PO/PR: 4–6 mg/kg × 1
IM: 2–3 mg/kg × 1
Induction of General Anesthesia:
IV: 0.5–3 mg/kg
Adults:
IV: 1–4.5 mg/kg
IM: 3–8 mg/kg

Contraindicated in elevated ICP, hypertension, aneurysms, thyrotoxicosis, CHF, angina, and psychotic disorders. May cause hypertension, hypotension, emergence reactions, tachycardia, laryngospasm, respiratory depression, and stimulation of salivary secretions. Benzodiazepine may be added to prevent emergence phenomenon. Anticholinergic agent may be added to decrease hypersalivation. Rate of IV infusion should **not** exceed 0.5 mg/kg/min or be administered in less than 60 seconds. For additional information including onset and duration of action, see p. 905.

KETOCONAZOLE
Nizoral
Antifungal agent
Tabs: 200 mg
Suspension: 100 mg/5 ml
Cream: 2% (15, 30, 60 g)
Shampoo: 2%

No ? C

Oral:
Children ≥2 yr: 3.3–6.6 mg/kg/24 hr QD
Adult: 200–400 mg/24 hr QD
Max dose: 800 mg/24 hr ÷ BID
Topical: 1–2 applications/24 hr
Shampoo: Twice weekly for 4 weeks with at least 3 days between applications; intermittently as needed to maintain control
Suppressive therapy against mucocutaneous candidiasis in HIV:
Children: 5–10 mg/kg/24 hr ÷ QD-BID PO
Adolescents and Adults: 200 mg/dose QD PO

Monitor liver function tests in long-term use. Drugs that decrease gastric acidity will decrease absorption. May cause nausea, vomiting, rash, headache, pruritus, and fever. Inhibits CYP 450 3A4. Cardiac arrhythmias may occur when used with cisapride, terfenadine, astemizole. Concomitant administration of ketoconazole with any of these drugs is **contraindicated.** May increase levels/effects of phenytoin, digoxin, cyclosporin, corticosteroids, protease inhibitors, and warfarin. Phenobarbital, rifampin, isoniazide, H₂ blockers, antacids, and omeprazole can decrease levels of ketoconazole.

KETOROLAC

Toradol, Accular (ophth)
Nonsteroidal anti-inflammatory agent
Injection: 15, 30 mg/ml
Tab: 10 mg
Ophthalmic: 0.5% (5 ml)

Yes   **1**   **C**

IM/IV:
  Children: 0.5 mg/kg/dose IM/IV Q6 hr. **Max dose:** 30 mg Q6 hr or 120 mg/24 hr
  Adults: 30 mg IM/IV Q6 hr. **Max dose:** 120 mg/24 hr
PO:
  Children >50 kg and adults: 10 mg PRN Q6 hr; **max dose:** 40 mg/24 hr
Ophthalmic:
  Adults: Instill 1 drop in each affected eye QID for up to 7 days

Ketorolac therapy is **not** to exceed 5 days (IM, IV, PO). May cause GI bleeding, nausea, dyspepsia, drowsiness, decreased platelet function, and interstitial nephritis. **Not** recommended in patients at increased risk of bleeding. Do **not** use in hepatic or renal failure. The **IV** route of administration in children is **not** yet recommended by the manufacturer, although it is well supported in the literature and in practice.

LABETALOL

Normodyne, Trandate
Adrenergic antagonist (alpha and beta), antihypertensive
Tabs: 100, 200, 300 mg
Injection: 5 mg/ml
Suspension: 10 mg/ml

No   **1**   **C/D**

Children:
PO: Initial: 4 mg/kg/24 hr ÷ BID.
May increase up to 40 mg/kg/24 hr
IV: Hypertensive emergency:
Intermittent dose: 0.2–1 mg/kg/dose
Q10 min PRN; **max:** 20 mg/dose
Infusion: 0.4–1 mg/kg/hr, to **max** of 3
mg/kg/hr; may initiate with a 0.2–1
mg/kg bolus; **max bolus:** 20 mg
Adults:
PO: 100 mg BID, increase by 100
mg/dose Q2–3 days PRN to **max** of 2.4
g/24 hr
IV: Hypertensive emergency:
Intermittent dose: 20–80 mg/dose
(begin with 20 mg) Q10 min PRN;
max: 300 mg total dose
Infusion: 2 mg/min, increase to titrate
to response

Contraindicated in asthma,
pulmonary edema, cardiogenic
shock, and heart block. May cause
orthostatic hypotension, edema, CHF,
bradycardia, AV conduction disturbances,
bronchospasm, urinary retention, and skin
tingling. Patient should remain supine for
up to 3 hours after IV administration.
Pregnancy category changes to "D" if used
in 2nd or 3rd trimesters.
Onset of action: PO: 1–4 hours; IV:
5–15 minutes.

LACTULOSE
Cephulac, and others
Ammonium detoxicant, laxative
Syrup: 10 g/15 ml

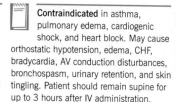

No   ?   B

Chronic constipation:
Children: 7.5 ml/24 hr PO after
breakfast
Adults: 15–30 ml/24 hr PO to max of
60 ml/24 hr
Portal systemic encephalopathy (adjust
dose to produce 2–3 soft stools/day):
Infants: 2.5–10 ml/24 hr PO ÷ TID-QID
Children: 40–90 ml/24 hr PO ÷ TID-QID
Adults: 30–45 ml/dose PO TID-QID;
acute episodes 30–45 ml Q1–2 hr until
2–3 soft stools/day
Rectal (adults): 300 ml diluted in 700
ml water or NS in 30–60 min retention
enema; may give Q4–6 hr

Contraindicated in galactosemia.
Use with **caution** in diabetes
mellitus. GI discomfort and
diarrhea may occur. For portal systemic
encephalopathy, monitor serum ammonia,
serum potassium, and fluid status.
Adjust dose to achieve 2–3 soft stools
per day. Do **not** use with antacids.

For explanation of icons, see p. 600.

LAMIVUDINE
Epivir, Epivir-HBV, 3TC
Antiviral agent, nucleoside analogue reverse transcriptase inhibitor
Tabs: 100 mg (Epivir-HBV), 150 mg
Oral solution: 5 mg/ml (Epivir-HBV), 10 mg/ml
In combination with Zidovudine (AZT) as Combivir: #Tabs: 150 mg lamivudine + 300 mg zidovudine

 Yes   3   C

 Neonate (<30 days): 2 mg/kg/dose PO BID
Children (3 mon-12 yrs): 4 mg/kg/dose PO BID; **max dose:** 150 mg/dose
Adolescents and Adults:
    <50 kg: 2 mg/kg/dose PO BID
    ≥50 kg: 150 mg/dose PO BID
Needle stick prophylaxis: 150 mg/dose PO BID × 28 days. Use in combination with zidovudine (AZT) 200 mg/dose PO TID or 300 mg/dose PO BID, and indinavir 800 mg/dose PO TID × 28 days.
Chronic Hepatitis B (see remarks):
    Children (dosage based on pharmacokinetics): 3 mg/kg/dose PO QD
    ≥13 yrs and Adults: 100 mg/dose PO QD

May cause headache, fatigue, nausea, diarrhea, skin rash, pancreatitis and abdominal pain. Peripheral neuropathy, decreased neutrophil count, and increased liver enzymes may occur in advanced disease with combination therapy. Concomitant use with co-trimoxazole (TMP/SMX) may result in increase lamivudine levels.

CHRONIC HEPATITIS B: Use Epivir-HBV product for this indication. Safety and effectiveness in children and in adults treated beyond 1 year have **not** been studied. Patients with both HIV and hepatitis B should use the higher HIV doses along with an appropriate combination regimen.

May be administered with food. **Adjust dose in renal impairment (see p. 933).**

LAMOTRIGINE
Lamictal
Anticonvulsant
Tabs: 25, 100, 150, 200 mg

 Yes   ?   C

Children (2–16 yr):

WITH enzyme inducing anti-epileptic drugs (AEDs) WITHOUT valproic acid: Start with 2 mg/kg/24 hr PO ÷ BID × 2 weeks, then 5 mg/24 hr PO ÷ BID × 2 weeks, followed by 10 mg/kg/24 hr PO ÷ BID. Usual dosage range: 5–15 mg/kg/24 hr

Max dose: 15 mg/kg/24 hr or 400 mg/24 hr

WITH enzyme inducing AEDs WITH valproic acid: Start with 0.2 mg/kg/24 hr PO QD × 2 weeks, then 0.5 mg/kg/24 hr PO QD × 2 weeks, followed by 1 mg/kg/24 hr PO QD

Max dose: 5 mg/kg/24 hr ÷ QD-BID or 250 mg/24 hr

WITHOUT enzyme inducing AEDs WITH valproic acid: Start with 0.1–0.2 mg/kg/24 hr PO QD × 2 weeks, then 0.2–0.5 mg/kg/24 hr PO QD × 2 weeks, followed by 0.5–1 mg/kg/24 hr PO QD

Max dose: 2 mg/kg/24 hr or 150 mg/24 hr

≥16 yr and Adults:

WITHOUT valproic acid: 50 mg QD PO × 2 weeks, then increase to 50 mg BID × 2 weeks; may increase to 300–500 mg/24 hr ÷ BID

WITH valproic acid: 25 mg QOD PO × 2 weeks, then increase to 25 mg QD × 2 weeks; may increase to 100–150 mg/24 hr ÷ BID

Enzyme inducing anti-epileptic drugs (AEDs) include carbamazepine, phenytoin, and phenobarbital. Stevens-Johnson syndrome, toxic epidermal necrolysis, and other potentially life-threatening rashes have been reported in children and adults (incidence higher in children). May cause fatigue, drowsiness, ataxia, rash (especially with valproic acid), headache, nausea, vomiting, and abdominal pain. Diplopia, nystagmus, alopecia have also been reported. Reduce dose in renal failure. Withdrawal symptoms may occur if discontinued suddenly.

Acetaminophen, carbamazepine and phenytoin may decrease levels of lamotrigine. Valproic acid may increase levels.

LEVOTHYROXINE (T$_4$)

Synthroid, Levothroid
Thyroid product

No   1   A

Tabs: 25, 50, 75, 88, 100, 112, 125, 137, 150, 175, 200, 300 mcg
Injection: 200, 500 mcg
Suspension: 25 mcg/ml

For explanation of icons, see p. 600.

Children PO dosing:
0–6 mo: 8–10 mcg/kg/dose QD
6–12 mo: 6–8 mcg/kg/dose QD
1–5 yr: 5–6 mcg/kg/dose QD
6–12 yr: 4–5 mcg/kg/dose QD
>12 yr: 2–3 mcg/kg/dose QD
IM/IV dose: 50%–75% of oral dose QD
Adults:
  PO:
  Initial: 12.5–50 mcg/dose QD
  Increment: Increase by 25–50 mcg/24 hr at intervals of Q2–4 wk
  Average adult dose: 100–200 mcg/24 hr
IM/IV dose: 50% of oral dose QD
Myxedema coma or stupor: 200–500 mcg × 1, then 100–300 mcg the next day if needed IV

Contraindications include acute MI, thyrotoxicosis uncomplicated by hypothyroidism, and uncorrected adrenal insufficiency. May cause hyperthyroidism, rash, growth disturbances, hypertension, arrythmias, diarrhea, and weight loss.

Total replacement dose may be used in children unless there is evidence of cardiac disease; in that case, begin with ¼ of maintenance and increase weekly. Titrate dosage with clinical status and serum T_4 and TSH. Increases the effects of warfarin. Phenytoin, carbamazepine may decrease levothyroxine levels.

100 mcg levothyroxine = 65 mg thyroid USP. Administer oral doses on an empty stomach. Excreted in low levels in breast milk; preponderance of evidence suggest no clinically significant effect in infants.

LIDOCAINE

Xylocaine and others
Antiarrhythmic class Ib, local anesthetic

No 1 C

Injection: 0.5%, 1%, 1.5%, 2%, 4%, 10%, 20% (1% sol = 10 mg/ml)
Injection with 1:50,000 epi: 2%
Injection with 1:100,000 epi: 1%, 2%
Injection with 1:200,000 epi: 0.5%, 1%, 1.5%, 2%
Ointment: 2.5% (37.5 g), 5% (50 g)
Cream: 0.5% (120 g)

Jelly: 2% (30 ml)
Liquid (viscous): 2% (20, 100 ml)
Solution (topical): 2% (15, 240 ml), 4% (50 ml)
Oral Spray: 10% (26.8 ml aerosol)
Topical 2.5% (with 2.5% prilocaine): See EMLA and p. 899.

Anesthetic:
Injection:
   Without epi: **max dose** of 4.5 mg/kg/dose (up to 300 mg)
   With epi: **max dose** of 7 mg/kg/dose (up to 500 mg); do **not** repeat within 2 hours
Topical: 3 mg/kg/dose no more frequently than Q2 hr
Antiarrhythmic: Bolus with 1 mg/kg/dose slowly IO, IV; may repeat in 10–15 minutes × 2; **max total dose** 3–5 mg/kg within the first hour
ETT dose = 2–2.5 × IV dose
Continuous Infusion: 20–50 mcg/kg/min IV; see inside cover for infusion preparation

Contraindicated in Stokes-Adams attacks, SA, AV, or intraventricular heart block without a pacemaker. Side effects include hypotension, asystole, seizures, and respiratory arrest.

Decrease dose in hepatic failure or decreased cardiac output. Do **not** use topically for teething. Prolonged infusion may result in toxic accumulation of lidocaine, especially in infants. Do **not** use epinephrine-containing solutions for treatment of arrhythmias.

Therapeutic levels 1.5–5 mg/L. Toxicity occurs at >7 mg/L. Toxicity in neonates may occur at >5 mg/L. Elimination $T_{1/2}$: premature infant: 3.2 hrs, adult: 1.5–2 hrs.

LINDANE
Kwell, Scabene, G-well, Gamma benzene hexachloride
Scabicidal agent, pediculoside
Shampoo: 1% (30, 60, 473, 3800 ml)
Lotion: 1% (30, 60, 473, 3800 ml)
Cream: 1% (60 g)

No   ?   B

Scabies: Apply thin layer of cream or lotion to skin. Bathe and rinse off medication in adults after 8–12 hr; children 6–8 hr. May repeat × 1 in 7 days PRN.
Pediculosis capitis: Apply 15–30 ml of shampoo, lather for 4–5 minutes, rinse hair and comb with fine comb to remove nits. May repeat × 1 in 7 days PRN.
Pediculosis pubis: May use lotion or shampoo (applied locally) as above.

Avoid contact with face, urethral meatus, damaged skin, or mucous membranes. Systemically absorbed. Risk of toxic effects is greater in young children; use other agents (permethrin) in infants, young children, and during pregnancy. May cause a rash; rarely may cause seizures or aplastic anemia. For scabies, change clothing and bedsheets after starting treatment and treat family members. For pediculosis pubis, treat sexual contacts.

For explanation of icons, see p. 600.

LITHIUM

Eskalith, Lithane, Lithonate, Lithotabs, Lithobid, Cibalith-S
Antimanic agent

Yes   X   D

Carbonate:

300 mg carbonate = 8.12 mEq lithium
Caps: 150, 300, 600 mg
Tabs: 300 mg
Controlled-release tabs: 450 mg
Slow-release tabs: 300 mg

Citrate:

Syrup: 8 mEq/5 ml (10, 480 ml); 5 ml is equivalent to 300 mg Li carbonate
Cibalith-S is citrate; all other brands are carbonate.

Children:
Initial: 15–60 mg/kg/24 hr ÷ TID-QID PO. Adjust as needed (weekly) to achieve therapeutic levels.

Adults:
Initial: 300 mg TID PO. Adjust as needed to achieve therapeutic levels. Usual dose is about 300 mg TID-QID.
Max dose: 2.4 g/24 hr

Contraindicated in severe cardiovascular or renal disease. Increased sodium intake will depress lithium levels. Decreased sodium intake or increased sodium wasting will increase lithium levels. May cause goiter, nephrogenic diabetes insipidus, hypothyroidism, arrhythmias, or sedation at therapeutic doses.

Therapeutic levels: 0.6–1.5 mEq/L. In either acute or chronic toxicity, confusion, and somnolence may be seen at levels of 2–2.5 mEq/L. Seizures or death may occur at levels >2.5 mEq/L. Recommended serum sampling: trough level within 30 minutes prior to the next scheduled dose. Steady-state is achieved within 4–6 days of continuous dosing.

Adjust dose in renal failure (see p. 939).

LOPERAMIDE

Imodium, Imodium AD, and others
Antidiarrheal

No   1   B

Caps: 2 mg
Tabs: 2 mg
Caplets: 2 mg
Liquid: 1 mg/5 ml (60, 90, 120 ml)

Active diarrhea:
Children (Initial doses within the first 24 hrs):
2–6 yr (13–20 kg): 1 mg PO TID
6–8 yr (20–30 kg): 2 mg PO BID
8–12 yr (>30 kg): 2 mg PO TID
Max single dose 2 mg
Follow initial day's dose with 0.1 mg/kg/dose after each loose stool (not to exceed the above initial doses).
Adults: 4 mg/dose × 1, followed by 2 mg/dose after each stool up to **max dose** of 16 mg/24 hr
Chronic diarrhea:
Children: 0.08–0.24 mg/kg/24 hr ÷ BID-TID **Max dose:** 2 mg/dose

May cause nausea, rash, vomiting, constipation, cramps, dry mouth, CNS depression. **Avoid** use in children <2 yr. **Discontinue** use if no clinical improvement is observed within 48 hr. Naloxone may be administered for CNS depression.

LORACARBEF
Lorabid
Antibiotic, carbacephem
Susp: 100 mg/5 ml, 200 mg/5 ml (50, 100 ml)
Caps: 200, 400 mg

Yes   1   B

Infants and Children: (6 mo–12 yr):
Acute Otitis Media: 30 mg/kg/24 hr ÷ Q12 hr PO
Pharyngitis, Skin/soft tissue infection: 15 mg/kg/24 hr ÷ Q12 hr PO
≥13 yr and adults:
Uncomplicated cystitis: 200 mg PO Q24 hr
Sinusitis/uncomplicated pyelonephritis: 400 mg PO Q12 hr
Pharyngitis, Skin/soft tissue infection: 200 mg PO Q12 hr
Lower respiratory infections: 200–400 mg PO Q12 hr

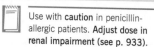

Use with **caution** in penicillin-allergic patients. **Adjust dose in renal impairment (see p. 933).** Use suspension for acute otitis media due to higher peak plasma levels. Adverse effects similar to other orally administered beta-lactam antibiotics. Administer on an empty stomach 1 hour before or 2 hours after meals.

LORATADINE
Claritin, Claritin RediTabs, Claritin-D 12 Hour, Claritin-D 24 Hour
Antihistamine, less sedating

No ? B

Tabs: 10 mg
Disintegrating Tabs (RediTabs): 10 mg
Syrup: 1 mg/ml
Time release tabs in combination with pseudoephedrine (PE):
  Claritin-D 12 Hour: 5 mg loratidine + 120 mg PE
  Claritin-D 24 Hour: 10 mg loratidine + 240 mg PE

Loratadine:
  >3 yr - Adults:
    <30 kg: 5 mg PO QD
    ≥30 kg: 10 mg PO QD
In hepatic failure, prolong dosage
interval of the above dosage to QOD.
*Time release tabs of loratidine and
pseudoephedrine:*
  ≥12 yr and Adults:
    Claritin-D 12 Hour: 1 tablet PO BID
    Claritin-D 24 Hour: 1 tablet PO QD

May cause drowsiness, fatigue, dry
mouth, headache, palpitations,
dermatitis, and dizziness. Has not
been implicated in causing cardiac
arrhythmias when used with other drugs
that are metabolized by hepatic
microsomal enzymes (e.g., ketoconazole,
erythromycin). Administer doses on an
empty stomach.

LORAZEPAM
Ativan
Benzodiazepine anticonvulsant

No 3 D

Tabs: 0.5, 1, 2, mg
Injection: 2, 4 mg/ml (each contains 2% benzyl alcohol)
Oral Sol conc: 2 mg/ml

Status Epilepticus:
Neonates, Infants, Children, and
Adolescents:
0.05–0.1 mg/kg/dose IV over 2–5 min. May repeat 0.05 mg/kg × 1 in 10–15 min.
Max dose: 4 mg/dose.
Adult:
4 mg/dose given slowly over 2–5 minutes. May repeat in 5–15 minutes. Usual **total max dose** in 12 hour period = 8 mg.
Antiemetic adjunct therapy:
Children:
0.04–0.08 mg/kg/dose IV Q6 hr PRN.
Max single dose: 4 mg
Anxiolytic/Sedation:
Children:
0.05 mg/kg/dose Q4–8 hr PO/IV; **max dose:** 2 mg/dose.

May also give IM for preprocedure sedation
Adults:
1–10 mg/24 hr PO ÷ BID-TID

Contraindicated in narrow-angle glaucoma and severe hypotension.
May cause respiratory depression, especially in combination with other sedatives. May also cause sedation, dizziness, mild ataxia, mood changes, rash, and GI symptoms. Injectable product may be given rectally. Benzyl alcohol may be toxic to newborns in high doses.
Onset of action for sedation: PO, 20–30 minutes; IM, 30–60 minutes; IV, 1–5 minutes. Duration of action: 6–8 hrs. **Flumazenil is the antidote.**

LOW MOLECULAR WEIGHT HEPARIN
See Enoxaparin

LYPRESSIN
Diapid, 8-lysine vasopressin
Posterior pituitary hormone
Nasal spray: 185 mcg/ml (8 ml); each spray delivers 7 mcg or 2 posterior pituitary (pressor) units.

No   ?   C

Diabetes insipidus:
1–2 sprays into each nostril QID and HS. If patient requires more than 2–3 sprays per dose, increase frequency of doses rather than amounts/dose.

Titrate dose to thirst, urinary frequency. Coronary vasoconstriction may occur with large doses. May cause nasal congestion, headache, conjunctivitis, and abdominal cramps. Allergic rhinitis or nasal congestion may interfere with absorption. Carbamazepine or chlorpropamide may potentiate effect.

For explanation of icons, see p. 600.

MAGNESIUM CITRATE
Evac-Q-Mag, 16.17% Elemental Mg
Laxative/cathartic
Sol: (300 ml): 5 ml = 3.9–4.7 mEq Mg

Yes   1   B

 Children:
<6 yr: 2–4 ml/kg/24 hr PO ÷ QD-BID
6–12 yr: 100–150 ml/24 hr PO ÷ QD-BID
>12 yr: 150–300 ml/24 hr PO ÷ QD-BID

Use with **caution** in renal insufficiency and patients receiving digoxin. May cause hypermagnesemia, diarrhea, muscle weakness, hypotension, respiratory depression. Up to about 30% of dose is absorbed. May decrease absorption of H_2 antagonists, phenytoin, iron salts, tetracycline, steroids, benzodiazepines, and ciprofloxacin.

MAGNESIUM HYDROXIDE
Milk of magnesia, 41.69% Elemental Mg
Antacid, laxative
Liquid: 390 mg/5 ml, 400 mg/5 ml (Milk of Magnesia), 800 mg/5 ml (Milk of Magnesia concentrate)
Susp: 2.5 g/30 ml
Chewable Tabs: 311 mg
Combination product with Aluminum Hydroxide: see Aluminum Hydroxide

Yes   1   B

All doses based on 400 mg/5 ml Magnesium hydroxide
Laxative:
Children:
 Dose/24 hr ÷ QD-QID PO
 <2 yr: 0.5 ml/kg
 2–5 yr: 5–15 ml
 6–12 yr: 15–30 ml
 ≥12 yr: 30–60 ml

Antacid:
 Children: 2.5–5 ml/dose QD-QID PO
 Adults:
  Liquid: 5–15 ml/dose QD-QID PO
  Tabs: 622–1244 mg/dose QD-QID PO

See Magnesium citrate.

MAGNESIUM OXIDE

Maox, 60.32% Elemental Mg
Oral Magnesium salt
Tabs: 400, 420, 500 mg
Caps: 140 mg
400 mg Magnesium Oxide is equivalent to 241.3 mg Elemental Mg or 20 mEq Mg

Yes   1   B

Doses expressed in Mg oxide salt
Magnesium suplementation:
Children: 5–10 mg/kg/24 hr ÷
TID-QID PO
Adults: 400–800 mg/24 hr ÷ BID-QID
PO
Hypomagnesemia:
Children: 65–130 mg/kg/24 hr ÷ QID
PO
Adults: 2000 mg/24 hr ÷ QID PO

See Mg citrate. For RDA for
Magnesium, see p. 486.

MAGNESIUM SULFATE

Epsom salts, 9.9% Elemental Mg
Magnesium salt
Inj: 100 mg/ml (0.8 mEq/ml), 125 mg/ml (1 mEq/ml), 250 mg/ml (2 mEq/ml), 500 mg/ml (4 mEq/ml)
Oral Sol: 50% (500 mg/ml)
Granules: approx 40 mEq Mg per 5 g (240 g)
500 mg Magnesium Sulfate is equivalent to 49.3 mg Elemental Mg or 4.1 mEq Mg

Yes   1   B

All doses expressed in MgSO₄ salt
Cathartic:
Child: 0.25 g/kg/dose PO Q4–6 hr
Adult: 10–30 g/dose PO Q4–6 hr
Hypomagnesemia or hypocalcemia:
IV/IM: 25–50 mg/kg/dose Q4–6 hr ×
3–4 doses; repeat PRN. **Max single
dose: 2 g**
PO: 100–200 mg/kg/dose QID PO
Daily Maintenance:
30–60 mg/kg/24 hr or 0.25–0.5 mEq/
kg/24 hr IV
Max dose: 1 g/24 hr
*Adjunctive therapy for moderate to severe
reactive airway disease exacerbation
(bronchodilation):*
Children: 25 mg/kg/dose (**max dose:
2 g**) × 1 IV over 20 minutes
Adult: 2 g/dose × 1 IV over 20 minutes

When given IV **beware** of hypotension, respiratory depression,
complete heart block, hypermagnesemia. Calcium gluconate (IV)
should be available as **antidote**. Use with
caution in patients with renal insufficiency
and with patients on digoxin. **Serum
level–dependent toxicity** include the
following: >3 mg/dl: CNS depression; >5
mg/dl: decreased deep tendon reflexes,
flushing, somnolence; and >12 mg/dl:
respiratory paralysis, heart block.
Maximum IV intermittent infusion rate:
1 mEq/kg/hr or 125 mg MgSO₄ salt/kg/hr.

MANNITOL
Osmitrol, Resectisol
Osmotic diuretic
Inj: 50, 100, 150, 200, 250 mg/ml (5%, 10%, 15%, 20%, 25%)

 Yes ? C

Anuria/Oliguria:
Test Dose: to assess renal function:
0.2 g/kg/dose IV; **max:** 12.5 g over
3–5 min. If there is no diuresis within
2 hr, discontinue mannitol.
Initial: 0.5–1 g/kg/dose
Maintenance: 0.25–0.5 g/kg/dose Q4–
6 hr IV
Cerebral Edema:
0.25 g/kg/dose IV over 20–30 min. May
increase gradually to 1 g/kg/dose if
needed. (May give furosemide 1 mg/kg
concurrently or 5 min before mannitol.)

Contraindicated in severe renal
disease, active intracranial bleed,
dehydration, and pulmonary
edema. May cause circulatory overload
and electrolyte disturbances. For
hyperosmolar therapy, keep serum
osmolality at 310–320 mOsm/kg.
Caution: may crystallize with
concentration ≥20%; use in-line filter.
May cause hypovolemia, headache, and
polydipsia. Reduction in ICP occurs in
15 minutes and lasts 3–6 hours.

MEBENDAZOLE
Vermox
Anthelmintic
Chewable tabs: 100 mg (May be swallowed whole or chewed)

No   1   C

 Children and Adults:
Pinworms:
100 mg PO × 1, repeat in 2 wk if not cured
Hookworms, roundworms (Ascaris), and whipworm (Trichuris):
100 mg PO BID × 3 days. Repeat in 3–4 wk if not cured.
Capillariasis:
200 mg PO BID × 20 days

Experience in children <2 yr is limited. May cause diarrhea and abdominal cramping in cases of massive infection. Family may need to be treated as a group. Therapeutic effect may be decreased if administered to patients receiving carbamazepine or phenytoin. Administer with food.

MEFLOQUINE HCl
Lariam
Antimalarial
Tabs: 250 mg (228 mg base)

No   ?   C

 Doses expressed in mg Mefloquine HCl salt
Malaria Prophylaxis (start 1 week prior to exposure and continue for 4 weeks after leaving edemic area):
Children (PO, administered Q weekly):
15–19 kg: 62.5 mg (¼ tablet)
20–30 kg: 125 mg (½ tablet)
31–45 kg: 187.5 mg (¾ tablet)
>45 kg: 250 mg (1 tablet)
Adult: 250 mg PO Q weekly
Malaria Treatment:
>15 kg: 15–25 mg/kg/dose PO × 1;
max dose: 1250 mg/dose. See latest edition of the Red Book for additional information.

Use with **caution** in cardiac dysrhythmias and neurologic disease. May cause dizziness, headache, syncope, seizures, ocular abnormalities, GI symptoms, leukopenia, and thrombocytopenia. Monitor liver enzymes and ocular exams during prolonged therapy. Metoclopramide may increase peak mefloquine levels. Mefloquine may reduce valproic acid levels.

Do **not** take on an empty stomach. Administer with at least 240 ml (8 oz) water.

For explanation of icons, see p. 600.

MEPERIDINE HCl
Demerol and others
Narcotic, analgesic
Tabs: 50, 100 mg
Syrup, elixir: 50 mg/5 ml
Inj: 10, 25, 50, 75, and 100 mg/ml

Yes　2　B/D

 PO, IM, IV, and SC:
Children:
　1–1.5 mg/kg/dose Q3–4 hr PRN
　Max dose: 100 mg
Adults:
　50–150 mg/dose Q3–4 hr PRN

See p. 897 for details of use and equianalgesic dosing. **Contra-indicated** in cardiac arrhythmias, asthma, increased ICP. Potentiated by MAO inhibitors, tricyclic antidepressants, phenothiazines, other CNS-acting agents. Meperidine may increase the adverse effects of isoniazid. May cause nausea, vomiting, respiratory depression, smooth muscle spasm, pruritus, palpatations, hypotension, constipation, and lethargy.

Drug is metabolized by the liver and its metabolite (normeperidine) is renally eliminated. **Caution:** in renal failure, sickle cell disease, and seizure disorders, accumulation of normeperidine metabolite may precipitate seizures. **Adjust dose in renal failure (see p. 939).** Pregnancy category changes to "D" if used for prolonged periods or in high doses at term.
Onset of action: PO/IM/SC, 10–15 minutes; IV, 5 minutes.

1983 MP statement lists as compatible with breastfeeding; no reevaluations in subsequent statements.

MEROPENEM
Merrem
Carbapenem antibiotic
Inj: 0.5, 1 g; Each 1 g contains 3.92 mEq Na.

Yes　?　B

Infants >3 months and Children:
Mild to Moderate infections: 60 mg/kg/24 hr IV ÷ Q8 hr; **max dose:** 3 g/24 hr
Meningitis and Severe infections: 120 mg/kg/24 hr IV ÷ Q8 hr; **max dose:** 6 g/24 hr
Adults:
Mild to Moderate infections: 1.5–3 g/24 hr IV ÷ Q8 hr
Meningitis and Severe infections: 6 g/24 hr IV ÷ Q8 hr

Contraindicated in patients sensitive to carbapenems, or with a history of anaphylaxis to beta-lactam antibiotics. Drug penetrates well into the CSF. May cause diarrhea, rash, vomiting, oral moniliasis, glossitis, pain and irritation at the IV injection site, and headache. Hepatic enzyme and bilirubin elevation, leukopenia, and neutropenia have been reported. **Adjust dose in renal impairment (see p. 933).**

METAPROTERENOL

Metaprel, Alupent, and others
Beta-2-adrenergic agonist

No ? C

Syrup: 10 mg/5 ml
Tabs: 10, 20 mg
Inhaler: 650 mcg/actuation (5, 10 ml) Approx 100 actuations/5 ml
Inhalant solution: 5% (50 mg/ml) (0.3, 10, 30 ml)
Single-dose inhalant solution: 0.4% (4 mg/ml), 0.6% (6 mg/ml) (2.5 ml)

Inhalation:
Aerosol:
2–3 puffs Q3–4 hr to max dose of 12 puffs/24 hr
Nebulized Solution:
Dilute 0.1–0.3 ml of 5% solution in 2.5 ml NS; administer Q4–6 hr PRN
Single-dose solutions:
Infants: 2.5 ml of 0.4%
Children: 2.5 ml of 0.6%
Usual dose: Q4–6 hr. May give more frequently for acute bronchospasm.
Oral:
Children
<2 yr: 0.4 mg/kg/dose Q6–8 hr
2–6 yr: 0.33–0.85 mg/kg/dose Q6–8 hr
6–9 yr: 10 mg/dose Q6–8 hr
>9 yr and Adults: 20 mg/dose Q6–8 hr

Contraindicated in cardiac arrhythmias, or narrow angle glaucoma. Adverse reactions as with other beta-adrenergic agents. Excessive use may result in cardiac arrhythmias and death. Also causes tachycardia, increased myocardial O_2 consumption, hypertension, nervousness, headaches, nausea, palpitations, and tremor. The use of tube spacers may enhance efficacy of administering doses via metered dose inhaler. Nebulizers may be given more frequently in the acute setting.

METHADONE HCl

Dolophine
Narcotic, analgesic

Yes 1 B/D

Tabs: 5, 10 mg
Tabs (dispersible): 40 mg
Sol: 5, 10 mg/5 ml
Conc. Sol: 10 mg/ml
Inj: 10 mg/ml

For explanation of icons, see p. 600.

Children: 0.7 mg/kg/24 hr ÷ Q4–6 hr PO, SC, IM, or IV PRN pain.
Max dose: 10 mg/dose
Adults: 2.5–10 mg/dose Q3–4 hr PO, SC, IM, or IV PRN pain.
Detoxification or maintenance: See package insert

May cause respiratory depression, sedation, increased intracranial pressure, hypotension, and bradycardia. Average $T_{1/2}$: children 19 hr, adults 35 hr. Oral duration of action is 6–8 hours initially and 22–48 hours after repeated doses. Respiratory effects last longer than analgesia. Accumulation may occur with continuous use, making it necessary to adjust dose. See p. 896 for equianalgesic dosing and onset of action. **Adjust dose in renal insufficiency (see p. 939).** Pregnancy category changes to "D" if used for prolonged period or in high doses at term.

METHICILLIN
Staphcillin
Antibiotic, penicillin (penicillinase-resistant)
Inj: 1, 4, 6, 10 g (2.6–3.1 mEq Na/g)

Yes ? B

Neonates: IM/IV
≤7 days:
  <2 kg: 50–100 mg/kg/24 hr ÷ Q12 hr
  ≥2 kg: 75–150 mg/kg/24 hr ÷ Q8 hr
>7 days:
  <1.2 kg: 50–100 mg/kg/24 hr ÷ Q12 hr
  1.2–2 kg: 75–150 mg/kg/24 hr ÷ Q8 hr
  ≥2 kg: 100–200 mg/kg/24 hr ÷ Q6 hr
Infants >1 mo and children: 150–400 mg/kg/24 hr ÷ Q4–6 hr IV/IM
Adults: 4–12 g/24 hr ÷ Q4–6 hr IV/IM
Max dose: 12 g/24 hr

Allergic cross-reactivity with and same toxicity as penicillin. May cause bone marrow suppression, positive Coombs' test, hairy tongue, and phlebitis at infusion site. Methicillin has been associated with interstitial nephritis and hemorrhagic cystitis.

Use higher end of dosage range for serious infections and meningitis. **Adjust dose in renal failure (see p. 933).** Alternative agents are oxacillin and nafcillin.

METHIMAZOLE
Tapazole
Anithyroid agent
Tabs: 5, 10 mg

No 1 D

 Children:
Initial: 0.4–0.7 mg/kg/24 hr or
15–20 mg/m²/24 hr PO ÷ Q8 hr
Maintenance: 1/3–2/3 of initial dose PO
÷ Q8 hr
Max dose: 30 mg/24 hr PO
Adults:
Initial: 15–60 mg/24 hr PO ÷ TID
Maintenance: 5–15 mg/24 hr PO ÷
TID
Max dose: 30 mg/24 hr

Readily crosses placental
membranes and distributes into
breast milk. Blood dyscrasias,
dermatitis, hepatitis, arthralgia, CNS
reactions, pruritus, nephritis, hypopro-
thrombonemia, agranulocytosis, headache, fever, hypothyroidism may occur.
Switch to maintenance dose when patient
is euthyroid. Administer doses with food.

METHSUXIMIDE
Celontin Kapseals
Anticonvulsant
Caps: 150, 300 mg

No ? C

Children PO:
10–15 mg/kg/24 hr ÷ Q6–8 hr.
Increase weekly up to **max** 30 mg/
kg/24 hr
Adults PO:
Initial: 300 mg/24 hr ÷ BID-QID for
1 wk. May increase by 300 mg/24 hr
each wk to **max dose** of 1.2 gm/24 hr
÷ BID-QID

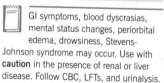 GI symptoms, blood dyscrasias,
mental status changes, periorbital
edema, drowsiness, Stevens-
Johnson syndrome may occur. Use with
caution in the presence of renal or liver
disease. Follow CBC, LFTs, and urinalysis.
Avoid abrupt withdrawal.
Measure therapeutic range for
metabolite, N-desmethylmethsuximide.
Therapeutic reference range: 10–40
mg/L. Recommended serum sampling
time at steady-state: obtain trough level
within
30 minutes of the next scheduled dose
after 5–7 days of continuous dosing.

For explanation of icons, see p. 600.

METHYLDOPA

Aldomet

Central alpha-adrenergic blocker, antihypertensive

Yes   1   C

Tabs: 125, 250, 500 mg
Inj: 50 mg/ml
Susp: 250 mg/5 ml

 Hypertension:
Children: 10 mg/kg/24 hr ÷
Q6–12 hr PO; increase PRN Q2
days. **Max dose:** 65 mg/kg or 3 g/24 hr,
whichever is less.
Adults: 250 mg/dose BID-TID PO.
Increase PRN Q2 days to max: 3 g/
24 hr
Hypertensive Crisis:
Children: 2–4 mg/kg/dose IV to **max** of
5–10 mg/kg/dose IV Q6–8 hr. Max dose
(whichever is less): 65 mg/kg/24 hr or
3 g/24 hr.
Adults: 250–1000 mg IV Q6–8 hr.
Max: 4 g/24 hr

Contraindicated in
pheochromocytoma and active liver
disease. Use with **caution** if patient
is receiving haloperidol, propranolol,
lithium, sympathomimetics. Positive
Coombs' test rarely associated with
hemolytic anemia, fever, leukopenia,
sedation, memory impairment, hepatitis,
GI disturbances, orthostatic hypotension,
black tongue, and gynecomastia may
occur. May interfere with lab tests for
creatinine, urinary catecholamines, uric
acid, AST.
Adjust dose in renal failure (see p.
940).

METHYLENE BLUE

Urolene Blue

Antidote, drug-induced methemoglobinemia, and cyanide toxicity

Yes   ?   C/D

Tabs: 65 mg
Inj: 10 mg/ml (1%)

Methemoglobinemia:
Adults and Children:
1–2 mg/kg/dose or 25–50 mg/m^2/
dose IV over 5 min. May repeat in 1 hr
if needed.

At high doses, may cause
methemoglobinemia. Avoid
subcutaneous or intrathecal routes
of administration. Use with caution in
G6PD deficiency or renal insufficiency.
May cause nausea, vomiting, dizziness,
headache, diaphoresis, stained skin, and
abdominal pain. Causes blue-green
discoloration of urine and feces.
Pregnancy category changes to "D" if
injected intraamniotically.

METHYLPHENIDATE HCl

Ritalin, Ritalin SR, others
CNS stimulant
Tabs: 5, 10, 20 mg
Slow-release tabs: 20 mg (8-hr duration)

No ? C

Attention deficit hyperactivity disorder:
≥6 yr:
Initial: 0.3 mg/kg/dose (or 2.5–5 mg/dose) given before breakfast and lunch. May increase by 0.1 mg/kg/dose PO (or 5–10 mg/24 hr) weekly until maintenance dose achieved. May give extra afternoon dose if needed.
Maintenance dose range: 0.3–1 mg/kg/24 hr
Max dose: 2 mg/kg/24 hr or 60 mg/24 hr.

Contraindicated in glaucoma, anxiety disorders, motor tics and Tourette's syndrome. Medication should generally not be used in children <5 yr old as diagnosis of ADHD in this age group is extremely difficult and should be made only in consultation with a specialist. Use with **caution** in patients with hypertension and epilepsy. Insomnia, weight loss, anorexia, rash, nausea, emesis, abdominal pain, hyper- or hypotension, tachycardia, arrhythmias, palpitations, restlessness, headaches, fever, tremor, thrombocytopenia may occur. High dose may slow growth by appetite suppression.

May increase serum concentrations of tricyclic antidepressants, phenytoin, phenobarbital, and warfarin. Effect of methylphenidate may be potentiated by MAO inhibitors.

METHYLPREDNISOLONE

Medrol, Solu-Medrol, Depo-Medrol, and others
Corticosteroid
Tabs: 2, 4, 8, 16, 24, 32 mg
Tabs, dose pack: 4 mg (21s)
Inj: Na succinate (Solu-Medrol) 40, 125, 500, 1000, 2000 mg (IV/IM use)
Inj: Acetate 20, 40, 80 mg/ml (IM repository) (Depo-Medrol)

No ? C

*Antiinflammatory/
immunosuppressive:*
PO/IM/IV: 0.5–1.7 mg/kg/24 hr ÷
Q6–12 hr
Status Asthmaticus:
Children: IM/IV:
Loading dose: 2 mg/kg/dose × 1
Maintenance: 2 mg/kg/24 hr ÷ Q6 hr
Adults: 10–250 mg/dose Q4–6 hr IM/IV
Acute spinal cord injury:
30 mg/kg IV over 15 minutes followed
in 45 minutes by a continuous infusion
of 5.4 mg/kg/hr × 23 hr

See pp. 908-909 for relative,
steroid potencies and doses based
on body surface area. Not all
practitioners use loading dose for status
asthmaticus. Acetate form may be used
for intramuscular, intra-articular, and
intralesional injection; it should **not** be
given IV. Like all steroids, may cause
hypertension, pseudotumor cerebri, acne,
Cushing's syndrome, adrenal axis
suppression, GI bleeding, hyperglycemia,
and osteoporosis.

METOCLOPRAMIDE
Clopra, Maxolon, Reglan, and others
Antiemetic, prokinetic agent
Tabs: 5, 10 mg
Inj: 5 mg/ml
Syrup (sugar-free): 5 mg/5 ml
Conc sol: 10 mg/ml

 Yes 3 B

*Gastroesophageal reflux (GER) or
GI dysmotility:*
Infants and Children: 0.1–0.2 mg/
kg/dose up to QID IV/IM/PO; **max dose:**
0.8 mg/kg/24 hr
Adult: 10–15 mg/dose QAC and QHS
IV/IM/PO
Antiemetic:
1–2 mg/kg/dose Q2–6 hr IV/IM/PO.
Premedicate with diphenhydramine to
reduce EPS.

Contraindicated in GI obstruction,
seizure disorder, pheochromocytoma, or in patients receiving
drugs likely to cause extrapyramidal
symptoms (EPS). May cause EPS,
especially at higher doses. Sedation,
headache, anxiety, leukopenia, and
diarrhea may occur.
For GER, give 30 min before meals and
at bedtime. **Adjust dose in renal
impairment (see p. 940).**

METOLAZONE
Zaroxolyn, Diulo, Mykrox
Diuretic
Tabs: 0.5 (Mykrox), 2.5, 5, 10 mg
Susp: 1 mg/ml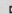

   No 1 D

Dosage based on Zaroxolyn (for Mykrox or oral suspension, see remarks):

Children: 0.2–0.4 mg/kg/24 hr ÷ QD-BID PO

Adults:

  Hypertension: 2.5–5 mg QD PO

  Edema: 5–20 mg QD PO

Contraindicated in patients with anuria, hepatic coma.

Electrolyte imbalance, GI disturbance, hyperglycemia, marrow suppression, chills, hyperuricemia, chest pain, hepatitis, and rash may occur. Mykrox and oral suspension have increased bioavailability; therefore lower doses may be necessary when using these dosage forms.

METRONIDAZOLE

Flagyl, Protostat, Metro, and others

Antibiotic, antiprotozoal

Yes 3 B

Tabs: 250, 500 mg

Caps: 375 mg

Susp: 100 mg/5 ml, or 50 mg/ml

Inj: 500 mg

Ready to use inj: 5 mg/ml (28 mEq Na/g)

Gel, topical: 0.75%

Cream, topical: 0.75%

Gel, vaginal: 0.75%

For explanation of icons, see p. 600.

Amebiasis:
Children: 35–50 mg/kg/24 hr PO ÷ TID × 10 days
Adults: 750 mg/dose PO TID × 10 days
Anaerobic Infection:
Neonates: PO/IV:
<7 days: <1.2 kg: 7.5 mg/kg Q48 hr
1.2–2 kg: 7.5 mg/kg Q24 hr
≥2 kg: 15 mg/kg/24 hr ÷ Q12 hr
≥7 days: <1.2 kg: 7.5 mg/kg Q48 hr
1.2–2 kg: 15 mg/kg/24 hr ÷ Q12 hr
≥2 kg: 30 mg/kg/24 hr ÷ Q12 hr
Infants/Children/Adults:
IV/PO: 30 mg/kg/24 hr ÷ Q6 hr
Max dose: 4 g/24 hr
Bacterial Vaginosis:
Adolescents and Adults: 500 mg PO BID × 7 days or 2 g PO × 1 dose
Giardiasis:
Children: 15 mg/kg/24 hr PO ÷ TID × 5 days
Adults: 250 mg PO TID × 5 days
Trichomoniasis: Treat sexual contacts
Children: 15 mg/kg/24 hr PO ÷ TID × 7 days
Adolescents/Adults: 2 g PO × 1 or 250 mg PO TID or 375 mg PO BID × 7 days
C. difficile infection:
Children: 30 mg/kg/24 hr ÷ Q6 hr PO/IV (IV may be less efficacious) × 10 days
Adults: 250–500 mg TID-QID × 10–14 days

Helicobacter pylori infection:
Use in combination amoxicillin and bismuth subsalicylate.
Children: 15–20 mg/kg/24 hr ÷ BID PO × 4 weeks
Adults: 250–500 mg TID PO × 14 days
Inflammatory bowel disease (as alternative to sulfasalazine):
Adults: 400 mg BID PO
Perianal Disease: 20 mg/kg/24 hr PO in 3–5 divided doses

Avoid use in first-trimester pregnancy. Use with **caution** in patients with CNS disease, blood dyscrasias, severe liver or renal disease (GFR <10 ml/min); see p. 933. Nausea, diarrhea, urticaria, dry mouth, leukopenia, vertigo, metallic taste, peripheral neuropathy may occur. Candidiasis may worsen. May discolor urine. Patients should **not** ingest alcohol for 24–48 hr after dose (disulfuram-type reaction).

May increase levels or toxicity of phenytoin, lithium, and warfarin. Phenobarbital and rifampin may increase metronidazole metabolism.

IV infusion must be given slowly over 1 hr. For intravenous use in all ages, some references recommend a 15 mg/kg loading dose.

MEZLOCILLIN
Mezlin
Antibiotic, penicillin (extended spectrum)
Inj: 1, 2, 3, 4, 20 g (contains 1.85 mEq Na/g)

Yes   2   B

Neonates, IM/IV:
<1.2 kg: 150 mg/kg/24 hr ÷ Q12 hr
≥1.2 kg:
    ≤ 7 days: 150 mg/kg/24 hr ÷ Q12 hr
    >7 days: 225 mg/kg/24 hr ÷ Q8 hr
Infants and Children, IM/IV: 200–300 mg/kg/24 hr ÷ Q4–6 hr
Cystic Fibrosis, IM/IV: 300–450 mg/kg/24 hr ÷ Q4–6 hr; **max dose:** 24 g/24 hr
Adults, IM/IV: 1.5–4 g/dose Q4–6 hr; **max dose:** 24 g/24 hr

Use with **caution** in biliary obstruction and renal impairment (see p. 933). May cause seizures, nausea, diarrhea, vomiting, bone marrow suppression, blood dyscrasias, elevated BUN/Cr, and elevated LFTs. Causes false-positive direct Coombs' test, urinary protein, prolonged bleeding time, and electrolyte abnormalities.

MICONAZOLE
Monistat
Antifungal agent
Cream: 2% (15, 30, 90 g)
Lotion: 2% (30, 60 ml)
Topical solution: 2% with alcohol (7.4, 29.6 ml)
Vaginal cream: 2% (45 g)
Vaginal suppository: 100 mg (7's), 200 mg (3's)
Powder: 2% (45, 90 g)
Spray: 2% (105 ml)
Inj: 1% (10 mg/ml)

No   ?   C

Topical: Apply BID × 2–4 wk
Vaginal: 1 applicator full of cream or 100 mg suppository QHS × 7 days or 200 mg suppository QHS × 3 days
IV:
    Neonates: 5–15 mg/kg/24 hr ÷ Q8–24 hr
    Infants and Children: 20–40 mg/kg/24 hr ÷ Q8 hr
    Adult: 1.2–3.6 g/24 hr ÷ Q8 hr

Use with **caution** in liver disease. Side effects include phlebitis (IV route), pruritus, rash, nausea, vomiting, fever, drowsiness, diarrhea, anemia, lipemia, thrombocytopenia, anorexia, tremors, and flushing. CN XII nerve palsy and arachnoiditis have been reported.

MIDAZOLAM
Versed
Benzodiazepine
Inj: 1, 5 mg/ml
Oral sol: 2.5 mg/ml, 3 mg/ml
Oral syrup: 2 mg/ml
Liquid gelatin sol: 1 mg/ml

Yes 3 D

 Titrate to effect under controlled conditions.
See p. 902 for additional routes of administration.
Sedation for procedures:
Children:
IV:
6 months–5 yrs: 0.05–0.1 mg/kg/dose over 2–3 min. May repeat dose PRN in 2–3 min intervals up to a **max total dose** of 6 mg. A total dose up to 0.6 mg/kg may be necessary for desired effect.
6–12 yrs: 0.025–0.05 mg/kg/dose over 2–3 min. May repeat dose PRN in 2–3 min intervals up to a **max total dose** of 10 mg. A total dose up to 0.4 mg/kg may be necessary for desired effect.
>12–16 yrs: Use adult dose; up to a **max total dose** of 10 mg
Adults:
IV: 0.5–2 mg/dose over 2 min. May repeat PRN in 2–3 min intervals until desired effect. Usual total dose: 2.5–5 mg.
Sedation with mechanical ventilation:
Intermittent:
Infants and Children: 0.05–0.15 mg/kg/dose Q1–2 hr PRN

Continuous IV infusion (initial doses, titrate to effect):
Neonates:
<32 weeks gestation: 0.5 mcg/kg/min
≥32 weeks gestation: 1 mcg/kg/min
Infants and Children: 1–2 mcg/kg/min
See inside front cover for infusion preparation.

Contraindicated in patients with narrow angle glaucoma and shock.
Causes respiratory depression, hypotension and bradycardia. Cardiovascular monitoring is recommended. Use lower doses or reduce dose when given in combination with narcotics or in patients with respiratory compromise.
Drug is a substrate for CYP 450 3A4 (see p. 924). Serum concentrations may be increased by cimetidine, erythromycin, itraconazole, ketoconazole, and protease inhibitors. Sedative effects may be antagonized by theophylline. **Effects can be reversed by flumazenil.** For pharmacodynamic information, see p. 903.
Adjust dose in renal failure (see p. 940).

MILRINONE
Primacor
Inotrope
Inj: 1 mg/ml (5 ml)

Yes   ?   C

Children (limited data): 50 mcg/kg IV bolus over 10 minutes, followed by a continuous infusion of 0.5–1 mcg/kg/min and titrate to effect.
Adults: 50 mcg/kg IV bolus over 10 minutes, followed by a continuous infusion of 0.375–0.75 mcg/kg/min and titrate to effect.

Contraindicated in severe aortic stenosis, severe pulmonic stenosis, acute MI. May cause headache, dysrhythmias, hypotension, hypokalemia, nausea, vomiting, anorexia, abdominal pain, hepatotoxicity, and thrombocytopenia. Pediatric patients may require higher mcg/kg/min doses because of a faster elimination $T_{1/2}$ and larger volume of distribution, when compared to adults. Hemodynamic effects can last up to 3–5 hours after discontinuation of infusion in children. Reduce dose in renal impairment.

MINERAL OIL
Kondremul and others
Laxative, lubricant
Liquid: various sizes
Rectal preparation: 133 ml
Emulsion, oral: 1.4 g/5 ml; 2.5 ml/5 ml, 2.75 ml/5 ml, 4.75 ml/5 ml
Jelly, oral: 2.75 ml/5 ml

No   ?   C

Children 5–11 yr:
  PO: 5–15 ml/24 hr ÷ QD-TID
  Rectal: 30–60 ml as single dose
Children ≥12 yr and Adults:
  PO: 15–45 ml/24 hr ÷ QD-TID
  Rectal: 60–150 ml as single dose

May cause lipid pneumonitis (via aspiration), diarrhea, cramps.
  Onset of action is approximately 6–8 hrs. Higher doses may be necessary to achieve desired effect. Do **not** give QHS dose and use with **caution** in children <5 years to minimize risk of aspiration. May impair the absorption of fat-soluble vitamins, calcium, phosphorus, oral contraceptives, and warfarin. Emulsified preparations are more palatable.
  For disimpaction, doses up to 1 ounce (30 ml) per year of age (**maximum** of 8 ounces) BID can be given.

For explanation of icons, see p. 600.

MINOCYCLINE
Minocin and others
Antibiotic, tetracycline derivative
Tabs: 50, 100 mg
Caps: 50, 100 mg
Caps (pellet filled): 50, 100 mg
Oral susp: 50 mg/5 ml (60 ml); contains 5% alcohol
Inj: 100 mg

No   2   D

Children (8–12 yr): 4 mg/kg/dose × 1 PO/IV, then 2 mg/kg/dose Q12 hr PO/IV; **max dose:** 200 mg/24 hr
Adolescent and Adults: 200 mg/dose × 1 PO/IV, then 100 mg Q12 hr PO/IV

Nausea, vomiting, allergy, photophobia, injury to developing teeth. High incidence of vestibular dysfunction, 30%–90%. Do **not** take with milk or dairy products.

MINOXIDIL
Loniten, Rogaine, Minoxidil for Men
Antihypertensive agent, hair growth stimulant
Tabs: 2.5, 10 mg
Topical Solution (Rogaine, Minoxidil for Men): 2% (60 ml)

No   1   C

Children:
Start with 0.2 mg/kg/24 hr PO QD; **max. dose:** 5 mg/24 hr. Dose may be increased in increments of 0.1–0.2 mg/kg/24 hr at 3 day intervals. Usual effective range: 0.25–1 mg/kg/24 hr PO ÷ QD–BID; **max dose:** 5 mg/kg/24 hr up to 50 mg/24 hr.

>12 yr and Adults:
Oral: Start with 5 mg QD. Dose may be gradually increased at 3 day intervals. *Usual effective range:* 10–40 mg/24 hr ÷ QD–BID; **max dose:** 100 mg/24 hr. *Topical (Alopecia):* Apply 1 ml to the total affected areas of the scalp BID (QAM and QHS). **Max dose:** 2 ml/24 hr.

Contraindicated in acute MI, dissecting aortic aneurysm, pheochromocytoma. Concurrent use with a beta-blocker and diuretic to prevent reflex tachycardia and reduce water retention, respectively. May cause drowsiness, dizziness, CHF, pulmonary edema, pericardial effusion, pericarditis, thrombocytopenia, leukopenia, Stevens-Johnson syndrome, and hypertrichosis (reversible) with systemic use. Concurrent use of guanethidine may cause profound orthostatic hypotension; use with other antihypertensive agents may cause additive hypotension. Antihypertensive onset of action within 30 minutes and peak effects within 2–8 hours.

TOPICAL USE remarks: local irritation, contact dermatitis may occur. Do **not** use in conjunction with other topical agents including topical corticosteroids, retinoids and petrolatum or agents that are known to enhance cutaneous drug absorption. Onset of hair growth (topical use) is 4 months.

MITHRAMYCIN
See Plicamycin

For explanation of icons, see p. 600.

MONTELUKAST

Singulair

Anti-asthmatic, leukotriene receptor antagonist

No ? B

Tabs: 10 mg

Chewable Tabs: 5 mg; contains phenylalanine

 Children (6–14 yrs): Chew 5 mg (chewable tablet) QHS
>15 yrs and Adults: 10 mg PO QHS

 Chewable tablet dosage form is **contraindicated** in phenylketonuric patients. Side effects include: headache, abdominal pain, dyspepsia, fatigue, dizziness, cough, and elevated liver enzymes. Diarrhea, laryngitis, pharyngitis, nausea, otitis, sinusitis, and viral infections have been reported in children. Drug is a substrate for CYP 450 3A4 and 2C9 (see p. 924). Phenobarbital and rifampin may induce hepatic metabolism to increase the clearance of montelukast.

MORPHINE SULFATE

various brand names

Narcotic, analgesic

Yes 2 B/D

Oral Sol: 10 mg/5 ml, 20 mg/5 ml

Conc. Oral Sol: 100 mg/5 ml

Tabs: 15, 30 mg

Controlled release tabs: 15, 30, 60, 100 mg

Sustained release tabs: 30, 60, 100 mg

Soluble tabs: 10, 15, 30 mg

Rectal suppository: 5, 10, 20, 30 mg

Inj: 0.5, 1, 2, 3, 4, 5, 8, 10, 15, 25 mg/ml

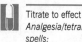 Titrate to effect
Analgesia/tetralogy (cyanotic) spells:
Neonates: 0.05–0.2 mg/kg/dose IM, slow IV, SC Q4 hr
Neonatal opiate withdrawal: 0.08–0.2 mg/dose Q3–4 hr PRN
Infants and Children:
PO: 0.2–0.5 mg/kg/dose Q4–6 hr PRN (immediate release) or 0.3–0.6 mg/kg/dose Q12 hr PRN (controlled release)
IM/IV/SC: 0.1–0.2 mg/kg/dose Q2–4 hr PRN; **max dose:** 15 mg/dose.
Adults:
PO: 10–30 mg Q4 hr PRN (immediate release) or 15–30 mg Q8–12 hr PRN (controlled release)
IM/IV/SC: 2–15 mg/dose Q2–6 hr PRN
Continuous IV infusion: (Dosing ranges, titrate to effect)
Neonates: 0.01–0.02 mg/kg/hr
Infants and Children: Postoperative pain: 0.01–0.04 mg/kg/hr; sickle cell and cancer: 0.04–0.07 mg/kg/hr
Adults: 0.8–10 mg/hr

Dependence, CNS and respiratory depression, nausea, vomiting, urinary retention, constipation, hypotension, bradycardia, increased ICP, miosis, biliary spasm, allergy may occur. **Naloxone may be used to reverse effects,** especially respiratory depression. Causes histamine release resulting in itching and possible bronchospasm. Neonates may require higher doses due to decreased amounts of active metabolites. See p. 896 for equianalgesic dosing. Pregnancy category changes to "D" if used for prolonged periods or in higher doses at term. Rectal dosing is same as oral dosing but is not recommended due to poor absorption.

Adjust dose in renal failure (see p. 940).

MUPIROCIN

Bactroban
Topical antibiotic
Ointment: 2% (15, 30 g)
Cream: 2% (15, 30 g)
Nasal Ointment: 2% (1 g), as calcium salt

No ? B

Topical: apply small amount TID to affected area × 5–14 days
Intranasal: apply small amount intranasally 2–4 times/24 hr for 5–14 days

If clinical response is not apparent in 3–5 days with topical use, reevaluate infection. Intranasal administration may be used to eliminate carriage of *S. aureus.* May cause minor local irritation.

MYCOPHENOLATE MOFETIL

Yes ? C

CellCept
Immunosuppressant agent
Tabs: 500 mg
Caps: 250 mg
Inj: 500 mg

Children (from initial pharmacokinetic studies; and in combination with other immunosuppressants): 600 mg/m^2/dose PO BID
Adults (in combination with corticosteroids and cyclosporine):
IV: 2000–3000 mg/24 hr ÷ BID
Oral: 2000–3000 mg/24 hr ÷ BID; doses as high as 3500–4000 mg/24 hr ÷ BID have been given to liver and renal transplant patients.

Check specific transplantation protocol for specific dosage. Mycophenolate mofetil is a pro-drug for mycophenolic acid. Common side effects may include: headache, hypertension, diarrhea, vomiting, bone marrow suppression, anemia, fever, opportunistic infections, and sepsis. May also increase the risk for lymphomas or other malignancies.

Use with **caution** in patients with active GI disease or renal impairment (GFR <25 ml/min/1.73 m^2) outside of the immediate post-transplant period. In adults with renal impairment, **avoid** doses >2 g/24 hr and observe carefully. No dose adjustment is needed for patients experiencing delayed graft function postoperatively.

Drug interactions: (1) Displacement of phenytoin or theophylline from protein binding sites will decrease total serum levels and increase free serum levels of these drugs. Salicylates displaces myco-phenolate to increase free levels of mycophenolate. (2) Competition for renal tubular secretion results in increase serum level of acyclovir, ganciclovir, probenecid, and mycophenolate (when any of these are used together). Administer oral doses on an empty stomach. Cholestyramine and antacid use may decrease myco-phenolic acid levels. Infuse intravenous doses over 2 hours.

NAFCILLIN

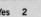

Yes 2 B

Unipen, Nafcil, Nallpen, and others
Antibiotic, penicillin (penicillinase resistant)
Tabs: 500 mg
Caps: 250 mg
Oral Sol: 250 mg/5 ml
Inj: 0.5, 1, 2, 4, 10 g; contains 2.9 mEq Na/g

Neonates: IM/IV
  ≤7 days:
    <2 kg: 50 mg/kg/24 hr ÷ Q12 hr
    ≥2 kg: 75 mg/kg/24 hr ÷ Q8 hr
  >7 days:
    <1.2 kg: 50 mg/kg/24 hr ÷ Q12 hr
    1.2–2 kg: 75 mg/kg/24 hr ÷ Q8 hr
    ≥2 kg: 100 mg/kg/24 hr ÷ Q6 hr
Infants and Children:
  PO: 50–100 mg/kg/24 hr ÷ Q6 hr
  IM/IV: (mild to moderate infections):
    50–100 mg/kg/24 hr ÷ Q6 hr
    (severe infections): 100–200
    mg/kg/24 hr ÷ Q4–6 hr
Adults:
  PO: 250–1000 mg Q4–6 hr
  IV: 500–2000 mg Q4–6 hr
  IM: 500 mg Q4–6 hr
  Max dose: 12 g/24 hr

Allergic cross-sensitivity with penicillin. Oral route **not** recommended due to poor absorption. High incidence of phlebitis with IV dosing. CSF penetration is poor unless meninges are inflamed. Use with **caution** in patients with combined renal and hepatic impairment (reduce dose by 33-50%). Nafcillin may increase elimination of warfarin. Acute interstitial nephritis is rare. May cause rash and bone marrow suppression.

NALOXONE
Narcan
Narcotic antagonist
Inj: 0.4, 1 mg/ml
Neonatal Inj: 0.02 mg/ml

No   ?   B

Opiate intoxication:
Neonates, Infants, Children <20 kg: IM/IV/SC/ETT: 0.1 mg/kg/dose.
May repeat PRN Q2–3 min.
Children ≥20 kg or >5 yr: 2 mg/dose.
May repeat PRN Q2–3 min.
Continuous Infusion (Children and Adults): 0.005 mg/kg loading dose followed by infusion of 0.0025 mg/kg/hr has been recommended. A range of 0.0025–0.16 mg/kg/hr has been reported. Taper gradually to avoid relapse.
Adults: 0.4–2 mg/dose. May repeat PRN Q2–3 min. Use 0.1–0.2 mg increments in opiate dependent patients.

Does **not** cause respiratory depression. Short duration of action may necessitate multiple doses. For severe intoxication, doses of 0.2 mg/kg may be required. If no response is achieved after a cumulative dose of 10 mg, reevaluate diagnosis. In the non-arrest situation, use the lowest dose effective (may start at 0.001 mg/kg/dose). See p. 906. The neonatal concentration (0.02 mg/ml) is **no** longer recommended in most instances due to large volumes of administration, 2 mg = 100 ml. Will produce narcotic withdrawal syndrome in patients with chronic dependence. Use with **caution** in patients with chronic cardiac disease. Abrupt reversal of narcotic depression may result in nausea, vomiting, diaphoresis, tachycardia, hypertension, and tremulousness.

NAPROXEN/NAPROXEN SODIUM

Naprosyn, Anaprox, Aleve [OTC]
Nonsteroidal antiinflammatory agent   **Yes   1   B/D**
Tabs (Naproxen): 250, 375, 500 mg
Tabs (Naproxen sodium):
  Anaprox: 275 mg (250 mg base), 550 mg (500 mg base); contains 1 mEq, 2 mEq Na, respectively
  Aleve: 220 mg (200 mg base); contains 0.87 mEq Na
Susp: Naproxen 125 mg/5 ml; conatins 0.34 mEq Na/1 ml

All doses based on naproxen base
  Children >2 yr:
    Analgesia: 5–7 mg/kg/dose Q8–12 hr PO
  JRA: 10–20 mg/kg/24 hr ÷ Q12 hr PO
  Usual max dose range: 1250 mg/24 hr
Rheumatoid arthritis, ankylosing spondylitis:
  Adults: 250–500 mg BID PO
Dysmenorrhea:
  500 mg × 1, then 250 mg Q6–8 hr PO; **max dose:** 1250 mg/24 hr.

May cause GI bleeding, thrombocytopenia, heartburn, headache, drowsiness, vertigo, tinnitus. Use with **caution** in patients with GI disease, cardiac disease, renal or hepatic impairment, and those receiving anticoagulants. See Ibuprofen for other side effects.

Pregnancy category changes to "D" if used in 3rd trimester or near delivery. Administer doses with food or milk to reduce GI discomfort.

NEDOCROMIL SODIUM

Tilade
Antiallergic agent   **No**   **?**   **B**
Aerosol Inhaler: 1.75 mg/actuation (112 actuations/inhaler, 16.2 g)

Children >12 yr and adults:
2 puffs QID. May reduce dosage to
BID-TID once clinical response is
obtained.

May cause dry mouth/pharyngitis,
unpleasant taste, cough, nausea,
headache, and rhinitis. Therapeutic
response often occurs within 2 weeks,
however, a 4–6 week trial may be needed
to determine maximum benefit.

NELFINAVIR

Viracept, NFV
Antiviral, protease inhibitor   **No**   **3**   **B**
Powder, oral: 200 mg/ level teaspoonful or 50 mg/ level scoop (50 mg/gram
powder); contains 11.2 mg phenylalanine/gram powder)
Tabs: 250 mg

Neonates (investigational dose
from ACTG 353): 40 mg/kg/dose
PO BID
Children (>3 months): 25–30
mg/kg/dose PO TID; **max dose:** 750
mg/dose TID
Adolescents and Adults: 750 mg PO TID
or 1250 mg PO BID

Avoid use of oral powder dosage
form in patients with phenylketouria
since it contains phenylalanine.
Diarrhea is the most common side effect.
Asthenia, abdominal pain, rash, hyperglycemia, and exacerbation of chronic liver
diesease may occur. Spontaneous bleeding
episodes in hemophiliacs have been
reported.
Nelfinavir is a substrate and inhibitor of
CYP 450 3A4 (see p. 924). The following
drugs should **NOT** be coadministered with
nelfinavir: terfenadine, astemizole,

cisapride, midazolam, triazolam, ergot
derviatives, amiodarone, or quinidine.
Rifampin, phenobarbital, phenytoin, and
carbamazepine can decrease nelfinavir
levels. Nelfinavir can increase rifabutin
levels; decrease delavirdine levels; and
decrease oral contraceptive effectiveness
(use alternative methods). When used in
combination with other protease inhibitors
(PI), nelfinavir and other PI levels may
increase. **Always check the potential for
other drug interactions when either
initiating therapy or adding new drugs
onto an existing regimen.**
Administer all doses with food; avoid
mixing with acidic foods or juice. If
didanosine is part of the antiviral regimen,
nelfinavir should be administered at least
2 hours prior or 1 hour after didanosine.
Oral powder dosage form may be mixed
with water, milk, pudding, or formula (up
to 6 hours). **Non-compliance can quickly
promote resistant HIV strains.**

For explanation of icons, see p. 600.

NEOMYCIN SULFATE

Mycifradin

Antibiotic, aminoglycoside; ammonium detoxicant

Yes ? C

Tabs: 500 mg
Sol: 125 mg/5 ml (contains parabens)
Cream: 0.5%
Ointment: 0.5%

 Diarrhea:
Preterm and newborns: 50 mg/kg/24 hr ÷ Q6 hr PO
Hepatic Encephalopathy:
Infants and Children: 50–100 mg/kg/24 hr ÷ Q6–8 hr PO × 5–6 days. **Max dose:** 12 g/24 hr
Adults: 4–12 g/24 hr ÷ Q4–6 hr PO × 5–6 days
Bowel prep:
Children: 90 mg/kg/24 hr PO ÷ Q4 hr × 2–3 days
Adults: 1 g Q1 hr PO × 4 doses, then 1 g Q4 hr PO × 5 doses. (Many other regimens exist)
Topical: Apply QD–QID to infected area.

Contraindicated in intestinal obstruction. Monitor for nephrotoxicity and ototoxicity. Oral absorption is limited, but levels may accumulate. Consider dosage reduction in the presence of renal failure. May cause itching, redness, edema, colitis, candidiasis, or poor wound healing if applied topically.

NEOMYCIN/POLYMYXIN B/± BACITRACIN

Neosporin, Neosporin GU Irrigant, and others

No ? C

Topical antibiotic

Ointment (topical): 3.5 mg neomycin sulfate, 400 U bacitracin, 5000 U polymyxin B/g
Cream: 3.5 mg neomycin sulfate, 10,000 U polymyxin B/g
Ointment (ophthalmic): 3.5 mg neomycin sulfate, 400 U bacitracin, 10,000 U polymyxin B/g
Solution, Genitourinary Irrigant: 40 mg neomycin sulfate, 200, 000 U polymyxin B/ ml (1, 20 ml); contains methylparabens

Topical: apply to minor wounds and burns TID
Ophthalmic: apply small amount to conjunctiva QD–QID

Do **not** use for extended periods. May cause superinfection, delayed healing. See Neomycin. Ophthalmic preparation may cause stinging and sensitivity to bright light.

NEOSTIGMINE
Prostigmin and others
Anticholinesterase (cholinergic) agent
Tabs: 15 mg (bromide)
Inj: 0.25, 0.5, 1 mg/ml (methylsulfate)

Yes   ?   C

Myasthenia gravis-Diagnosis: **Use with atropine (see comments).**
Children: 0.025–0.04 mg/kg IM × 1
Adults: 0.022 mg/kg IM × 1
Myasthenia gravis—Treatment:
Children:
　IM, IV, SC: 0.01–0.04 mg/kg/dose Q2–3 hr PRN
　PO: 2 mg/kg/24 hr ÷ Q3–4 hr
Adults: IM, IV, SC: 0.5–2.5 mg/dose Q1–3 hr PRN
　PO: 15 mg/dose TID. May increase every 1–2 days. Dosage requirements may vary from 15–375 mg/24 hr.
Reversal of nondepolarizing neuromuscular blocking agents:
Administer with atropine or glycopyrrolate.
Infants: 0.025–0.1 mg/kg/dose IV
Children: 0.025–0.08 mg/kg/dose IV
Adults: 0.5–2.5 mg/dose IV
Max dose: 5 mg/dose

Contraindicated in GI and urinary obstruction. **Caution** in asthmatics.
　May cause cholinergic crisis, bronchospasm, salivation, nausea, vomiting, diarrhea, miosis, diaphoresis, lacrimation, bradycardia, hypotension, fatigue, confusion, respiratory depression, seizures. Titrate for each patient, but **avoid** excessive cholinergic effects.
　For diagnosis of myasthenia gravis (MG), administer atropine 0.011 mg/kg/dose IV immediately before or IM (0.011 mg/kg/dose) 30 minutes before neostigmine. For treatment of MG, patients may need higher doses of neostigmine at times of greatest fatigue.
　Antidote: Atropine 0.01–0.04 mg/kg/dose. Atropine and epinephrine should be available in the event of a hypersensitivity reaction.
　Adjust dose in renal failure (see p. 940).

NEVIRAPINE
Viramine, NVP
Antiviral, non-nucleoside reverse transcriptase inhibitor
Tabs: 200 mg
Suspension: 10 mg/ml (240 ml)

Yes   3   C

Neonate-3 months (investigational dose from ACTG 356): Start with 5 mg/kg/dose QD PO × 14 days, followed by 120 mg/m^2/dose Q12 hr PO × 14 days, then 200 mg/m^2/dose Q12 hr PO

Children: Start with 120 mg/m^2/dose QD PO × 14 days, then increase dose to 120 mg/m^2/dose Q12 hr PO if no rash or other side effects. Usual maintenance dose: 120–200 mg/m^2/dose Q12 hr PO; **max dose:** 200 mg/dose Q12 hr PO

Adults: Start with 200 mg/dose QD PO × 14 days, then increase to 200 mg/dose Q12 hr if no rash or other side effects.

Use with **caution** in patients with hepatic or renal dysfunction. Most frequent side effects include: skin rash (may be life-threatening, including Stevens-Johnson), sedation, headache, and GI discomfort. **Discontinue therapy** if a severe rash or a rash with fever, blistering, oral lesions, conjunctivitis, and muscle aches occurs. Monitor liver function tests and CBCs.

Nevirapine induces the CYP450 3A4 drug metabolizing isoenzyme to cause an autoinduction of its own metabolism within the first 2-4 weeks of therapy and has the potential to interact with many drugs. The drug can decrease levels of indinavir, ritonavir, and saquinavir. Rifampin and rifabutin can lower serum levels of nevirapine. Cimetidine, clarithromycin, erythromycin, ketoconazole can increase serum levels of nevirapine. **Carefully review the patients' drug profile for other drug interactions each time** nevirapine **is initiated or when a new drug is added to a regimen containing nevirapine.**

Doses can be administered with food and concurrently with didanosine.

NICARDIPINE
Cardene, Cardene SR
Calcium channel blocker, antihypertensive
Caps (immediate release): 20, 30 mg
Sustained Release Caps: 30, 45, 60 mg
Inj: 2.5 mg/ml (10 ml)

Yes 3 C

Children:
Hypertension: 0.5–3 mcg/kg/min via continuous IV infusion
Adult:
Angina: 20 mg PO (immediate release) TID, dose may be increased after 3 days to 40 mg PO TID
Hypertension:
Oral:
Immediate release: 20 mg PO TID, dose may be increased after 3 days to 40 mg PO TID if needed.
Sustained release: 30 mg PO BID, dose may be increased after 3 days to 60 mg PO BID if needed.
Continuous IV infusion: Start at 5 mg/hr, increase dose as needed by 2.5 mg/hr Q5–15 min up to a **maximum** of 15 mg/hr. Following attainment of desired BP, decrease infusion to 3 mg/hr and adjust rate as needed to maintain desired response.

Reported use in children has been limited to a small number pre-term infants, infants and children up to 11 years old. **Contraindicated** in advanced aortic stenosis. Use with **caution** in hepatic or renal dysfunction by carefully titrating dose. The drug undergoes significant first pass metabolism through the liver and is excreted in the urine (60%). May cause headache, dizziness, asthenia, peripheral edema, and GI symptoms. **See nifedipine for drug and food interactions.** Onset of action for PO administration is 20 minutes with peak effects in 0.5–2 hours. IV onset of action is 1 minute. Duration of action following a single IV or PO dose is 3 hours. For additional information, see p. 12.

NIFEDIPINE
Adalat, Adalat CC, Procardia, Procardia XL, and others
Calcium channel blocker, antihypertensive
Caps: (Adalat, Procardia): 10 mg (0.34 ml), 20 mg (0.45 ml)
Sustained Release Tabs: (Adalat CC, Procardia XL): 30, 60, 90 mg.

No 1 C

Children:
Hypertension/Hypertensive
Urgency: 0.25–0.5 mg/kg/dose
Q4–6 hr PRN PO/SL. **Max dose:** 10
mg/dose or 3 mg/kg/24 hr
Hypertrophic Cardiomyopathy: 0.5–
0.9 mg/kg/24 hr ÷ Q6–8 hr PO/SL
Adults:
Hypertension:

Caps: Start with 10 mg/dose PO TID.
May increase to 30 mg/dose PO TID-
QID.

Max dose: 180 mg/24 hr
Sustained Release: Start with 30–
60 mg PO QD. May increase to **max
dose:** 120 mg/24 hr

Use with **caution** in patients with
CHF and aortic stenosis. May
cause severe hypotension,
peripheral edema, flushing, tachycardia,
headaches, dizziness, nausea,
palpitations, syncope. Nifedipine is a
substrate for CYP 450 3A3/4 (see p.
924). Do **not** administer with grapefruit
juice; may increase bioavailability and
effects. Nifedipine may increase
phenytoin, cyclosporine, and digoxin
levels. For hypertensive emergencies, see
p. 12.

For sublingual administration, capsule
must be punctured and liquid expressed
into mouth. A small amount is absorbed
via the SL route. The majority of effects
are due to swallowing and oral absorption.
Do **not** crush or chew sustained release
tablet dosage form.

NITROFURANTOIN

Furadantin, Macrodantin, Macrobid, and others
Antibiotic　　　　　　　　　　　　　　　　Yes　1　B
Caps (Macrocrystals): 25, 50, 100 mg
Caps (Dual release, Macrobid): 100 mg (25 mg macrocrystal/75 mg monohydrate)
Caps, extended release: 100 mg
Susp: 25 mg/5 ml

Children (>1 month):
Treatment: 5–7 mg/kg/24 hr ÷
Q6 hr PO; **max dose:** 400 mg/
24 hr
UTI Prophylaxis: 1–2 mg/kg/dose QHS
PO; **max dose:** 100 mg/24 hr
Adults:
(macrocrystals): 50–100 mg/dose
Q6 hr PO
(dual-release): 100 mg/dose Q12 hr PO
UTI Prophylaxis (macrocrystals):
50–100 mg/dose PO QHS

Contraindicated in severe renal
disease, G6PD deficiency, infants
<1 mo of age, and pregnant
women at term. May cause nausea,
hypersensitivity reactions, vomiting,
cholestatic jaundice, headache, polyneuropathy, and hemolytic anemia.
Causes false-positive urine glucose with
Clinitest. Administer doses with food or
milk.

NITROGLYCERIN

Tridil, Nitro-bid, Nitrostat, and others
Vasodilator, antihypertensive

Inj: 0.5, 0.8, 5, 10 mg/ml
Sublingual tabs: 0.3, 0.4, 0.6 mg
Buccal tabs (controlled release): 1, 2, 3 mg
Sustained release tabs: 2.6, 6.5, 9 mg
Sustained release caps: 2.5, 6.5, 9, 13 mg
Ointment, topical: 2%
Patch: 2.5, 5, 7.5, 10, 15 mg/24 hr
Spray, translingual: 0.4 mg per metered spray (13.8 g, delivers 200 doses per canister)

No   ?   B

Children:
Continuous IV infusion: Begin with
    0.25–0.5 mcg/kg/min; may
increase by 0.5–1 mcg/kg/min Q3–
5 min PRN. Usual dose: 1–5
mcg/kg/min. **Max dose:** 20 mcg/kg/min
Adults:
Continuous IV infusion: 5 mcg/min IV,
then increase Q3–5 min PRN by 5 mcg/
min up to 20 mcg/min. If no response,
increase by 10 mcg/min Q3–5 min
PRN up to a **maximum** of 200 mcg/
min.
Sublingual: 0.2–0.6 mg Q5 min. **Max**
of 3 doses in 15 min.
Oral: 2.5–9 mg BID-TID; up to 26 mg
QID
To prepare infusion: See inside front
cover.
**NOTE: the dosage units for adults are in
mcg/min; compared to mcg/kg/min for
children.**

Contraindicated in glaucoma and
severe anemia. In small doses
(1–2 mcg/kg/min) acts mainly on
systemic veins and decreases preload. At
3–5 mcg/kg/min acts on systemic
arterioles to decrease resistance. May
cause headache, flushing, GI upset,
blurred vision, methemoglobinemia. Use
with **caution** in severe renal impairment,
increased ICP, hepatic failure. IV
nitroglycerin may antagonize
anticoagulant effect of heparin.

Decrease dose gradually in patients
receiving drug for prolonged periods to
avoid withdrawal reaction. Must use
polypropylene infusion sets to avoid
adsorption of drug to plastic tubing.

NITROPRUSSIDE
Nipride and others
Vasodilator, antihypertensive
Inj: 50 mg

Yes   ?   C

 Children and Adults: IV, continuous infusion
Dose: Start at 0.3–0.5 mcg/kg/min, titrate to effect. Usual dose is 3–4 mcg/kg/min. **Max dose:** 10 mcg/kg/min.
To prepare infusion: See inside front cover.

Contraindicated in patients with decreased cerebral perfusion and in situations of compensatory hypertension (increased ICP). Monitor for hypotension and acidosis. Dilute with D5W and protect from light.

Nitroprusside is nonenzymatically converted to cyanide, which is converted to thiocyanate. Cyanide may produce metabolic acidosis and methemoglobinemia. Thiocyanate may produce psychosis and seizures. Monitor thiocyanate levels if used for >48 hrs or if dose ≥4 mcg/kg/min. **Thiocyanate levels should be <50 mg/L.** Monitor **cyanide levels (toxic levels >2 mcg/ml)** in patients with hepatic dysfunction and thiocyanate levels in patients with renal dysfunction.

NOREPINEPHRINE BITARTRATE
Levophed and others
Adrenergic agonist
Inj: 1 mg/ml as norepinephrine base

No   ?   C

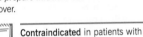

Children: Continuous IV infusion doses as norepinephrine base. Start at 0.05–0.1 mcg/kg/min. Titrate to effect. Max dose: 2 mcg/kg/min.
To prepare infusion: See inside front cover.
Adults: Continuous IV infusion doses as norepinephrine base. Start at 4 mcg/min and titrate to effect. Usual dosage range: 8–12 mcg/min. NOTE: the dosage units for adults are in mcg/min; compared to mcg/kg/min for children.

May cause cardiac arrhythmias, hypertension, hypersensitivity, headaches, vomiting, uterine contractions, and organ ischemia. May cause decreased renal blood flow and urine output. Avoid extravasation into tissues; may cause severe tissue necrosis. If this occurs, treat locally with phentolamine.

NORFLOXACIN

Noroxin, Chibroxin
Antibiotic, quinolone
Tabs: 400 mg
Ophthalmic drops: 3 mg/ml (5 ml)

Yes   3   C

Adults: 400 mg PO BID
N. gonorrheae: 800 mg once PO
Ophthalmic: 1–2 drops QID. May
give up to Q2 hr for severe infections.

Like other quinolones, there is
concern regarding arthropathy,
which has been shown in
immature animals. Norfloxacin does **not**
adequately treat chlamydia co-infections.
Use with **caution** in children <18 years.
Inhibits CYP 450 1A2, see p. 924. May
increase serum theophylline levels. May
prolong PT in patients on warfarin. See
Ciprofoxacin for common side effects and
drug interactions. Administer doses on an
empty stomach.

Adjust dose in renal failure (see p. 934).

NORTRIPTYLINE HYDROCHLORIDE

Pamelor, Aventyl, and others
Antidepressant, tricyclic
Caps: 10, 25, 50, 75 mg
Sol: 10 mg/5 ml (4% alcohol)

No   3   D

Depression:
Children 6–12 years: 1–3 mg/kg/
24 hr ÷ TID-QID PO or 10–20 mg/
24 hr ÷ TID-QID PO
Adolescents: 1–3 mg/kg/24 hr ÷ TID-
QID PO or 30–50 mg/24 hr ÷ TID-QID
PO
Adults: 75–100 mg/24 hr ÷ TID-QID
PO
Max dose: 150 mg/24 hr
Nocturnal Enuresis:
6–7 years (20–25 kg): 10 mg PO QHS
8–11 years (25–35 kg): 10–20 mg PO
QHS
>11 years (35–54 kg): 25–35 mg PO
QHS

See Imipramine for common side
effects. Less CNS and
anticholinergic side effects than
amitriptyline. Administer with food to
decrease GI upset. Therapeutic
antidepressant effects occur in 7–21 days.
Do **not** discontinue abruptly. Use lower
doses and titrate doses slower in hepatic
impairment.

**Therapeutic nortriptyline levels for
depression: 50–150 ng/ml.**
Recommended serum sampling time:
obtain a single level 8 or more hours after
an oral dose (following 4 days of
continuous dosing for children and after
9–10 days for adults).

NYSTATIN

Mycostatin, Nilstat, and others
Antifungal agent

No 1 B

Tabs: 500,000 U
Troches/pastilles: 200,000 U
Susp: 100,000 U/ml (60, 473 ml)
Cream/Ointment: 100,000 U/g (15, 30 g)
Topical powder: 100,000 U/g (15 g)
Vaginal Tabs: 100,000 U (15s, 30s)

Oral:
Preterm infants: 0.5 ml (50,000 U) to each side of mouth QID
Term infants: 1 ml (100,000 U) to each side of mouth QID
Children/Adults:
    Susp: 4–6 ml (400,000–600,000 U) swish and swallow QID
    Troche: 200,000–400,000 U 4–5 ×/ 24 hr
Vaginal: 1 tab QHS × 14 days
Topical: Apply BID-QID

May produce diarrhea and GI side effects. Treat until 48–72 hr after resolution of symptoms. Drug is poorly absorbed through the GI tract. Do **not** swallow troches whole (allow to dissolve slowly). Oral suspension should be swished about the mouth and retained in the mouth as long as possible before swallowing.

OCTREOTIDE ACETATE

Sandostatin
Somatostatin analog, antisecretory agent

No ? B

Inj (amps): 0.05, 0.1, 0.5 mg/ml (1 ml)
Inj (multi-dose vials): 0.2, 1 mg/ml (5 ml)

Infants and Children:
Diarrhea (IV/SC): 1–10 mcg/kg/24 hr ÷ Q12–24 hr. Dose may be increased within the recommended range by 0.3 mcg/kg/dose every 3 days as needed.
Max dose: 1500 mcg/24 hr

Cholelithiasis, hyperglycemia, hypoglycemia, nausea, diarrhea, abdominal discomfort, headache, pain at injection site may occur. Growth hormone suppression may occur with long-term use. Cyclosporine levels may be reduced in patients receiving this drug.

OFLOXACIN

Floxin, Floxin Otic, Ocuflox
Antibiotic, quinolone
Tabs: 200, 300, 400 mg
Inj: 4, 20, 40 mg/ml
Otic Solution: 0.3% (5 ml)
Ophthalmic Solution: 0.3% (1, 5 ml)

Yes   3   C

Adults:
Lower Respiratory Tract, Skin, and Skin Structure Infections: 400 mg PO/IV Q12 hr × 10 days
Uncomplicated Gonorrhea: 400 mg PO × 1, plus treatment for chlamydia.
Nongonococcal (Chlamydia) Urethritis, Cervicitis: 300 mg PO/IV Q12 hr × 10 days
UTI: 200 mg PO/IV Q12 hr × 3–10 days
Prostatitis: 300 mg PO/IV Q12 hr × 6 weeks; **maximum IV** use at 10 days, convert to PO
Otitic Use:
Otitis Externa:
1–12 yr: 5 drops to affected ear(s) BID × 10 days
>12 yr: 10 drops to affected ear(s) BID × 10 days
Chronic Suppurative Otitis Media:
≥12 yr: 10 drops to affected ear(s) BID × 14 days
Acute Otitis Media with Tympanostomy Tubes:
1–12 yr: 5 drops to affected ear(s) BID × 10 days
Ophthalmic Use:
>1 yr: 1 drop to affected eye(s) Q2–4 hr × 2 days, then QID for an additional 5 days

Like other quinolones, ofloxacin has caused arthropathy in immature animals; use with **caution** in children less than 18 years old. Common side effects with systemic use include nausea, diarrhea, headache, insomnia, dizziness. Rash, photosensitivity, pain, liver enzyme elevation, neutropenia have also been reported. Like most fluroquinolones, drug may inhibit CYP 450 1A2 (see p. 924) to increase theophylline serum levels. Antacids, didanosine, sucralfate, food may impair the oral absorption of ofloxacin. **Adjust dose in renal impairment (see p. 934).**

Pruritus, local irritation, taste perversion, dizziness, earache have been reported with otic use. Ocular burning/discomfort is frequent with ophthalmic use.

When using otic solution, warm solution by holding the bottle in the hand for 1–2 minutes. Cold solutions may result in dizziness. For otitis externa, patient should lie with affected ear upward before instillation and remain in the same position after dose administration for 5 minutes to enhance drug delivery. For acute otitis media with tympanostomy tubes, patient should lie in the same position prior to instillation and the tragus should be pumped 4 times after the dose to assist in drug delivery to the middle ear.

Administer oral doses on an empty stomach, 1 hour before or 2 hours after meals, and avoid antacids containing magnesium or aluminum or products containing iron or zinc within 4 hours before or 2 hours after dosing.

FORMULARY

OMEPRAZOLE

Prilosec
Gastric acid pump inhibitor
Caps, sustained release: 10, 20 mg
Oral Suspension: 2 mg/ml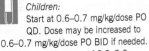

No 3 C

Children:
Start at 0.6–0.7 mg/kg/dose PO QD. Dose may be increased to 0.6–0.7 mg/kg/dose PO BID if needed. Effective dosage range of 0.3–3.3 mg/kg/24 hr has been reported.
Adults:
Duodenal ulcer: 20 mg/dose PO QD × 4–8 weeks
Gastric ulcer: 40 mg/24 hr PO ÷ QD-BID × 4–8 weeks
Pathological hypersecretory conditions: Start with 60 mg/24 hr PO QD. If needed, dose may be increased up to 120 mg/24 hr PO ÷ TID. Daily doses >80 mg should be administered in divided doses.

Common side effects: headache, diarrhea, nausea, and vomiting.
Drug induces CYP 450 1A2 and is also a substrate and inhibitor of CYP 2C19 (see p. 924). Increases $T_{1/2}$ of diazepam, phenytoin, and warfarin. May decrease absorption of itraconazole, ketoconazole, iron salts, and ampicillin esters.

Administer all doses before meals. Capsules contain enteric-coated granules to ensure bioavailability. Do **not** chew or crush capsule. For doses unable to be divided by 10 mg, capsule may be opened and intact pellets may be administered in an acidic beverage (i.e., apple juice, cranberry juice). The extemporaneously compounded oral suspension product may be less bioavailable due to the loss of the enteric-coating.

ONDANSETRON

Zofran
Antiemetic agent, 5-HT₃ antagonist
Inj: 2 mg/ml (2, 20 ml)
Premix Inj: 32 mg/50 ml
Tabs: 4, 8 mg
Oral Solution: 4 mg/5 ml (50 ml)

No ? B

Oral:
Children, dose based on body surface area:
<0.3 m²: 1 mg TID PRN nausea
0.3–0.6 m²: 2 mg TID PRN nausea
0.6–1 m²: 3 mg TID PRN nausea
>1 m²: 4–8 mg TID PRN nausea
Dose based on age:
<4 years: Use dose based on body surface area from above.
4–11 years: 4 mg TID PRN nausea
>12 years and adults: 8 mg TID PRN nausea
IV: Children and Adults:
Moderately emetogenic drugs:
0.15 mg/kg/dose at 30 min before, 4 and 8 hrs after emetogenic drugs. Then same dose Q4 hr PRN nausea.

Highly emetogenic drugs:
0.45 mg/kg/dose (**max:** 32 mg/dose) 30 min before emetogenic drugs. Then 0.15 mg/kg/dose Q4 hr PRN.

Bronchospasm, tachycardia, hypokalemia, seizures, headaches, lightheadedness, constipation or diarrhea, and transient increases in AST, ALT, and bilirubin may occur. Follow theophylline, phenytoin, or warfarin levels closely, if used in combination. Data limited for use in children <3 years old.
In severe hepatic impairment, extend internal up to QD and limit **max** dose to 8 mg/dose.

OPIUM TINCTURE
Deodorized tincture of opium
Narcotic, analgesic
No   2   B
Liquid: 10% opium. Contains 17%–21% alcohol (1 ml equivalent to 10 mg morphine)

Dilute 25-fold with water to make a final concentration of 0.4 mg/ml morphine equivalent. Dose for the **dilution** is equivalent to paregoric doses (see paregoric).

Use 25-fold dilution to treat neonatal abstinence syndrome (NAS). Doses for the **dilution** are equivalent to paregoric doses. Morphine may also be used to treat NAS. May cause respiratory depression, hypotension, bradycardia, and CNS depression. Pregnancy category changes to "D" if used for prolonged periods or in high doses at term.

For explanation of icons, see p. 600.

OXACILLIN

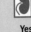

Bactocill, Prostaphlin
Antibiotic, penicillin (penicillinase resistant)

Yes   ?   B

Caps: 250, 500 mg
Oral Sol: 250 mg/5 ml
Inj: 0.25, 0.5, 1, 2, 4, 10 g; contains 2.8-3.1 mEq Na per 1 g drug

Neonates, IM/IV: doses are the same as for nafcillin.
Infants and Children:
Oral: 50–100 mg/kg/24 hr ÷ Q6 hr
IM/IV: 100–200 mg/kg/24 hr ÷ Q4–6 hr
Max dose: 12 g/24 hr
Adults:
Oral: 500–1000 mg/dose Q4–6 hr
IM/IV: 250–2000 mg/dose Q4–6 hr

Side effects include allergy, diarrhea, nausea, vomiting, leukopenia, and hepatotoxicity. CSF penetration is poor unless meninges are inflamed. Acute interstitial nephritis has been reported. Hematuria and azotemia have occurred in neonates and infants with high doses. Use the lower end of the usual dosage range for patients with creatinine clearances <10 ml/min. Oral form should be administered on an empty stomach.

OXYBUTYNIN CHLORIDE

Ditropan, Dridase
Anticholinergic agent, antispasmodic

No   ?   B

Tabs: 5 mg
Syrup: 1 mg/ml (473 ml)

Child ≤5 yr: 0.2 mg/kg/dose BID-QID PO
Child >5 yr: 5 mg/dose BID-TID PO
Adult: 5 mg/dose BID-QID PO

Anticholinergic side effects may occur, including drowsiness and hallucinations. **Contraindicated** in glaucoma, GI obstruction, megacolon, myasthenia gravis, severe colitis, hypovolemia, and GU obstruction.

OXYCODONE
Roxicodone, Oxycontin
Narcotic, analgesic
Sol: 1 mg/ml (8% alcohol), 20 mg/ml
Tabs: 5 mg
Controlled-release tabs (Oxycontin): 10, 20, 40 mg
Caps: 5 mg

Yes   2   B/D

Dose based upon oxycodone salt:
Children: 0.05–0.15 mg/kg/dose Q4–6 hr PRN up to 10 mg/dose PO
Adults: 5–10 mg Q4–6 hr PRN PO; see remarks for use of controlled release tablets.

Abuse potential, CNS and respiratory depression, increased ICP, histamine release, constipation, GI distress may occur. Use with **caution** in severe renal impairment.

Naloxone is the antidote. See p. 896 for equianalgesic dosing. Check dosages of acetaminophen or aspirin when using combination products (e.g., Tylox, Percodan). Aspirin is not recommended in children due to concerns of Reye's syndrome. When using controlled released tablets (Oxycontin), determine patients total 24 hr requirements and divide by 2 to administer on a Q12 hr dosing interval. Pregnancy category changes to "D" if used for prolonged periods or if high doses at term.

OXYCODONE AND ACETAMINOPHEN
Tylox, Roxilox, Percocet, and Roxicet 5/500
Combination analgesic with a narcotic
Capsule/Caplet: acetaminophen 500 mg, oxycodone HCl 5 mg
Tabs: acetaminophen 325 mg, oxycodone HCl 5 mg
Sol: acetaminophen 325 mg, oxycodone HCl 5 mg/5 ml (0.4% alcohol)

Yes   2   C

Dose based on amount of oxycodone and acetaminophen.

See oxycodone and acetaminophen.

For explanation of icons, see p. 600.

OXYCODONE AND ASPIRIN

Percodan, Percodan-Demi, Roxiprin
Combination analgesic (narcotic and salicylate)
Yes   2   D

Tabs:

(Percodan or Roxiprin): aspirin 325 mg, oxycodone HCl 4.5 mg and oxycodone tereph 0.38 mg

(Percodan-Demi): aspirin 325 mg, oxycodone HCl 2.25 mg, and oxycodone tereph 0.19 mg

Dose based on amount of oxycodone (combined salts) and aspirin.

See oxycodone and aspirin. Do **not** use in children <16 yr because of Reye's syndrome.

OXYMETAZOLINE

Nasal: Afrin, Allerest 12 Hour Nasal, Nostrilla, and others
Ophthalmic: OcuClear, Visine LR
Nasal decongestant, vasoconstrictor
No   ?   C

Nasal Drops: 0.025%, 0.05%
Nasal Spray: 0.05%
Ophthalmic Drops: 0.025% (15, 30 ml)

Nasal decongestant (**not to exceed 3 days in duration**):

2–5 yr: 2–3 drops of 0.025% solution in each nostril BID
≥ 6 yr–Adults: 2–3 sprays or 2–3 drops of 0.05% solution in each nostril BID
Ophthalmic:
≥6 yr–Adults: Instill 1–2 drops in the affected eye(s) Q6 hr

Contraindicated in patients on MAO inhibitor therapy. Rebound nasal congestion may occur with excessive use (>3 days) via the nasal route. Systemic absorption may occur with either route of administration. Headache, dizziness, hypertension, transient burning, stinging, dryness, nasal mucosa ulceration, sneezing, blurred vision, mydriasis have occurred. Do **not** use ophthalmic solution if it changes color or becomes cloudy.

PALIVIZUMAB

Synagis
Monoclonal antibody
No   ?   C

Inj: 100 mg

RSV Prophylaxis:
≤2 yrs with Chronic Lung Disease or Premature Infants (<35 weeks gestation) <12 months of age: 15 mg/kg/dose IM Q monthly during the RSV season.

RSV season typically November through April in the northern hemisphere but may begin earlier or persist later in certain communities. Use with caution in patients with thrombocytopenia or any coagulation disorder because of IM route of administration. IM is currently the only route of administration. The following adverse effects have been reported at slightly higher incidences when compared to placebo: rhinitis, rash, pain, increased liver enzymes, pharyngitis, cough, wheeze, diarrhea, vomiting, conjunctivitis, and anemia.

Advantages over intravenous RSV immune globulin include smaller fluid volume of drug, ease of IM injection (compared to lengthy IV infusion), and does not interfere with the response to routine childhood vaccines.

Each dose should be administered IM in the anterolateral aspect of the thigh. Avoid injection in the gluteal muscle because of risk for damage to the sciatic nerve. Reconstitute each vial with 1 ml sterile water for injection and gently swirl the contents. Dose should be administered within 6 hours of reconstitution.

PANCREATIC ENZYMES

No   ?   C

See pp. 916–917 for description and contents of lipase, protease, and amylase.

Initial doses: (actual requirements are patient specific)
Enteric-coated microspheres and microtabs:
Infants: 2000–4000 U lipase per 120 ml formula or per breast feeding
Children <4 yr: 1000 U lipase/kg/meal
Children ≥4 yr: 500 U lipase/kg/meal
The total daily dose should include approximately three meals and two to three snacks per day. Snack doses are approximately ½ meal doses.

May cause occult GI bleeding, allergic reactions to porcine proteins, hyperuricemia, and hyperuricosuria with high doses. Dose should be titrated to eliminate diarrhea and to minimize steatorrhea. Do not chew microspheres or microtabs. Concurrent administration with H_2 antagonists or gastric acid pump inhibitors may enhance enzyme efficacy. Doses higher than 6000 U lipase/kg/meal have been associated with colonic strictures in children <12 years of age. Powder dosage form is not preferred due to potential GI mucosal ulceration.

PANCURONIUM BROMIDE

Pavulon
Nondepolarizing neuromuscular blocking agent   **Yes   ?   C**
Injection: 1, 2 mg/ml (contains 1% benzyl alcohol)

Neonate:
Initial: 0.02 mg/kg/dose IV
Maintenance: 0.05–0.1 mg/kg/
dose Q 0.5–4 hr PRN
1 mo–adult:
Initial: 0.04–0.1 mg/kg/dose IV
Maintenance: 0.015–0.1 mg/kg/dose IV
Q30–60 min
Continuous IV infusion: 0.1 mg/kg/hr

Onset of action is 1–2 minutes.
Drug effects may be accentuated
by hypothermia, acidosis, neonatal
age, decreased renal function, halothane,
succinylcholine, hypokalemia, clindamycin, tetracycline, and aminoglycoside
antibiotics. May cause tachycardia,
salivation, and wheezing. Antidote is
neostigmine (with atropine or glycopyrrolate). **Avoid** use in severe renal
impairment (CrCl <10 ml/min).

PAREGORIC

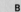

Camphorated opium tincture
Narcotic, antidiarrheal   **No   2   B**
Camphorated tincture: 2 mg (morphine equivalent)/5 ml (some
preparations contain up to 45% alcohol)

Analgesia/Antidiarrheal:
Children: 0.25–0.5 ml/kg/dose PO
QD-QID
Adults: 5–10 ml/dose PO QD-QID
Neonatal opiate withdrawal:
Start with 0.2–0.3 ml/dose Q3–4 hr,
increase dose by
0.05 ml/dose Q3–4 hr until symptoms
abate; **max dose:** 0.7 ml/dose

Each 5 ml paregoric contains 2 mg
morphine equivalent, 0.02 ml anise
oil, 20 mg benzoic acid, 20 mg
camphor, 0.2 ml glycerin, and alcohol. The
final concentration of morphine equivalent
is 0.4 mg/ml. This is 25-fold less potent
than undiluted deodorized tincture of
opium (DTO: 10 mg morphine equivalent/
ml). **If using DTO to treat neonatal
abstinence, must dilute 25-fold prior to
use.** Similar side effects to morphine. After
symptoms are controlled for several days,
dose for opiate withdrawal should be
decreased gradually over a 2- to 4-week
period (e.g., by 10% Q2–3 days).

PAROMYCIN SULFATE

Humatin
Amebicide, antibiotic (aminoglycoside)
Caps: 250 mg

No   ?   C

Intestinal Amebiasis (Entamoeba histolytica) *and* Dientamoeba fragilis *infection:*
Children and Adults: 25–35 mg/kg/ 24 hr PO ÷ Q8 hr × 7 days
Tapeworm (see comments):
Children: 11 mg/kg/dose Q15 min × 4 doses
Adults: 1 g Q15 min × 4 doses
Tapeworm (Hymenolepis nana):
Children and Adults: 45 mg/kg/dose PO QD × 5–7 days
Cryptosporidial diarrhea:
Adults: 1.5–3 g/24 hr PO ÷ 3–6 × daily. Duration varies from 10–14 days to 4–8 weeks. Maintenance therapy has also been used.

Tapeworms affected by short-duration therapy include *T. saginata, T. solium, D. latum,* and *D. caninum.* Drug is poorly absorbed and therefore not indicated for sole treatment of extraintestinal amebiasis. Side effects include GI disturbance, hematuria, rash, ototoxicity, and hypocholesterolemia.

PAROXETINE

Paxil
Antidepressant, selective serotonin reuptake inhibitor
Tabs: 10, 20, 30, 40 mg

Yes   3   B

For explanation of icons, see p. 600.

Children:
Depression (limited data, in an open labeled trial of 45 children (<14 yrs old—mean age 10.7 ± 2 yrs): Start with 10 mg PO QD. If needed adjust upwards. A mean dose of 16.2 mg/24 hr was used for an average of 8.4 months in the open label trial. Additional studies are needed.

Adult:
Depression: Start with 20 mg PO QAM × 4 weeks. If no clinical improvement, increase dose by 10 mg/24 hr Q 7 days PRN up to a **maximum** of 50 mg/24 hr.
Obsessive Compulsive Disorder: Start with 20 mg PO QD; increase dose by 10 mg/24 hr Q 7 days PRN up to a **maximum** of 60 mg/24 hr. Usual dose is 40 mg PO QD.
Panic Disorder: Start with 10 mg PO QD; increase dose by 10 mg/24 hr Q 7 days PRN up to a **maximum** of 60 mg/24 hr.

Contraindicated in patients taking MAO inhibitors or within 14 days of discontinuing MAO inhibitors. Common side effects include anxiety, nausea, anorexia, decreased appetite. Paroxetine is an inhibitor and substrate for CYP 450 2D6 (see p. 924). May increase the effects/toxicity of tricyclic antidepressants, theophylline, and warfarin. Cimetidine, ritonavir, MAO inhibitors (fatal serotonin syndrome), dextromethorphan, phenothiazines and type 1C antiarrhythmics may increase the effect/toxicity of paroxetine.

Patients with severe renal or hepatic impairment should initiate therapy at 10 mg/day and increase dose as needed up to a maximum of 40 mg/24 hr. Do **not** discontinue therapy abruptly, may cause sweating, dizziness, confusion and tremor.

PEMOLINE
Cylert
CNS stimulant
Tabs: 18.75, 37.5, 75 mg
Chewable tabs: 37.5 mg

Yes ? B

Children ≥6 yr:
Initial: 37.5 mg QAM PO
Increment: 18.75 mg/24 hr at weekly intervals
Maintenance: 0.5–3 mg/kg/24 hr (effective dose range: 56.25–75 mg/24 hr)
Max dose: 112.5 mg/24 hr
Effect may not be seen for 3–4 weeks. **Do not abruptly discontinue drug.**

May cause insomnia, headache, seizures, anorexia, hypersensitivity, depression, abdominal pain, movement disorders, hepatotoxicity, drug dependence. Use with **caution** in renal disease (~50% excreted in urine unchanged). **Contraindicated** in hepatic insufficiency and Tourette's syndrome. Long-term use associated with growth inhibition. **Not recommended for children <6 years old.**

PENICILLAMINE

Cuprimine, Depen
Heavy metal chelator
Tabs: 250 mg
Caps: 125, 250 mg
Susp: 50 mg/ml

Yes ? D

Lead chelation therapy (third-line therapy):
Children: 30–40 mg/kg/24 hr or 600–750 mg/m²/24 hr PO ÷ TID-QID. **Max dose:** 1.5 g/hr
Adults: 1–1.5 g/24 hr PO ÷ BID-TID
Durations of treatment vary from 1–6 months.
Wilson's disease (see remarks for titration information):
Infants and Children: 20 mg/kg/24 hr PO ÷ BID–QID. **Max dose:** 1 g/24 hr
Adults: 250 mg/dose PO QID. **Max dose:** 2 g/24 hr
Arsenic poisoning:
100 mg/kg/24 hr PO ÷ Q6 hr × 5 days. **Max dose:** 1 g/24 hr
Cystinuria (see remarks for titration information):
Infants and young children: 30 mg/kg/24 hr ÷ QID PO
Older children and adults: 1–4 g/24 hr ÷ QID PO
Primary biliary cirrhosis; Adults:
Initial: 250 mg/24 hr PO; increase by 250 mg Q2 wk to a total of 1 g/24 hr (given as 250 mg QID)
Juvenile Rheumatoid Arthritis:
5 mg/kg/24 hr ÷ QD-BID PO × 2 mo, then 10 mg/kg/24 hr ÷ QD-BID PO × 4 mo

Dose should be given 1 hr before or 2 hr after meals. **AAP relegates this drug as a third line agent** indicated only after unacceptable reaction with oral succimer and calcium EDTA (see p. 34). If used, must be in lead-free environment, since it can increase absorption of lead if present in GI tract. **Avoid** use if patient's creatinine clearance is <50 ml/min. Follow CBC, LFTs, and urine. Can cause optic neuritis, fever, rash, nausea, altered taste, vomiting, lupuslike syndrome, nephrotic syndrome, peripheral neuropathy, leukopenia, eosinophilia, thrombocytopenia. May reduce serum digoxin levels. **Avoid** concomitant administration with iron, antacids, and food.

Patients treated for Wilson's disease, rheumatoid arthritis, or cystinuria should be treated with pyridoxine 25–50 mg/24 hr. Titrate urinary copper excretion to >1 mg/24 hr for patients with Wilson's disease. Patients with cystinuria should have doses titrated to maintain urinary cystine excretion at <100–200 mg/24 hr.

For explanation of icons, see p. 600.

FORMULARY

PENICILLIN G PREPARATIONS— BENZATHINE

Permapen, Bicillin L-A

No   ?   B

Antibiotic, penicillin (very long-acting IM)

Inj: 300,000, 600,000 U/ml (may contain parabens and povidone).
Injection should be IM only.

 Group A streptococci:
Infants and Children:
25,000–50,000 U/kg/dose IM
× 1. **Max dose:** 1.2 million U/dose
Or
>1 month and <27 kg: 600,000
U/dose IM × 1
≥27 kg and Adults: 1.2 million U/dose
IM × 1
Rheumatic Fever prophylaxis:
Infants and Children: 25,000–50,000
U/kg/dose IM Q3–4 wk. **Max dose:**
1.2 million U/dose

Adults: 1.2 million U/dose IM Q3–4 wk
or 600,000 U/dose IM Q2 wk
*Syphilis: early acquired and >1 year
duration:* See p. 399.

Provides sustained levels for
2–4 weeks. Side effects same as
for Penicillin G. **Do not administer
intravenously; cardiac arrest and death
may occur. Not** recommended for
congenital syphilis.

PENICILLIN G PREPARATIONS— PENICILLIN G BENZATHINE AND PENICILLIN G PROCAINE

No   ?   B

Bicillin C-R, Bicillin C-R 900/300

Antibiotic, penicillin (very long acting)

Bicillin CR:
150,000 U PenG procaine + 150,000 U PenG benzathine/ml to provide
300,000 U penicillin per 1 ml (10 ml vial)
300,000 U PenG procaine + 300,000 U PenG benzathine/ml to provide
600,000 U penicillin per 1 ml (1, 2 ml tubex, 4 ml syringe)
Bicillin CR (900/300): 150,000 U PenG procaine + 450,000 U PenG
benzathine/ml (2 ml tubex)
Injection should be for IM only.

Acute streptococcal infection: Dose
such that PenG benzathine is given
in recommended amount (1997
Red Book, p. 488). See doses for PenG
benzathine.

This preparation provides early
peak levels in addition to prolonged
levels of penicillin in the blood. Do
not administer IV. The addition of procaine
penicillin has not been shown to be more
efficacious than benzathine alone.
However, it may reduce injection
discomfort.

PENICILLIN G PREPARATIONS— POTASSIUM AND SODIUM

Various trade names

Yes ? B

Antibiotic, aqueous penicillin

Inj (K+): 1, 5, 10, 20 million units (contains 1.7 mEq K and 0.3 mEq Na/1 million unit Pen G)

Inj (Na+): 5 million units (contains 2 mEq Na/1 million unit Pen G)

Conversion: 250 mg = 400,000 U

Neonates: IM/IV
≤7 days:
  ≤2 kg: 50,000–100,000 U/kg/ 24 hr ÷ Q12 hr
  >2 kg: 75,000–150,000 U/kg/24 hr ÷ Q8 hr
>7 days:
  <1.2 kg: 50,000–100,000 U/kg/ 24 hr ÷ Q12 hr
  1.2–2 kg: 75,000–150,000 U/kg/ 24 hr ÷ Q8 hr
  ≥2 kg: 100,000–200,000 U/kg/24 hr ÷ Q6 hr
Group B Streptococcal Meningitis:
  ≤7 days: 250,000–450,000 U/kg/ 24 hr ÷ Q8 hr
  >7 days: 450,000 U/kg/24 hr ÷ Q6 hr

Infants and Children:
  IM/IV: 100,000–400,000 U/kg/24 hr ÷ Q4–6 hr; **max dose:** 24 million U/24 hr
Adults:
  IM/IV: 4–24 million U/24 hr ÷ Q4–6 hr
Congenital Syphilis, Neurosyphilis: See p. 399.

Use penicillin V potassium for oral use. Side effects: anaphylaxis, urticaria, hemolytic anemia, interstitial nephritis, Jarisch-Herxheimer reaction (syphilis). $T_{1/2}$ = 30 min; may be prolonged by concurrent use of probenecid. For meningitis, use higher daily dose at shorter dosing intervals. **Adjust dose in renal impairment; see p. 934 for details.**

PENICILLIN G PREPARATIONS— PROCAINE

Wycillin, Cysticillin A.S., Pfizerpen-AS

No ? B

Antibiotic, penicillin (long-acting IM)

Inj: 300,000, 500,000, 600,000 U/ml (may contain parabens, phenol, providone, and formaldehyde).

Contains 120 mg procaine per 300,000 U.

Newborns: 50,000 U/kg/24 hr IM QD; see comments
Infants and Children:
25,000–50,000 U/kg/24 hr ÷ Q12–24 hr IM. **Max dose:** 4.8 million U/24 hr
Adults: 0.6–4.8 million U/24 hr ÷ Q12–24 hr IM
Congenital syphilis, Syphilis, Neurosyphilis: See p. 399.

Provides sustained levels for 2–4 days. Use with caution in neonates due to higher incidence of sterile abscess at injection site and risk of procaine toxicity. Side effects similar to penicillin G. In addition, may cause CNS stimulation and seizures. Do **not** administer IV; neurovascular damage may result. Large doses may be administered in two injection sites. No longer recommended for empiric treatment of gonorrhea due to resistant strains.

PENICILLIN V POTASSIUM

Pen Vee K, V-Cillin K, and others
Antibiotic, penicillin
Tabs: 125, 250, 500 mg
Oral Sol: 125 mg/5 ml, 250 mg/5 ml
250 mg = 400,000 U

Yes   ?   B

Children: 25–50 mg/kg/24 hr ÷ Q6–8 hr PO. Max dose: 3 g/24 hr
Adults: 250–500 mg/dose PO Q6–8 hr
Acute group A streptococcal pharyngitis:
  Children: 250 mg PO BID-TID × 10 days
  Adolescents and Adults: 500 mg PO BID-TID × 10 days
Secondary rheumatic fever/pneumococcal prophylaxis:
  ≤5 yr: 125 mg PO BID
  >5 yr: 250 mg PO BID

GI absorption is better than penicillin G. Note: Must be taken 1 hr before or 2 hr after meals. Penicillin will prevent rheumatic fever if started within 9 days of the acute illness. The BID regimen for streptococcal pharyngitis should be used only if good compliance is expected. **Adjust dose in renal failure (see p. 934).**

PENTAMIDINE ISETHIONATE

Pentam 300, Pentacarinat, NebuPent
Antibiotic, antiprotozoal
Inj: 300 mg (Pentam 300, Pentacarinat)
Inhalation: 300 mg (NebuPent)

Yes   ?   C

Treatment:
Pneumocystis carinii: 4 mg/kg/24 hr
IM/IV QD × 14–21 days
Trypanosomiasis (T. gambiense, T. rhodesiense): 4 mg/kg/24 hr IM QD × 10 days
Leishmaniasis (L. donovani): 2–4 mg/kg/dose IM QD or QOD × 15 doses
Prophylaxis:
Pneumocystis carinii:
IM/IV: 4 mg/kg/dose Q2–4 wk
Inhalation (≥5 yr): 300 mg in 6 ml H_2O via inhalation Q month (Respigard II nebulizer). See also p. 388 for indications.
Trypanosomiasis (T. gambiense, T. rhodesiense): 4 mg/kg/24 hr IM q3–6mo.
Max single dose: 300 mg

May cause hypoglycemia, hyperglycemia, hypotension (both IV and IM administration), nausea, vomiting, fever, mild hepatotoxicity, pancreatitis, megaloblastic anemia, nephrotoxicity, hypocalcemia, and granulocytopenia. Additive nephrotoxicity with aminoglycosides, amphotericin B, cisplatin, and vancomycin may occur. Aerosol administration may also cause bronchospasm, oxygen desaturation, dyspnea, and loss of appetite. Infuse IV over 1 hour to reduce the risk of hypotension. Sterile abscess may occur at IM injection site.

Adjust dose in renal impairment (see p. 934).

PENTOBARBITAL

Nembutal, others
Barbiturate
Caps: 50, 100 mg
Suppository: 30, 60, 120, 200 mg
Inj: 50 mg/ml
Elixir: 18.2 mg/5 ml

No   ?   D

Hypnotic
Children:
 PO/PR.
  <4 years: 3–6 mg/kg/dose QHS
  ≥4 years: 1.5–3 mg/kg/dose QHS
 IM: 2–6 mg/kg/dose. **Max dose:**
 100 mg
Pre-procedure Sedation
Children:
 PO/PR/IM: 2–6 mg/kg/dose. **Max**
 dose: 150 mg
 IV: 1–3 mg/kg/dose. **Max dose:**
 150 mg
Barbiturate coma
Children and Adults
 IV: Load: 10–15 mg/kg given slowly
 over 1–2 hr
 Maintenance: Begin at 1 mg/kg/hr.
 Dose range: 1–3 mg/kg/hr as needed.

Contraindicated in liver failure, CHF, and hypotension. No advantage over phenobarbital for control of seizures. Adjunct in treatment of ICP. May cause drug-related isoelectric EEG. Do **not** administer for >2 wk in treatment of insomnia. May cause hypotension, arrhythmias, hypothermia, respiratory depression, and dependence. Onset of action: PO/PR: 15–60 min; IM: 10–15 min; IV: 1 min. Duration of action: PO/PR: 1–4 hr; IV: 15 min.

Administer IV at a rate of <50 mg/min. Suppositories should **not** be divided.

Therapeutic serum levels: Sedation: 1–5 mg/L; Hypnosis: 5–15 mg/L; Coma: 20–40 mg/L (steady state is achieved after 4–5 days of continuous IV dosing).

PERMETHRIN

Elimite, Nix
Scabicidal agent

No   ?   B

Cream (Elimite-Rx): 5% (60 g)
Liquid cream rinse (Nix-OTC): 1% (60 ml)

Pediculus capitis, Phthirus pubis:
Head Lice: Saturate hair and scalp with 1% cream rinse after shampooing, rinsing, and towel drying hair. Leave on 10 minutes, then rinse. May repeat in 7–10 days. May be used for lice in other areas of the body (i.e., pubic lice) in same fashion.
Scabies: Apply 5% cream neck to toe (head to toe for infants and toddlers) wash off with water in 8–14 hours. May repeat in 7 days.

Ovicidal activity generally makes single dose regimen adequate.

Avoid contact with eyes during application. Shake well before using. May cause pruritus, hypersensitivity, burning, stinging, erythema, and rash. For either lice or scabies, instruct patient to launder bedding and clothing. For lice, treat symptomatic contacts only. For scabies, treat all contacts even if asymptomatic. The 5% cream has been used safely in children <1 month with neonatal scabies (a 6 hour application time was utilized). Topical cream dosage form contains formaldehyde. Dispense 60 gm per adult or 2 small children.

PHENAZOPYRIDINE HCl

Pyridium
Urinary analgesic
(OTC)

Yes ? B

Tabs: 95, 100, 200 mg
Oral Suspension: 10 mg/ml

Children 6–12 yr: 12 mg/kg/24 hr ÷ TID PO until symptoms of lower urinary tract irritation are controlled or 2 days.
Adults: 100–200 mg TID PO until symptoms are controlled or 2 days.

May cause hepatitis, GI distress, vertigo, headache, renal insufficiency, methemoglobinemia, hemolytic, anemia. Colors urine orange; stains clothing. May also stain contact lenses. Give doses after meals.

Adjust dose in renal impairment (see p. 940).

PHENOBARBITAL

Luminal, Solfoton, and others
Barbiturate

Yes 2 D

Tabs: 8, 15, 16, 16.2, 30, 32, 60, 65, 100 mg
Caps: 16 mg
Elixir: 15, 20 mg/5 ml (contains alcohol)
Inj: 30, 60, 65, 130 mg/ml (some injectable products may contain benzyl alcohol and propylene glycol)
Powder for Injection: 120 mg

Status epilepticus:
Loading dose, IV:
  Neonates, Infants, and Children:
  15–20 mg/kg/dose in a single or
  divided dose. May give additional
  5 mg/kg doses Q15–30 min to a
  maximum of 30 mg/kg.
Maintenance dose, PO/IV: Monitor
levels.
  Neonates: 3–5 mg/kg/24 hr ÷ QD-
  BID
  Infants: 5–6 mg/kg/24 hr ÷ QD-BID
  Children 1–5 yr: 6–8 mg/kg/24 hr ÷
  QD-BID
  Children 6–12 yr: 4–6 mg/kg/24 hr ÷
  QD-BID
  >12 yr: 1–3 mg/kg/24 hr ÷ QD-BID
Hyperbilirubinemia: <12 yr: 3–8 mg/kg/
24 hr PO ÷ BID-TID. Doses up to 12 mg/
kg/24 hr have been used.
Sedation, children: 6 mg/kg/24 hr PO ÷
TID
Pre-op sedation, children: 1–3
mg/kg/dose IM/IV/PO × 1. Give 60–90
minutes prior to procedure.

Contraindicated in porphyria,
severe respiratory disease with
dyspnea or obstruction. Use with
caution in hepatic or renal disease. IV
administration may cause respiratory
arrest or hypotension. Side effects include:
drowsiness, cognitive impairment, ataxia,
hypotension, hepatitis, skin rash,
respiratory depression, apnea,
megaloblastic anemia and anti-convulsant
hypersensitivity syndrome. Paradoxical
reaction in children (not dose-related) may
cause hyperactivity, irritability, insomnia.
Induces several liver enzymes (see p.
924), thus decreases blood levels of many
drugs (e.g., anticonvulsants). IV push not
to exceed 1 mg/kg/min.

$T_{1/2}$ is variable with age: neonates,
45–100 hr; infants, 20–133 hr; children,
37–73 hr. Due to long half-life, consider
other agents for sedation for procedures.

Therapeutic levels: 15–40 mg/L.
Recommended serum sampling time at
steady-state: trough level obtained within
30 minutes prior to the next scheduled
dose after 10–14 days of continuous
dosing.

**Adjust dose in renal failure (see
p. 940).**

PHENTOLAMINE MESYLATE

Regitine
Adrenergic blocking agent (alpha); antidote, extravasation
Inj: 5 mg vial (contains 25 mg mannitol)

No   ?   C

Treatment of alpha adrenergic drug extravasation (most effective within 12 hr of extravasation)

Neonates: Make a solution of 0.25–0.5 mg/ml with normal saline. Inject 1 ml (in 5 divided doses of 0.2 ml) SC around site of extravasation; **max total dose:** 0.1 mg/kg or 2.5 mg total.

Infants, Children, and Adults: Make a solution of 0.5–1 mg/ml with normal saline. Inject 1–5 ml (in 5 divided doses) SC around site of extravasation; **max total dose:** 0.1–0.2 mg/kg or 5 mg total.

Diagnosis of pheochromocytoma, IM/IV:
Children: 0.05–0.1 mg/kg/dose up to a **max** of 5 mg
Adults: 5 mg/dose

Hypertension, prior to surgery for pheochromocytoma, IM/IV:
Children: 0.05–0.1 mg/kg/dose up to a **max** of 5 mg 1–2 hrs prior to surgery, repeat Q2–4 hr PRN
Adults: 5 mg/dose 1–2 hrs prior to surgery, repeat Q2–4 hrs PRN

For diagnosis of pheochromocytoma, patient should be resting in a supine position. A blood pressure reduction of more than 35 mm Hg systolic and 24 mm Hg diastolic is considered a positive test for pheochromocytoma. For treatment of extravasation, use 27- to 30-gauge needle with multiple small injections and monitor site closely as repeat doses may be necessary.

PHENYLEPHRINE HCl
Neo-Synephrine and others
Adrenergic agonist

No ? C

Nasal drops: 0.125, 0.16, 0.25, 0.5% (15, 30 ml)
Nasal spray: 0.25, 0.5, 1% (15, 30 ml)
Ophthalmic drops: 0.12% (0.3, 15, 20 ml), 2.5% (2, 3, 5, 15 ml), 10% (1, 2, 5, 15 ml)
Inj: 10 mg/ml (1%)

For explanation of icons, see p. 600.

Hypotension:
Children:
IM/SC: 0.1 mg/kg/dose Q1–2 hr
PRN; **max dose:** 5 mg
IV bolus: 5–20 mcg/kg/dose Q10–
15 min PRN
IV drip: 0.1–0.5 mcg/kg/min; titrate to
effect
Adults:
IM/SC: 2–5 mg/dose Q1–2 hr PRN;
max dose: 5 mg
IV bolus: 0.1–0.5 mg/dose Q10–
15 min PRN
IV drip: Initial rate at 100–180 mcg/
min; titrate to effect. Usual
maintenance dose: 40–60 mcg/min.
To prepare infusion: See inside front
cover.
   NOTE: the dosage units for adults are in
mcg/min; compared to mcg/kg/min for
children.
Nasal decongestant (in each nostril; give
up to 3 days):
   Infants (>6 mon old): 1–2 drops of
0.16% sol Q3 hr PRN

<6 yr: 2–3 drops of 0.125% sol Q4 hr
PRN
6–12 yr: 2–3 drops or 1–2 sprays of
0.25% sol Q4 hr PRN
>12 yr–adult: 2–3 drops or 1–2 sprays
of 0.25% or 0.5% sol Q4 hr PRN
Pupillary dilation: 2.5% sol; 1 drop in
each eye 15 min before exam

Use **cautiously** in presence of
arrhythmias, hyperthyroidism, or
hyperglycemia. May cause tremor,
insomnia, palpitations. Metabolized by
MAO. **Contraindicated** in
pheochromocytoma and severe
hypertension. Nasal decongestants may
cause rebound congestion with excessive
use (>3 days). The 1% nasal spray can
be used in adults with extreme
congestion. Injectable product may
contain sulfites. Note: Phenylephrine is
found in a variety of combination cough
and cold products.

PHENYTOIN
Dilantin
Anticonvulsant, class Ib antiarrhythmic
Chewable tabs: 50 mg (Infatab)
Prompt caps: 30, 100 mg
Extended-release caps: 30, 100 mg
Susp: 125 mg/5 ml (240 ml)
Inj: 50 mg/ml

No   1   D

Status epilepticus: See p. 15
Loading dose (all ages): 15–20 mg/kg IV

Max dose: 1500 mg/24 hr

Maintenance for seizure disorders:
Neonates: start with 5 mg/kg/24 hr PO/IV ÷ Q12 hr; usual range 5–8 mg/kg/24 hr PO/IV ÷ Q8–12 hr
Infants/Children: start with 5 mg/kg/24 hr ÷ BID-TID PO/IV; usual dose range (doses divided BID-TID)
6 mo–3 yr: 8–10 mg/kg/24 hr
4–6 yr: 7.5–9 mg/kg/24 hr
7–9 yr: 7–8 mg/kg/24 hr
10–16 yr: 6–7 mg/kg/24 hr
Note: Use QD-BID dosing with extended release caps.
Adults: Start with 100 mg/dose Q8 hr IV/PO and carefully titrate to 300–600 mg/24 hr (or 6–7 mg/kg/24 hr) ÷ Q8–24 hr IV/PO

Anti-arrhythmic (secondary to digitalis intoxication):
Load (all ages): 1.25 mg/kg IV Q5 min up to a total of 15 mg/kg
Maintenance:
Children: IV/PO: 5–10 mg/kg/24 hr ÷ Q12 hr
Adults: 250 mg PO QID × 1 day, then 250 mg PO Q12 hr × 2 days, then 300–400 mg/24 hr ÷ Q6–24 hr

Contraindicated in patients with heart block or sinus bradycardia.

IM administration is not recommended because of erratic absorption and pain at injection site. Side effects: gingival hyperplasia, hirsutism, dermatitis, blood dyscrasia, ataxia, SLE-like and Stevens-Johnson syndromes, lymphadenopathy, liver damage, and nystagmus. Many drug interactions: levels may be increased by cimetidine, chloramphenicol, INH, sulfonamides, trimethoprim, etc. Levels may be decreased by some antineoplastic agents. Phenytoin induces hepatic microsomal enzymes (CYP 450 3A4, see p. 924) leading to decreased effectiveness of oral contraceptives, quinidine, valproic acid, and theophylline.

Oral absorption reduced in neonates. $T_{1/2}$ is variable (7–42 hr) and dose-dependent. Drug is highly protein-bound; free fraction of drug will be increased in patients with hypoalbuminemia. IV push/infusion rate: not to exceed 0.5 mg/kg/min in neonates, or 1 mg/kg/min infants, children and adults with max: 50 mg/min; may cause cardiovascular collapse.

For seizure disorders, therapeutic levels: 10–20 mg/L (free and bound phenytoin) OR, 1–2 mg/L (free only). Recommended serum sampling times: trough level (PO/IV) within 30 minutes prior to the next scheduled dose; peak or post load level (IV) 1 hour after the end of IV infusion. Steady state is usually achieved after 5–10 days of continuous dosing. For routine monitoring, measure trough.

PHOSPHORUS SUPPLEMENTS

NeutraPhos, NeutraPhos-K, K-PHOS Neutral, Uro-KP-Neutral,
Sodium Phos, Potassium Phos

Yes ? C

Oral: (reconstitute in 75 ml H$_2$O per capsule or packet)

Na and K Phosphate:
NeutraPhos; Caps, powder: 250 mg P, 7 mEq Na, 7 mEq K
Uro-KP-Neutral; Tabs: 250 mg P, 10.9 mEq Na, 1.27 mEq K
K-PHOS Neutral; Tabs: 250 mg P, 13 mEq Na, 1.1 mEq K

K Phosphate:
NeutraPhos-K; Caps, powder: 250 mg P, 14.25 mEq K
Inj:
Na Phosphate: 94 mg P, 4 mEq Na/ml
K Phosphate: 94 mg P, 4.4 mEq K/ml
CONVERSION: 31 mg P = 1 mM P

Acute hypophosphatemia: 5–10 mg/kg/dose IV over 6 hr
Maintenance/Replacement:
Children:
IV: 15–45 mg/kg over 24 hr
PO: 30–90 mg/kg/24 hr ÷ TID-QID
Adults:
IV: 1.5–2 g over 24 hr
PO: 3–4.5 g/24 hr ÷ TID-QID
Recommended infusion rate: ≤3.1 mg/kg/hr (0.1 mM/kg/hr) of phosphate. When potassium salt is used, the rate will be limited by the maximum potassium infusion rate. Do not co-infuse with calcium containing products.

May cause tetany, hyperphosphatemia, hyperkalemia, hypocalcemia. Use with caution in patients with renal impairment. Be aware of sodium and/or potassium load when supplementing phosphate. IV administration may cause hypotension, renal failure; or arrhythmias, heart block, cardiac arrest with potassium salt. PO dosing may cause nausea, vomiting, abdominal pain, or diarrhea. See p. 246 for daily requirements and additional information on hypo- and hyperphosphatemia.

PHYSOSTIGMINE SALICYLATE

Antilirium
Cholinergic agent

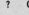

No ? C

Inj: 1 mg/ml (2 ml); contains 2% benzyl alcohol and 0.1% sodium bisulfite

For antihistamine overdose or anticholinergic poisoning (see p. 25).

Physostigmine antidote: Atropine always should be available.
Contraindicated in asthma, gangrene, diabetes, cardiovascular disease, GI or GU tract obstruction, any vagotonic state, patients receiving choline esters or depolarizing neuromuscular blocking agents (eg. decamethonium, succinylcholine).

PHYTONADIONE
See Vitamin K1

PILOCARPINE HCl

Akarpine, Isopto Carpine, Piligan, Ocusert Pilo, and others
Cholinergic agent   **No**   **?**   **C**
Ophthalmic sol: 0.25%, 0.5%, 1%, 2%, 3%, 4%, 5%, 6%, 8%, 10%
Ophthalmic gel: 4% (3.5 g)
Ocular therapeutic system (Ocusert Pilo): 20, 40 mcg/hr for 1 week (8 units)
Tab: 5 mg

For elevated intraocular pressure:
1–2 drops in each eye 4–6 ×/24 hr; adjust concentration and frequency as needed.
Gel: 0.5" ribbon applied to lower conjunctival sac QHS. Adjust dose as needed.
Xerostomia:
  Adults: 5 mg/dose PO TID, dose may be titrated to 10 mg/dose PO TID in patients who do not respond to lower dose and who are able to tolerate the drug.

Contraindicated in acute iritis or anterior chamber inflammation.
May cause stinging, burning, lacrimation, headache, retinal detachment. Use with **caution** in patients with corneal abrasion.

PIPERACILLIN

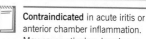

Pipracil
Antibiotic, penicillin (extended spectrum)   **Yes**   **?**   **B**
Inj: 2, 3, 4, 40 g
Contains 1.85 mEq Na/g

Neonates, IV:
≤7 days:
  ≤36 weeks gest: 150 mg/kg/24 hr
  ÷ Q12 hr
  >36 weeks gest: 225 mg/kg/24 hr ÷
  Q8 hr
>7 days:
  ≤36 weeks gest: 225 mg/kg/24 hr ÷
  Q8 hr
  >36 weeks gest: 300 mg/kg/24 hr ÷
  Q6 hr
Infants and Children:
  200–300 mg/kg/24 hr IM/IV ÷ Q4–
  6 hr.
  Max dose: 24 g/24 hr
Cystic Fibrosis:
  350–600 mg/kg/24 hr IM/IV ÷
  Q4–6 hr.
  Max dose: 24 g/24 hr
Adults: 2–4 g/dose IV Q4–6 hr or 1–2 g/
dose IM Q6 hr. **Max dose:** 24 g/24h

Similar to penicillin. Like other penicillins, CSF penetration occurs only with inflamed meninges. **Adjust dose in renal impairment (see p. 934).** May cause seizures, myoclonus, and fever. May falsely lower aminoglycoside serum level results if the drugs are infused close to one another; allow a minimum of 2 hours between infusions to prevent this interaction.

PIPERACILLIN/TAZOBACTAM

Zosyn
Antibiotic, penicillin (extended spectrum with beta-lactamase inhibitor)   **Yes   ?   B**
Inj: 2 g Piperacillin, 0.25 g Tazobactam; 3 g Piperacillin, 0.375 g Tazobactam; 4 g Piperacillin, 0.5 g Tazobactam (8:1 ratio of piperacillin to tazobactam)

All doses based on piperacillin component
  Infants <6 mo: 150–300 mg/kg/
24 hr IV ÷ Q6–8 hr
Infants >6 mo and Children: 300–400 mg/kg/24 hr IV ÷ Q6–8 hr
Adults: 3 g IV Q6 hr; doses as high as 18 g/24 hr IV ÷ Q4 hr have been used in nosocomial pneumonia.
Cystic Fibrosis: see piperacillin

Tazobactam is a beta-lactamase inhibitor, thus extending the spectrum of piperacillin. Like other penicillins, CSF penetration occurs only with inflamed meninges. **Adjust dose in renal impairment (see p. 935).** See Piperacillin and Penicillin for other comments.

PIPERAZINE
Vermizine
Anthelmentic
Tabs: 250 mg

Yes 2 B

Enterobius vermicularis *(pinworm):*
Adults and children: 65 mg/kg/
24 hr PO QD × 7 days. **Max dose:**
2.5 g/24 hr. May repeat in 1 wk if
necessary.
Ascaris lumbricoides *(roundworm):*
Children: 75 mg/kg/24 hr PO QD ×
2 days
Adults: 3.5 g PO QD × 2 days
Max dose: 3.5 g/24 hr

Contraindicated in seizure
disorders, liver or renal impairment.
Large doses may cause GI
irritation, blurred vision, urticaria, and
muscle weakness. Use with caution when
administering with chlorpromazine.

Other agents, mebendazole and pyrantel
pamoate, are considered first line therapy
for Ascaris and Enterobius infections. In
cases of intestinal obstruction due to
heavy worm load, piperazine may be
given through NG tube at doses
recommended *(Red Book,* 1997, pg.
143). **Pyrantel pamoate and piperazine
should not be administered together
because they are antagonistic.**
Breastfeeding mothers should take their
doses immediately following feeding infant
and then express and discard milk during
the next 8 hours.

PIRBUTEROL ACETATE
Maxair
Beta-2-adrenergic agonist
Aerosol inhaler: 0.2 mg/actuation (25.6 g, 300 actuations)
AUTOHALER: 0.2 mg/actuation (13.7 g, 400 actuations; 2.8 g, 80 actuations)
2.8 g is sample pack

No ? C

Children ≥12 yr and Adults: 1–2
inhalations Q4–6 hr.
Max dose: 12 inhalations/24 hr.

See albuterol. AUTOHALER is
breath actuated inhaler. See
package insert for directions.
Actuations are minimum amount/unit.
Onset of action: 3 minutes. Duration: 5 hr.

For explanation of icons, see p. 600.

PLICAMYCIN
Mithracin
Antidote, hypercalcemia; antineoplastic
Inj: 2.5 mg (contains 100 mg mannitol)

Yes   ?   D

Hypercalcemia: 25 mcg/kg/dose in 1 L D$_5$W or NS over 4–6 hours IV QD × 1–4 days. May repeat at intervals of 1 week PRN.

Contraindicated in clinical bleeding, bone marrow suppression. Use with **caution** in hepatic or **renal** impairment (see p. 940). Bone marrow suppression, hemorrhagic diathesis with coagulopathy, cellulitis with extravasation, nausea, vomiting, electrolyte imbalances, hepatotoxicity, renal toxicity may occur.

POLYETHYLENE GLYCOL—ELECTROLYTE SOLUTION
GoLYTELY, Co-Lav, Colovage, CoLyte, GoEvac, NuLYTELY, OCL
Colonic lavage solution
Powder for oral solution: (GoLYTELY): polyethylene glycol 3350 236 g, Na sulfate 22.74 g, Na bicarbonate 6.74 g, NaCl 5.86 g, KCl 2.97 g. Contents vary somewhat. See package insert for contents of other products.

No   ?   C

Children:
Oral: 25–40 ml/kg/hr until rectal effluent is clear
Nasogastric: 20–30 ml/min (1.2–1.8 L/hr) up to 4 L
Adults: 240 ml PO Q10 min up to 4 L or until rectal effluent is clear

Contraindicated in toxic megacolon, gastric retention, colitis, bowel perforation. Use with **caution** in patients prone to aspiration or with impaired gag reflex. Effect should occur within 1–2 hr. Solution generally more palatable if chilled. Monitor electrolytes, BUN, serum glucose, and urine osmolality with prolonged administration. Patients should be NPO 3–4 hours before administration.

POLYMYXIN B SULFATE AND BACITRACIN

No ? C

Ak-poly-BAC, Polysporin
Topical antibiotic
Ophthalmic ointment: Bacitracin 500 U and polymyxin B 10,000 U/g (3.5, 3.75 g)
Topical ointment: Bacitracin 500 U and polymyxin B 10,000 U/g (15, 30 g)
Topical powder: Bacitracin 500 U and polymyxin B 10,000 U/g (10 g)
Topical spray: Bacitracin 111 U and polymyxin B 2222 U/g (90 g)

Ophthalmic: Apply to affected eye 4–6 ×/24 hr
Topical: Apply ointment or powder to affected area QD-TID

Do **not** use ophthalmic ointment for longer than 1 wk. Do **not** use topical ointment in the eyes. Side effects: rash, itching, burning, conjunctival erythema, anaphylactoid reaction, swelling.

POLYMYXIN B SULFATE, NEOMYCIN SULFATE, HYDROCORTISONE

No ? C

Cortisporin, Otocort, and others
Topical antibiotic (otic preps listed)
Otic solution or suspension: Polymyxin B sulfate 10,000 U, Neomycin sulfate 5 mg, Hydrocortisone 10 mg/ml (10 ml)

Otitis externa: 3–4 drops TID-QID × 7–10 days. If preferred, a cotton wick may be saturated and inserted into ear canal. Moisten wick with antibiotic every 4 hours. Change wick Q24 hr.

Shake suspension well before use. **Contraindicated** in patients with active vaccinia, varicella, and herpes simplex. May cause cutaneous sensitization. Do **not** use in cases with perforated eardrum because of possible ototoxicity.

For explanation of icons, see p. 600.

POTASSIUM IODIDE

Pima, Potassium Iodide Enseals, SSKI, Iosat, Thyro Block, and others

No 1 D

Antithyroid agent

Tabs: 130 mg
Syrup (Pima): 325 mg/5 ml (473 ml)
Saturated Solution (SSKI): 1000 mg/ml (30, 240 ml)
Lugol's (Strong Iodine) Solution: Iodine 50 mg and Potassium Iodide 100 mg per ml (120, 473 ml)

Neonatal Graves' disease: 1 drop strong iodine (Lugol's sol) PO Q8 hr

Thyrotoxicosis:
Children: 50–250 mg PO TID (about 1–5 drops of SSKI TID)
Adults: 50–500 mg PO TID (1–10 drops SSKI PO TID)

Sporotrichosis:
Adults and Children: 65–325 mg PO TID. Daily doses may be increased by 150–250 mg/24 hr. **Max dose:** increase to tolerance or 4.5–9 g/24 hr.

Contraindicated in pregnancy. GI disturbance, metallic taste, rash, salivary gland inflammation, headache, lacrimation, and rhinitis are symptoms of iodism. Give with milk or water after meals. Monitor thyroid function tests. Onset of antithyroid effects: 1–2 days.

Continue sporotrichosis treatment for 4–6 wk after lesions have completely healed. Increase dose until either maximum dose is achieved or signs of intolerance appear.

POTASSIUM SUPPLEMENTS

Many brand names

Yes 1 A

Potassium chloride:
40 mEq K = 3 g KCl
Sustained-release caps: 8, 10 mEq
Sustained-release tabs: 6.7, 8, 10, 20 mEq
Powder: 15, 20, 25 mEq/packet
Sol: 10% (6.7 mEq/5 ml), 15% (10 mEq/5 ml), 20% (13.3 mEq/5 ml)
Concentrated Inj: 1.5, 2, 3 mEq/ml

Potassium gluconate:
40 mEq K = 9.4 g K gluconate
Tabs: 500 mg (2.15 mEq), 595 mg (2.56 mEq)
Elixir: 20 mEq/15 ml
Potassium acetate:
40 mEq K = 3.9 g K acetate
Concentrated Inj: 2, 4 mEq/ml
Potassium phosphate:
See Phosphorus supplements

Normal daily requirements: See p. 229.

Replacement: Determine based on maintenance requirements, deficit and ongoing losses. See pp. 240–241.
Hypokalemia:
Oral:
  Children: 1–4 mEq/kg/24 hr ÷ BID-QID. Monitor serum potassium.
  Adults: 40–100 mEq/24 hr ÷ BID-QID
IV: MONITOR SERUM K CLOSELY
  Children: 0.5–1 mEq/kg/dose given as an infusion of 0.5 mEq/kg/hr × 1–2 hr. **Max** IV infusion rate: 1 mEq/kg/hr. This may be used in critical situations (i.e., hypokalemia with arrhythmia).
  Adults:
    Serum K ≥2.5 mEq/L: Replete at rates up to 10 mEq/hr. Total dosage not to exceed 200 mEq/24 hr.

Serum K <2 mEq/L: Replete at rates up to 40 mEq/hr. Total dosage not to exceed 400 mEq/24 hr.
Max peripheral IV Sol conc: 40 mEq/L
Max conc for central line administration: 150–200 mEq/L

PO administration may cause GI disturbance and ulceration. Oral liquid supplements should be diluted in water or fruit juice prior to administration. Sustained-release tablets must be swallowed whole, and not dissolved in the mouth or chewed.

Do **not** administer IV potassium undiluted. IV administration may cause irritation, pain, phlebitis at the infusion site. **Rapid or central IV infusion may cause cardiac arrhythmias.** Patients receiving infusion >0.5 mEq/kg/hr (>20 mEq/hr for adults) should be placed on an ECG monitor.

PRALIDOXIME CHLORIDE

Protopam, 2-PAM
Antidote, organophosphate poisoning
Autoinj: 300 mg/ml (2 ml)
Inj: 1000 mg/20 ml

Yes   ?   C

Use with atropine
Children: 20–50 mg/kg/dose × 1 IM/IV/SC. May repeat in 1–2 hours if muscle weakness is not relieved.
Adults: 1–2 g/dose × 1 IM/IV/SC. May repeat in 1–2 hours if muscle weakness is not relieved.

Removal of secretions and maintaining a patent airway is critical. For IV administration, dilute to 50 mg/ml or less and infuse over 15–30 minutes (not to exceed 200 mg/minute). Drug is generally ineffective if administered 36–48 hours after exposure. Additional doses may be necessary. May cause muscle rigidity, laryngospasm, and tachycardia after rapid IV infusion. Reduce dosage in renal impairment since 80–90% of the drug is excreted unchanged in the urine 12 hours after administration.

For explanation of icons, see p. 600.

PRAZIQUANTEL

Biltricide
Anthelmintic
Tab: 600 mg (tri-scored)

No ? B

Children and Adults:
Schistosomiasis: 20 mg/kg/dose
PO BID-TID × 1 day
Flukes: 25 mg/kg/dose PO Q8 hr × 1
day (× 2 days for *P. westermani*)
Cysticercosis: 50 mg/kg/24 hr PO ÷
Q8 hr × 15 days (dexamethasone may
be added to regimen for 2–3 days to
minimize inflammatory response)
Tapeworms: 5–10 mg/kg/dose PO ×
1 dose (25 mg/kg/dose × 1 dose for
H. nana)

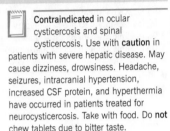
Contraindicated in ocular
cysticercosis and spinal
cysticercosis. Use with **caution** in
patients with severe hepatic disease. May
cause dizziness, drowsiness. Headache,
seizures, intracranial hypertension,
increased CSF protein, and hyperthermia
have occurred in patients treated for
neurocysticercosis. Take with food. Do **not**
chew tablets due to bitter taste.

PRAZOSIN HCl

Minipress
Adrenergic blocking agent (alpha-1), antihypertensive,
vasodilator
Caps: 1, 2, 5 mg

No ? C

Children:
Initial: 5 mcg/kg PO test dose
Maintenance: 25–150 mcg/kg/
24 hr ÷ Q6 hr
Max dose: 15 mg/24 hr or 0.4 mg/kg/
24 hr
Adults:
1 mg PO BID-TID initially. Increase PRN
to **max dose** of 20 mg/24 hr PO ÷ BID-
TID

May cause syncope, tachycardia,
hypotension, dizziness, nausea,
headache, drowsiness, fatigue,
anticholinergic effects. Marked orthostatic
hypotension, syncope, and loss of
consciousness may occur with first dose.

PREDNISOLONE

Delta-Cortef, Prelone, Pediapred, and others
Corticosteroid

No   1   B

Tabs: 5 mg
Syrup: 15 mg/5 ml (Prelone, 5% alcohol) (240 ml)
Syrup: 5 mg/5 ml (Pediapred) (120 ml)
Inj (as acetate): 25, 50 mg/ml (not for IV use)
Inj (as Na phosphate): 20 mg/ml
Inj (as tebutate): 20 mg/ml (not for IV use)
Ophthalmic Suspension (as acetate): 0.12%, 0.125%, 1% (5, 10 ml)
Ophthalmic Solution (as Na phosphate): 0.125%, 1% (5, 10, 15 ml)

See Prednisone (equivalent dosing)
Ophthalmic:
Children and Adults: Start with 1–2 drops Q1 hr during the day and Q2 hr during the night until favorable response, then reduce dose to 1 drop Q4 hr. Dose may be further reduced to 1 drop TID-QID.

See pp. 908–909 for relative steroid potencies.

PREDNISONE

Many brand names
Corticosteroid

No   1   B

Tabs: 1, 2.5, 5, 10, 20, 50 mg
Syrup/Solution: 1 mg/ml (5% alcohol)
Conc Sol: 5 mg/ml (30% alcohol)

Children:
Anti-inflammatory/immunosuppressive: 0.5–2 mg/kg/24 hr PO ÷ QD-QID
Acute Asthma: 2 mg/kg/24 hr PO ÷ QD-BID × 5 days; **Max dose:** 80 mg/24 hr
Nephrotic Syndrome: Starting doses of 2 mg/kg/24 hr PO (**Max dose:** 80 mg/24 hr) are recommended. Further treatment plans are individualized. Consult a nephrologist.

See p. 907 for physiologic replacement, relative steroid potencies, and doses based on body surface area. Methylprednisolone is preferable in hepatic disease because prednisone must be converted to methylprednisolone in the liver.

Side effects may include: mood changes, seizures, hyperglycemia, diarrhea, nausea, abdominal distension, GI bleeding, and HPA axis suppression, cushingoid effects, cataracts with prolonged use. Barbiturates, carbamazepine, phenytoin, rifampin, isoniazid, may reduce the effects of prednisone; whereas estrogens may enhance the effects.

For explanation of icons, see p. 600.

PRIMIDONE
Mysoline
Anticonvulsant, barbiturate
Tabs: 50, 250 mg
Susp: 250 mg/5 ml

Yes   2   D

<8 yr	≥8yr and adults
DAY 1–3	
50mg PO QHS	100–125mg PO QHS
DAY 4–6	
50mg PO BID	100–125mg PO BID
DAY 7–9	
100mg PO BID	100–125mg PO TID
Thereafter	
125-250mg PO TID or	250mg PO TID-QID; **Max dose:** 2g/24hr
10–25mg/kg/24hr ÷ TID-QID	

Use with **caution** in renal or hepatic disease and pulmonary insufficiency. Primidone is metabolized to phenobarbital and has the same drug interactions and toxicities (see phenobarbital, p. 810). Additionally, primidone may cause vertigo, nausea, leukopenia, malignant lymphoma-like syndrome, diplopia, nystagmus, systemic lupus-like syndrome. **Adjust dose in renal failure (see p. 941).**

Follow both primidone and phenobarbital levels. Therapeutic levels: 5–12 mg/L of primidone and 15–40 mg/L of phenobarbital. Recommended serum sampling time at steady-state: trough level obtained within 30 minutes prior to the next scheduled dose after 1–4 days of continuous dosing.

PROBENECID
Benemid
Penicillin therapy adjuvant, uric acid lowering agent
Tabs: 500 mg

Yes   ?   B

Use with penicillin
Children (2–14 yr): 25 mg/kg PO ×
1, then 40 mg/kg/24 hr ÷ QID;
max dose: 500 mg/dose
Adults (>50 kg): 500 mg PO QID
Hyperuricemia: 250 mg PO BID × 1
week, then 500 mg PO BID; may
increase Q4 weeks PRN up to 2–3 g/
24 hr ÷ BID.

Use with **caution** in patients with
peptic ulcer disease.
Contraindicated in children
<2 years old and patients with renal
insufficiency. Do not use if GFR <30 ml/
min.

Increases uric acid excretion. Inhibits
renal tubular secretion of acyclovir,
organic acids, penicillins, cephalosporins,
AZT, dapsone, methotrexate, non-steroidal
anti-inflammatory agents, benzodiazepines. Salicylates may decrease
probenecid's activity. Alkalinize urine in
patients with gout. May cause headache,
GI symptoms, rash, anemia, and
hypersensitivity. False-positive glucosuria
with Clinitest can occur.

PROCAINAMIDE
Pronestyl, Procan SR, and others
Antiarrhythmic, class Ia
Tabs: 250, 375, 500 mg
Sustained Release Tabs: 250, 500, 750, 1000 mg
Caps: 250, 375, 500 mg
Inj: 100, 500 mg/ml
Susp: 5, 50, 100 mg/ml

Yes   1   C

Children:

IM: 20–30 mg/kg/24 hr ÷ Q4–6 hr; **max dose:** 4 g/24 hr (peak effect in 1 hr).

IV: Load: 2–6 mg/kg/dose over 5 min (max dose: 100 mg/dose); repeat dose Q5–10 min PRN up to a total **maximum** of 15 mg/kg. Do not exceed 500 mg in 30 minutes.

Maintenance: 20–80 mcg/kg/min by continuous infusion; **max dose:** 2 g/24 hr

PO: 15–50 mg/kg/24 hr ÷ Q3–6 hr; **max dose:** 4 g/24 hr

Adults:

IM: 50 mg/kg/24 hr ÷ Q3–6 hr

IV: Load: 50–100 mg/dose; repeat dose Q5 min PRN to max of 1000–1500 mg

Maintenance: 1–6 mg/min by continuous infusion

PO: Usual dose: 50 mg/kg/24 hr

Immediate Release: 250–500 mg/dose Q3–6 hr

Sustained Release: 500–1000 mg/dose Q6 hr

Contraindicated in myasthenia gravis, complete heart block, SLE, torsade de pointes. Use with caution in asymtomatic premature ventricular contractions, digitalis intoxication, CHF, renal or hepatic dysfunction. **Adjust dose in renal failure (see p. 941).**

May cause lupus-like syndrome, positive Coombs' test, thrombocytopenia, arrhythmias, GI complaints, confusion. Monitor BP's, ECG when using IV. QRS widening by >0.02 sec suggests toxicity.

Cimetidine, ranitidine, amiodarone, beta-blockers, trimethoprim may increase procainamide levels. Procainamide may enhance the effects of skeletal muscle relaxants and anticholinergic agents. Therapeutic levels: 4–10 mg/L of procainamide or 10–30 mg/L of procainamide and NAPA levels combined.

Recommended serum sampling times: M/PO intermittent dosing: trough level within 30 minutes prior to the next scheduled dose after 2 days of continuous dosing (steady-state). IV continuous infusion: 2 and 12 hours after start of infusion and at 24 hour interval thereafter.

PROCHLORPERAZINE
Compazine and others
Antiemetic, phenothiazine derivative
Tabs: 5, 10, 25 mg
Slow-release caps: 10, 15, 30 mg
Syrup: 5 mg/5 ml (120 ml)
Suppository: 2.5, 5, 25 mg
Inj: 5 mg/ml (2, 10 ml)

No   2   C

Antiemetic doses:
Children (>10 kg or >2 yr):
PO or PR: 0.4 mg/kg/24 hr ÷ TID-QID
IM: 0.1–0.15 mg/kg/dose TID-QID
Adults:
PO:
Immediate Release: 5–10 mg/dose TID-QID
  Extended Release: 10 mg/dose BID or 15 mg/dose QD
PR: 25 mg/dose BID
IM: 5–10 mg/dose Q4–6 hr
IV: 5–10 mg/dose may repeat Q3–4 hr
Max IM/IV dose: 40 mg/24 hr

Toxicity as for other phenothiazines (see chlorpromazine). Extra-pyramidal reactions (reversed by diphenhydramine) or orthostatic hypotension may occur. Do **not** use IV route in children. **Use only in management of prolonged vomiting of known etiology.**

PROMETHAZINE

Phenergan, Provigan, and others
Antihistamine, antiemetic, phenothiazine derivative
Tabs: 12.5, 25, 50 mg
Syrup: 6.25 mg/5 ml, 25 mg/5 ml
Suppository: 12.5, 25, 50 mg
Inj: 25, 50 mg/ml

No   ?   C

Antihistaminic:
Children: 0.1 mg/kg/dose Q6 hr and 0.5 mg/kg/dose QHS PO PRN
Adults: 12.5 mg PO TID and 25 mg QHS.
Nausea and vomiting PO/IM/IV/PR:
Children: 0.25–1 mg/kg/dose Q4–6 hr PRN.
Adults: 12.5–25 mg Q4–6 hr PRN.
Motion sickness: (1st dose 0.5–1 hr before departure):
Children: 0.5 mg/kg/dose Q12 hr PO PRN.
Adults: 25 mg PO BID PRN.

Toxicity similar to other phenothiazines (see chlor-promazine). **Use only in management of prolonged vomiting of known etiology.** Administer with meals to decrease GI irritation (PO route). May cause profound sedation, blurred vision, and dystonic reactions (reversed by diphenhydramine).

For explanation of icons, see p. 600.

PROPRANOLOL

Inderal

Adrenergic blocking agent (beta), antiarrhythmic, class II

  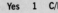

Yes   1   C/D

Tabs: 10, 20, 40, 60, 80, 90 mg
Extended-release caps: 60, 80, 120, 160 mg
Sol: 20, 40 mg/5 ml
Conc. Sol: 80 mg/ml
Inj: 1 mg/ml
Susp: 1 mg/ml

Arrhythmias:
Children:
　IV: 0.01–0.1 mg/kg/dose IV push over 10 minutes, repeat Q6–8 hr PRN. **Max dose:** 1 mg/dose for infants; **Max dose:** 3 mg/dose for children.
　PO: Start at 0.5–1 mg/kg/24 hr ÷ Q6–8 hr; increase dosage Q3–5 days PRN. Usual dosage range: 2–4 mg/kg/24 hr ÷ Q6–8 hr. **Max dose:** 60 mg/24 hr or 16 mg/kg/24 hr.
Adults:
　IV: 1 mg/dose Q5 min up to total 5 mg
　PO: 10–30 mg/dose TID-QID. Increase PRN. Usual range 40–320 mg/24 hr ÷ TID-QID.
Hypertension:
Children:
　PO: Initial: 0.5–1 mg/kg/24 hr ÷ Q6–12 hr. May increase dose Q3–5 days PRN; **max dose:** 8 mg/kg/24 hr
Adults:
　PO: 40 mg/dose PO BID or 60–80 mg/dose (sustained release capsule) PO QD. May increase 10–20 mg/dose Q3–5 days; **max dose:** 640 mg/24 hr
Migraine Prophylaxis:
Children:
　<35 kg: 10–20 mg PO TID
　≥35 kg: 20–40 mg PO TID
Adults: 80 mg/24 hr ÷ Q6–8 hr PO; increase dose Q3–4 weeks PRN. Usual effective dose range: 160–240 mg/24 hr.
Tetralogy Spells:
　IV: 0.15–0.25 mg/kg/dose slow IV push. May repeat in 15 min × 1.

　PO: Start at 2–4 mg/kg/24 hr PRN. Usual dose range: 4–8 mg/kg/24 hr ÷ Q6 hr PRN. Doses as high as 15 mg/kg/24 hr have been used with careful monitoring.
Thyrotoxicosis:
　Neonates: 2 mg/kg/24 hr PO ÷ Q6–12 hr
Adolescents and Adults:
　IV: 1–3 mg/dose over 10 min. May repeat in 4–6 hr.
　PO: 10–40 mg/dose PO Q6 hr

Contraindicated in asthma, Raynaud's syndrome, heart failure, and heart block. Use with **caution** in presence of obstructive lung disease, diabetes mellitus, renal or hepatic disease. May cause hypoglycemia, hypotension, nausea, vomiting, depression, weakness, impotence, bronchospasm, and heart block.

Therapeutic levels: 30–100 ng/ml. Drug is metabolized by multiple CYP 450 isoenzymes. Concurrent administration with barbiturates, indomethacin, or rifampin may cause decreased activity of propranolol. Concurrent administration with cimetidine, hydralazine, flecainide, quinidine, chlorpromazine, or verapamil may lead to increased activity of propranolol. Avoid IV use of propranolol with calcium channel blockers; may increase effect of calcium channel blocker.

Note: Oral bioavailability is 30%–60% of dose (may be increased in Down syndrome). Pregnancy category changes to "D" if used in 2nd or 3rd trimesters.

PROPYLTHIOURACIL
PTU
Antithyroid agent
Tabs: 50 mg
100 mg PTU = 10 mg Methimazole

Yes   1   D

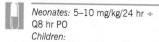

Neonates: 5–10 mg/kg/24 hr ÷ Q8 hr PO
Children:
Initial: 5–7 mg/kg/24 hr ÷ Q8 hr PO
OR by age:
   6–10 yr: 50–150 mg/24 hr ÷ Q8 hr PO
   >10 yr: 150–300 mg/24 hr ÷ Q8 hr PO
Maintenance: Generally begins after 2 months. Usually 1/3–2/3 the initial dose when the patient is euthyroid.
Adults:
Initial: 300–450 mg/24 hr ÷ Q8 hr PO; some may require larger doses of 600–1200 mg/24 hr
Maintenance: 100–150 mg/24 hr ÷ Q8 hr PO

May cause blood dyscrasias, fever, liver disease, dermatitis, urticaria, malaise, CNS stimulation or depression, arthralgias. Monitor thyroid function. Dosages should be adjusted as required to achieve and maintain T_3, T_4, TSH levels in normal ranges. **Adjust dosage in renal impairment (see p. 941).** For neonates, crush tablets, weigh appropriate dose, and mix in formula/breast milk.

PROSTAGLANDIN E$_1$
PGE$_1$, Alprostadil, Prostin VR
Prostaglandin E$_1$, vasodilator
Inj: 500 mcg/ml

No   ?   X

Neonates:
Initial: 0.05–0.1 mcg/kg/min. Advance to 0.2 mcg/kg/min if necessary.
Maintenance: When increase in PaO_2 is noted, decrease immediately to lowest effective dose. Usual dosage range: 0.01–0.4 mcg/kg/min; doses above 0.4 mcg/kg/min not likely to produce additional benefit.
To prepare infusion: see inside front cover.

For palliation only. Continuous vital sign monitoring essential. **May cause apnea,** fever, seizures, flushing, bradycardia, hypotension, diarrhea, gastric outlet obstruction, and reversible cortical proliferation of long bones (with prolonged use). Decreases platelet aggregation.

For explanation of icons, see p. 600.

PROTAMINE SULFATE

No ? C

Antidote, heparin
Inj: 10 mg/ml

 Heparin antidote, IV:
1 mg protamine will neutralize
115 U porcine intestinal or 90 U
beef lung heparin.
Consider time of heparin and antidote
administration:
*If protamine given immediately after
heparin:* give 1–1.5 × doses above
If within 0.5–1 hr: give 50% of above
dose
If ≥2 hr: give 25% of above dose
Max dose: 50 mg IV
Max rate: 5 mg/min

 May cause hypotension,
bradycardia, dyspnea, and
anaphylaxis. Monitor aPTT or ACT.
Heparin rebound with bleeding has been
reported to occur 8–18 hours later.

PSEUDOEPHEDRINE

Yes 1 C

Sudafed, Novafed, and others
Sympathomimetic, nasal decongestant
Tabs: 30, 60 mg
Extended release tab: 120 mg
Caps: 60 mg
Sustained release caps: 120 mg
Liquid: 15, 30 mg/5 ml
Drops: 7.5 mg/0.8 ml

 Children <12 yr: 4 mg/kg/24 hr ÷
Q6 hr PO
Children ≥12 yr and adults:
Immediate release: 30–60 mg/dose
Q6–8 hr PO; **max dose:** 240 mg/24 hr
Sustained release: 120 mg PO Q12 hr

Use with **caution** in hypertension,
hyperglycemia, hyperthyroidism,
cardiac disease. May cause
nervousness, restlessness, insomnia,
arrhythmias. Pseudoephedrine is a
common component of OTC cough and
cold preparations. Since drug and active
metabolite are primarily excreted renally,
doses should be adjusted in renal
impairment.

PSYLLIUM

Metamucil, Fiberall, Seraton, Konsyl, and many others
Bulk-forming laxative

No 1 C

Granules: 2.5 g/rounded teaspoonful (480 g), 4.03 g/rounded tea-spoonful (100, 250 g)
Powder: 50% psyllium, 50% dextrose (sugar-free version available); 100% psyllium (6 g/ rounded teaspoon; Konsyl)
Wafers: 3.4 g
Effervescent Powder: 3.4 g/rounded teaspoonful (single dose packet, 141 g, 261 g, 387 g, 621 g)
Chewable squares: 1.7 g, 3.4 g

Children (granules or powder must be mixed with a full glass of water or juice):
<6 yr: 1.25–2.5 g/dose PO QD-TID;
max dose 7.5 g/24 hr
6–11 yr: 2.5–3.75 g/dose PO QD-TID;
max dose 15 g/24 hr
≥12 yr: 2.5–7.5 g/dose PO QD-TID;
max dose: 30 g/24 hr

Contraindicated in cases of fecal impaction or GI obstruction.
Phenylketonurics should be aware that certain preparations may contain aspartame. Should be taken with a full glass of liquid. Onset of action: 12–72 hr.

PYRANTEL PAMOATE

Antiminth, Reese's Pinworm medicine, Pin-Rid, Pin-X
Anthelmintic

No ? C

Susp: 50 mg/ml (60 ml)
Liquid: 50 mg/ml, 144 mg/ml (30 ml)
Caps: 180 mg (62.5 mg base)

Adults and Children:
Ascariasis *(roundworm):* 11 mg/kg/dose PO × 1
Enterobius *(pinworm):* 11 mg/kg/dose PO × 1. Repeat same dose 2 weeks later.
Hookworm or Eosinophilic Enterocolitis: 11 mg/kg/dose PO QD × 3 days
Max single dose (all indications): 1 g/dose

May cause nausea, vomiting, anorexia, transient AST elevations, headaches, rash, muscle weakness. Use with **caution** in liver dysfunction. Do **not** use in combination with piperazine because of antagonism. Drug may be mixed with milk or fruit juices and may be taken with food.

For explanation of icons, see p. 600.

PYRAZINAMIDE

Pyrazinoic acid amide
Antituberculous agent
Yes ? C
Tab: 500 mg
Suspension: 100 mg/ml

Children:
Daily dose: 20–40 mg/kg/24 hr PO ÷ QD-BID; **max dose:** 2 g/24 hr
Twice weekly dose: 50–70 mg/kg/dose PO 2 ×/week;
max dose: 4 g/dose
Adults:
Daily dose: 15–30 mg/kg/24 hr PO ÷ QD-QID; **max dose:** 2 g/24 hr
Twice weekly dose: 50–70 mg/kg/dose PO 2 ×/week;
max dose: 4 g/dose

See pp. 402–403 for recommended treatment for tuberculosis. **Contraindicated** in severe hepatic damage. Hepatoxicity is most common side effect. Hyperuricemia, maculopapular rash, arthralgia, fever, acne, porphyria, dysuria, photosensitivity may occur. Use with **caution** in patients with renal failure (dosage reduction have been recommended), gout, or diabetes mellitus.

PYRETHRINS

A-200 Pyrinate, Pyrinayl, Pronto Plus, RID, and others
Pediculicide
No ? C
Available as gel, shampoo, and liquid, all in combination with piperonyl butoxide. All products are available without a prescription.

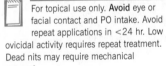

Pediculosis: Apply to hair or affected body area for 10 min, then wash thoroughly; repeat in 7–10 days.

For topical use only. **Avoid** eye or facial contact and PO intake. Avoid repeat applications in <24 hr. Low ovicidal activity requires repeat treatment. Dead nits may require mechanical removal.

PYRIDOSTIGMINE BROMIDE

Mestinon, Regonol
Cholinergic agent
No 1 C
Syrup: 60 mg/5 ml (480 ml)
Tabs: 60 mg
Inj: 5 mg/ml
Sustained release tab: 180 mg

Myasthenia Gravis:
Neonates:
  PO: 5 mg/dose Q4–6 hr
  IM/IV: 0.05–0.15 mg/kg/dose Q4–6 hr;
  max single IM/IV dose: 10 mg
Children:
  PO: 7 mg/kg/24 hr in 5–6 divided
  doses
  IM/IV: 0.05–0.15 mg/kg/dose Q4–6 hr;
  max single IM/IV dose: 10 mg
Adults:
  PO (immediate release): 60 mg TID.
  Increase Q48 hr PRN. Usual effective
  dose: 60–1500 mg/24 hr.
  PO (sustained release): 180–540 mg
  QD-BID
  IM/IV: 2–5 mg/dose Q2–3 hr

Changes in oral dosages may take
several days to show results. Use
with **caution** in patients with
epilepsy, asthma, bradycardia, hyperthyroidism, arrhythmias, or peptic ulcer.
May cause nausea, vomiting, diarrhea,
rash, headache, and muscle cramps.
Atropine is the antidote for autonomic.

PYRIDOXINE

Vitamin B$_6$
Vitamin, water soluble
No 1 A/C
Tabs: 25, 50, 100 mg
Tabs, extended release: 100 mg
Inj: 100 mg/ml

For explanation of icons, see p. 600.

Deficiency, IM/IV/PO (PO preferred):
Children: 5–25 mg/24 hr × 3 weeks, followed by 1.5—2.5 mg/24 hr as maintenance therapy (via multivitamin preparation)
Adult: 10–20 mg/24 hr × 3 weeks, followed by 2–5 mg/24 hr as maintenance therapy (via multivitamin preparation)
Drug induced neuritis, PO:
Prophylaxis:
Children: 1–2 mg/kg/24 hr
Adults: 25–100 mg/24 hr
Treatment:
Children: 10–50 mg/24 hr
Adults: 100–200 mg/24 hr
Sideroblastic anemia, PO: 200–600 mg/24 hr × 1–2 months. If adequate response, dose may be reduced to 30–50 mg/24 hr.
Pyridoxine dependent seizures:
Initial: 50–100 mg/dose IM or rapid IV × 1
Maintenance: 50–100 mg/24 hr PO
Recommended daily allowance: See p. 485.

Chronic administration has been associated with sensory neuropathy. Nausea, headache, increased AST, decreased serum folic acid level, and allergic reaction may occur. See p. 473 for management of neonatal seizures. Pregnancy category changes to "C" if used in doses above the RDA.

PYRIMETHAMINE
Daraprim
Antiparasitic agent
Tabs: 25 mg
Susp: 1, 2 mg/ml

No 1 C

Congenital Toxoplasmosis (administer with sulfadiazine):
Load: 2 mg/kg/24 hr PO ÷ Q12 hr × 2 days
Maintenance: 1 mg/kg/24 hr PO QD × 2–6 months, then 1 mg/kg/24 hr 3 ×/week to complete total 12 months of therapy.
Toxoplasmosis (administer with sulfadiazine or trisulfapyrimidines)
Children:
Load: 2 mg/kg/24 hr PO ÷ BID × 3 days; **max dose:** 100 mg/24 hr
Maintenance: 1 mg/kg/24 hr PO ÷ QD-BID × 4 weeks; **max dose:** 25 mg/24 hr

Adults: 50–75 mg/24 hr × 1–3 weeks depending on response. After response, decrease dose by 50% and continue for an additional 4–5 weeks.

Pyrimethamine is a folate antagonist. Supplementation with folinic acid leucovorin at 5–10 mg/24 hr is recommended. Pyrimethamine can cause glossitis, seizures, rash, and photosensitivity. For congenital toxoplasmosis, see *Clin Infect Dis* 1994; 18:38–72.

QUINIDINE
Many brand names
Antiarrhythmic, class Ia

Yes   1   C

As gluconate (62% quinidine):
Slow release tabs: 324 mg
Inj: 80 mg/ml

As sulfate (83% quinidine):
Tabs: 200, 300 mg
Slow release tab: 300 mg
Susp: 10 mg/ml

As polygalacturonate (80% quinidine):
Tabs: 275 mg
Equivalents: 200 mg sulfate = 267 mg
gluconate = 275 mg
polygalacturonate

All doses expressed as salt forms.
Antiarrhythmia:
Children (Give PO as sulfate. Give
IM/IV *as gluconate):*
Test dose: 2 mg/kg × 1 IM/PO; **max
dose:** 200 mg
Therapeutic dose:
IV (as gluconate): 2–10 mg/kg/dose
Q3–6 hr PRN
PO (as sulfate): 15–60 mg/kg/24 hr
÷ Q6 hr
Adults:
Test dose: 200 mg × 1 IM/PO. Give
PO as sulfate, IM as gluconate.
Therapeutic dose
As sulfate:
PO, Immediate Release: 100–
600 mg/dose Q4–6 hr. Begin at
200 mg/dose and titrate to desired
effect.
PO, Sustained Release: 300–
600 mg/dose Q 8–12 hr.
As gluconate:
IM: 400 mg/dose Q4–6 hr
IV: 200–400 mg/dose, infused at a
rate of ≤10 mg/min.
PO: 324–972 mg Q8–12 hr
As polygalacturonate:
PO: 275 mg Q8–12 hr

Test dose is given to assess for
idiosyncratic reaction to quinidine.
Toxicity indicated by increase of
QRS interval by ≥0.02 sec (skip dose or
stop drug). May cause GI symptoms,
hypotension, tinnitus, TTP, rash, heart
block, blood dyscrasias. When used
alone, may cause 1:1 conduction in atrial
flutter leading to ventricular fibrillation.
May get idiosyncratic ventricular
tachycardia with low levels, especially
when initiating therapy.

Can cause increase in digoxin levels.
Quinidine potentiates the effect of
neuromuscular blocking agents, beta-
blockers, anticholinergics, and warfarin.
Amiodarone, antacids, delavirdine,
saquinavir, ritonavir, verapamil, or
cimetidine may enhance the drug's effect.
Barbiturates, phenytoin, cholinergic drugs,
nifedipine, sucralfate, or rifampin may
reduce quinidine's effect. Use with
caution in renal insufficiency (15–25% of
drug is eliminated unchanged in the
urine). **Adjust dose in renal failure (se p.
941).**

Therapeutic levels: 3–7 mg/L.
Recommended serum sampling times at
steady-state: trough level obtained within
30 minutes prior to the next scheduled
dose after 1–2 days of continuous dosing
(steady-state).

RANITIDINE HCl

Zantac, Zantac 75[OTC]
Histamine-2-antagonist

Yes   1   B

Tabs: 75(OTC), 150, 300 mg
Effervescent Tabs: 150 mg
Syrup: 15 mg/ml
Effervescent Granules: 150 mg
Carbohydrate-free Oral Solution: 5,
10 mg/ml [dissolve 150 mg
effervescent granules with 30 ml
(5 mg/ml) or 15 ml (10 mg/ml) water;
solution good for 24 hrs]

Caps, GELdose: 150, 300 mg
Inj: 25 mg/ml
Inj (pre-mixed): 0.5 mg/ml
(preservative-free in ½ normal saline,
100 ml)

Neonates:
  PO: 2–4 mg/kg/24 hr ÷ Q8–12 hr
  IV: 2 mg/kg/24 hr ÷ Q6–8 hr
Infants and Children:
  PO: 4–5 mg/kg/24 hr ÷ Q8–12 hr
    Max dose: 6 mg/kg/24 hr
  IM/IV: 2–4 mg/kg/24 hr ÷ Q6–8 hr
Adults:
  PO: 150 mg/dose BID or 300 mg/dose
  QHS
  IM/IV: 50 mg/dose Q6–8 hr
    Max dose: 400 mg/24 hr
Continuous infusion, all ages: Administer
daily IV dosage over 24 hrs (may be
added to parenteral nutrition solutions)

May cause headache and GI
disturbance, malaise, insomnia,
sedation, arthralgia, hepatotoxicity.
May increase levels of nifedipine. May
decrease levels of ketoconazole,
itraconazole, delavirdine.
Extemporaneously compounded
carbohydrate-free oral solution dosage
form useful for patients receiving the
ketogenic diet. **Adjust dose in renal
failure (see p. 941).**

RESPIRATORY SYNCYTIAL VIRUS IMMUNE GLOBULIN

Respigam
Immune Globulin, RSV (high titer)
Injection: 50 mg/ml (1000 mg/20 ml, 2,500 mg/50 ml)

No   ?   C

RSV Prophylaxis:
Children <2 yrs: 750 mg/kg/dose IV Q monthly during the RSV season (typically November through April in the northern hemisphere but may begin earlier or persist later in certain communities).

Although this product has a broad indication for use in children <2 yrs old with BPD or history of prematurity (<35 weeks' gestation), see latest version of the AAP Redbook for specific use recommendations. **Con-**traindicated in Ig A deficiency. Should **not** be used in patients with cyanotic heart disease. Use with **caution** in patients with fluid restrictions. Frequent side effects include fever, respiratory distress, vomiting, and wheezing. Monitor heart rate, blood pressure, temperature, respiratory rate. Parenteral live virus vaccines (i.e., MMR, measles, varicella) should be deferred for 9–10 months after the last dose of RSVIG. Gradually increase IV infusion (if tolerated) by starting at 1.5 ml/kg/hr for 15 minutes, increase to 3 ml/kg/hr the next 15 minutes, then to 6 ml/kg/hr to the end of infusion.

Rh$_o$ (D) IMMUNE GLOBULIN INTRAVENOUS (HUMAN)

WinRho-SD
Immune Globulin
Inj: 600, 1500 IU
Conversion: 1 mcg = 5 IU

No   ?   C

Immune Thrombocytopenic Purpura (nonsplenectomized Rh$_o$(D)-positive patients):
Initial dose (may given in two divided doses on separate days or as a single dose):
  Hemoglobin ≥10 mg/dl: 250 IU/kg/dose IV × 1
  Hemoglobin <10 mg/dl: 125–200 IU/kg/dose IV × 1
Additional doses: 125–300 IU/kg/dose IV; actual dose and frequency of adminstration is determined from the patient's response.

WinRho SD is currently the only Rh$_o$ (D) immune globulin product compatable for intravenous administration. **Contraindicated** in Ig A deficiency. Use with **extreme caution** in patients with a hemoglobin <8 mg/dl. Adverse events associated with ITP include headache, chills, fever, and reduction in hemoglobin (due to the destruction of Rho (D) antigen-positive red cells). May interfere with immune response to live virus vaccines (i.e., MMR, varicella). Administer IV doses over 3–5 minutes.

RIBAVIRIN
Virazole, Rebetol
Antiviral agent

Yes ? X

Aerosol (Virazole): 6 g
Oral Caps (Rebetol): 200 mg [only available in combination with Interferon Alfa-2b as a kit (Rebetron)]

Inhalation:
Continuous: Administer 6 g by aerosol over 12–18 hr QD for 3–7 days. The 6 g ribavirin vial is diluted in 300 ml preservative-free sterile water to a final concentration of 20 mg/ml. Must be administered with Viratek Small Particle Aerosol Generator (SPAG-2).
Intermittent (For non-ventilated patients): Administer 2 g by aerosol over 2 hours TID for 3–7 days. The 6 g ribavirin vial is diluted in 100 ml preservative-free sterile water to a final concentration of 60 mg/ml. Use not recommended in patients with endotracheal tubes.
Hepatitis C:
Adults (in combination with interferon alfa-2b at 3 million units 3 ×/week SC):
≤75 kg (PO): 400 mg QAM and 600 mg QPM
>75 kg (PO): 600 mg BID

Use of ribavirin in RSV is controversial. Ribavirin aerosol therapy is a consideration for selected infants and young children at high risk for serious RSV disease (see Red Book for details). Most effective if begun early in course of RSV infection; generally in the first 3 days. May cause worsening respiratory distress, rash, conjunctivitis, mild bronchospasm, hypotension, anemia, and cardiac arrest. Respiratory therapy and nursing personnel should be trained in ribavirin administration because of its teratogenic effects in animals. Drug can precipitate in the respiratory equipment.

ORAL RIBAVIRIN: With oral use, administer with caution in patients with creatinine clearance <50 ml/min; **not recommended in severe renal impairment.** Anemia (most common), insomnia, depression, irritability, and suicidal behavior have been reported with the oral route of administration. Reduce dose to 600 mg/24 hr if hemoglobin <10 g/dL but discontinue use of drug if hemoglobin drops below 8.5 g/dL.

RIBOFLAVIN
Riobin
Vitamin B$_2$
Tabs: 25, 50, 100 mg

No 1 A/C

Riboflavin deficiency:
Children: 2.5–10 mg/24 hr ÷ QD-BID PO
Adults: 5–30 mg/24 hr ÷ QD-BID PO
RDA requirements: see p. 485.

Hypersensitivity may occur. Administer with food. Causes yellow to orange discoloration of urine. For multi-vitamin information, see p. 517.
Pregnancy category changes to "C" if used in doses above the RDA.

RIFABUTIN
Mycobutin
Antituberculous agent
Caps: 150 mg
Susp: 10 mg/ml

Yes ? B

MAC Prophylaxis for 1st episode of opportunistic disease in HIV:
Children:
    <6 yrs: 5 mg/kg/24 hr PO QD; **max dose:** 300 mg/24 hr
    ≥6 yrs: 300 mg PO QD with food
Adolescents and Adults: 300 mg PO QD or 150 mg PO BID with or without azithromycin.
MAC Prophylaxis for Recurrence of opportunistic disease in HIV (in combination with a multidrug regimen which includes a macrolide antibiotic):
Infants and Children: 5 mg/kg/24 hr PO QD; **max dose:** 300 mg/24 hr
Adolescents and Adults: 300 mg PO QD or 150 mg PO BID with food
MAC Treatment:
Children: 5–10 mg/kg/24 hr PO QD; **max dose:** 300 mg/24 hr as part of a multi-drug regimen.
Adult: 300–600 mg/24 hr PO ÷ QD-BID as part of a multi-drug regimen. Do **not** exceed 300 mg/24 hr if given in combination with a macrolide antibiotic or fluconazole.

May cause GI distress, discoloration of skin and body fluids (brown-orange color), and marrow suppressive effects. Use with **caution** in renal failure (53% renal excretion). May permanently stain contact lenses. Uveitis can occur when using high doses (>300 mg/24 hr in adults) in combination with macrolide antibiotics. Rifabutin is structurally similar to rifampin, thus anticipated to have similar drug interactions as rifampin (see Rifampin). Clarithromycin and fluconazole increase rifabutin levels. May decrease effectiveness of dapsone, AZT, oral contraceptives, warfarin, oral contraceptives, digoxin, cyclosporin, ketoconazole, and narcotics. Doses may be administered with food if patient experiences GI intolerance.

RIFAMPIN
Rimactane, Rifadin
Antibiotic, antituberculous agent
Caps: 150, 300 mg
Susp: 10 mg/ml, 15 mg/ml
Inj: 600 mg

Yes 1 C

Tuberculosis: (see pp. 402–403 for duration of therapy and combination therapy). Twice weekly therapy may be used after 1–2 months of daily therapy

Children:
  Daily therapy: 10–20 mg/kg/24 hr ÷ Q12–24 hr IV/PO
  Twice weekly therapy: 10–20 mg/kg/24 hr PO twice weekly
  Max daily dose: 600 mg/24 hr
Adults:
  Daily therapy: 10 mg/kg/24 hr QD PO
  Twice weekly therapy: 10 mg/kg/24 hr QD twice weekly
  Max daily dose: 600 mg/24 hr
Prophylaxis for N. meningitidis:
  0–1 mo: 10 mg/kg/24 hr ÷ Q12 hr PO × 2 days
  >1 mo: 20 mg/kg/24 hr ÷ Q12 hr PO × 2 days
  Adults: 600 mg PO Q12 hr × 2 days
  Max dose (all ages): 1200 mg/24 hr
Prophylaxis for H. influenzae:
  0–1 mo: 10 mg/kg/dose PO QD × 4 days

>1 mo: 20 mg/kg/dose PO QD × 4 days
Adults: 600 mg PO QD × 4 days
Max dose (all ages): 600 mg/24 hr

May cause GI irritation, allergy, headache, fatigue, ataxia, confusion, fever, hepatitis, blood dyscrasias, interstital nephritis, and elevated BUN and uric acid. Causes red discoloration of body secretions such as urine, saliva, and tears (which can permanently stain contact lenses). Induces hepatic enzymes (CYP 450 2C9, 2C19, and 3A4) which may decrease plasma concentration of digoxin, corticosteroids, benzodiazepines, calcium channel blockers, beta-blockers, cyclosporine, oral anticoagulants, barbiturates, and theophylline. May reduce the effectiveness of oral contraceptives. Reduce dose in hepatic impairment. Give 1 hour before or 2 hour after meals. **Adjust dose in renal failure (see p. 935).**

RIMANTADINE
Flumadine
Antiviral agent
Syrup: 50 mg/ 5 ml
Tabs: 100 mg

Yes ? C

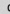

Influenza A prophylaxis:
  Children <10 yr: 5 mg/kg/24 hr
  PO QD; **max dose:** 150 mg/24 hr
  Children ≥10 yr and adults: 100 mg PO
  BID
Influenza A treatment:
  Children <10 yr: 5 mg/kg/24 hr PO ÷
  QD-BID; **max dose:** 150 mg/24 hr
  Children ≥10 yr (<40 kg): 5 mg/kg/
  24 hr PO ÷ QD-BID
  Children ≥10 yr (≥40 kg) and adults:
  100 mg PO BID

During influenza season, use
prophylaxis for 2–3 weeks after
influenza vaccination in order for
patient to develop protective antibody
response. Alternatively may be used for
10 days after patient has been exposed.
Duration of treatment is generally
5–7 days. Attempt to begin medication
within the first 48 hours of illness. May
cause GI disturbance, dizziness,
headache, urinary retention. CNS
disturbances are less than with
amantadine. Use with **caution** in renal or
hepatic insufficiency; dosage reduction
may be necessary. A dosage reduction of
50% have been recommended in severe
hepatic or renal impairment.

RITONAVIR
Norvir
Antiviral, protease inhibitor
Caps: 100 mg
Oral Solution: 80 mg/ml (240 ml)

No   3   B

For explanation of icons, see p. 600.

Children ≤12 yrs: Start at 250 mg/m^2/dose Q12 hr PO, then increase dose at 2–3 day intervals by 50 mg/m^2/dose Q12 hr up to 400 mg/m^2/dose Q12 hr. Dosage range: 350–400 mg/m^2/dose Q12 hr.

Max dose: 600 mg/dose BID

Adolescent and Adults: Start at 300 mg/dose Q12 hr PO. To minimize nausea and vomiting, increase stepwise to 600 mg/dose Q12 hr over 5 days as tolerated. If used in combination with saquinavir, increase dose to only to 400 mg/dose Q12 hr PO.

Dose titration schedule is recommended to minimize risk for side effects. Use with **caution** in liver impairment.

Most frequent side effects include nausea, vomiting, diarrhea, headache, abdominal pain, anorexia. Paresthesias, and increases in liver enzymes, triglycerides, cholesterol, serum glucose may also occur. Spontaneous bleeding in hemophiliacs has been reported.

Inhibits and is metabolized by the CYP3A4 microsomal enzyme to cause many drug interactions (see p. 924). Do **NOT** use concurrently with amiodarone, astemizole, bepridil, bupropion, cisapride, clozapine, dihydroergotamine, ergotamine, flecainide, encainide, meperidine, pimozide, piroxicam, propafenone, propoxyphene, quinidine, rifabutin, rifampin, terfenadine, and benzo-diazepines (except for lorazepam). Drug may increase the levels of clarithromycin, desipramine, warfarin, and digoxin. Theopylline and digoxin levels may be reduced. Always check the potential for other drug interactions when either initiating therapy or adding new drugs onto an existing regimen.

Administer doses with food to assure absorption. If didanosine is included in the anti-retroviral regimen, space the administration of two drug by 2 hours. Store both capsules and oral solution in the refrigerator. Oral solution can be kept at room temperature if used within 30 days. Oral solution must be kept in original container. Administering doses with milk, chocolate milk, pudding, or ice cream can enhance compliance in children. Non-compliance can quickly promote resistant HIV strains.

ROCURONIUM
Zemuron
Nondepolarizing neuromuscular blocking agent
Inj: 10 mg/ml (5, 10 ml)

No   ?   B

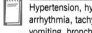

Children and Adults:
IV: Start with 0.6–1.2 mg/kg/dose × 1, if needed, maintenance doses at 0.1–0.2 mg/kg/dose Q 20–30 min.
Continuous IV Infusion: Start at 10–12 mcg/kg/min and titrate to effect. Maintenance infusion rates have ranged from 4–16 mcg/kg/min in adults.

Hypertension, hypotension, arrhythmia, tachycardia, nausea, vomiting, bronchospasm, wheezing, hiccups, rash, and edema at the injection site may occur. Increased neuromuscular blockade may occur with concomitant use of aminoglycosides, clindamycin, tetracycline, magnesium sulfate, quinine, quinidine, succinylcholine, and inhalation anesthetics. Carbamazepine, phenytoin, phenylephrine, azathioprine, and theophylline may reduce neuromuscular blocking effects.

Peak effects occur in 0.5–1 min for children and in 1–3.7 min for adults. Duration of action: 30–40 minutes in children and 20–94 minutes in adults (longer in geriatrics). Recovery time in children 3 months to 1 year is simular to adults. In obese patients, use actual body weight for dosage calculation.

SALMETEROL
Serevent, Serevent Diskus
Beta-2-adrenergic agonist (long acting)

No   ?   C
Aerosol Metered dose inhaler (MDI): 21 mcg/actuation (6.5 g, 13 g; 6.5 g = 60 actuations)
Dry powder inhalation (DPI; Diskus): 50 mcg/inhalation (28, 60 inhalations)

Chronic Asthma:
MDI:
    Children: 1–2 puffs (21–42 mcg) Q12 hr
    >12 yr and adults: 2 puffs (42 mcg) Q12 hr
DPI (>4 yr and adults): 1 inhalation (50 mcg) Q12 hr
Exercise Induced Asthma (>12 yrs):
MDI: 2 puffs 30–60 minutes before exercise. Additional doses should not be used for another 12 hours.
DPI: 1 inhalation 30–60 minutes before exercise. Additional does should not be used for another 12 hours.

Should **not** be used to relieve symptoms of acute asthma. It is long acting and has its onset of action in 10–20 minutes with a peak effect at 3 hours. May be used QHS (1–2 MDI puffs or 1 DPI) for nocturnal symptoms. Salmeterol is a chronic medication and is not used in similar fashion to short acting beta agonists (i.e., albuterol). Patients already receiving salmeterol Q12 hr (MDI or DPI) should not use additional doses for prevention of exercise-induced bronchospasm; consider alternative therapy. Proper patient education is essential. Side effects similar to albuterol.

For explanation of icons, see p. 600.

SAQUINAVIR
Invirase (mesylate salt), Fortovase
Antiviral agent, protease inhibitor
Caps, hard gel: (Invirase): 200 mg
Caps, soft gel: (Fortovase): 200 mg

No 3 B

Children (investigational dose from ACTG 397):
Fortovase: 50 mg/kg/dose PO TID
Adolescent and Adults:
Single protease inhibitor regimen:
Invirase: 600 mg/dose PO TID
Fortovase: 1200 mg/dose PO TID
In combination with Ritonavir:
Invirase or Fortovase: 400 mg/dose PO TID

Most frequent adverse effects include diarrhea, GI discomfort, nausea and headache.
Spontaneous bleeding in hemophiliacs, hyperglycemia, and body fat redistribution without serum lipid abnormalities have been reported.

Drug inhibis and is metabolized by the CYP450 3A4 drug metabolizing enzyme (see p. 924). Do **not** use in combination with astemizole, terfenadine, cisapride, ergot alkaloids, and benzodiazepines (except lorazepam). Increased levels and/or toxicity may occur with the following concurrent medications: calcium channel blockers, clindamycin, dapsone, quinidine. Rifampin, rifabutin, niverapine, carbamazepine, dexamethasone, phenobarbital, and phenytoin can decrease saquinavir levels. Whereas, delavirdine, ketoconazole, grapefruit juice, and other protease inhibitors may increase saquinavir levels. Always carefully review patient's medication profile for other potential drug-drug interactions.

Administer each dose with food or within 2 hours after a meal. Fortovase capsules are usually stored in the refrigerator; their stability will decrease to 3 months once they are brought to room temperature. Non-compliance can quickly promote resistant HIV strains.

SCOPOLAMINE HYDROBROMIDE
Hyoscine, Transderm Scop, Isopto
Anticholinergic agent
Inj: 0.3, 0.4, 0.86, 1 mg/ml
Transdermal: 1.5 mg/patch; delivers 0.5 mg over 3 days
Ophthalmic sol: 0.25% (5, 15 ml)

No 1 C

Antiemesis (SC/IM/IV):
Children: 6 mcg/kg/dose Q6–8 hr
PRN; **max dose:** 300 mcg/dose
Adults: 0.2–1 mg/dose Q6–8 hr PRN
Transdermal (≥12 yr): Apply patch behind
the ear at least 4 hr prior to exposure to
motion; use for 72 hr.
Ophthalmic:
Children refraction: 1 drop BID for 2 days
before procedure.
Children iridocyclitis: 1 drop up to TID.

Toxicities similar to atropine.
Contraindicated in urinary or GI
obstruction and glaucoma. May
cause dry mouth, drowsiness, blurred
vision. Transdermal route should not be
used in children <12 yr. Systemic effects
have been reported with both topical and
ophthalmic preparations. Compress
nasolacrimal ducts to minimize systemic
effects when using ophthalmic
preparations.

SELENIUM SULFIDE
Selsun, Exsel (Rx)
Topical antiseborrheic agent
Lotion/Shampoo: 1% (OTC), 2.5% (Rx & OTC)
Shampoo: 1% (OTC)

No ? C

 Seborrhea/Dandruff: massage
5–10 ml of 1% or 2.5% into wet
scalp and leave on scalp × 2–3
min. Rinse thoroughly and repeat.
Shampoo twice weekly × 2 weeks.
Maintenance applications once every 1–4
weeks.
Tinea versicolor: apply 2.5% to affected
areas of skin. Allow to remain on skin ×
30 minutes. Rinse thoroughly. Repeat QD
× 7 days. Follow with monthly
applications for 3 months to prevent
recurrences.

Rinse hands and body well after
treatment. May cause local irritation, hair loss, and hair discoloration. **Avoid** eyes and genital area.
Shampoo may be used for tinea capitis to
reduce risk of transmission to others (does
not eradicate tinea infection).

For explanation of icons, see p. 600.

SENNA
Senokot, Senna-Gen, and others
Laxative, stimulant
Granules: 326 mg/tsp
Rectal suppository: 652 mg
Syrup: 218 mg/5 ml (60 ml, 240 ml)
Tab: 187, 217, 374, 600 mg
Liquid: 33.3 mg/ml (contains 3.5% or 4.9% alcohol)

No 1 C

Children:
Oral: 10–20 mg/kg/dose PO QHS.
Max doses as shown below or
1 mo–1 yr: 55–109 mg PO QHS to
max: 218 mg/24 hr
1–5 yr: 109–218 mg PO QHS to
max: 436 mg/24 hr
5–15 yrs: 218–436 mg PO QHS to
max: 872 mg/24 hr
Rectal: Children >27 kg: 326 mg (½
supp.) PR QHS
Adults:
Oral:
   Granules: 1 tsp at bedtime; **max dose:** 2 tsp BID.

Syrup: 2–3 tsp (10–15 ml) at
bedtime; **max dose:** 3 tsp BID.
Tablet: 2 tabs (187 mg × 2) at
bedtime; **max dose:** 4 tabs (187 mg
× 4) BID.
Rectal: 652 mg (1 supp.) PR QHS;
may repeat dose × 1 in 2 hours if
needed.

Effects occur within 6–24 hr after
oral administration. May cause
nausea, vomiting, diarrhea,
abdominal cramps. Active metabolite
stimulates Auerbach's plexus.

SERTRALINE HCl
Zoloft
Antidepressant (selective serotonin reuptake inhibitor)
Tabs: 25, 50, 100 mg
Caps: 25, 50, 100 mg

Yes 3 B

Depression:
Adults: Start at 50 mg PO QD. May increase dosage in 1 week intervals up to **max dose:** 200 mg/24 hr
Obsessive Compulsive Disorder:
Children:
Initial dose: 6–12 yrs start at 25 mg PO QD; *≥13 yrs* start at 50 mg PO QD
Maintenance dose: if needed, initial dose may be increased at 1 week intervals up to a **max dose:** 200 mg/24 hr.

This drug should **not** be used in combination with an MAO inhibitor or within 14 days of discontinuing an MAO inhibitor. Use with **caution** in patients with hepatic or renal impairment. Adverse effects include nausea, diarrhea, tremor, increased sweating. Hyponatremia and platelet dysfunction have been reported. Concurrent administration with warfarin may increase PT. Inhibits the CYP450 2D6 drug metabolizing enzyme; see p. 924 for potential interacting drugs (substrates metabolized by the same enzyme).

SILVER SULFADIAZINE
Silvadene, Thermazene, SSD Cream, SSD AF Cream
Topical antibiotic
Cream: 1% (20, 25, 50, 85, 400, 1000 g)

No ? C

Cover affected areas completely QD–BID. Apply cream to a thickness of ⅟₁₆" using sterile technique.

Contraindicated in premature infants and infant ≤ to 2 months of age due to concerns of kernicterus. Discard product if cream has darkened. Adverse effects include pruritus, rash, bone marrow suppression, and hemolytic anemia, as well as interstitial nephritis. See p. 89 for more information.

SIMETHICONE
Mylicon, Phazyme, Mylanta Gas, Gas-X, and others
Antiflatulent
Oral drops: 40 mg/0.6 ml (15, 30 ml)
Caps: 125 mg
Tabs: 60, 95 mg
Chewable Tabs: 40, 80, 125 mg

No ? C

Infants and Children <2 yrs:
20 mg PO QID; **max dose:** 240 mg/24 hr
2–12 yrs: 40 mg PO QID
>12 yrs: 40–125 mg PO QAC and QHS PRN; **max dose:** 500 mg/24 hr

Avoid carbonated beverage and gas-forming foods. Oral liquid may be mixed with water, infant formula, or other suitable liquids for ease of oral administration.

SODIUM PHOSPHATE

Yes ? C

Fleet, Fleet Phospho-soda
Laxative, enema/oral
Enema (Fleet): 6 g Na phos and 16 g Na biphosphate/100 ml
  Pediatric size: 67.5 ml
  Adult size: 133 ml

Oral Solution (Fleet Phospho Soda): 18 g Na phos and 48 g Na biphosphate/100 ml (30, 45, 90, 237 ml); contains 96.4mEq Na per 20 ml

Not to be used for phosphorus supplementation. See phosphorus.
Enema:
2–12 yr: 67.5 ml enema × 1. May repeat × 1
>12 yr and adults: 133 ml enema × 1. May repeat × 1
Oral Laxative (mix with equal volume of water):
  5–9 yr: 5 ml PO × 1
  10–12 yr: 10 ml PO × 1
  >12 yr: 20 to 30 ml PO × 1

Contraindicated in patients with severe renal failure, congenital megacolon, and congestive heart failure. May cause hyperphosphatemia, hypernatremia, hypocalcemia, hypotension, dehydration, and acidosis. Avoid retention of enema solution, as this may lead to severe electrolyte disturbances due to enhanced systemic absorption. Onset of action: PO: 3–6 hr; PR: 2–5 min.

SODIUM POLYSTYRENE SULFONATE

Yes ? C

Kayexalate, SPS
Potassium removing resin
Powder: 454 g
Susp: 15 g/60 ml (contains 21.5 ml sorbitol/60 ml) (60, 120, 200, 500 ml)
Contains 4.1 mEq Na$^+$/g drug

Children:
Usual dose: 1 g/kg/dose Q6 hr PO
or Q2–6 hr PR
Adults:
PO: 15–60 g QD-QID
PR: 30–50 g Q6 hr
Note: Suspension may be given PO or PR.
Practical exchange ratio is 1 mEq K per
1 g resin. May calculate dose according to
desired exchange.

1 mEq Na delivered for each mEq K
removed. Use **cautiously** in presence of renal failure. May cause
hypokalemia, hypomagnesemia, and
hypocalcemia. Do **not** administer with
antacids or laxatives containing Mg or Al.
Systemic alkalosis may result. Retain
enema in colon for at least 30–60 minutes.

SPECTINOMYCIN
Trobicin
Antibiotic, aminoglycoside
Inj: 2 g with 3.2 ml diluent which contains 0.9% benzyl alcohol

Yes   ?   B

Uncomplicated Gonorrhea:
Children <45 kg: 40 mg/kg IM × 1
≥45 kg and adults: 2 g IM × 1
Max dose: 2 g/dose IM
Disseminated Gonorrhea:
≥45 kg and adults: 2 g IM Q12 hr ×
7 days. Alternatively may treat × 24–
48 hr and switch to oral alternative.

Not effective for syphilis. Drug is
primarily used to treat gonorrhea in
patients who cannot tolerate
cephalosporins or fluoroquinolones.
Vertigo, malaise, nausea, anorexia, chills,
fever, urticaria may occur. Repeated
dosing of the drug will accumulate in
renal failure. IM use only.

SPIRONOLACTONE
Aldactone
Diuretic, potassium sparing
Tabs: 25, 50, 100 mg
Susp: 1, 2, 5 mg/ml

Yes   1   D

For explanation of icons, see p. 600.

Diuretic:
Children: 1–3.3 mg/kg/24 hr ÷ BID-QID PO
Adults: 25–200 mg/24 hr ÷ BID-QID PO
Max dose: 200 mg/24 hr
Diagnosis of primary aldosteronism:
Children: 125–375 mg/m²/24 hr ÷ BID-QID PO
Adults: 400 mg QD PO × 4 days (short test) or 3–4 weeks (long test), then 100–400 mg QD maintenance.

Contraindicated in acute renal failure (see p. 941). May cause hyperkalemia, GI distress, rash, gynecomastia. May potentiate ganglionic blocking agents and other antihypertensives. Monitor potassium levels and be aware of other K⁺ sources, K⁺ sparing diuretics, and angiotensin-converting enzyme inhibitors (all can increase K⁺).

STAVUDINE
Zerit, d4T
Antiviral agent, nucleoside analogue reverse transcriptase inhibitor
Caps: 15, 20, 30, 40 mg
Oral Solution: 1 mg/ml

Yes 3 C

Children:
<30 kg: 1 mg/kg/dose PO Q12 hr
Adolescents and Adults:
30–60 kg: 30 mg PO Q12 hr
>60 kg: 40 mg PO Q12 hr

Active against most AZT-resistant viral strains. Common side effects include headache, GI discomfort, and rash. Peripheral neuropathy, pancreatitis, and elevated liver enzymes have been reported. **Adjust dosage in renal impairment (see p. 935).** Should not be given in combination with zidovudine (AZT) because of poor antiviral effect.

Doses can be administered with food. Oral solution: shake well before measuring each dose and keep refrigerated (30 day stability after initial reconstitution).

STREPTOKINASE
Kabikinase, Streptase
Thrombolytic enzyme
Inj: 250,000; 600,000; 750,000; 1,500,000 IU

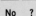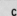

No ? C

DVT: **Should be used in consultation with a hematologist.**
Duration of therapy will depend on clinical response and generally does not exceed 3 days.

Children: 3500–4000 U/kg over 30 min, followed by 1000–1500 U/kg/hr; OR 2000 U/kg load over 30 min followed by 2000 U/kg/hr. Duration of infusion is individualized based on response.

 Contraindicated with intracranial or intraspinal surgery, hx of internal bleeding, recent streptococcus infection, CVA within 2 months. May cause hemorrhage, urticaria, itching, flushing, musculoskeletal pain, bronchospasm, and anaphylaxis. Pediatric safety and efficacy information is limited.

STREPTOMYCIN SULFATE

Antibiotic, aminoglycoside; antituberculous agent
Inj: 400 mg/ml (2.5 ml)

Yes   1   D

 Tuberculosis: (see p. 403 for duration of therapy and combination therapy)

Children:
Daily therapy: 20–40 mg/kg/24 hr IM QD
Max daily dose: 1 g/24 hr
Twice weekly therapy: 20–40 mg/kg/dose IM twice weekly
Max daily dose: 1.5 g/24 hr

Adults:
Daily therapy: 15 mg/kg/24 hr IM QD
Max daily dose: 1 g/24 hr
Twice weekly therapy: 25–30 mg/kg/dose IM twice weekly
Max daily dose: 1.5 g/24 hr

Use with caution in pre-existing vertigo, tinnitus, hearing loss, neuromuscular disorders. **Adjust dose in renal insufficiency (see p. 935).** Drug is administered via deep IM injection only. Follow auditory status. May cause CNS depression or other neurologic problems, myocarditis, serum sickness.

Therapeutic levels: peak 15–40 mg/L, trough: <5 mg/L. Recommended serum sampling time at steady-state: trough within 30 minutes prior to the 3rd consecutive dose and peak 30–60 minutes after the administration of the 3rd consecutive dose. Therapeutic levels are not achieved in CSF.

For explanation of icons, see p. 600.

SUCCIMER
Chemet, DMSA [dimercaptosuccinic acid]
Chelating agent
Cap: 100 mg

Yes ? C

 Lead Chelation, Children:
10 mg/kg/dose (or 350 mg/m^2/dose) PO Q8 hr × 5 days, then 10 mg/kg/dose (or 350 mg/m^2/dose) PO Q12 hr × 14 days.
Manufacturer recommends:

Wt (kg)	Dose (mg)
8–15	100
16–23	200
24–34	300
35–44	400
≥45	500

Give dose above every 8 hr for 5 days.
Then same dose Q12 hr for 14 days.

Use **caution** in patients with compromised renal function. Repeated courses may be necessary. Follow serum lead levels (see p. 34). Min: 2 wk between courses, unless blood levels require more aggressive management. Side effects: GI symptoms, increased LFTs (10%), rash, headaches, dizziness. **Co-administration with other chelating agents is not recommended.** Treatment of iron deficiency is recommended as well as environmental remediation. Contents of capsule may be sprinkled on food for those who are unable to swallow capsule.

SUCCINYLCHOLINE
Anectine, Quelicin, and others
Neuromuscular blocking agent
Inj: 20 mg/ml (10 ml), 50 mg/ml (10 ml), 100 mg/ml (5, 10 ml)
Powder for inj: 100, 500, 1000 mg

No ? C

Paralysis for intubation:
Infants and Children:
Initial:
IV: 1–2 mg/kg/dose × 1
IM: 3–4 mg/kg/dose × 1
Max dose: 150 mg/dose
Maintenance: 0.3–0.6 mg/kg/dose IV Q5–10 min PRN. **Continuous infusion not recommended**
Adults:
Initial:
IV: 0.3–1.1 mg/kg/dose × 1
IM: 3–4 mg/kg/dose × 1
Max dose: 150 mg/dose
Maintenance: 0.04–0.07 mg/kg/dose IV Q5–10 min PRN

Pretreatment with atropine is recommended to reduce incidence of bradycardia. For rapid sequence intubation, see p. 7. May cause malignant hyperthermia, bradycardia, hypotension, arrhythmia, and hyperkalemia. Use with **caution** in patients with severe burns, paraplegia, or crush injuries and in patients with preexisting hyperkalemia. Beware of prolonged depression in patients with liver disease, malnutrition, pseudocholinesterase deficiency, hypothermia, and those receiving aminoglycosides, phenothiazines, quinidine, beta-blockers, amphotericin b, cyclophosphamide, diuretics, lithium, acetylcholine, and anticholinesterases. Diazepam may decrease neuromuscular blocking effects.Duration of action 4–6 minutes
IV, 10–30 minutes IM. Must be prepared to intubate within 1 minute.

SUCRALFATE
Carafate
Oral anti-ulcer agent
Tabs: 1 g
Susp: 100 mg/ml (420 ml)

Yes ? B

Children: 40–80 mg/kg/24 hr ÷ Q6 hr PO
Adults: 1 g PO QID 1 hr AC and QHS

May cause vertigo, constipation, dry mouth. Aluminum may accumulate in patients with renal failure. This may be augmented by the use of aluminum-containing antacids. Decreases absorption of phenytoin, digoxin, theophylline, cimetidine, fat soluble vitamins, ketoconazole, quinolones, and oral anticoagulants. Administer these drugs at least 2 hours before or after sucralfate doses.

For explanation of icons, see p. 600.

SULFACETAMIDE SODIUM

Sulamyd and others
Ophthalmic antibiotic, sulfonamide derivative

No   2   B/D

Ophth Sol: 10% (1, 2, 2.5, 5, 15 ml), 15% (2, 5, 15 ml), 30% (5, 15 ml)
Ophth Ointment: 10% (3.5 g)

 >2 months and Adults:
Ophthalmic ointment: Apply ribbon QID and QHS

Drops: 1–2 drops Q2–3 hr to affected eye.

See sulfisoxazole. 10% solution is used most frequently. May cause local irritation, stinging, burning, toxic epidermal necrolysis (rarely). Local irritation occurs more frequently with higher strength preparations. Pregnancy category changes to "D" if administered near term.

SULFADIAZINE

Various trade names
Antibiotic, sulfonamide derivative

Yes   2   B/D

Tabs: 500 mg
Susp: 100 mg/ml ✅

Congenital toxoplasmosis
(administer with pyrimethamine and folinic acid) (From *Clin Infect Dis* 18:38, 1994):
Infants: 100 mg/kg/24 hr PO ÷ BID × 12 months
Toxoplasmosis (administer with pyrimethamine and folinic acid):
Children: 100–200 mg/kg/24 hr ÷ Q6 hr PO × 3–4 weeks
Adults: 4–6 g/24 hr PO ÷ Q6 hr × 3–4 weeks
Rheumatic Fever Prophylaxis:
≤27 kg: 500 mg PO QD
>27 kg: 1000 mg PO QD

Contraindicated in porphyria and hypersensitivity to sulfonamides. Use with **caution** in premature infants and infants <2 mo because of risk of hyperbilirubinemia; and in hepatic or renal dysfunction (30–44% eliminated in urine). Maintain hydration. May cause increased effects of warfarin, methotrexate, and sulfonylureas due to drug displacement from protein binding sites. May cause fever, rash, hepatitis, SLE-like syndrome, vasculitis, bone marrow suppression, hemolysis in patients with G6PD deficiency, and Stevens-Johnson syndrome. Pregnancy category changes to "D" if administered near term.

SULFASALAZINE

Salicylazo-sulfapyridine, SAS, Azulfidine
Anti-inflammatory agent
Tabs: 500 mg
Enteric-coated Tabs: 500 mg
Oral Susp: 250 mg/5 ml

Yes 2 B/D

Ulcerative Colitis:
Children >2 yr:
Initial:
Moderate/severe: 50–70 mg/kg/24 hr ÷ Q4–6 hr PO; **max dose:** 6 g/24 hr
Mild: 40–50 mg/kg/24 hr ÷ Q4–6 hr PO
Maintenance: 30 mg/kg/24 hr ÷ QID PO; **max dose:** 2 g/24 hr
Adults:
Initial: 3–4 g/24 hr ÷ Q4–6 hr PO
Maintenance: 2 g/24 hr ÷ Q6–12 hr PO
Max dose: 6 g/24 hr

Use with **caution** in renal impairment. Maintain hydration. May cause orange-yellow discoloration of urine and skin. May permanently stain contact lenses. May cause photosensitivity, hypersensitivity, blood dyscrasias, CNS changes, nausea, vomiting, anorexia, diarrhea, and renal damage. May cause hemolysis in patients with G6PD deficiency. Decreases folic acid absorption; and reduces serum digoxin, cyclosporine levels. Slow acetylators may require lower dosage due to accumulation of active sulfapyridine metabolite. Pregnancy category changes to "D" if administered near term.

SULFISOXAZOLE

Gantrisin
Antibiotic, sulfonamide derivative
Tabs: 500 mg
Susp: 500 mg/5 ml (480 ml)
Syrup: 500 mg/5 ml (480 ml)
Ophthalmic sol: 4% (40 mg/ml) (15 ml)

Yes 2 B/D

For explanation of icons, see p. 600.

Otitis media prophylaxis: 50 mg/kg/dose QHS PO
Rheumatic fever prophylaxis:
<27 kg: 500 mg PO QD
≥27 kg: 1000 mg PO QD
Meningicoccus prophylaxis (for susceptible strains):
<1 yr: 500 mg PO QD × 2 days
1–12 yrs: 500 mg PO BID × 2 days
>12 yrs: 1 g PO BID × 2 days
Ophthalmic sol: 1–2 drops Q1–4 hr; increase the time interval between doses as the condition responds.

Contraindicated in urinary obstruction, near-term pregnant or nursing mothers. Use with **caution** in infants <2 mo, the presence of renal or liver disease, or G6PD deficiency. **Adjust dose in renal failure (see p. 935).** Maintain adequate fluid intake. See Sulfadiazine for toxicities and drug interactions. Interferes with folate absorption. Pregnancy category changes to "D" if administered near term. For combination with erythromycin, see p. 708.

SUMATRIPTAN SUCCINATE

Imitrex
Antimigraine agent, selective serotonin agonist
Inj: 12 mg/ml
Unit use syringe: 6 mg/syringe (2 syringes per box)
Tabs: 25, 50 mg
Nasal Spray (as a unit-dose spray device): 5 mg dose in 100 micro-liters (6 units per pack); 20 mg dose in 100 micro-liters (6 units per pack)

Yes   ?   C

Adolescents and adults:
PO: 25 mg as soon as possible after onset of headache. If no relief in 2 hours, give 25–100 mg Q 2 hr up to a **daily maximum** of 200 mg. **Max single dose:** 100 mg/dose.
Max daily dose: 200 mg/24 hr
SC: 6 mg × 1 as soon as possible after onset of headache. If no response, may give an additional dose of ≤6 mg one hour later. **Max daily dose:** 12 mg/24 hr.
Nasal: 5–20 mg/dose into one nostril or divided into each nostril. If headache returns, dose may be repeated in 2 hours up to a **maximum** of 40 mg/24 hr.

Contraindicated with concomitant administration of ergotamine derivatives, MAO inhibitors (and use within the past 2 weeks), or other vasoconstrictive drugs. Not for migraine prophylaxis. Use with **caution** with renal or hepatic impairment. Acts as selective agonist for serotonin receptor. May cause coronary vasospasm if administered IV. **Use injectable form SC only.** Flushing, dizziness, chest, jaw, and neck tightness may occur after injection. Onset of action is 10–120 min SC, and 60–90 min PO. For nasal use, the safety of treating more than 4 headaches in a 30 day period has not been established.

SURFACTANT, PULMONARY/ BERACTANT

Survanta
Bovine lung surfactant
Susp: 200 mg/ 8 ml (8 ml)

No

Prophylatic therapy: 4 ml/kg/dose intratracheally as soon as possible; up to 4 doses may be given at intervals no shorter than Q6 hr during the first 48 hr of life.
Rescue therapy: 4 ml/kg/dose intratracheally, immediately following the diagnosis of respiratory distress syndrome (RDS). May repeat dose as needed Q6 hr to maximum of 4 doses total.
Method of administration for above therapies: Each dose is divided into four 1 ml/kg aliquots; administer 1 ml/kg in each of four different positions (slight downward inclination with head turned to the right, head turned to the left; slight upward inclination with the head turned to the right, head turned to the left).

All doses are administered intratracheally. If the suspension settles during storage, gently swirl the contents—do not shake.

Transient bradycardia, O_2 desaturation, pallor, vasoconstriction, hypotension, endotracheal tube blockage, hypercarbia, hypercapnea, apnea, and hypertension may occur during the administration process. Other side effects may include pulmonary interstitial emphysema, pulmonary air leak, and post-treatment nosocomial sepsis. Monitor heart rate and transcutaneous O_2 saturation during dose administration; and arterial blood gases for post-dose hyperoxia and hypocarbia after administration.

SURFACTANT, PULMONARY/ COLFOSCERIL PALMITATE

Exosurf Neonatal
Synthetic lung surfactant
Intratracheal susp: 108 mg/10 ml (10 ml)

No

Prophylaxis therapy: 5 ml/kg intratracheally as soon as possible; 2 additional doses are given to infants remaining on ventilators at 12 and 24 hrs later.
Rescue therapy: 5 ml/kg intratracheally as soon as the diagnosis of RDS is made. A second 5 ml/kg dose should be administered 12 hr later as two 2.5 ml/kg aliquots.

For intratracheal use only.
Pulmonary hemorrhage, apnea, mucous plugging, and decrease in transcutaneous O_2 of >20% may occur. Drug needs to be reconstituted with preservative-free sterile water for injection. Suction infant prior to administration. Suction only if necessary until 2 hours after administration. Monitor O_2 saturation, EKG, and blood pressure during dose administration; and arterial blood gases for post-dose hyperoxia and hypocarbia after administration.

For explanation of icons, see p. 600.

TACROLIMUS

Prograf, FK506
Immunosuppressant

Yes   ?   C

Caps: 1, 5 mg
Suspension: 0.5 mg/ml
Inj: 5 mg/ml (1 ml); contains alcohol and polyoxyl 60 hydrogenaed castor oil

Children:
Liver transplantation without pre-existing renal or hepatic dysfunction (initial doses; titrate to therapeutic levels):

IV: 0.05–0.15 mg/kg/24 hr by continuous infusion

PO: 0.15–0.3 mg/kg/24 hr ÷ Q12 hr

Adults (initial doses; titrate to therapeutic levels):

IV: 0.05–0.1 mg/kg/24 hr by continuous infusion

PO:
Liver transplantation: 0.1–0.15 mg/kg/24 hr ÷ Q12 hr
Kidney transplantation: 0.2 mg/kg/24 hr ÷ Q12 hr

IV dosage form **contraindicated** in patients allergic to polyoxyl 60 hydrogenated caster oil. Experience in pediatric kidney transplantation is limited. Pediatric patients have required higher mg/kg doses than adults. **For BMT** use (beginning 1 day before BMT), dose and therapeutic levels similar to those in liver transplantation have been used.

Major adverse events include tremor, headache, insomnia, diarrhea, constipation, hypertension, nausea, and renal dysfunction. Hypokalemia, hypomagnesemia, hyperglycemia, confusion, depression, infections, lymphoma, liver enzyme elevation, and coagulation disorders may also occur. Tacrolimus is a substrate of the CYP450 3A4 drug metabolizing enzyme, see p. 924. Calcium channel blockers, imidazole antifungals (ketoconazole, itraconazole, fluconazole, clotrimazole), macrolide antibiotics (erythromycin, clarithromycin, troleandomycin), cisapride, cimetidine, cyclosporine, danazol, methyl-prednisolone, and grapefruit juice can increase tacrolimus serum levels. Carbamazepine, phenobarbital, phenytoin, rifampin, and rifabutin may can decrease levels. Reduce dose in renal or hepatic insufficeincy.

Monitor trough levels (just prior to a dose at steady-state). Steady-state is generally achieved after 2–5 days of continuous dosing. Interpretation will vary based on treatment protocol and assay methodology (Whole blood ELISA vs. MEIA vs. HPLC). Whole blood trough concentrations of 5–20 ng/ml have been recommended in liver transplantation. Trough levels of 7–20 ng/ml for the first 3 months and 5–15 ng/ml after 3 months have been recommended in renal transplantation.

Tacrolimus therapy generally should be initiated 6 hours or more after transplantation. PO is the preferred route of administration and should be administered on an empty stomach.

TERBUTALINE

Brethine, Bricanyl
Beta-2-adrenergic agonist
Tabs: 2.5, 5 mg

Yes 1 B

Suspension: 1 mg/ml
Inj: 1 mg/ml
Aerosol Inhaler: 200 mcg/actuation (300 actuations per inhaler, 10.5 g)

PO: ≤12 yr: Initial: 0.05 mg/kg/dose TID, increase as required. **Max dose:** 0.15 mg/kg/dose TID or total of 5 mg/24 hr.

>12 yr and adults: 2.5–5 mg/dose PO Q6–8 hr. **Max dose:** 12–15 yr, 7.5 mg/24 hr: *>15 yr,* 15 mg/24 hr

Nebulization:
<2 yr: 0.5 mg in 2.5 ml NS Q4–6 hr
2–9 yr: 1 mg in 2.5 ml NS Q4–6 hr
>9 yr: 1.5–2.5 mg in 2.5 ml NS Q4–6 hr

SC: ≤12 yr: 0.005–0.01 mg/kg/dose Q15–20 min × 2; **max dose:** 0.4 mg/dose.

>12 yr–adult: 0.25 mg/dose Q15–30 min PRN × 2; **max dose:** 0.5 mg/4 hr period

Inhalations: 1–2 inhalations Q4–6 hr
Continuous Infusion, IV: 2–10 mcg/kg loading dose followed by infusion of 0.1–0.4 mcg/kg/minute. May titrate in increments of 0.1–0.2 mcg/kg/minute Q30 min depending on clinical response. To prepare infusion: see inside front cover.

Nervousness, tremor, headache, nausea, tachycardia, arrhythmias, palpitations may occur. Paradoxical bronchoconstriction may occur with excessive use; if it occurs, discontinue drug immediately. Injectable product may be used for nebulization. For acute asthma, nebulizations may be given more frequently than Q4–6 hr. **Adjust dose in renal failure (see p. 941).**

TETRACYCLINE HCl

Many brand names: Achromycin, Terramycin, Sumycin, Panmycin
Antibiotic

Yes 2 D

Tabs: 250, 500 mg
Caps: 100, 250, 500 mg
Suspension: 125 mg/5 ml (473 ml)
Ointment: Ophthalmic: 1% (3.5 g)
Ointment: Topical: 3% (14.2, 30 g)
Ophthalmic drops: 1% (0.5, 1, 4 ml)
Topical Solution: 2.2 mg/ml (70 ml); contains 40% ethanol

Do **not** use in children <8 yr:
Older children: PO: 25–50 mg/kg/24 hr ÷ Q6 hr.
Max dose: 3 g/24 hr
Adults: PO: 1–2 g/24 hr ÷ Q6 hr
Chlamydia infection: 500 mg PO QID × 7 days. See also p. 394.
Ophthalmic:
  Neonatal prophylaxis: 1% ointment × 1 in both eyes.
  Solution: 2 drops into affected eye BID-QID
Acne Vulgaris: Apply topical solution to affected areas BID

Not recommended in patients <8 yr due to tooth staining and decreased bone growth. Also not recommended for use in pregnancy because these side effects may occur in the fetus. The risk for these adverse effects are highest with long-term use. May cause nausea, GI upset, hepatotoxicity, stomatitis, rash, fever, and superinfection. Photosensitivity reaction may occur. Avoid prolonged exposure to sunlight. Never use use outdated tetracyclines because they may cause Fanconi-like syndrome. Do not give with dairy products or with any divalent cations (i.e., Fe^{++}, Ca^{++}, Mg^{++}). Give 1 hr before or 2 hr after meals. **Adjust dose in renal failure (see p. 935).**

THEOPHYLLINE

TheoDur, Slo-bid Gyrocaps, Slo-Phyllin Gyrocaps, and many others

No 1 C

Bronchodilator, methylxanthine
Other dosage forms may exist
Immediate Release:
  Tabs: 100, 125, 200, 250, 300 mg
  Caps: 100, 200 mg
  Elixir/Solution/Syrup: 80 mg/15 ml, 150 mg/15 ml. Some elixirs contain up to 20% alcohol. Some syrups and solutions are alcohol and dye free.
  Inj: 0.4, 0.8, 1.6, 2, 3.2, 4 mg/ml

Sustained Release:
  Tabs: 100, 200, 250, 300, 400, 450, 500, 600 mg
  Caps: 50, 60, 65, 75, 100, 125, 130, 200, 250, 260, 300 mg
  Sustained release forms should not be chewed or crushed. Capsules may be opened and contents may be sprinkled on food.

Dosing intervals are for immediate release preparations.

For sustained release preparations divide daily dose QD-TID based on product.

Neonatal apnea:

Load: 5 mg/kg/dose PO × 1

Maintenance: 3–6 mg/kg/24 hr PO ÷ Q6–8 hr

Bronchospasm: PO:

Loading dose: 1 mg/kg/dose for each 2 mg/L desired increase in serum theophylline level.

Maintenance, infants (<1 yr):

Preterm:

<24 days old (postnatal): 1 mg/kg/dose PO Q12 hr

≥24 days old (postnatal): 1.5 mg/kg/dose PO Q12 hr

Full-term up to 1 yr old: Total daily dose (mg) = $[(0.2 \times$ age in weeks) + $5] \times$ (kg body weight)

≤26 weeks old: divide daily dose Q8 hr

>26 weeks old: divide daily dose Q6 hr

Maintenance, children >1 yr and adults without risk factors for altered clearance:

<45 kg: Begin therapy at 12–14 mg/kg/24 hr ÷ Q4–6 hr up to **max** of 300 mg/24 hr. If needed based on serum levels, gradually increase to 16–20 mg/kg/24 hr ÷ Q4–6 hr. **Max dose:** 600 mg/24 hr

≥45 kg: Begin therapy with 300 mg/24 hr ÷ Q6–8 hr. If needed based on serum levels, gradually increase to 400–600 mg/24 hr ÷ Q6–8 hr.

Drug metabolism varies widely with age, drug formulation, and route of administration. Most common side effects and toxicities are nausea, vomiting, anorexia, abdominal pain, gastroesophageal reflux, nervousness, tachycardia, seizures, and arrhythmias.

Serum levels should be monitored. Therapeutic levels: bronchospasm: 10–20 mg/L; apnea: 7–13 mg/L. Half-life is age-dependent: 30 hr (newborns); 6.9 hr (infants); 3.4 hr (children); 8.1 hr (adults). See aminophylline for guidelines for serum level determinations. Theophylline is a substrate for CYP 450 1A2. Levels increased with allopurinol, alcohol, ciprofloxacin, cimetidine, clarithromycin, disulfiram, erythromycin, estrogen, propranolol, thiabendazole, and verapamil. Levels decreased with carbamazepine, isoproterenol, phenobarbital, phenytoin, and rifampin.

Use ideal body weight in obese patients when calculating dosage because of poor distribution into body fat. Risk factors for increased clearance include: smoking, cystic fibrosis, hyperthyroidism, and high protein carbohydrate diet. Factors for decreased clearance include: CHF, fever, viral illness, and sepsis. Compatible in breastfeeding but may cause irritability in infant.

Suggested Dosage Intervals for Sustained Released Products:

For explanation of icons, see p. 600.

THEOPHYLLINE SUSTAINED RELEASE PRODUCTS

Trade name	Available strengths (mg)	Dosage interval (hr)
Capsules		
Aerolate	130, 260	Q8–12
Slo-bid Gyrocaps	50, 75, 100, 125, 200, 300	Q8–12
Slo-Phyllin Gyrocaps	60, 125, 250	Q8–12
Theo 24	100, 200, 300	Q24
Theobid Jr. Duracaps	130	Q12
Theobid Duracaps	260	Q12
Theoclear-LA or Theospan-SR	130, 260	Q12
Theovent	125, 250	Q12
Tablets		
Theophylline SR	100, 200, 300	Q12–Q24
Quibron-T/SR Dividose	300	Q8–12
Respid	250, 500	Q8–12
Sustaire	100, 300	Q8–12
Theo Dur	100, 200, 300, 450	Q8–24
Theocron	100, 200, 300	Q12–24
Theolair SR	200, 250, 300, 500	Q8–12
Theo-Sav	100, 200, 300	Q8–24
T-phyl	200	Q8–12
Uni-Dur or Uniphyl	400, 600	Q24

THIABENDAZOLE

Mintezol
Anthelmintic
Susp: 500 mg/5 ml
Chew Tabs: 500 mg

Yes ? C

 PO, Adults and Children: 50 mg/kg/24 ÷ BID; max dose: 3 g/24 hr
Duration of therapy (consecutive days)
Strongyloides: × 2 days (5 days for dissiminated disease)
Intestinal Nematodes: × 2 days
Cutaneous Larva Migrans: × 2–5 days
Visceral Larva Migrans: × 5–7 days
Trichinosis: × 2–4 days

 Use with **caution** in renal or hepatic impairment.
Nausea, vomiting, and vertigo are frequent side effects. May cause rash, hypersensitivity, erythema multiforme, leukopenia, and hallucinations. May increase serum levels of theophylline or caffeine. Clinical experience in children weighing <13.6 kg (30 lbs) is limited.

THIAMIN (VITAMIN B₁)

Betalin S, and others
Water soluble vitamin
Tabs: 25, 50, 100, 250, 500 mg
Enteric coated Tabs: 20 mg
Inj: 100 mg/ml, 200 mg/ml

No   1   A/C

For US RDA, see p. 485.
Beriberi (thiamin deficiency):
Children: 10–25 mg/dose IM/IV
QD (if critically ill) or 10–50 mg/dose
PO QD × 2 wk, followed by 5–10
mg/dose QD for 1 mo.
Adults: 5–30 mg/dose IM/IV TID ×
2 wk, followed by 5–30 mg/24 hr PO ÷
QD or TID for 1 mo.
Wernicke's encephalopathy syndrome:
100 mg IV × 1, then 50–100 mg IM/IV
QD until patient resumes a normal diet.
(Administer thiamin before starting
glucose infusion.)

Multivitamin preparations contain
amounts meeting RDA
requirements. Allergic reactions
and anaphylaxis may occur, primarily with
IV administration. Therapeutic range:
1.6–4 mg/dL. High carbohydrate diets or
IV dextrose solutions may increase
thiamin requirements. Large doses may
interfere with serum theophylline assay.
Pregnancy category changes to "C" if used
in doses above the RDA.

THIOPENTAL SODIUM

Pentothal
Barbiturate
Inj: 250, 400, 500 mg, 1, 2.5, 5 g (reconstituted to 20 mg/ml or
25 mg/ml)
Rectal Susp: 400 mg/g (2 g)

Yes   1   C

Cerebral edema: 1.5–5
mg/kg/dose IV. Repeat PRN for
increased ICP.
Anesthesia induction, children and adults:
IV: 2–6 mg/kg: Use lower doses in
patients with hemodynamic instability.
See p. 6 for rapid sequence intubation.
Deep Sedation:
Children: 30 mg/kg PR × 1; **max:** 1 g/
dose

Contraindicated in acute
intermittent porphyria. May cause
respiratory depression, hypotension, anaphylaxis, decreased cardiac
output. Deep sedation is used for
diagnostic imaging studies.
Onset of action: 30–60 sec for IV;
7–10 min for PR. Duration of action:
5–30 min for IV; 90 min for PR. **Adjust
dose in renal failure (see p. 941).**

THIORIDAZINE

Mellaril and others
Antipsychotic, phenothiazine derivative
Tabs: 10, 15, 25, 50, 100, 150, 200 mg
Oral conc: 30, 100 mg/ml (120 ml)
Susp.: 25 mg/5 ml, 100 mg/5 ml (480 ml)

No ? C

Children 2–12 yr: 0.5–3 mg/kg/24 hr PO ÷ BID-TID. **Max dose:** 3 mg/kg/24 hr
>12 yr and adults:
Initial dose: 75–300 mg/24 hr PO ÷ TID
Increase PRN to **max dose** 800 mg/24 hr ÷ BID-QID

Contraindicated in severe CNS depression, brain damage, severe hypotension or hypertension. May cause drowsiness, extrapyramidal reactions, autonomic symptoms, ECG changes, arrhythmias, paradoxical reactions, endocrine disturbances. Long-term use may cause tardive dyskinesia. Pigmentary retinopathy may occur with higher doses; a periodic eye exam is recommended. More autonomic symptoms and less extrapyramidal effects than chlorpromazine. Concurrent use with epinephrine can cause hypotension. Increased cardiac arrhythmias may occur with tricyclic antidepressants.

TIAGABINE

Gabitril Filmtab
Anticonvulsant
Tabs: 4, 12, 16, 20 mg

No ? C

Adjunctive therapy for partial seizures:

≥12 yrs and Adults: Start at 4 mg PO QD × 7 days. If needed, increase dose to 8 mg/24 hr PO ÷ BID. Dosage may be increased further by 4–8 mg/24 hr at weekly intervals (daily doses may be divided BID-QID) until a clinical response is achieved or up to specified maximum dose.

Maximum Dose:
  12–18 yrs: 32 mg/24 hr
  Adults: 56 mg/24 hr

Use with **caution** in hepatic insufficiency (may need to reduce dose and/or increase dosing interval). Most common side effects include: dizziness, asthenia, nausea, nervousness, temor, abdominal pain, confusion, and difficulty in concentrating.

Tiagabine's clearance is increased by concurrent hepatic enzyme-inducing antiepileptic drugs (i.e., phenytoin, carbamazepine, and barbiturates). Lower doses or a slower titration for clinical response may be necessary for patients receiving non-enzyme inducing drugs (i.e., valproate, gabapentin, and lamotrigine).

Doses should be administered with food.

TICARCILLIN
Ticar
Antibiotic, penicillin (extended spectrum)
Inj: 1, 3, 6, 20, 30 g
Each gram contains 5.2–6.5 mEq Na.

Yes   1   B

Neonates, IM/IV:
≤7 days:
  <2 kg: 150 mg/kg/24 hr ÷ Q12 hr
  ≥2 kg: 225 mg/kg/24 hr ÷ Q8 hr
>7 days:
  <1.2 kg: 150 mg/kg/24 hr ÷ Q12 hr
  1.2–2 kg: 225 mg/kg/24 hr ÷ Q8 hr
  >2 kg: 300 mg/kg/24 hr ÷ Q6–8 hr
Infants and Children (IM/IV): 200–300 mg/kg/24 hr ÷ Q4–6 hr. **Max dose:** 24 g/24 hr
Cystic Fibrosis (IM/IV): 300–600 mg/kg/24 hr ÷ Q4–6 hr. **Max dose:** 24 g/24 hr
Adults (IM/IV): 1–4 g/dose Q4–6 hr
Uncomplicated UTI, IM/IV:
  Adult: 1 g/dose Q6 hr

May cause decreased platelet aggregation, bleeding diathesis, hypernatermia, hematuria, hypokalemia, hypocalcemia, allergy, rash, increased AST. Like other penicillins, CSF penetration occurs only with inflamed meninges. Do not mix with aminoglycoside in same solution. **Adjust dose in renal failure; see p. 935.**

For explanation of icons, see p. 600.

TICARCILLIN/CLAVULANATE

Timentin
Antibiotic, penicillin (extended spectrum with beta-lactamase Yes 1 B
inhibitor)
Inj: 3.1 g (3 g ticarcillin and 0.1 g clavulanate); contains 4.75 mEq
Na$^+$ and 0.15 mEq K$^+$ per 1 g drug

Doses should be based on tiarcillin
component; see Ticarcillin.
Max dose: 18–24 g/24 hr

Activity similar to ticarcillin except
that beta-lactamase inhibitor
broadens spectrum to include S.
aureus and H. influenzae. Like other
penicillins, CSF penetration occurs only
with inflamed meninges. May interfere
with urine protein measurement. **Adjust
dosage in renal impairment (see p. 935).**

TOBRAMYCIN

Nebcin, Tobrex, TOBI, and others
Antibiotic, aminoglycoside Yes ? C
Inj: 10, 40 mg/ml
Powder for inj: 1.2 g
Ophthalmic ointment: 0.3% (3.5 g)
Ophthalmic solution: 0.3% (5 ml)
Nebulizer solution (TOBI): 300 mg/5 ml (preservative free) (56's)

Neonates, IM/IV:
Child: 6–7.5 mg/kg/24 hr ÷ Q8 hr IV/IM
Cystic Fibrosis: 7.5–10 mg/kg/24 hr ÷ Q8 hr IV
Adults: 3–6 mg/kg/24 hr ÷ Q8 hr IV/IM
Ophthalmic: Apply thin ribbon of ointment to affected eye BID-TID; or 1–2 drops of solution to affected eye Q4 hr
Inhalation:
Cystic Fibrosis prophylaxis therapy (TOBI):
≥6 yr and Adults: 300 mg Q12 hr administered in repeated cycles of 28 days on drug followed by 28 days off drug.

Use with **caution** in patients receiving anesthetics or neuromuscular blocking agents, and in patients with neuromuscular disorders. May cause ototoxicity, nephrotoxicity, myelotoxicity, allergy.

Ototoxic effects synergistic with furosemide. Higher doses are recommended in patients with cystic fibrosis neutropenia, or burns. **Adjust dose in renal failure (see p. 935).** Monitor peak and trough levels.
Therapeutic peak levels:
6–10 mg/L in general
8–10 mg/L in pulmonary infections, neutropenia, and severe sepsis
Therapeutic trough levels: <2 mg/L. Recommended serum sampling time at steady-state: trough within 30 minutes prior to the 3rd consecutive dose and peak 30–60 minutes after the administration of the 3rd consecutive dose.
For inhalation use with other medications in cystic fibrosis, use the following order of administration: bronchodilator first, chest physiotherapy, other inhaled medications, then tobramycin last.

Postconceptional age (wk)	Postnatal age (days)	Dose (mg/kg/dose)	Interval (hr)
≤29*	0 to 28	2.5	24
	>28	3	24
30–36	0 to 14	3	24
	>14	2.5	12
≥37	0 to 7	2.5	12
	>7	2.5	8

*Or significant asphyxia.

TOLAZOLINE
Priscoline
Adrenergic blocking agent (alpha)
Inj: 25 mg/ml (4 ml)

Yes   ?   C

Pulmonary hypertension, newborn:
Test dose: 1–2 mg/kg IV over
10 minutes
Maintenance infusion: 0.5–2 mg/kg/hr
IV
Administer via upper extremity or scalp
vein.
Dissolve 50 mg/kg × (wt in kg) in 50 ml
of D_5W (ml/hr = mg/kg/hr)
Acute Vasospasm: 0.25 mg/kg/hr IV (no
loading dose)

Monitor BP, renal function, and
CBC. May cause GI and pulmonary
hemorrhage. If hypotension occurs,
use dopamine (not epinephrine or
norepinephrine). Reduce dose in renal
impairment (decrease dose 50% if urinary
output is <0.9 ml/kg/hr).

TOLMETIN SODIUM
Tolectin
Nonsteroidal anti-inflammatory agent
Tabs: 200, 600 mg
Caps: 400 mg
Contains 0.8 mEq Na per 200 mg drug

No   1   C/D

Children ≥ 2 yr:
Anti-inflammatory:
Initial: 20 mg/kg/24 hr ÷ TID-QID
PO. May increase in increments of 5
mg/kg/24 hr to **max dose** of 30
mg/kg/24 hr or 2 g/24 hr
Analgesic: 5–7 mg/kg/dose PO Q6–8 hr.
Max dose: 30 mg/kg/24 hr or 2 g/24 hr
Adults:
Initial: 400 mg TID PO
Maintenance: Titrate to desired effect.
Usually, 600–1800 mg/24 hr ÷ TID
PO. **Max dose:** 2 g/24 hr

May cause GI irritation or bleeding,
CNS symptoms, platelet dysfunction, false positive proteinuria.
Take with food or milk. May increase the
effects of warfarin and methotrexate.
Pregnancy category changes to "D" if used
in 3rd trimester or near delivery.

TOLNAFTATE
Tinactin, Aftate, and others
Antifungal agent

No   ?   C

Topical aerosol liquid: 1% (113 g)
Aerosol powder: 1% (100, 150 g)
Cream: 1% (15, 30, 45 g)
Gel: 1% (15 g)
Powder: 1% (45, 67.5, 70.9, 90 g)
Topical Sol: 1% (10, 60 ml)

Topical:
Apply 1–2 drops of solution or small amount of gel, liquid, cream, or powder to affected areas BID for 2–6 wk.

May cause mild irritation and sensitivity. Avoid eye contact. Do **not** use for nail or scalp infections.

TRAZODONE
Desyrel
Antidepressant, triazolopyridine-derivative
Tabs: 50, 100, 150, 300 mg

No   3   C

Depression (titrate to lowest effective dose):
Children (6–18 yr): Start at 1.5–2 mg/kg/24 hr PO ÷ BID-TID; if needed, gradually increase dose Q3–4 days up to a **maximum** of 6 mg/kg/24 hr ÷ TID
Adolescents: Start at 25–50 mg/24 hr PO QD, increase to 100–150 mg/24 hr ÷ BID-TID
Adults: Start at 150 mg/24 hr PO ÷ TID; if needed, increase by 50 mg/24 hr Q 3–4 days up a **maximum** of 600 mg/24 hr for hospitalized patients (400 mg/24 hr for ambulatory patients).

Use with **caution** in pre-existing cardiac disease, initial recovery phase of MI, and electroconvulsive therapy. Common side effects include dizziness, drowsiness, dry mouth, diarrhea. Seizures, tardive dyskinesia, EPS, arrhythmias, priaprism, blurred vision, neuromuscular weakness, anemia, orthostatic hypotension, and rash has been reported. Trazodone may increase digoxin levels and increase CNS effects of alcohol, barbiturates, and other CNS depressants. Maximum antidepressant effect is seen at 2–6 weeks.

For explanation of icons, see p. 600.

TRETINOIN

Retin-A, Retin-A Micro, Avita
Retinoic acid derivative, topical acne product

No ? C

Cream: 0.025%, 0.05%, 0.1% (20, 45 g)
Topical Gel: 0.01%, 0.025%; contains 90% alcohol (15, 45 g)
Topical Gel (Retin-A Micro): 0.1%; contains glycerin, propylene glycol, benzyl alcohol (20, 45 g)
Topical Liquid: 0.05%; contains 55% alcohol (28 ml)

Topical:
Children >12 yr and Adults:
Gently wash face with a mild soap, pat the skin dry, and wait 20 to 30 minutes before use. Initiate therapy with either 0.025% cream or 0.01% gel and apply to the affected areas of the face QHS.

Contraindicated in sunburns. Avoid excessive sun exposure. If stinging or irritation occurs, decrease frequency of administration to QOD. **Avoid** contact with eyes, ears, nostrils, mouth, or open wounds. Local adverse effects include irritation, erythema, excessive dryness, blistering, crusting, hyper- or hypo-pigmentation, and acne flare-ups. Concomitant use of other topical acne products may lead to significant skin irritation. Onset of therapeutic benefits may be experienced within 2–3 weeks with optimal effects in 6 weeks.

TRIAMCINOLONE

Azmacort, Nasacort, Nasacort AQ, Kenalog, Aristocort, and others
Corticosteroid

No ? C

Nasal inhaler (Nasacort): 55 mcg/actuation (100 actuations per 10 g)
Nasal spray (Nasacort AQ): 55 mcg/actuation (120 actuations per 16.5 g)
Oral inhaler: 100 mcg/actuation (240 actuations per 20 g)
Tabs: 1, 2, 4, 8 mg
Oral syrup: 4 mg/5 ml (120 ml)
Cream: 0.025%, 0.1%, 0.5%
Ointment: 0.025%, 0.1%, 0.5%

Lotion: 0.025%, 0.1%
Topical aerosol: 0.2 mg/2 second spray (23, 63 g)
Dental paste: 0.1% (5 g)
See Special Drug Topics for potency rankings and sizes of topical preparations.
Inj as acetonide: 3, 10, 40 mg/ml
Inj as diacetate: 25, 40 mg/ml
Inj as hexacetonide: 5, 20 mg/ml

Oral Inhalation:
Children 6–12 yr: 1–2 puffs TID-QID or 2–4 puffs BID; **max dose:** 12 puffs/24 hr
≥12 yr and adults: 2 puffs TID-QID or 4 puffs BID; **max dose:** 16 puffs/24 hr
NIH-National Heart Lung and Blood Institute recommendations (divide daily doses BID-QID): see pp. 911–912.
Intranasal (always titrate to lowest effective dose after symptoms are controlled):
Nasacort:
Children 6–11 yr: 2 sprays in each nostril QD
≥12 yr and adults: 2 sprays in each nostril QD. May increase to 4 sprays/nostril/24 hr ÷ QD-QID
Nasacort AQ:
Children 6–11 yr: Start with 1 spray in each nostril QD. If no benefit in one week, dose may be increased to 2 sprays in each nostril QD.
≥12 yr and adults: Start with 2 sprays in each nostril QD.

Max AQ dose: 2 sprays in each nostril/24 hr
Topical: Apply to affected areas QD-TID
Systemic Use: Use ⅙ of Cortisone dose. See p. 907.
Intralesional, ≥12 yr and Adults (as diacetate or acetonide): 1 mg/site at intervals of 1 week or more. May give separate doses in sites >1 cm apart, not to exceed 30 mg.

Rinse mouth thoroughly with water after each use of the oral inhalation dosage form. Nasal preparations may cause epistaxis, cough, fever, nausea, throat irritation, and dyspepsia. Topical preparations may cause dermal atrophy, telangiectasias, and hypopigmentation. Topical steroids should be used with caution on the face and in intertriginous areas. See p. 907.

Dosage adjustment for hepatic failure with systemic use may be necessary.

TRIAMTERENE
Dyrenium
Diuretic, potassium sparing
Caps: 50, 100 mg

Yes   ?   B

Children: 2–4 mg/kg/24 hr ÷ QD-BID PO. May increase up to a **maximum** of 6 mg/kg/24 hr or 300 mg/24 hr.
Adults: 100–300 mg/24 hr ÷ QD-BID PO; **max dose:** 300 mg/24 hr

Do not use if GFR <10 ml/hr. Adjust dose in renal impairment (see p. 941). Monitor serum electrolytes. May cause hyperkalemia, hyponatremia, hypomagnesemia, and metabolic acidosis. Interstitial nephritis, thrombocytopenia, and anaphylaxis have been reported.

Concurrent use of ACE inhibitors may increase serum potassium. Use with **caution** when administering medications with high potassium load (e.g., some penicillins) and in patients on high potassium diets. Cimetidine may increase effects. This drug is also available as a combination product with hydrochlorothiazide.

TRIETHANOLAMINE POLYPEPTIDE OLEATE

No ? C

Cerumenex
Otic cerumenolytic
Solution: 10% (6, 12 ml)

Children and adults: Fill ear canal, insert cotton plug. After 15–30 minutes, flush ear with warm water. May repeat dose in the presence of unusually hard impactions.

Contraindicated with perforated tympanic membrane.
Hypersensitivity and localized dermatitis may occur.

TRIMETHOBENZAMIDE HCl

No ? C

Tigan
Antiemetic
Caps: 100, 250 mg
Suppository: 100, 200 mg
Inj: 100 mg/ml

Children:
<15 kg: PR: 100 mg/dose TID-QID.
15–40 kg: PO/PR: 100–200 mg/dose TID-QID
Adults:
PO: 250 mg/dose TID-QID
PR/IM: 200 mg/dose TID-QID

Do **not** use in premature or newborn infants. Avoid use in patients with hepatotoxicity, acute vomiting, or allergic reaction. CNS disturbances are common in children (extrapyramidal symptoms, drowsiness, confusion, dizziness). Hypotension, especially with IM use, may occur. Suppository contains 2% benzocaine. **IM not recommended in children.**

TRIMETHOPRIM-SULFAMETHOXAZOLE

See Co-Trimoxazole

UROKINASE

Abbokinase, Abbokinase Open Cath
Thrombolytic enzyme
Inj: 5,000 U/ml (Abbokinase Open Cath); 250,000 U (both products are preservative-free)

No   ?   B

Deep vein thrombosis and pulmonary emboli: **Should be used in consultation with a hematologist.** 4400 U/kg over 10 min, followed by 4400 U/kg/hr for 12–72 hr. Titrate to effect.

Occluded IV catheter:

Aspiration method: Use 5,000 U/ml conc. Instill into catheter a volume equal to the internal volume of catheter over 1–2 min, leave in place for 1–4 hr, then aspirate; may repeat with 10,000 U/ml in each lumen if no response. **DO NOT infuse into patient.**

IV infusion method: 150–200 U/kg/hr in each lumen for 8–48 hr at a rate of at least 20 ml/hr.

For dialysis patients: 5,000 U in each lumen administered over 1–2 min; leave drug in for 1–2 days, then aspirate.

 Contraindicated for patients with active internal bleeding, bacterial endocarditis, intracranial neoplasm, arteriovenous malformation, or aneurysm, history of cerebrovascular accident, or recent trauma/surgery. Monitor hematocrit, platelets, PT, and aPTT before and during continuous infusion therapy.

Discontinue administration if signs of bleeding occur. Side effects include allergic reactions, fever, rash, and bronchospasm.

URSODIOL
Actigall
Gallstone solubilizing agent, cholelitholytic agent
Susp: 60 mg/ml
Caps: 300 mg

No ? B

 Children: 10–15 mg/kg/24 hr QD PO
Adults: 8–10 mg/kg/24 hr ÷ BID-TID PO

Cystic Fibrosis (to improve fatty acid metabolism in liver disease): 15–30 mg/kg/24 hr ÷ QD-TID PO

 Contraindicated in calcified cholesterol stones, radiopaque stones, bile pigment stones, or stones >20 mm in diameter. May cause

GI disturbance, rash, arthralgias, anxiety, headache, and elevated liver enzymes. Aluminum-containing antacids, cholestyramine, and oral contraceptives decrease ursodiol effectiveness. Dissolution of stones may take several months. Stone recurrence occurs in 30–50% of patients.

Limited data for use in TPN induced cholestasis at 30 mg/kg/24 hr ÷ TID PO (see *Gastroenterology* 1996; 111(3):716-719).

VALACYCLOVIR

Valtrex
Antiviral agent
Tablets: 500, 1000 mg

Yes   1   B

Adults (Immunocompetent):
Herpes Zoster: 1 gm/dose PO TID × 7 days within 48–72 hours of onset of rash.
Genital Herpes:
  Initial Episodes: 1 gm/dose PO BID × 10 days.
  Recurrent Episodes: 500 mg/dose PO BID × 5 days.
  Suppressive Therapy: 500–1000 mg/dose PO QD

This pro-drug is metabolized to acyclovir and L-valine with better oral absorption than acyclovir. Use with **caution** in hepatic or renal insufficiency. **Adjust dose in renal insufficiency (see p. 936).** Thrombotic thrombocytopenic purpura/hemolytic uremic syndrome (TTP/HUS) has been reported in patients with advanced HIV infection and in bone marrow and renal transplant recipients. Probenecid or cimetidine can reduce the rate of conversion to acyclovir. See acyclovir for additional drug interactions and adverse effects.

For initial episodes of genital herpes, therapy is most effective when initiated within 48 hours of symptom onset. Therapy should be initiated immediately after the onset of symptoms in recurrent episodes (no efficacy data when initiating therapy >24 hrs after onset of symptoms). Data is not available for use as suppressive therapy for periods >1 yr. Doses may be administered with or without food.

VALPROIC ACID

Depakene, Depacon
[Depakote—See Divalproex sodium]
Anticonvulsant
Caps: 250 mg
Syrup: 250 mg/5 ml (473 ml)
Inj (Depacon): 100 mg/ml (5ml)

No   1   D

Oral:
Initial: 10–15 mg/kg/24 hr ÷ QD-TID
Increment: 5–10 mg/kg/24 hr at weekly intervals to **max dose** of 60 mg/kg/24 hr
Maintenance: 30–60 mg/kg/24 hr ÷ BID-TID. Due to drug interactions, higher doses may be required in children on other anticonvulsants.
Intravenous (use only when PO is not possible):
Use same PO daily dose ÷ Q6 hr. Convert back to PO as soon as possible.
Rectal (Use syrup, diluted 1:1 with water, given PR as a retention enema):
Load: 20 mg/kg/dose
Maintenance: 10–15 mg/kg/dose Q8 hr

Contraindicated in hepatic disease. May cause GI, liver, blood, CNS toxicity, weight gain, transient alopecia, pancreatitis, nausea, sedation, vomiting, headache, thrombocytopenia, platelet dysfunction, and rash. Can cause hyperammonemia. Hepatic failure has occurred especially in children <2 yrs. Valproic acid increases phenytoin, diazepam, and phenobarbital levels. Phenytoin, phenobarbital, and carbamazepine decrease valproic acid levels.

Do not give syrup with carbonated beverages. Use of IV route has not been evaluated for >14 days of continuous use. Infuse IV over 1 hr up to a maximum rate of 20 mg/min.

Therapeutic levels: 50–100 mg/L. Recommendations for serum sampling at steady-state: obtain trough level within 30 minutes prior to the next scheduled dose after 2–3 days of continuous dosing. Monitor CBC, LFTs prior to and during therapy.

VANCOMYCIN
Vancocin and others
Antibiotic
Inj: 500, 1000 mg; 2, 5, 10 g
Caps: 125, 250 mg
Sol: 1, 10 g (reconstitute to 500 mg/6 ml)

Yes   ?   C/B

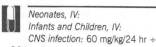

Neonates, IV:
Infants and Children, IV:
 CNS infection: 60 mg/kg/24 hr ÷ Q6 hr
Other infections: 40 mg/kg/24 hr ÷ Q6–8 hr
Max dose: 1 g/dose
Adults: 2 g/24 hr ÷ Q6–12 hr IV
C. difficile *Colitis:*
 Children: 40–50 mg/kg/24 hr ÷ Q6 hr PO × 7–10 days
 Max dose: 500 mg/24 hr
 Adults: 125 mg/dose PO Q6 hr × 7–10 days
Endocarditis prophylaxis: See p. 163.

Ototoxicity and nephrotoxicity may occur and may be exacerbated with concurrent aminoglycoside use.
Adjust dose in renal failure (see p. 936).
Low concentrations of the drug may appear in CSF with inflamed meninges. "Red man syndrome" associated with rapid IV infusion. Infuse over 60 min (may infuse over 120 min if 60 min infusion is not tolerated). Note: diphenhydramine is used to reverse red man syndrome. Allergic reactions have been reported.

Although the monitoring of serum levels is controversial, the following guidelines are recommended. Therapeutic levels: peak: 25–40 mg/L; trough: <10 mg/L. Recommended serum sampling time at steady-state: trough within 30 minutes prior to the 3rd–5th consecutive dose and peak 60 minutes after the administration of the 3rd–5th consecutive dose.

Elimination $T_{1/2}$: Newborn, 4–10 hours; 3 mo–4 yr, 4 hours; >3 yr, 2.2–3 hours; adults, 5–8 hours.

Metronidazole (PO) is the drug of choice for *C. difficile* colitis; vancomycin should be avoided due to the emergence of vancomycin resistant enterococcus. Pregnancy category "B" is assigned with the oral route of administration.

Weight (kg)	Postnatal age	
	<7days	≥7days
<1.2	15mg/kg/dose Q24hr	15mg/kg/dose Q24hr
1.2–2	10–15mg/kg/dose Q12–18hr	10–15mg/kg/dose Q8–12hr
>2	10–15mg/kg/dose Q8–12hr	15–20mg/kg/dose Q8hr

VARICELLA-ZOSTER IMMUNEGLOBULIN (HUMAN)
VZIG
No ? C
Hyperimmune globulin
1 vial = 125 U (volume in each vial will vary but is typically 2.5 ml or less)

For explanation of icons, see p. 600.

≤10 kg: 125 U IM
10.1–20 kg: 250 U IM
20.1–30 kg: 375 U IM
30.1–40 kg: 500 U IM
>40 kg: 625 U IM (not >2.5 ml per inj site)

Contraindicated in severe thrombocytopenia due to IM injection. See pp. 372–373 for indications. Dose should be given within 48 hr of exposure and no later than 96 hr post exposure. Local discomfort, redness, swelling at the injection site may occur. **May induce anaphylactic reactions in immunoglobulin A deficient individuals.** Interferes with immune response to live virus vaccines such as measles, mumps, and rubella; defer administration of live vaccines 5 months after VZIG dose.

VASOPRESSIN
Pitressin
Antidiuretic hormone analog
Inj: 20 U/ml (aqueous) (0.5, 1 ml)

No ? B

Diabetes Insipidus: Titrate dose to effect
  SC/IM:
  Children: 2.5–10 U BID-QID
  Adults: 5–10 U BID-QID
Continuous infusion, adults and children: Start at 0.5 mU/kg/hr (0.0005 U/kg/hr). Double dosage every 30 minutes PRN up to **max dose** of 10 mU/kg/hr (0.01 U/kg/hr)
Growth hormone and corticotropin provocative tests:
  Children: 0.3 U/kg IM; **max dose:** 10 U
  Adult: 10 U IM
GI hemorrhage (IV):
  Children: Start at 0.002–0.005 U/kg/min. Increase dose as needed to 0.01 U/kg/min.
  Adults: Start at 0.2–0.4 U/min. Increase dose as needed to **max dose** of 1 U/min.

Side effects include tremor, sweating, vertigo, abdominal discomfort, nausea, vomiting, urticaria, anaphylaxis, hypertension, and bradycardia. May cause vasoconstriction, water intoxication, and bronchoconstriction. Drug interactions: lithium, demeclocycline, heparin, and alcohol reduce activity; carbamazepine, tricyclic antidepressants, fludrocortisone, and chlorpropamide increase activity.

Do **not** abruptly discontinue IV infusion (taper dose). Patients with variceal hemorrhage and hepatic insufficiency may respond to lower dosages. Monitor fluid intake and output, urine specific gravity, urine and serum osmolality and sodium.

VECURONIUM BROMIDE
Norcuron
Nondepolarizing neuromuscular blocking agent
Inj: 10 mg

Yes **?** **C**

 Neonates:
Initial: 0.1 mg/kg/dose IV
Maintenance: 0.03–0.15 mg/kg/
dose IV Q1–2 hr PRN
>7 wk–1 yr:
Initial: 0.08–0.1 mg/kg/dose IV
Maintenance: 0.05–0.1 mg/kg/dose IV
Q1 hr PRN;
>1 yr–adults:
Initial: 0.08–0.1 mg/kg/dose IV
Maintenance: 0.05–0.1 mg/kg/dose IV
Q1 hr PRN; may administer via
continuous infusion at 0.1 mg/kg/hr IV

 Use with **caution** in patients with
renal or hepatic impairment, and
neuromuscular disease. Infants
from 7 wk to 1 yr are more sensitive to
the drug and may have a longer recovery
time. Children (1–10 yr) may require
higher doses and more frequent
supplementation than adults. Enflurane,
isoflurane, aminoglycosides, magnesium
salts, tetracyclines, bacitracin, and
clindamycin may increase the potency
and duration of neuromuscular blockade.
May cause arrythmias, rash, and
bronchospasm.

Neostigmine, pyridostigmine, or
edrophonium are antidotes. Onset of
action within 1–3 minutes. Duration is
30–90 minutes. See p. 7 for rapid
sequence intubation.

VERAPAMIL
Isoptin, Calan, and others
Calcium channel blocker
Tabs: 40, 80, 120 mg
Sustained release tabs: 120, 180, 240 mg
Sustained release caps: 120, 180, 240, 360 mg
Inj: 2.5 mg/ml
Susp: 50 mg/ml

Yes **1** **C**

IV: Give over 2–3 minutes. May repeat once after 30 mins.
0–1 yr: 0.1–0.2 mg/kg, using continuous ECG monitoring.
1–15 yr: 0.1–0.3 mg/kg; **max dose:** 5 mg 1st dose, 10 mg 2nd dose.
Adults: 5–10 mg (0.075–0.15 mg/kg), 10 mg 2nd dose.
PO: Children: 4–8 mg/kg/24 hr ÷ TID
Adults: 240–480 mg/24 hr ÷ TID-QID Divide QD-BID for sustained release preparations.
Adult antianginal dose: 80 mg/dose Q6–8 hr PO; **max dose:** 480 mg/24 hr

Contraindications include hypersensitivity, cardiogenic shock, severe CHF, sick-sinus syndrome, or AV block. Due to negative inotropic effects, verapamil should **not** be used to treat SVT in an emergency setting in infants. **Avoid** IV use in neonates and young infants due to apnea, bradycardia, hypotension. Monitor ECG. Have calcium and isoproterenol available to reverse myocardial depression.

Like other calcium channel antagonists, drug is a substrate of CYP 450 3A4 (see p. 924). Barbiturates, sulfinpyrazone, phenytoin, vitamin D, and rifampin may decrease serum levels/effects of verapamil; quinidine may increase serum levels/effects. Verapamil may increase effects of beta-blockers (severe myocardial depression), carbamazepine, cyclosporine, digoxin, fentanyl, nondepolarizing musclerelaxants, and prazosin. Reduce dose in renal insufficiency, see p. 941.

VIDARABINE
Adenine arabinoside, ara-A, Vira-A
Antiviral agent
Ophthalmic ointment: 3% monohydrate (2.8% vidarabine base) (3.5 g)

No ? C

 Keratoconjunctivitis (HSV, VZV): Apply ½ in. ribbon of ointment to lower conjunctival sac Q3 hr, 5 ×/24 hr until complete re-epithelialization has occurred, then decrease dose to BID for an additional 7 days.

If there are no signs of improvement after 7 days, or if complete re-epithelialization has not occurred in 21 days, consider other forms of therapy.

Ophthalmic product may cause burning, lacrimation, keratitis, photophobia, blurred vision.

VITAMIN A
Aquasol A and others

No   ?   A/X

Drops: 5000 IU/0.1 ml (30 ml)
Caps: 10,000, 25,000, 50,000 IU
Tabs: 5000 IU
Inj: 50,000 IU/ml (2 ml)

US RDA: See p. 485.
Supplementation in measles
(6 months to 2 years)
6 months–1 yr: 100,000 IU/dose QD
PO × 2 days. Repeat 1 dose at 4 weeks.
1–2 yr: 200,000 IU/dose QD PO ×
2 days. Repeat 1 dose at 4 weeks.
Malabsorption syndrome prophylaxis:
Children >8 yr and adults:
10,000–50,000 IU/24 hr PO of water
miscible product.

High doses above the U.S. RDA
are teratogenic (category X). The
use of vitamin A in measles is
recommended in children 6 months to 2
years of age who are either hospitalized or
who have any of the following risk factors:
immunodeficiency, ophthalmologic
evidence of vitamin A deficiency, impaired
GI absorption, moderate to severe
malnutrition, and recent immigration from
areas with high measles mortality. May
cause GI disturbance, rash, headache,
increased ICP (pseudotumor cerebri),
papilledema, and irritability. The following
products will reduce vitamin A absorption:
mineral oil, cholestyramine, and
neomycin. May reverse the anti-coagulant
effects of warfarin if used in large doses.
See pp. 513–515 for multivitamin
preparations.

VITAMIN B₁
See Thiamin

VITAMIN B₂
See Riboflavin

VITAMIN B₃/NIACIN
Many brand names

No   ?   A/C

Tabs: 25, 50, 100, 250, 500 mg
Timed or extended release tabs: 150, 250, 375, 500, 750, 1000 mg
Timed release caps: 125, 250, 300, 400, 500 mg
Elixir: 50 mg/5 ml (14% alcohol)
Inj: 100 mg/ml

US RDA: See p. 485.
Pellagra PO/IM/IV/SC:
Children: 50–100 mg/dose TID
Adults: 50–100 mg/dose TID-QID
Max dose: 500 mg/24 hr

Contraindicated in hepatic dysfunction, active peptic ulcer, and severe hypotension. Adverse reactions of flushing, pruritus, GI distress may occur with PO administration. May cause hyperglycemia, hyperuricemia, blurred vision, abnormal liver function tests, dizziness, and headaches. Pregnancy category changes to "C" if used in doses above the RDA. See pp. 513–515 for multivitamin preparations.

VITAMIN B₆
See Pyridoxine

VITAMIN B₁₂/CYANOCOBALMIN
Many brand names

No   1   A/C

Tabs: 25, 50, 100, 250, 500, 1000 mcg
Inj: 30, 100, 1000 mcg/ml

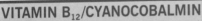

US RDA: See p. 485.

Vitamin B12 deficiency, treatment:
Children: 100 mcg/24 hr IM/deep
SC × 10–15 days

Maintenance: at least 60 mcg/month
IM/deep SC

Adults: 30–100 mcg/24 hr × 5–10 days
IM/deep SC

Maintenance: 100–200 mcg/month
IM/deep SC

Pernicious anemia:
Children: 30–50 mcg/24 hr for at least
14 days to total dose of 1000–5000 mcg
IM/deep SC

Maintenance: 100 mcg/month
IM/deep SC

Adults: 100 mcg/24 hr × 7 days IM/
deep SC, followed by 100 mcg/dose
QOD × 14 days, then 100 mcg/dose Q
3–4 days until remission is complete.

Maintenance: 100 mcg/month
IM/deep SC

Contraindicated in optic nerve atrophy. May cause hypokalemia, hypersensitivity, pruritus, and vascular thrombosis. Pregnancy category changes to "C" if used in doses above the RDA.

Protect product from light. Oral route of administration is generally not recommended for pernicious anemia and B12 deficiency due to poor absorption. IV route of administration is not recommended because of a more rapid elimination. See pp. 513–515 for multivitamin preparations.

VITAMIN C
See Ascorbic Acid

VITAMIN D₂
See Ergocalciferol

For explanation of icons, see p. 600.

VITAMIN E/ALPHA-TOCOPHEROL
Aquasol E, Liqui-E, and others

Yes ? A/C

Tabs: 200, 400 IU
Caps: 100, 200, 400, 500, 600, 1000 IU
Caps, water miscible: 73.5, 147, 165, 330 mg; 100, 200, 400 IU
Drops: 50 IU/ml (water miscible)
Liquid: 400 IU/15 ml (water miscible)

 US RDA: See p. 485.
Vitamin E deficiency, PO: Follow levels
Use water miscible form with malabsorption
Neonates: 25–50 IU/24 hr
Children: 1 IU/kg/24 hr
Adults: 60–75 IU/24 hr
Cystic Fibrosis (use water miscible form): 5–10 IU/kg/24 hr PO QD; **max dose:** 400 IU/24 hr.

 Adverse reactions include GI distress, rash, headache, gonadal dysfunction, decrease serum thyroxine and triiodothyronine, and blurred vision. Necrotizing enterocolitis has been associated with large doses (>200 units/24 hr).

One unit of vitamin E = 1 mg of dl-alphatocopherol acetate. In malabsorption, water miscible preparations are better absorbed. Therapeutic levels: 6–14 mg/L.
Pregnancy category changes to "C" if used in doses above the RDA. See pp. 513–515 for multivitamin preparations.

VITAMIN K₁/PHYTONADIONE
Aqua-Mephyton, Mephyton

No 1 C

Tabs: 5 mg
Inj: 2, 10 mg/ml; contans benzyl alcohol

Neonatal hemorrhagic disease:
  Prophylaxis: 0.5–1 mg IM × 1
  Treatment: 1–2 mg/24 hr IM/SC/IV
Oral anticoagulant overdose:
  Infants: 1–2 mg/dose Q4–8 hr IM/SC/IV
  Children and adults: 2.5–10 mg/dose PO/IM/SC/IV
  Dose may be repeated 12–48 hr after PO dose or 6–8 hr after parenteral dose
Vitamin K deficiency:
  Infants and Children:
    PO: 2.5–5 mg/24 hr
    IM/SC/IV: 1–2 mg/dose × 1
  Adults:
    PO: 5–25 mg/24 hr
    IM/SC//IV: 10 mg/dose × 1

Monitor PT/aPTT. Large doses (10–20 mg) in newborns may cause hyperbilirubinemia and severe hemolytic anemia. Blood coagulation factors increase within 6–12 hours after oral doses and within 1–2 hours following parenteral administration.

IV injection rate not to exceed 3 mg/m^2/min or 1 mg/min. IV doses may cause flushing, dizziness, hypotension, anaphylaxis. IV administration is indicated only when other routes of administration are not feasible (or in emergency situations).

Mineral oil may decrease GI absorption of vitamin K with concurrent oral administration. See pp. 513–515 for multivitamin preparations.

WARFARIN
Coumadin, Sofarin
Anticoagulant
Tabs: 1, 2, 2.5, 3, 4, 5, 6, 7.5, 10 mg
Inj: 5 mg

Yes   1   D

Infants and Children:
Loading dose:
Baseline INR 1–1.3: 0.1–0.2 mg/kg/dose PO QD × 2 days; **max dose:** 10 mg/dose

Liver Dysfunction: 0.1 mg/kg/dose PO QD × 2 days; **max dose:** 5 mg/dose
Maintenance dose: 0.1 mg/kg/24 hr PO QD. Adjust dose to achieve the desired INR or PT. Maintenance dose range: 0.05–0.34 mg/kg/24 hr PO QD.
Adults: 5–15 mg PO QD × 2–5 days. Adjust dose to achieve the desired INR or PT. Maintenance dose range: 2–10 mg/24 hr PO QD.

Contraindicated in severe liver or kidney disease, uncontrolled bleeding, GI ulcers, and malignant hypertension. Acts on vitamin-K dependent coagulation factors II, VII, IX, and X. Side effects include: fever, skin lesions, skin necrosis (especially in protein C deficiency), anorexia, nausea, vomiting, diarrhea, hemorrhage, and hemoptysis.

Warfarin is a substrate for CYP 450 1A2 and 2C9, (see p. 924). Chloramphenicol, chloral hydrate, cimetidine, delavirdine, fluconazole, metronidazole, indomethacin, non-steroidal antiinflammatory agents, omeprazole, quinidine, salicylates, sulfonamides, zafirlukast, zileuton may increase warfarin's effect. Ascorbic acid, barbituates, carbamazepine, cholestyramine, dicloxacillin, griseofulvin, oral contraceptives, rifampin, spironolactone, sucralfate, and vitamin K (including foods with high content) may decrease warfarin's effect.

Younger children generally require higher doses to achieve desired effect. The INR (international ratio) is the recommended test to monitor warfarin anticoagulant effect. Monitor INR after 5–7 days of new dosage. The particular INR desired is based upon the indication. An INR of 2–3 has been recommended for prophylaxis and treatment of DVT, pulmonary emboli, and bioprosthetic heart valves. An INR of 2.5–3.5 has been recommended for mechanical prosthetic heart valves and the prevention of recurrent systemic emboli. If PT is monitored, it should be 1.5–2 times the control.

Onset of action occurs within 36–72 hours and peak effects occur within 5–7 days. The antidote is vitamin K and fresh frozen plasma.

ZAFIRLUKAST
Accolate
Anti-asthmatic, leukotriene receptor antagonist
Tabs: 20 mg

No   3   B

Asthma:
Children ≥12 yr and Adults: 20 mg PO BID

Use with **caution** in hepatic insufficiency; **50–60% reduction in clearance occurs in alcoholic cirrhosis.** May cause headache, dizziness, nausea, diarrhea, abdominal pain, vomiting, generalized pain, asthenia, myalgia, fever, ALT elevation, and dyspepsia.

Inhibits CYP 450 2C9 and 3A4 isoenzymes, see p. 924). Erythromycin, terfenadine, and theophylline decrease zafirlukast levels; Aspirin increases levels. Zafirlukast may increase the effects of warfarin. Administer doses on an empty stomach, at least 1 hour prior or 2 hours after eating.

ZALCITABINE

Hivid, ddC

Antiviral agent, nucleoside analogue reverse transcriptase inhibitor   **Yes   3   C**
Tabs: 0.375, 0.75 mg
Syrup (available only by compassionate use program via Roche Pharmaceuticals): 0.1 mg/ml

Children <13 yr (NIH Pediatric HIV Working Group Guidelines):
Usual dose: 0.01 mg/kg/dose PO TID
Dosage range: 0.005–0.01 mg/kg/dose PO TID
Adolescents and Adults: 0.75 mg PO TID

Use with **caution** in patients with liver disease, pancreatitis, or severe myelosuppression. Peripheral neuropathy, headaches, GI disturbances, and malaise are common side effects. Other side effects include bone marrow suppression, hepatitis, pancreatitis,

hypertension, rash, oral and esophageal ulcers, myalgias, and fatigue.

Amphotericin, cimetidine, foscarnet, and aminoglycosides may reduce clearance and increase chances of peripheral neuropathy. In addition, drugs which cause peripheral neuropathy (ddI) should not be used in combination with ddC. Concurrent use of IV pentamidine can increase risk of pancreatitis. Antacids can decrease absorption. **Adjust dose in renal dysfunction (see p. 936).**
Administer doses on an empty stomach; 1 hour before or 2 hours after meals.

For explanation of icons, see p. 600.

FORMULARY

ZIDOVUDINE
Retrovir, AZT
Antiviral agent, nucleoside analogue reverse transcriptase inhibitor   **Yes   3   C**

Caps: 100 mg
Liquid: 50 mg/5 ml
Inj: 10 mg/ml
In combination with Lamivudine (3TC) as Combivir:
   Tabs: 300 mg zidovudine + 150 mg lamivudine

See p. 390 for indications.
Dosages may differ in separate
protocols.
Children 3 mo–12 yr:
   PO: 160 mg/m^2/dose Q8 hr. Dose can
   range from 90–180 mg/m^2/dose Q6–
   8 hr.
   Intermittent IV: 120 mg/m^2/dose Q6 hr
   Continuous IV infusion: 20 mg/m^2/hr
≥12 yr and adults:
   PO:
      Symptomatic HIV: 200 mg/dose TID,
      or 300 mg/dose BID; **max dose:** 600
      mg/24 hr.
      Asymptomatic HIV: 100 mg/dose
      Q4 hr while awake (500 mg/24 hr)
   IV:
      Symptomatic HIV: 1 mg/kg/dose
      Q4 hr
Prevention of vertical transmission:
   14–34 weeks of pregnancy:

   Until labor: 100 mg PO 5 × /24 hr or
   600 mg/24 hr PO ÷ BID-TID
   During labor: 2 mg/kg/dose IV over
   1 hour followed by 1 mg/kg/hr IV
   infusion until umbilical cord clamped.
   Neonate: 2 mg/kg/dose Q6 hr PO or
   1.5 mg/kg/dose Q6 hr IV over 60 min.
   Begin within 12 hr of birth and
   continue until 6 wk of age.
   *Premature Infant (investigational dose
   from ACTG 331):* 1.5 mg/kg/dose IV/PO
   Q12 hr from birth to 2 weeks of age;
   then increase to 2 mg/kg/dose IV/PO Q8
   hr thereafter.
Needle stick prophylaxis: 200 mg/dose
PO TID or 300 mg/dose PO BID × 28
days. Use in combination with lamivudine
150 mg/dose PO BID, and indinavir 800
mg/dose PO TID × 28 days.

Use with **caution** in patients with impaired renal or hepatic function. Dosage reduction is recommended in severe renal impairment and may be necessary in hepatic dysfunction. Drug penetrates well into the CNS. Most common side effects include: anemia, granulocytopenia, nausea, and headache (dosage reduction, erythropoietin, filgrastim/GCSF or discontinuance may be required depending on event). Seizures, confusion, rash, myositis, myopathy (use >1 yr), hepatitis and elevated liver enzymes have been reported. Macrocytosis is noted after 4 weeks of therapy and can be used as an indicator of compliance.

Do **not** use in combination with stavudine because of poor antiretroviral effect. Effects of interacting drugs include: increased toxicity (acyclovir, trimethoprim-sulfamethoxazole); increased hematological toxicity (ganciclovir, interferon-alpha, marrow suppressive drugs); and granulocytopenia (drugs which affect glucuronidation). Methadone, atovaquone, cimetidine, valproic acid, probenecid, fluconazole may increase levels of zidovudine. Rifampin, rifabutin, clarithromycin may decrease levels.

Some NIH Pediatric HIV Working Group participants use 180 mg/m^2/dose Q12 hr PO when using other antiretroviral combinations in children 3 months–12 years (data is limited).

Do **not** administer IM. IV form is incompatible with blood product infusions and should be infused over 1 hour (intermittent IV dosing). Despite manufacturer recommendations of administering oral doses 30 minutes prior to or 1 hour after meals, doses may be administered with food.

ZILEUTON
Zyflo
Anti-asthmatic, 5-lipoxygenase inhibitor
Tabs: 600 mg

No   ?   C

Asthma:
Children ≥12 yr and Adults:
600 mg PO QID (with meals and at bedtime)

Contraindicated in active liver disease. Major adverse effects include headache, dyspepsia, nausea, abdominal pain, and elevated transaminase levels. Fatigue, dizziness, insomnia, paresthesia, and rash have been reported.

Zileuton is a substrate for CYP 450 1A2, 2C9, and 3A4 isoenzymes. May increase the effects and/or toxicity of alprazolam, astemizole (contraindicated), clozapine, digoxin, propranolol, terfenadine (contraindicated), theophylline, and warfarin. Doses may be administered with or without food.

For explanation of icons, see p. 600.

FORMULARY

ZINC SALTS

No ? C

Tabs as sulfate, 23% elemental: 66, 110, 200 mg
Caps as sulfate, 23% elemental: 110, 220 mg
Tabs as gluconate, 14.3% elemental: 10, 15, 50, 78 mg
Liq as acetate: 5, 10 mg elemental Zn/ml
Inj as sulfate: 1 mg, 5 mg elemental Zn/ml
Inj as chloride: 1 mg elemental Zn/ml

Zinc deficiency:
Infants and Children: 0.5–1 mg elemental Zn/kg/24 hr PO ÷ QD-TID.
Adults: 25-50 mg elemental Zn/dose (100–220 mg Zn sulfate/dose) PO TID
US RDA: See p. 486.
For supplementation in parenteral nutrition, see p. 516.

Nausea, vomiting, GI disturbances, leukopenia, diaphoresis may occur. Gastric ulcers, hypotension, and tachycardia may occur at high doses. Patients with excessive losses (burns) or impaired absorption require higher doses. Approximately 20% to 30% of oral dose is absorbed. Oral doses may be administered with food if GI upset occurs.

VII. BIBLIOGRAPHY

1. Package inserts of medications.
2. Committee on Drugs. The transfer of drugs and other chemicals into human milk. *Pediatrics* 1994; 93:137.
3. Briggs GG, Freeman RK, Yaffe SJ. *A reference guide to fetal and neonatal risk: drugs in pregnancy and lactation,* 5th edn. Baltimore: Williams & Wilkins; 1998.
4. *The Medical Letter on drugs and therapeutics.* The Medical Letter, Inc, New Rochelle, NY, 10801.
5. Peter G et al. 1997 *red book: report of the Committee on Infectious Diseases,* 24th edn. Elk Grove Village, IL: American Academy of Pediatrics; 1997.
6. Gilbert DN, Moellering RC, Sande MA. *The Sanford guide to antimicrobial therapy,* 28th edn. Vienna, VA: Antimicrobial Therapy, Inc; 1998.
7. Nelson JD. *1998–1999 pocket book of pediatric antimicrobial therapy,* 13th edn. Baltimore: Williams & Wilkins; 1998.
8. Bartlett JG. *1998 medical management of HIV infection.* Baltimore: Port City Press; 1998.
9. Young TE, Mangum OB. *Neofax: a manual of drugs used in neonatal care,* 11th edn. Raleigh, NC: Acorn Publishing; 1998.
10. McEvoy GK. *AHFS 98 drug information.* Bethesda, MD: American Society of Health-System Pharmacists; 1998.
11. Boyd JR. *Facts and Comparisons: loose leaf drug information service,* Philadelphia: JB Lippincott, updated monthly.
12. Micromedex, Inc. *Drug dex,* vol. 99, 1974–1999.

13. Taketomo CK, Hodding JH, Kraus DM. *Pediatric dosage handbook*, 5th edn. Hudson, OH: Lexi-Comp, Inc; 1998.

14. Benitz WE, Tatro DS. *The pediatric drug handbook,* 3rd edn. St Louis: Mosby; 1995.

15. Ellsworth AJ, Witt DM, Dugdale DC, Oliver LM. *Mosby's 1998 medical drug reference.* St Louis: Mosby; 1998.

16. Pagliaro LA, Pagliaro AM. *Problems in pediatric drug therapy,* 3rd edn. Hamilton, IL: Drug Intelligence Publications; 1995.

17. Dipchand AI. *The Hospital for Sick Children handbook of pediatrics,* 9th edn. St Louis: Mosby; 1997.

18. Centers for Disease Control and Prevention. Recommendations and reports: guidelines for the use of antiretroviral agents in pediatric HIV infection. *MMWR* 1998; 47(RR-4):1–43.

18. National Institutes of Health: National Heart, Lung, and Blood Institute—Expert Panel Report 2. *Clinical practice guidelines: guidelines for the diagnosis and management of asthma.* NIH Publ. No. 97–4051; April 1997.

19. Borowitz DS, Grand RJ, Durie PR: The Consensus Committee. Use of pancreatic enzyme supplements for patients with cystic fibrosis in the context of fibrosing colonopathy. *J Pediatr* 1995; 127:681–684.

20. Nichols DG, Yaster M, Lappe DG, Haller JA Jr. *Golden hour: the handbook of advanced pediatric life support,* 2nd edn. St Louis: Mosby; 1996.

21. Yaster M, Krane EJ, Kaplan RF, Cote CJ, Lappe DG. *Pediatric pain management and sedation handbook.* St Louis: Mosby; 1997.

22. Chameides L, Hazinski MF: *Textbook of pediatric advanced life support,* Dallas: American Heart Association; 1994.

ANALGESIA AND SEDATION

Beverley Robin, MD

I. ASSESSMENT OF PAIN

Observe behavior and physiologic changes that may accompany pain. Consider the child's self-report as the most reliable indicator of the existence and intensity of acute pain. At regular intervals monitor the child to determine the intensity and location of the pain and effectiveness of analgesia.

A. INFANT

1. **Physiologic response:** Seen primarily in early onset of acute pain; subsides with continuing or chronic pain. Increase in blood pressure, heart rate, respiratory rate, oxygen desaturation, crying, diaphoresis, flushing, pallor.
2. **Behavioral response:** Observe characteristics and duration of cry, facial expressions, visual tracking, body movements, and response to stimuli. Trust parents' and nurses' interpretations.

B. PRESCHOOLER:
In addition to physiologic and behavioral responses use the 'FACES' pain rating scale to assess the intensity of the pain (Fig. 30.1). Identify what word the child uses for pain.

C. SCHOOL-AGE AND ADOLESCENT:
Evaluate physiologic responses. Ask the patient to describe and locate the pain. Use a pain rating scale where 0 is no pain and 10 is the worst pain ever experienced by the patient.

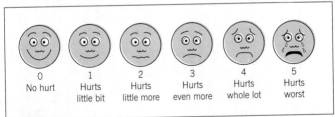

0	1	2	3	4	5
No hurt	Hurts little bit	Hurts little more	Hurts even more	Hurts whole lot	Hurts worst

FIG. 30.1
FACES pain rating scale. (From Wong[1].)

TABLE 30.1
NONNARCOTIC ANALGESICS

Drug	Dose	Route	Interval	GI irritation	Platelet inhibition
Acetaminophen[a]	10–15mg/kg, max. 75mg/kg/day, adult dose 325–650mg/dose, max. 4g/day	PO/PR	Q4–6hr	No	No
Ibuprofen	5–10mg/kg, max. 40mg/kg/day, adult dose 200–800mg/dose. max. 3.2g/day	PO	Q6–8hr	Yes	Yes
Indomethacin	0.5mg/kg, max. 4mg/kg/day, adult dose 50–150mg/day	PO/PR	Q6hr	Yes	Yes
Ketorolac	0.5mg/kg, max. dose 30mg or 120mg/day	IV/IM	Q6hr	Yes	Yes
	Children >50kg and adults: 10mg/dose, max. dose 40mg/day	PO	Q6hr	Yes	Yes
Naproxen	5–10mg/kg, adult dose 250–500mg, max. 1250mg/day	PO	Q8–12hr	Yes	Yes
Choline MG trisalicylate[b]	7.5–15mg/kg, adult dose 500mg–1.5g (dose based on salicylate content)	PO	Q6–8hr Q8–24hr	Yes	No
Salicylate[b]	10–15mg/kg, max. 4g/day	PO/PR	Q4hr	Yes	Yes

PR, by rectum.

[a]Does not have antiinflammatory properties. Initial rectal dose: 25–40mg/kg.

[b]Contraindicated in patients <16 years of age with varicella or influenza because there is an association with Reye syndrome. May be used for the treatment of rheumatic pain.

II. ANALGESICS

A. NONNARCOTIC ANALGESICS (Table 30.1): Commonly used in the management of mild-to-moderate pain of nonvisceral origin. Administered alone or in combination with opiates.

1. **Weak analgesic with antipyretic activity:** Acetaminophen.
2. **Nonsteroidal antiinflammatory drugs (NSAIDs):** Especially useful for sickle cell, bony, rheumatic, and inflammatory pain. Recommend use of H_2-receptor blocker concomitantly.

B. OPIATES

1. **Definition:** Drugs that are not opium derivatives but that are opium-like or morphine-like in their effects.
2. **Commonly used opioids** (Table 30.2).

C. LOCAL ANESTHETICS: Reversibly block conduction of nerve impulses along peripheral and central nerve pathways. Used primarily to anesthetize areas for minor procedures, they are administered topically, subcutaneously, into peripheral nerves, or centrally (epidural/spinal).

1. **Injectable local anesthetics** (Table 30.3)

a. Local infiltration: Infiltration of the skin at the site; used for painful procedures such as wound closure, blood drawing, IV placement, lumbar puncture. To reduce stinging from injection, alkalinize the anesthetic; add 1mL (or 1mEq) sodium bicarbonate to 9mL lidocaine, or 1mL sodium bicarbonate to 29mL bupivacaine. To enhance intensity and duration, add epinephrine in concentrations of 5mcg/mL, but never use epinephrine at areas supplied by end-arteries (e.g., pinna, digits, and penis).

b. Peripheral nerve blocks

　1) *Digital nerve block:* Indicated in finger or toe laceration repair, setting a fracture, paronychia drainage, nail removal.

　　a) *Technique:* Cleanse the skin. Insert 25G needle at the metacarpophalangeal junction on either side of the digit. Keep the needle perpendicular to the plane of the hand or foot and advance from dorsal to palmar surface while injecting slowly. Use 1–3mL **epinephrine-free** anesthetic. This block should not be performed if there is uncertainty regarding the blood supply to the digit (Fig. 30.2).

　2) *Penile nerve block:* Indicated in circumcision, meatotomy, and hypospadias repair.

　　a) *Technique:* Cleanse the skin. The nondominant hand holds the penis forward and down. A 25G needle is inserted at the 10:30 and 1:30 o'clock positions at the base of the penis. Inject 0.5–3mL **epinephrine-free** anesthetic in Buck's fascia, 3–5mm below the surface of the skin (Fig. 30.3).

30

ANALGESIA AND SEDATION

TABLE 30.2
COMMONLY USED OPIOIDS

Drug	Equianalgesic doses (mg/kg/dose)	Route	Onset (min)	Duration (hr)	Side effects	Comments
Codeine	1.2	PO	30–60	3–4	Nausea/vomiting	Use with acetaminophen for synergy.
Oxycodone	0.1	PO	30–60	3–4	May contain Na metabisulfite, which can precipitate anaphylaxis	Much less nauseating than codeine.
Morphine	0.1	IV	5–10 (IV)	3–4	Nausea, sedation, pruritus, constipation, seizures in neonates	—
	0.1–0.2	IM/SC	10–30	4–5		
	0.3–0.5	PO	30–60	4–5		
Methadone	0.1	IV	5–10	4–24	—	Intial dose may produce analgesia for 3–4hr; duration of action is increased with repeated dosing.
	0.1	PO	30–60	4–24		

Hydromorphone	0.015	IV/SC	5–10 (IV)	3–4	Less sedation, nausea, pruritus than morphine.
	0.02–0.1	PO	30–60		
Hydrocodone	0.1	PO	30–60	3–4	Much less nauseating than codeine. May contain Na metabisulfite, which can precipitate anaphylaxis
Meperidine	1.0	IV	5–10	3–4	Tachycardia, catastrophic interaction with MAO inhibitors, metabolite can cause seizures, can induce asthma attacks (from Na bisulfite)
	1.5–2.0	PO	30–60	2–4	Euphoric effects are greater than with morphine. Low doses stop shivering (0.1–0.25mg/kg)
Fentanyl	0.001	IV	1–2	0.5–1	Bradycardia, chest wall rigidity with high boluses (>5mcg/kg but can occur with low doses)
	0.01	Transmucosal	15		Levels of unbound drug are higher in newborns than older patients.

aWhen converting to methadone as part of an opioid taper, give 30% of the total converted dose initially and assess the need for a higher dose at subsequent intervals.

30

ANALGESIA AND SEDATION

TABLE 30.3

COMMONLY USED INJECTABLE LOCAL ANESTHETICS

Agent	Concentration (%)	Max. dose (mg/kg)	Onset (min)	Duration alone (hr)	Duration with epinephrine (hr)
Lidocaine	0.5–2	4.5–7	3	0.5–2	1–3
Bupivacaine	0.25	1.5–2.5	15	2–4	4–8

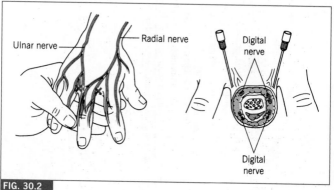

FIG. 30.2
Digital nerve block. (From Yaster[2].)

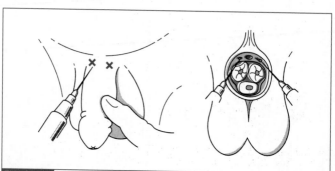

FIG. 30.3
Penile nerve block. (From Yaster[3].)

2. **Topical local anesthetics**
a. **EMLA (Eutectic Mixture of Local Anesthetics):** Topical emulsion of lidocaine (2.5%) and prilocaine (2.5%) applied to intact skin to produce anesthesia. Applied, then covered with an occlusive dressing; onset of complete anesthesia in 60–90 minutes. Indicated for procedures in which intact skin is punctured, such as venipuncture, circumcision, lumbar puncture, and bone marrow aspiration. Contraindicated in patients at risk of developing methemoglobinemia.
b. **Viscous lidocaine:** Provides analgesia for mucosal trauma and stomatitis. Not recommended in young children who cannot expectorate. Systemic toxicity can occur with mucosal absorption. Maximum dose is 3mg/kg per dose every 2 hours as needed.
c. **Lidocaine jelly:** Useful for decreasing pain with nasogastric tube placement or urethral catheterization.
d. **LET (Lidocaine, Epinephrine, Tetracaine):** Provides topical local anesthetic for dermal lacerations, applied to open wound either in a gel or liquid form. Can be prepared as 4% lidocaine, 1:2000 epinephrine, 0.5% tetracaine in hydroxyethyl cellulose gel. 1–3mL is applied with a cotton-tipped applicator/cotton ball (not gauze) and held in place for 20–30 minutes. Contraindicated in areas supplied by end-arteries (e.g., pinna, nose, penis, fingers, and toes). Maximum dose for topical lidocaine is 3mg/kg per dose.
e. **TAC (Tetracaine, Adrenaline [epinephrine], Cocaine):** 1–3mL provides topical local anesthetic for dermal lacerations, applied to open wound in either a gel or liquid form. Can be prepared as 1% tetracaine, 1:4000 epinephrine, and 4% cocaine HCl solution. A few drops are applied directly to the wound, and the remainder of the 3mL is applied by cotton-tipped applicator/cotton ball and held in place with firm pressure for 10 minutes. Contraindicated in areas supplied by end-arteries, on mucous membranes or on areas adjacent to mucous membranes, and in patients taking MAO (monoamine oxidase) inhibitors. Reapplication is contraindicated because cocaine is a controlled substance, and in addition, seizures have been reported even with appropriate dosing. Maximum dose for cocaine is 3mg/kg.

III. PATIENT-CONTROLLED ANALGESIA (PCA)
A. **DEFINITION:** Device that enables a patient to self-administer small doses of analgesics. May also be administered by parent or nurse in some situations.
B. **INDICATIONS:** Acute/chronic pain such as sickle cell, postoperative, burns, posttraumatic, and cancer. Also for preemptive pain management to facilitate dressing changes or for patients with mucositis secondary to radiation or chemotherapy.

30

ANALGESIA AND SEDATION

C. **ROUTES OF ADMINISTRATION:** IV, SC, epidural.
D. **PATIENT SELECTION CRITERIA:** Willingness on the part of the child and family to use the device appropriately, understanding of the instructions, absence of medical history in which opiates are contraindicated or restricted, children 4–6 years or older who are able to play hand-held computer games. Children who are under 5 years of age, or those who are physically or developmentally unable to push the button should be assessed on an individual basis for nurse- or parent-controlled analgesia.
E. **AGENTS** (Table 30.4)

IV. SEDATION (Fig. 30.4)

A. **DEFINITIONS**
1. **Conscious sedation:** Controlled state of depressed consciousness during which the child retains airway reflexes and a patent airway, responds to age-appropriate commands, and tolerates a noxious procedure.
2. **Deep sedation:** Controlled state of depressed consciousness during which airway reflexes and a patent airway may not be retained and the child is unable to respond to physical or verbal stimuli. Conscious sedation can easily progress to deep sedation, and most procedures performed on children under 5 years of age require deep sedation.
B. **PRINCIPLES AND INDICATIONS:** Minimize pain and discomfort, produce amnesia, behavior control, and immobility. In conscious sedation there is a rapid return to a state of alertness; used during diagnostic and therapeutic procedures.
C. **PREPARATION**
1. NPO for solids and nonclear liquids for 4–6 hours; clear liquids for 2–3 hours. Classification of breast milk as a clear liquid vs solid remains controversial.

TABLE 30.4

ORDERS FOR PCA

Drug	Basal rate (mcg/kg/hr)	Bolus dose (mcg/kg)	Lockout period (min)	Boluses/hr	Max. dose/hr (mcg/kg)
Morphine	10–30	10–30	6–10	4–6	100–150
Hydromorphone	3–5	3–5	6–10	4–6	15–20
Fentanyl	0.5–1.0	0.5–1.0	6–10	2–3	2–4

Adapted from Yaster[2].

2. **Intravenous access.**
3. **Airway equipment**

S Suction.

O Oxygen.

A Airway equipment: Oral/nasal airway, laryngoscope and appropriate-sized blades, appropriate-sized endotracheal tubes (ETT). with stylet, tape, bag-valve with appropriate-sized mask, suction.

P Pharmacy.

1) *Intubation medications:* Atropine, anesthetic, sedative/hypnotic, paralytic (see pp. 5–7).
2) *Emergency medications:* Epinephrine, atropine, lidocaine, glucose.
3) *Reversal agents:* Naloxone, flumazenil.

D. **MONITORING**
1. **Vital signs:** Baseline vital signs should be obtained initially; heart rate and oxygen saturation should be monitored continuously. Blood pressure and respiratory rate should be monitored intermittently. Vital signs should be recorded at 5–15-minute intervals.
2. **Airway:** Airway patency should be checked frequently.

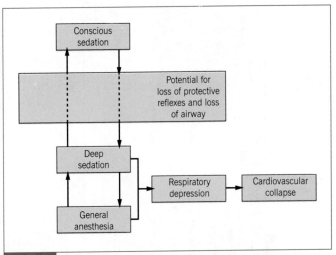

FIG. 30.4

American Academy of Pediatrics sedation continuum. (From Yaster[2].)

TABLE 30.5

COMMONLY USED BENZODIAZEPINES

Drug	Routes	Onset (min)	Dose (mg/kg/dose)	Duration (hr)
Diazepam (Valium)	IV/PO/PR	IV 1.5–3	IV 0.1–0.2	0.25–1
MEDIUM ACTION		PO 30–60	PO 0.2–0.3	2–3
		PR 7–15	PR 0.2–0.3	2–3
Lorazepam (Ativan)	IV/IM/PO/PR	IV 1–5	IV 0.05 (max. single dose 2mg)	3–4
LONG ACTION		IM 10–20	IM 0.05 (max. single dose 4mg)	3–6
		PO 30–60	PO 0.05 (max. single dose 4mg)	3–6
Midazolam (Versed)	IV/IM/PO/PR/IN	IV 1–3	IV 0.05 titrated to effect (max. dose 0.2mg/kg)	1–2
		IM 5–10	IM 0.1–0.2 (max. dose 10mg)	1–2
SHORT ACTION		PO[a] 10–30	PO 0.5–0.75 (max. dose 20mg)	1–2
		PR[a] 10	PR 0.3–1.0 (max. 20mg)	1–2
		IN[a] 5–10	IN 0.2–0.3 (max. 7.5mg)	1–2

IN, intranasal.
[a] Use IV solution for PO, PR, and IN administration.

E. **GENERAL GUIDELINES:** Determine a treatment plan. Combine drugs to potentiate their effects (also causes more respiratory depression than when either drug is used alone). Titrate to effect.

F. **PHARMACOLOGIC AGENTS**

1. **Benzodiazepines:** Sedative, anxiolytic, anterograde amnestic, skeletal muscle relaxant, anticonvulsant. No analgesic effects.

   a. Indications: Preprocedure sedation; anxiolysis and anterograde amnesia for painful and nonpainful procedures; sedation/anxiolysis of the critically ill child; induction of, or adjuvant to, general anesthetic; and anticonvulsant.

   b. Interactions: Sedative effects, as well as respiratory and circulatory depression, are potentiated by opiates, extremes of age, alcohol, and other CNS depressants.

   c. Side effects: Respiratory depression, upper airway obstruction, apnea, hypotension, coma.

   d. Common benzodiazepines (Table 30.5).

2. **Barbiturates:** Global CNS depression, sedation to general anesthetic, anticonvulsant. No intrinsic analgesic effects.

   a. Indications: Sedation and immobility for nonpainful procedures (e.g., radiologic imaging), preprocedure sedation, induction of general anesthesia, anticonvulsant, and alcohol and opiate withdrawal.

   b. Interactions: Sedative and circulatory depressant effects are potentiated by opiates, other CNS depressants, extremes of age.

   c. Side effects: Respiratory depression, upper airway obstruction, apnea, coma, residual sedation, hypotension, decreased intracranial pressure.

   d. Commonly used barbiturates.

      1) Pentobarbital (Table 30.6): Most commonly used to produce immobility in patients undergoing nonpainful procedures such as radiologic imaging. When given IV must be titrated slowly to effect;

30

ANALGESIA AND SEDATION

TABLE 30.6

ONSET, DURATION, AND DOSAGE OF PENTOBARBITAL

Route	Onset (min)	Duration (hr)	Dose
IV	1–10	1–4	Initial dose: 0.5–1.0mg/kg
			Titrate to max. dose of 6mg/kg or 150–200mg
IM	5–15	2–4	Initial dose: 2–6mg/kg
			Max. dose: 6mg/kg or 150mg
PO	15–60	2–4	Initial dose: 2–6mg/kg
			Max. dose: 6mg/kg or 200mg
PR	15–60	2–4	Initial dose: 2–6mg/kg
			Max. dose: 6mg/kg or 200mg

Adapted from Yaster[2].

respiratory depression, airway obstruction, apnea, and hypotension most commonly occur when given rapidly.

2) Thiopental IV: Reserved for induction of general anesthesia.
   a) Route of administration: Rectally only for sedation. Produces general anesthesia, hypotension, apnea, when given IV.
   b) Dose: 20–30mg/kg per dose rectally (patients on anticonvulsants chronically may need higher doses).
   c) Onset: 7–10 minutes.
   d) Duration: 30–90 minutes.

3. **Opioids:** Sedation and analgesia (Table 30.2). Withdrawal symptoms may develop if opioids are stopped after 7–10 days of frequent or continuous use. Therefore the dose should be tapered by 10% per day.

4. **Miscellaneous agents**

a. Chloral hydrate: Hypnotic, without analgesic activity; used to achieve immobility for nonpainful procedures such as radiologic imaging or EEG. Fails to provide adequate immobility approximately 30–40% of the time.
   1) Route: Oral or rectal.
   2) Dose: 25–100mg/kg. (Max. dose 2g.)
   3) Onset: 30–60 minutes.
   4) Side effects: Residual sedation, paradoxical excitement, ataxia, headache, nausea, diarrhea, emesis, acute intermittent porphyria, leukopenia. Sedative effects can cause airway obstruction; therefore patients should be monitored to the same degree as with other sedative/hypnotics.

b. Ketamine: Nonbarbiturate that causes a dissociative anesthesia with potent analgesia. Reserved for use by anesthesiologists.
   1) Indications: Induction of general anesthesia and sedation for painful procedures, especially in patients with reactive airways disease, congenital heart disease, burns, hemodynamic instability, trauma.
   2) Contraindications: Increased intracranial pressure, psychosis or personality disorder, or patients in whom the fasting status is unknown.
   3) Interactions: Sedative and circulatory depressant effects are potentiated by opiates, alcohol, extremes of age, and CNS depressants.
   4) Precautions: Emergence phenomenon associated with visual-auditory illusions that can progress to delirium (Table 30.7).

Note: A benzodiazepine and an antisialagogue such as atropine or glycopyrrolate should be given concomitantly to counteract the hallucinogenic and increased mucous/salivary gland secretion effects of ketamine, respectively.

TABLE 30.7
KETAMINE DOSING AND EFFECTS

Dose (mg/kg)	Onset (min)	Duration (min)	CNS effects	Cardiovascular effects	Respiratory effects	Other effects
SEDATION						
IM 2–3	5–15	30–90	Increased intracranial pressure Emergence delirium	Increased heart rate, blood pressure, cardiac output, systemic and pulmonary vascular resistance (can reverse right to left shunt particularly during 'Tet' spells in patients with tetralogy of Fallot) Direct myocardial depressant	Apnea with rapid IV infusion Bronchodilation	Increased muscle tone, jerking movements
PO/PR 4–6	20–45	60–120+	Potent hallucinogen		Increased secretions Laryngospasm and coughing secondary to increased secretions	Increased intraocular pressure Nausea and emesis
INDUCTION OF GENERAL ANESTHESIA						
IV 0.5–3.0	0.5–2	20–60				

These effects apply regardless of the route of administration.

30

ANALGESIA AND SEDATION

c. Antihistamines: Mild sedative hypnotics used for preprocedure sedation and treatment of opiate side effects.
   1) Diphenhydramine: 0.5–1.0mg/kg per dose given PO/IV/IM Q4–6hr. Adult dose 10–50mg/dose. (Max. dose 50mg.)
   2) Hydroxyzine: 0.5–1.0mg/kg per dose given PO/IM Q4–6hr. Adult dose 25–100mg/dose. (Max. dose 600mg/24hr.)

5. **Reversal agents**
a. Naloxone: Opioid antagonist.
   1) Indications: Opioid overdose, respiratory depression, newborn with acute maternal opiate exposure (caution: can precipitate withdrawal), pruritus, urinary retention, biliary spasm.
   2) Dose and administration: 0.001–0.1mg/kg/dose to maximum 2mg dose, given IV/IM/IO/ETT. May repeat every 2–3 minutes as needed. In the nonarrest situation use the lowest effective dose (start at 0.001mg/kg) to reverse respiratory depression and not analgesia.
   3) Onset and duration: Onset 1–2 minutes IV, 2–5 minutes by other routes. **Duration is 45 minutes, which may be shorter than the duration of action of the opiate. Patients may require repeated doses. Monitor for the return of respiratory depression.**
b. Flumazenil: Benzodiazepine antagonist.
   1) Dose and administration: 0.1mg given IV. If no response in 1–2 minutes, repeat every 2 minutes to maximum total dose of 1mg.
   2) Onset and duration: Onset usually within 1–3 minutes. **Duration is 45–60 minutes, which may be shorter than the duration of benzodiazepine. Monitor for the return of respiratory depression for at least 2 hours.**
   3) Caution: May precipitate seizures, particularly in patients with an underlying seizure disorder, or in those with tricyclic antidepressant overdose.

V. REFERENCES

1. Wong DL. *Whaley and Wong's essentials of pediatric nursing,* 5th edn. St Louis: Mosby, 1995.
2. Yaster M, Krane EJ, Kaplan RF, Coté CJ, Lappe DG. *Pediatric pain management and sedation handbook.* St Louis: Mosby; 1997.
3. Yaster M, Maxwell LG. Pediatric regional anesthesia. *Anesthesiology* 1989; **70:**324–338.

SPECIAL DRUG TOPICS

Diana C. Alexander, MD, MPH

I. TOPICAL CORTICOSTEROIDS (Table 31.1)

a. Table 31.1 provides a listing of topical steroids from the most potent (group I) to the least potent (group VII). Use intermediate- and low-potency steroids (groups IV–VII) for pediatric patients. Topical steroid use is contraindicated in varicella.

b. Occlusive dressings (including waterproof diapers) increase systemic absorption of topical steroids and should not be used with high-potency preparations. Topical steroids should be used with caution in intertriginous areas and on the face.

c. Apply once or twice daily. Penetration of the skin is greatest with ointments with decreasing effectiveness in gels, creams, and lotions. Prolonged use may result in cutaneous and systemic side effects.

d. A gram of topical cream or ointment should cover a 10 × 10cm area. A 30–60g tube will cover the entire body of an adult once.

31

II. COMMON INDICATIONS AND DOSES OF SYSTEMIC CORTICOSTEROIDS

A. ENDOCRINE

1. **Physiologic replacement**
a. Cortisone acetate: PO: 24–36mg/m²/24hr ÷ Q8hr (mean 30); IM: 12–18mg/m²/dose QD (mean 15).
b. Hydrocortisone: PO: 18–30mg/m²/24hr ÷ Q8hr (mean 24); IM: 9–18mg/m²/dose.
c. Prednisolone/prednisone: PO: 4–6mg/m²/24hr ÷ Q12hr (mean 5).
d. Dexamethasone: PO/IM/IV: 0.5–0.75mg/m²/24hr ÷ Q6–12hr.

2. **Stress dosing:** Consider for patients on glucocorticoid therapy >1 month.
a. PO/IM: 2–4 times the physiologic replacement dose. Give preoperatively and postoperatively with gradual decrease to maintenance.
b. IV: Hydrocortisone sodium succinate (Solu-Cortef): 25–50mg/m²/24hr (give as a continuous infusion). If IV access not available, 50mg/m²/dose IM Q12hr.

3. **Adrenal insufficiency**
a. Chronic: See 'Physiologic replacement' above.
b. Acute
   1) Fluids: Bolus with 20mL/kg D₅ NS then 60mL/kg D₅NS administered over 24 hours.
   2) Steroids: Hydrocortisone sodium succinate (Solu-Cortef) 25–50mg/m² IV bolus, then begin continuous infusion over 24 hours as per 'stress dosing' protocol above.

TABLE 31.1

TOPICAL STEROID POTENCY RANKING

Group	Brand	Generic name	Sizes (in grams unless otherwise specified)
I	Temovate cr, ot 0.05%	Clobetasol propionate	15, 30, 45
	Diprolene ot 0.05% cr 0.05%	Betamethasone dipropionate	15, 45
MOST POTENT	Diprolene AF		15, 45
	Psorcon ot 0.05%	Diflorasone diacetate	15, 30, 60
	Ultravate cr, ot 0.05%	Halobetasol dipropionate	15, 45
II	Cyclocort ot 0.1%	Amcinonide	15, 30, 60
	Diprosone ot 0.05%	Betamethasone dipropionate	15, 45
	Elocon ot 0.1%	Mometasone furoate	15, 45
	Florone ot 0.05%	Diflorasone diacetate	15, 30, 60
	Halog cr, ot, sl 0.1%	Halcinonide	15, 30, 60, 240 sl: 20, 60mL
	Lidex cr, gl, ot, sl 0.05%	Fluocinonide	15, 30, 60, 120 sl: 20, 60mL
	Maxiflor ot 0.05%	Diflorasone diacetate	15, 30, 60
	Maxivate cr, ot 0.05%	Betamethasone dipropionate	15, 45
	Topicort cr, ot 0.25%	Desoximetasone	15, 60, 120
	Topicort gl 0.05%		15, 60
III	Aristocort A ot 0.1%	Triamcinolone acetonide	15, 60
	Cyclocort cr, lt 0.1%	Amcinonide	15, 30, 60 lt: 20, 60mL
	Diprosone cr 0.05%	Betamethasone dipropionate	15, 45
	Florone cr 0.05%	Diflorasone diacetate	15, 30, 60
	Lidex E cr 0.05%	Fluocinonide	15, 30, 60, 120
	Maxiflor cr 0.05%	Diflorasone diacetate	15, 30, 60
	Maxivate lt 0.05%	Betamethasone dipropionate	60mL
	Valisone ot 0.1%	Betamethasone valerate	14, 45

From Ferndale Laboratories, Ferndale, MI.
cr, cream; ot, ointment; gl, gel; sl, solution; lt, lotion.
There are other topical steroid preparations containing dexamethasone, flumethasone, prednisolone, and methylprednisolone.

TABLE 31.1

TOPICAL STEROID POTENCY RANKING—cont'd

Group	Brand	Generic name	Sizes (in grams unless otherwise specified)
IV	Aristocort ot 0.1%	Triamcinolone acetonide	15, 60, 240, 454
	Cordran ot 0.05%	Flurandrenolide	15, 30, 60, 225
	Elocon cr, lt 0.1%	Mometasone furoate	15, 45 lt: 30, 60mL
	Kenalog cr, ot 0.1%	Triamcinolone acetonide	15, 60, 80, 240
	Synalar ot 0.025%	Fluocinolone acetonide	15, 30, 60, 120, 425
	Topicort LP cr 0.05%	Desoximetasone	15, 60
V	Cordran cr 0.05%	Flurandrenolide	15, 30, 60, 225
	Kenalog lt 0.1%	Triamcinolone acetonide	15, 60mL
	Kenalog ot 0.025%		15, 60, 80, 240
	Locoid cr, ot 0.1%	Hydrocortisone butyrate	15, 45
	Synalar cr 0.025%	Fluocinolone acetonide	15, 30, 60, 425
	Tridesilon ot 0.05%	Desonide	15, 60
	Valisone cr, lt 0.1%	Betamethasone valerate	15, 45, 110, 430 lt: 20, 60mL
	Westcort cr, ot 0.2%	Hydrocortisone valerate	15, 45, 60 cr only: 120
VI	Aclovate cr, ot 0.05%	Alclometasone dipropionate	15, 45
	Aristocort cr 0.1%	Triamcinolone acetonide	15, 60, 240, 2520
	Kenalog cr, lt 0.025%	Triamcinolone acetonide	15, 60, 80, 240, 2520 lt: 60mL
	Locoid sl 0.1%	Hydrocortisone butyrate	20, 60mL
	Locorten cr 0.03%	Flumethasone pivalate	15, 60
	Synalar cr, sl 0.01%	Fluocinolone	15, 45, 60, 425 sl: 20, 60mL
	Tridesilon cr 0.05%	Desonide	15, 60
VII (LEAST POTENT)	Hytone cr, ot, lt 1%	Hydrocortisone	cr, ot: 30 cr, lt: 120mL
	Hytone cr, ot, lt 2.5%		cr, ot: 30 cr, lt: 60mL

4. **Congenital adrenal hyperplasia**
a. Non–salt losing: See 'Physiologic replacement' on p. 907.
b. Salt losing: Fludrocortisone acetate (Florinef): PO: Usually 0.1mg/24 hours, range of 0.05–0.2mg/24 hours in addition to physiologic glucocorticoid replacement.

B. PULMONARY

1. **Airway edema**
a. Dexamethasone: PO/IV/IM: 0.5–2mg/kg/24hr ÷ Q6hr. Begin 24 hours before extubation and continue for 4–6 doses after extubation.
b. Croup: Dexamethasone 0.6mg/kg/dose IM/IV ×1.

2. **Acute asthma**
a. Prednisone/prednisolone
   1) PO: 1–2mg/kg/24hr ÷ Q12–24hr ×3–5 days.
   2) **Max. dose:** 80mg/24hr.
b. Methylprednisolone (pediatric dosage)
   1) IV/IM: Load (optional) 2mg/kg/dose ×1.
   2) Maintenance: 2mg/kg/24hr ÷ Q6hr.
c. Hydrocortisone
   1) IV: Load (optional) 4–8mg/kg/dose; **max. dose:** 250mg.
   2) Maintenance: 8mg/kg/24hr ÷ Q6hr.

3. **Spinal cord injury**
a. Methylprednisolone: 30mg/kg bolus dose over 15 minutes, followed 45 minutes later by a continuous infusion of 5.4 mg/kg/hr ×23 hours.[10]

C. MISCELLANEOUS

1. **Antiemetic (chemotherapy induced)**
a. Dexamethasone
   1) IV: Initial: 10mg/m^2/dose (**max. dose:** 20mg/dose).
   2) Subsequent: 5mg/m^2/dose Q6hr.

2. **Cerebral edema**
a. Dexamethasone
   1) PO/IM/IV: Loading dose: 1–2mg/kg/dose ×1.
   2) Maintenance: 1–1.5mg/kg/24hr ÷ Q4–6hr (**max. dose:** 16mg/24 hours).

3. **Bacterial meningitis[9]**
a. Indications
   1) Dexamethasone is recommended for children >6 weeks old with Hib meningitis.
   2) Dexamethasone should be considered for children >6 weeks old with pneumococcal meningitis, but this is still controversial.
b. Dose: Dexamethasone—0.15mg/kg/dose IV Q6hr ×48 hours.
c. Timing: Ideally given with or just before first parenteral antibiotic dose. Initiation >4 hours after parenteral antibiotics is unlikely to be effective.

III. INHALED CORTICOSTEROIDS FOR AIRWAY INFLAMMATION
(Table 31.2)

TABLE 31.2

ESTIMATED COMPARATIVE DAILY DOSAGES FOR INHALED CORTICOSTEROIDS

Drug	Low dose	Medium dose	High dose
CHILDREN			
Beclomethasone dipropionate	84–336mcg	336–672mcg	>672mcg
42mcg/puff	(2–8 puffs)	(8–16 puffs)	(>16 puffs)
84mcg/puff	(1–4 puffs)	(4–8 puffs)	(>8 puffs)
Budesonide	100–200mcg	200–400mcg	>400mcg
DPI: 200mcg/dose		(1–2 inhalations)	(>2 inhalations)
Flunisolide	500–750mcg	1000–1250mcg	>1250mcg
250mcg/puff	(2–3 puffs)	(4–5 puffs)	(>5 puffs)
Fluticasone	88–176mcg	176–440mcg	>440mcg
MDI: 44mcg/puff	(2–4 puffs)	(4–10 puffs)	—
110mcg/puff	—	2–4 puffs)	(>4 puffs)
220mcg/puff	—	(1–2 puffs)	(>2 puffs)
DPI: 50, 100, 250mcg/dose	(2–4 inhalations – 50mcg)	(2–4 inhalations – 100mcg)	(>4 inhalations – 100mcg)
			(>2 inhalations – 250mcg)
Triamcinolone acetonide	400–800mcg	800–1200mcg	>1200mcg
100mcg/puff	(4–8 puffs)	(8–12 puffs)	(>12 puffs)

From Expert Panel II[1].

NOTE: The most important determinant of appropriate dosing is the clinician's and judgment of the patient's response to therapy. The clinician must monitor the patient's response on several clinical parameters and adjust the dose accordingly. The stepwise approach to therapy emphasizes that once control of asthma is achieved, the dose of medication should be carefully titrated to the minimum dose required to maintain control, thus reducing the potential for adverse effect. The reference point for the range of doses in children is data on the safety of inhaled corticosteroids in children, which in general, suggest that the dose ranges are equivalent to those of beclomethasone dipropionate 200–400mcg/day (low dose), 400–800mcg/day (medium dose), and >800mcg/day (high dose). Metered-dose inhaler (MDI) dosages are expressed as the activator dose (the amount of drug leaving the activator and delivered to the patient), which is the labeling required in the United States. Dry-powder inhaler (DPI) doses are expressed as the amount of drug in the inhaler after activation.

Continued

SPECIAL DRUG TOPICS 31

TABLE 31.2
ESTIMATED COMPARATIVE DAILY DOSAGES FOR INHALED CORTICOSTEROIDS—cont'd

Drug	Low dose	Medium dose	High dose
ADULTS			
Beclomethasone dipropionate	168–504mcg	504–840mcg	>840mcg
42mcg/puff	(4–12 puffs)	(12–20 puffs)	(>20 puffs)
84mcg/puff	(2–6 puffs)	(6–10 puffs)	(>10 puffs)
Budesonide	200–400mcg	400–600mcg	>600mcg
DPI: 200mcg/dose	(1–2 inhalations)	(2–3 inhalations)	(>3 inhalations)
Flunisolide	500–1000mcg	1000–2000mcg	>2000mcg
250mcg/puff	(2–4 puffs)	(4–8 puffs)	(>8 puffs)
Fluticasone	—	264–660mcg	>660mcg
MDI: 44mcg/puff	(2–6 puffs)	—	—
110mcg/puff	(2 puffs)	(2–6 puffs)	(>6 puffs)
220mcg/puff	—	—	(>3 puffs)
DPI: 50, 100, 250mcg/puff	(2–6 inhalations—50mcg)	(3–6 inhalations—100mcg)	(>6 inhalations—100mcg) **or** (>2 inhalations—250mcg)
Triamcinolone acetonide	400–1000mcg	1000–2000mcg	>2000mcg
100mcg/puff	(4–10 puffs)	(10–20 puffs)	(>20 puffs)

From Expert Panel II[1].

IV. DOSE EQUIVALENCE OF COMMONLY USED STEROIDS (Table 31.3)

TABLE 31.3
DOSE EQUIVALENCE OF COMMONLY USED STEROIDS[a]

Drug	Glucocorticoid effect equivalent to 100mg cortisol PO	Mineralocorticoid (mg): Na retention effect equivalent to 0.1mg Florinef[b]
Cortisone	125	20
Cortisol (Hydrocortisone)	100	20
Prednisone	25	50
Prednisolone	20–25	50
Methylprednisolone	15–20	No effect
Triamcinolone	10–20	No effect
9α-Fluorocortisol	6.5	0.1
Dexamethasone	1.5–3.75	No effect

Adapted from Kappy[11].

[a]The doses give approximately equivalent clinical effects. When using this table, select equipotent doses based on glucocorticoid or mineralocorticoid effect, since this is different for each drug.

[b]Total physiologic replacement for salt retention is usually 0.1mg Florinet, regardless of size.

V. OXIDIZING AGENTS AND GLUCOSE-6-PHOSPHATE DEHYDROGENASE (G6PD) DEFICIENCY (Table 31.4)

TABLE 31.4
OXIDIZING AGENTS AND G6PD DEFICIENCY

p-Aminosalicylic acid	Naphthalene[a]
Acetaminophen (Phenacetin)[a]	Nitrofurantoin (Furadantin)
Acetylsalicylic acid	Primaquine
Aniline dyes	Probenecid
Antipyrine	Salicylazosulfapyridine (Azulfidine)
Ascorbic acid[b]	Sulfacetamide (Sulamyd)
Chloramphenicol[c]	Sulfanilamide
Dapsone (diaminodiphenylsulfone)	Sulfisoxazole (Gantrisin)[a]
Fava beans	Sulfoxone[a]
Furazolidone (Furoxone)	Trisulfapyrimidine (Sultrin)
Methylene blue[a]	Vitamin K, water-soluble analogs only

The drugs and chemicals may cause hemolysis of 'reacting' (primaquine-sensitive) red blood cells (e.g., in patients with G6PD deficiency).

[a]Only slightly hemolytic to G6PD A patients in very large doses.

[b]Hemolytic in G6PD Mediterranean but not in G6PD A or Canton.

[c]In massive doses.

VI. MATERNAL DRUGS AND BREAST-FEEDING[2–4]
(Tables 31.5 and 31.6)

Drug exposure is minimized by maternal drug administration after breast-feeding. It is safer to use shorter-acting medications rather than drugs with sustained action.

TABLE 31.5

MATERNAL DRUGS CONTRAINDICATED IN BREAST-FEEDING[a]

Bromocriptine	Amphetamine
Cyclophosphamide	Cocaine
Cyclosporine	Heroin
Doxorubicin	Marijuana
Dextroamphetamine	Nicotine (smoking)
Ergotamine	Phencyclidine (PCP)
Lithium	
Methotrexate	
Phenindione	

[a]This list is not comprehensive. Please consult ch. 29 (formulary) or references[2-5] for pregnancy risk category and specific effects of drugs on the nursing infant.

TABLE 31.6

RADIOPHARMACEUTICALS AND BREAST-FEEDING

Drug	Duration radioactivity present in milk
Copper-64	50hr
Gallium-67	2wk
Indium-111	Small amount at 20hr
Iodine-123	Up to 36hr
Iodine-125	12days (risk of thyroid cancer)
Iodine-131	2–14days (depending on study)
Radioactive sodium	96hr
Technetium-99m	15hr–3days

NOTE: A nuclear medicine physician should be consulted before the diagnostic study so that the radionuclide with the shortest excretion time in breast milk can be used. Before the study, the mother should pump her breasts and store enough milk in the freezer for feeding the infant. After the study, the mother should pump her breasts to maintain milk production, but discard all the milk pumped for the required time that radioactivity is present in it. Milk samples can be screened by radiology departments for radioactivity before resumption of nursing.

VII. INSULIN (Table 31.7)

All preparations are available as human, purified pork, pork/beef, and beef. The human and more purified preparations produce less subcutaneous atrophy and less insulin resistance. For the management of diabetic ketoacidosis, see p. 207. See also Table 31-7.

TABLE 31.7

PHARMACOKINETICS OF INSULINS

Insulin	Onset (hr)	Peak (hr)	Effective duration (hr)	Maximum duration (hr)
ANIMAL				
Regular	0.5–2	3–4	4–6	6–8
Semi-Lente	1–1.5	5–10	12–16	20–24
NPH[a]	4–6	8–14	16–20	20–24
Lente	4–6	8–14	16–20	24–36
Ultralente	8–14	Minimal	24–36	
HUMAN				
Lispro[b]	0.15–0.25	0.5–1.5	3	4
Regular	0.5–1	2–3	3–6	4–6
NPH[a]	2–4	4–10	10–16	14–18
Lente	3–4	4–12	12–18	16–20
Ultralente	6–10	None	18–20	20–30

Adapted from American Diabetes Association[6].

All preparations are available as U-100 (100 U/mL) except for those that follow. Dilutions may be necessary to accurately deliver small doses.

U-500 (purified pork): 500U regular/mL.

U-70/30 (human or purified pork): 70U/mL NPH, 30U/mL regular.

U-50/50 (human): 50U/mL NPH, 50U/mL regular.

[a]Human neutral protamine Hagedorn (NPH) may have a slightly decreased duration of action compared with pork-derived NPH. Therefore the dose conversion may not be 1:1.

[b]Give 15min before a meal and use in conjunction with longer-acting form of insulin.

VIII. PANCREATIC ENZYME SUPPLEMENTS (Tables 31.8 and 31.9)

TABLE 31.8
PANCRELIPASE[a]

Product	Dosage form	Lipase (USP) units	Amylase (USP) units	Protease (USP) units
Cotazym	Capsule	8000	30,000	30,000
Cotazym-S	Capsule, enteric-coated sphere	5000	20,000	20,000
Pancrease	Capsule, delayed release	4000	20,000	25,000
Pancrease MT	Capsule,			
4	enteric-coated	4000	12,000	12,000
10	microtabs	10,000	30,000	30,000
16		16,000	48,000	48,000
20		20,000	56,000	44,000
Pancreacarb MS 8	Delayed-release capsule, enteric-coated, microsphere	8000	40,000	45,000
Ultrase	Capsule, enteric-coated, microsphere	4500	20,000	25,000
Ultrase MT	Capsule,			
6	enteric-coated	6000	19,500	19,500
12	minitab	12,000	39,000	39,000
18		18,000	58,500	58,500
20		20,000	65,000	65,000
Viokase	Powder	16,800/0.7g	70,000/0.7g ¼tsp = 0.7g	70,000/ 0.7g
	Tablet	8000	30,000	30,000

Adapted from Taketomo[7]; and from Solvay Pharmaceuticals, Inc. 1994; Fact and Comparisons: September, 1998; Scandipharm Product Information: July 1994 and May 1995.
[a]See formulary (ch. 29) for side effects associated with administration.

TABLE 31.9

PANCREATIN

Product	Dosage form	Lipase (USP) units	Amylase (USP) units	Protease (USP) units
Creon 5	Capsule, delayed release with enteric-coated microsphere	5000	16,000	18,750
Creon 10	Same as Creon 5	10,000	33,200	62,500
Creon 20	Same as Creon 5	20,000	66,400	75,000

IX. DRUGS COMMONLY USED IN HIV INFECTION (Table 31.10)[5]

TABLE 31.10

DRUGS COMMONLY USED IN HIV INFECTION

Drug name	Abbreviation	Trade name
NUCLEOSIDASE REVERSE TRANSCRIPTASE INHIBITORS		
Zidovudine	AZT, ZDV	Retrovir
Didanosine	ddI	Videx
Zalcitabine	ddC	Hivid
Stavudine	d4T	Zerit
Lamivudine	3TC	Epivir
Zidovudine/Lamivudine	AZT/3TC	Combivir
Abacavir	1592, 1592U89	Ziagen
NONNUCLEOSIDE INHIBITORS		
Nevirapine	BI-RG-587	Viramune
Delavirdine	U-901525/DLV	Rescriptor
Efavirenz	DMP 266	Sustiva
PROTEASE INHIBITORS		
Saquinavir	SQV/RO31-8959	Invirase, Fortovase
Ritonavir	RTV/ABT538	Norvir
Indinavir	IDV	Crixivan
Nelfinavir	NFV/AG 1343	Viracept
Amprenavir	141 W94/VB11103	Agenerase

X. CHEMOTHERAPEUTIC AGENTS (Table 31.11)

31

SPECIAL DRUG TOPICS

TABLE 31.11

CHARACTERISTICS OF CHEMOTHERAPEUTIC AGENTS

Drug name (drug class in italics)	Acute toxicity (DLT[a])	Long-term toxicity
Asparaginase (L-ASP, Elspar, PEG-ASP) *Enzyme*	DLT: Pancreatitis, seizures, hypersensitivity reactions (both acute and delayed; less with PEG modified), encephalopathy Other: Nausea, pancreatitis, hyperglycemia, azotemia, fever, coagulopathy, sagittal sinus thromboses and other venous thromboses, hyperammonemia	Neurologic deficits secondary to stroke
Bleomycin (Blenoxane) *DNA strand breaker*	DLT[b]: Anaphylaxis, pneumonitis Other: Pain, fever, chills, mucositis, skin reactions	Pulmonary fibrosis related to cumulative dose
Busulfan (Myleran) *Alkylator*	DLT: Myelosuppression, mucositis, seizures, hepatic venoocclusive disease Other: Hyperpigmentation, hypotension	Infertility, endocardial fibrosis, secondary malignancy
Carboplatin (CBDCA, Paraplatin) *DNA cross-linker*	DLT[b]: Thrombocytopenia, nephrotoxicity Other: Severe emesis, ototoxicity, peripheral neuropathy, optic neuritis (rare)	Renal insufficiency (less than cisplatin), hearing loss
Carmustine (bis-chloronitrosourea, BCNU, BiCNU) *Alkylator*	DLT: Myelosuppression (prolonged cumulative) Other: Vesicant, brownish discoloration of skin, hepatic and renal toxicity, severe emesis	Pulmonary fibrosis, infertility, secondary malignancy
Cisplatin (Platinol, *cis-platinum*, CDDP) *DNA cross-linker*	DLT[b]: Tubular and glomerular nephrotoxicity (related to cumulative dose), peripheral neuropathy Other: Severe emesis, myelosuppression, ototoxicity, SIADH (rare), papilledema and retrobulbar neuritis (rare)	Renal insufficiency, hearing loss, peripheral neuropathy
Cladribine (2-CdA, Leustatin) *Antimetabolite or nucleotide analog*	Myelosuppression, nausea and vomiting, headache, fever, chills, fatigue	

Agent / Class	Toxicities	Delayed / long-term toxicities
Cyclophosphamide (CTX, Cytoxan) *Alkylator prodrug*	DLT: Leukopenia, cardiomyopathy Other: Hemorrhagic cystitis (improved by mesna), emesis, direct ADH effect	Infertility, cardiomyopathy, secondary malignancy Leokoencephalopathy
Cytarabine (Ara-C) *Antimetabolite or nucleotide analog*	DLT[b]: Myelosuppression, cerebellar toxicity Other: Nausea and vomiting, anorexia, diarrhea, metallic taste, severe gastrointestinal ulceration, conjunctivitis, lethargy, ataxia, nystagmus, slurred speech, respiratory distress rapidly progressing to pulmonary edema, influenza-like syndrome, fever	Leukoencephalopathy
Dacarbazine (DIC, DTIC, imidazole carboxamide) *Alkylator*	DLT: Myelosuppression Other: Severe emesis, transaminitis, facial paresthesias (rare), rash	Infertility
Dactinomycin (actinomycin-D) *Antibiotic*	DLT: Myelosuppression, severe diarrhea Other: Vesicant, nausea, acne, erythema, radiation recall, hepatic venoocclusive disease	Secondary malignancy Secondary malignancy
Daunorubicin (daunomycin) *Anthracycline*	DLT[c]: Leukopenia, arrhythmia, congestive heart failure (related to cumulative dose) Other: Stomatitis, emesis, vesicant, red urine, radiation recall	Cardiomyopathy
Doxorubicin (Adriamycin) *Anthracycline*	Refer to daunorubicin	Cardiomyopathy

SIADH, syndrome of inappropriate antidiuretic hormone; ADH, antidiuretic hormone; AML, acute myeloid leukemia; SGOT, serum glutamic-oxaloacetic transaminase; MAOI, monoamine oxidase inhibitors.

[a]The dose-limiting toxicity (DLT) is the toxicity most likely to require adjustment or withholding of drug.

[b]Dose must be adjusted in renal insufficiency.

[c]Dose must be adjusted in hyperbilirubinemia.

[d]Dose must be adjusted in renal insufficiency and in patients with third spacing.

Continued

31

SPECIAL DRUG TOPICS

TABLE 31.11

CHARACTERISTICS OF CHEMOTHERAPEUTIC AGENTS—cont'd

Drug name (drug class in italics)	Acute toxicity (DLT[a])	Long-term toxicity
Etoposide (VP-16, VePesid) *Topoisomerase inhibitor*	DLT: Leukopenia, anaphylaxis (rare), transient cortical blindness Other: Hyperbilirubinemia, transaminitis, peripheral neuropathy (rare), hypotension	Secondary malignancy (AML)
Fludarabine (Fludara) *Purine antimetabolite or nucleotide analog*	Myelosuppression[b], anorexia, increased SGOT, somnolence, fatigue	Peripheral neuropathy, immune suppression
Fluorouracil (5-FU, Adrucil) *Nucleotide analog*	DLT: Myelosuppression (reversible with uridine), mucositis, severe diarrhea Other: Hand–foot syndrome, tear duct stenosis, hyperpigmentation, loss of nails; cerebellar syndrome (rare), and anaphylaxis	—
Hydroxyurea (Hydrea) *Ribonucleotide reductase inhibitor*	DLT: Leukopenia, pulmonary edema (rare) Other: Megaloblastic erythropoiesis, hyperpigmentation, azotemia, transaminitis, radiation recall	—
Idarubicin (Idamycin) *Anthracycline*	DLT: Arrhythmia, cardiomyopathy (cumulative) Other: Vesicant, diarrhea, mucositis, enterocolitis	Cardiomyopathy
Ifosfamide (isophosphamide, Ifex) *Alkylator prodrug*	DLT:[b] Myelosuppression, encephalopathy (rarely progressing to death), renal tubular damage Other: Emesis, hemorrhagic cystitis (improved with Mesna), direct ADH effect	Secondary malignancy, infertility
Liposomal doxorubicin (Doxil) *Anthracycline*	Refer to Daunorubicin	Refer to Daunorubicin
Lomustine (CCNU) *Alkylating agent*	Myelosuppression, nausea and vomiting, disorientation, fatigue	Secondary malignancy (leukemia)

Mechlorethamine (nitrogen mustard, HN₂ [mustine], Mustargen)	DLT: Leukopenia, thrombocytopenia
Alkylator	Other: Severe emesis, vesicant (antidote sodium thiosulfate), peptic ulcer (rare)	Secondary malignancy, infertility
Melphalan (L-PAM, Alkeran)	DLT: Prolonged leukopenia (6–8wk), mucositis, diarrhea
Alkylator	Other: Pruritus, emesis	Pulmonary fibrosis, secondary malignancy, infertility, cataracts
Mercaptopurine (6-MP)	DLT: Hepatic necrosis and encephalopathy (especially doses >2.5mg/kg per day)	Cirrhosis
Nucleotide analog	Other: Vesicant, headache, diarrhea, nausea
Methotrexate (MTX, Folex, Mexate, amethopterin)	DLT:ᵈ Stomatitis, diarrhea, renal dysfunction, encephalopathy, cortical blindness, ventriculitis (intrathecal)	Leukoencephalopathy, cirrhosis, pulmonary fibrosis, aseptic necrosis of bone, osteoporosis
Folate antagonist	Other: Photosensitivity, erythema, excessive lacrimation, transaminitis
Mitoxantrone (Novantrone, DHAD, DHAQ, dihydroxyanthracenedione)	DLT: Myelosuppression, cumulative cardiomyopathy	Cardiomyopathy
DNA intercalator	Other: Stomatitis, blue-green urine and serum
Paclitaxel (Taxol)	DLT: Neutropenia, anaphylaxis, ventricular tachycardia and myocardial infarction (rare)	Too soon to know
Tubulin inhibitor	Other: Mucositis, peripheral neuropathy, bradycardia, hypertriglyceridemia

SIADH, syndrome of inappropriate antidiuretic hormone; ADH, antidiuretic hormone; AML, acute myeloid leukemia; SGOT, serum glutamic-oxaloacetic transaminase; MAOI, monoamine oxidase inhibitors.

ᵃThe dose-limiting toxicity (DLT) is the toxicity most likely to require adjustment or withholding of drug.

ᵇDose must be adjusted in renal insufficiency.

ᶜDose must be adjusted in hyperbilirubinemia.

ᵈDose must be adjusted in renal insufficiency and in patients with third spacing.

Continued

SPECIAL DRUG TOPICS

31

TABLE 31.11

CHARACTERISTICS OF CHEMOTHERAPEUTIC AGENTS—cont'd

Drug name (drug class in italics)	Acute toxicity (DLT[a])	Long-term toxicity
Procarbazine (Matulane) *Alkylator*	DLT: Encephalopathy; pancytopenia, especially thrombocytopenia Other: Emesis, paresthesias, dizziness, ataxia, hypotension; adverse effects with tyramine-rich foods, ethanol, MAOIs, meperidine, and many other drugs	Secondary malignancy, infertility
Teniposide (VM-26) *Topoisomerase inhibitor*	DLT: Leukopenia, anaphylaxis (rare) Other: Hyperbilirubinemia, transaminitis	Secondary malignancy (AML)
Thioguanine (6-TG, 6-thioguanine) *Nucleotide analog*	DLT: Myelosuppression, bronchospasm and shock with rapid IV infusion, stomatitis, diarrhea Other: Hyperbilirubinemia, transaminitis, decreased vibratory sensation, ataxia, dermatitis	—
Thiotepa *Alkylating agent*	DLT: Cognitive impairment, leukopenia Other: Increased SGOT, headache, dizziness, rash, desquamation	Secondary malignancy (leukemia) impaired fertility, weakness of lower extremities
Topotecan (Hycamptamine) *Topoisomerase inhibitor*	DLT: Leukopenia, peripheral neuropathy (rare), and Horner's syndrome Other: Nausea, diarrhea, transaminitis, headache	Too soon to know
Vinblastine (Velban, VBL, vincaleukoblastine) *Microtubule inhibitor*	DLT[c]: Leukopenia Other: Vesicant (improved by hyaluronidase and applied heat), constipation, bone pain (especially in the jaw), peripheral and autonomic neuropathy, rarely SIADH	—
Vincristine (VCR, Oncovin) *Microtubule inhibitor*	DLT[c]: Peripheral and autonomic neuropathy, encephalopathy Other: Vesicant, bone pain, constipation, SIADH (rare)	—

ADJUNCTS TO CHEMOTHERAPY

Drug	Role	Toxicity
Amifostine	Reduces the toxicity of radiation and alkylating agents	Hypotension (62%), severe nausea and vomiting, flushing, chills, dizziness, somnolence, hiccups, sneezing, hypocalcemia in susceptible patients (<1%), short-term reversible loss of consciousness (rare), rigors (<1%), mild skin rash
Dexrazoxane	Protective agent for doxorubicin-induced cardiotoxicity	Myelosuppression
Leucovorin	Reduces methotrexate toxicity	Allergic sensitization (rare)
Mesna	Reduces risk of hemorrhagic cystitis	Headache, limb pain, abdominal pain, diarrhea, rash

SIADH, syndrome of inappropriate antidiuretic hormone; ADH, antidiuretic hormone; AML, acute myeloid leukemia; SGOT, serum glutamic-oxaloacetic transaminase; MAOI, monoamine oxidase inhibitors.

[a]The dose-limiting toxicity (DLT) is the toxicity most likely to require adjustment or withholding of drug.
[b]Dose must be adjusted in renal insufficiency.
[c]Dose must be adjusted in hyperbilirubinemia.
[d]Dose must be adjusted in renal insufficiency and in patients with third spacing.

31

SPECIAL DRUG TOPICS

XI. COMMON INDUCERS AND INHIBITORS OF THE CYTOCHROME P450 SYSTEM (Table 31.12)

TABLE 31.12

INDUCERS AND INHIBITORS OF THE CYTOCHROME P450 SYSTEM

Isoenzyme	Substrate (drug metabolized by that isoenzyme)	Inhibitors	Inducers
CYP1A2	Caffeine, tacrine, theophylline, lidocaine, R-warfarin	Cimetidine, ciprofloxacin, erythromycin, tacrine	Omeprazole, smoking, phenobarbital
CYP2B6	Cocaine, ifosphamide, cyclophosphamide	Chloramphenicol	Phenobarbital
CYP2C9/10	S-Warfarin, phenytoin, tolbutamide, diclofenac, piroxicam	Amiodarone, fluconazole, lovastatin	Rifampin, phenobarbital
CYP2C19	Diazepam, omeprazole, mephenytoin	Fluvoxamine, fluoxetine, omeprazole, felbamate	Rifampin, phenobarbital
CYP2D6	Codeine, haloperidol, dextromethorphan, tricyclic antidepressants, phenothiazines, metoprolol, propranolol (4-OH), venlafaxine, risperidone, encainide, paroxetine, sertraline	Quinidine, fluoxetine, sertraline, amiodarone, propoxyphene	None known
CYP2E1	Acetaminophen, alcohol	Disulfiram	Isoniazid, alcohol
CYP3A3/4	Nifedipine, verapamil, cyclosporine, carbamazepine, terfenadine, cisapride, astemizole, tacrolimus, midazolam, alfentanil, diazepam, loratadine, ifosphamide, cyclophosphamide, ritonavir, indinavir	Erythromycin, cimetidine, clarithromycin, fluvoxamine, fluoxetine, ketoconazole, itraconazole, grapefruit juice, metronidazole, ritonavir, indinavir, mibefradil	Rifampin, phenytoin, phenobarbital, carbamazepine

Adapted from Hansten[8].

CYP, cytochrome P450.

The cytochrome P450 enzyme system is composed of different isoenzymes. Each isoenzyme metabolizes a unique group of drugs or substrates. When an *inhibitor* of a particular isoenzyme is introduced, the serum concentration of any drug or *substrate* metabolized by that particular isoenzyme will *increase*. When an *inducer* of a particular isoenzyme is introduced, the serum concentration of drugs or *substrates* metabolized by that particular isoenzyme will *decrease*.

XII. ACNE THERAPEUTIC REGIMENS (Table 31.13)

TABLE 31.13
ACNE THERAPEUTIC REGIMENS

Clinical acne appearance	Treatment
Comedones only	Topical keratolytic: topical retinoid, benzoyl peroxide, salicylic acid
Comedones + mild inflammatory acne (papules and pustules)	Combination of topical keratolytics $\pm$ topical antibiotic (erythromycin, clindamycin, metronidazole) or topical azelaic acid
Moderate inflammatory acne (papules, pustules, cysts)	Oral antibiotic (clindamycin, doxycycline, minocycline, tetracycline, erythromycin, metronidazole) + topical keratolytics
Cystic acne (numerous cysts and pustules)	Isotretinoin orally, 1mg/kg per day (Caution in women of child-bearing age because of teratogenicity. Contraindicated in pregnancy.)

31

SPECIAL DRUG TOPICS

XIII. REFERENCES

1. Expert Panel Report II. *Guidelines for the diagnosis and management of asthma.* National Institutes of Health Publ. No. 97-4051. Bethesda, Md: National Asthma Education and Prevention Program; 1997.
2. American Academy of Pediatrics Committee on Drugs. The transfer of drugs and other chemicals into human milk. *Pediatrics* 1994; **93(1)**:137–150.
3. Hale TW. *Medications and mother's milk,* 6th edn. Amarillo, TX: Pharmasoft; 1997.
4. Briggs G, Freeman RK, Yaffer SJ. *Drugs in pregnancy and lactation,* 5th edn. Baltimore: Williams & Wilkins; 1998.
5. *Physician's desk reference,* 53rd edn. Montvale, NJ: Medical Economics, 1999.
6. American Diabetes Association. *Physician's guide to insulin dependent (type I) diabetes: diagnosis and treatment.* Alexandria, VA: The Association; 1988.
7. Taketomo CK, Hodding JH, Kraus DM. *American Pharmaceutical Association pediatric dosage handbook.* Hudson, OH: Lexi-Comp; 1998.
8. Hansten PD, Horn JR. *Hansten and Horn's drug interaction analysis and management.* Vancouver, British Columbia, Canada: Applied Therapeutics; 1997.
9. Peter G, ed. *1997 red book: report of the Committee on Infectious Diseases,* 24th edn. Elk Grove Village, IL: American Academy of Pediatrics, 1997.

10. Bracken MB, Shepherd MU, Collins WF, Holford TR, Young W, Baskin DS, Eisenberg HM, Flamm E, Leo-Summers L, Maroon J et al. A randomized controlled trial of methylprednisolone or naloxone in the treatment of acute spinal cord injury: results of the Second National Acute Spinal Cord Injury Study. *N Engl J Med* 1990; **322(20):**1405–1411.

11. Kappy MS, Blizzard RM. Migeon CJ, eds. *The diagnosis and treatment of endocrine disorders in childhood and adolescence,* 4th edn. Springfield, IL: Charles C Thomas, 1994.

DRUGS IN RENAL FAILURE

Manaji M. Suzuki, MD

I. DOSE ADJUSTMENT METHODS

A. **MAINTENANCE DOSAGE:** In patients with renal insufficiency, the dose may be adjusted using the following methods:

1. **Interval extension (I):** Lengthen the intervals between individual doses, keeping the dosage size normal. For this method, the suggested interval is shown.
2. **Dose reduction (D):** Reduce the amount of individual doses, keeping the interval between the doses normal. This method is recommended particularly for drugs in which a relatively constant blood level is desired. For this method the percentage of the usual dose is shown.
3. **Interval and dose reduction (DI):** Lengthen the interval, **and** reduce the dose.
4. **Interval *or* dose reduction:** In some instances, either the dose or the interval can be changed. In these instances the D and I are listed vertically in the tables.

Note: These dosage adjustments are for beyond the neonatal period. These dosage modifications are only approximations. Each patient must be monitored closely for signs of drug toxicity, and serum levels must be measured when available. Drug dose and interval should be monitored accordingly.

B. **DIALYSIS:** The quantitative effects of hemodialysis (He) and peritoneal dialysis (P) on drug removal are shown. 'Y' indicates the need for a supplemental dose with dialysis. 'N' indicates no need for adjustment. The designation 'No' does not preclude the use of dialysis or hemoperfusion for drug overdose.

II. ANTIMICROBIALS REQUIRING ADJUSTMENT IN RENAL FAILURE
(Table 32.1)

III. NONANTIMICROBIALS REQUIRING ADJUSTMENT IN RENAL FAILURE (Table 32.2)

IV. DRUGS REQUIRING NO ADJUSTMENT IN RENAL IMPAIRMENT
Most require adjustment in hepatic failure (Table 32.3).

32

TABLE 32.1

ANTIMICROBIALS REQUIRING ADJUSTMENT IN RENAL FAILURE

Drug	Pharmacokinetics			Adjustments in renal failure				Supplemental dose for dialysis
	Route of excretion[a]	Normal $t_{1/2}$ (hr)	Normal dose interval		Creatinine clearance (mL/min)			
				Method	>50	10–50	<10	
acyclovir (IV)	Renal	2–4	Q8hr	DI	Q8hr	Q12–24hr	50% and Q24hr	Y (He) N (P)
amantidine	Renal	10–28	Q12–24hr	I	Q12–24hr	Q24–48hr	Q7days	N (He) N (P)
amikacin[b]	Renal	1.5–3	Q8–12hr	I	Q8–12hr	Q12–18hr	Q24–48hr	Y (He) Y (P)
amoxicillin	Renal	1–3.7	Q8hr	I	Q8hr	Q8–12hr	Q12–24hr	Y (He) N (P)
amoxicillin–clavulanate	Renal	1	Q8–12hr	I	Q8hr	Q8–12hr	Q12–24hr	Y (He) Y (P)
amphotericin B	Renal 40% up to 7 days	Up to 15 days	QD	I	Dosage adjustments are unnecessary with preexisting renal impairment; if decreased renal function is due to amphotericin B, the daily dose can be decreased by 50% or the dose given QOD.			N (He) N (P)
amphotericin B cholesteryl sulfate (Amphotec)	?	28–29	QD	I	No guidelines established			N (He)

							?
mphotericin B lipid complex (Abelcet)	Renal 1%	170	QD	I	No guidelines established		?
mphotericin B liposomal (AmBisome)	Renal ≤10%	100–173	QD	I	No guidelines established		?
mpicillin	Renal	1–4	Q6hr	I	Q6hr	Q6–12hr	Y (He)
							N (P)
mpicillin/sulbactam	Renal	1–1.8	Q4–6hr	I	Q4–6hr	Q12hr	Y (He)
							N (P)
ztreonam	Renal (hepatic)	1.3–2.2	Q6–12hr	D	100%	25%	Y (He)
arbenicillin[c]	Renal (hepatic)	0.8–1.8	Q6hr	I	Q8–12hr	Q12–24hr	Y (He)
efaclor	Renal	0.5–1	Q8–12hr	D	100%	50%	Y (He)
							Y (P)
efadroxil	Renal	1–2	Q12hr	I	Q12hr	Q24–48hr	Y (He)
							N (P)
efamandole	Renal	1	Q4–8hr	I	Q6hr	Q6–8hr	Y (He)
efazolin	Renal	1.5–2.5	Q8hr	I	Q8hr	Q12hr	Y (He)
							N (P)

He, hemodialysis; P, peritoneal dialysis.
[a]Route in parentheses indicates secondary route of excretion.
[b]Subsequent doses are best determined by measurement of serum levels and assessment of renal insufficiency.
[c]May inactivate aminoglycosides in patients with renal impairment.

Continued

TABLE 32.1

ANTIMICROBIALS REQUIRING ADJUSTMENT IN RENAL FAILURE—cont'd

	Pharmacokinetics			Adjustments in renal failure				
					Creatinine clearance (mL/min)			
Drug	Route of excretion[a]	Normal $t_{1/2}$ (hr)	Normal dose interval	Method	>50	10-50	<10	Supplemental dose for dialysis
Cefepime	Renal	1.8–2	Q8–12hr	DI	Q12hr regimens: Est CrCl (mL/min)			Y (He)
					30–60	50mg/kg/dose Q24hr		
					11–29	25mg/kg/dose Q24hr		
					≤10	12.5mg/kg/dose Q24hr		
					Q8hr regimens: Est CrCl (mL/min)			
					30–50	50mg/kg/dose Q12hr		
					10–30	50mg/kg/dose Q24hr		
					<10	50mg/kg/dose Q24–48hr		
Cefixime	Renal (hepatic)	3–4	Q12–24hr	D	100%	75% (CrCl 21–60)	50% (CrCl <20)	N (He, P)
Cefotaxime	Renal	1–3.5	Q6–12hr	D	100%	CrCl <20 = → dose by 50%		Y (He) N (P)
Cefotetan	Renal (hepatic)	3.5	Q12hr	I	Q12hr	CrCl 10–30 = Q24hr	Q48	Y (He, P)

Drug	Route of elimination	Half-life normal (hr)	Normal interval	Method	Normal	CrCl 30–50 = Q8–12hr; CrCl 10–30 = Q12–24hr	CrCl <10 / Q24–48hr	Dialysis Y (He) N (P)
Cefoxitin	Renal	0.75–1.5	Q4–8hr	I		Q8–12hr / Q12–24hr	Q24–48hr	Y (He) N (P)
Cefpodoxime proxetil	Renal	2.2	Q12hr	I	Q12hr	Q12–24hr	Q24hr	Y (He) N (P)
Cefprozil	Renal	1.3	Q12hr	D	100%	50–100%	50%	Y (He)
Ceftazidime	Renal	1–2	Q8–12hr	I	Q8–12hr	Q12–24hr	Q24–48hr	Y (He, P)
Ceftibuten	Renal	1.5–2.5	Q24hr	D	100%	50–25%	25%	Y (He) N (P)
Ceftizoxime	Renal	1.6	Q6–12hr	I	Q8–12hr	Q36–48hr	Q48–72hr	Y (He)
Cefuroxime (IV)	Renal	1.6–2.2	Q8–12hr	I	Q8–12hr	Q8–12hr	Q24hr	Y (He) N (P)
Cephalexin	Renal	0.5–1.2	Q6hr	I	Q6hr	Q8–12hr	Q12–24hr	Y (He) N (P)
Cephalothin[a]	Renal (hepatic)	0.5–1	Q4–6hr	I	Q4–6hr	Q6–8hr	Q12hr	Y (He) N (P)
Cephradine	Renal	0.7–2	Q6–12hr	I	100%	50%	25%	Y (He)
Ciprofloxacin	Renal (hepatic)	1.2–5	Q8–12hr	D	100%	50–75%	50%	Y (He, P)

CrCl, creatinine clearance.

[a] May add to peritoneal dialysate to obtain adequate serum levels.

Continued

TABLE 32.1

ANTIMICROBIALS REQUIRING ADJUSTMENT IN RENAL FAILURE—cont'd

Drug	Pharmacokinetics			Adjustments in renal failure				Supplemental dose for dialysis
	Route of excretion[a]	Normal $t_{1/2}$ (hr)	Normal dose interval	Method	Creatinine clearance (mL/min)			
					>50	10–50	<10	
Clarithromycin	Renal/hepatic	3–7	Q12hr	DI	No change	CrCl <30 = ↓ dose by 50% and administer BID–QD		?
Co-trimoxazole (sulfamethoxazole/ trimethoprim)	Sulfamethoxazole: Hepatic (renal) Trimethoprim: Renal (hepatic)	Sulfamethoxazole: 9–11 Trimethoprim: 8–15	Q12hr	I	Q12hr	Q18hr	Q24hr	Y (He) N (P)
Erythromycin	Hepatic (renal)	1.5–2	Q6–8hr	D	100%	100%	50–75%	N (He)
Ethambutol	Renal (hepatic)	2.5–3.6	Q24hr	I	Q24hr	Q24–36hr	Q48hr ± ↓ dose	Y (He) N (P)
Famciclovir	Renal (hepatic)	2–3	500mg Q8hr	DI		CrCl 40–59 = 500mg Q12hr CrCl 20–39 = 500mg Q24hr <20 = 250 mg Q48hr		Y (He)
Fluconazole[d]	Renal	19–25	Q24hr	D	100%	25–50%	25%	Y (He, P)
Flucytosine[b]	Renal	3–8	Q6hr	I	Q6hr	Q12hr	Q24hr	Y (He, P)
Foscarnet	Renal	3–4.5	Q8–12hr	D		See package insert		Y (He)

			IV: Q12hr PO: TID	IV: DI PO: DI	IV: 50-100% and Q12hr PO: 50-100% and TID	25-50% and Q24hr	25% and Q24hr 50% and QD	Y (He, P)
Ganciclovir	Renal	2.5-3.6						
Gentamicin[b,d]	Renal	1.5-3	Q8-12hr	I	Q8-12hr	Q12-18hr	Q24-48hr	Y (He, P)
Imipenem/cilastatin	Renal	1-1.4	Q6-8hr	DI	50-100% and Q6-8hr	25-50% and Q8hr	25% and Q12hr	Y (He)
Isoniazid	Hepatic (renal)	2-4 (slow)[e] 0.5-1.5 (fast)	Q24hr	D	100%	100%	50%	Y (He, P)
Kanamycin	Renal	2-3	Q8hr	I	Q8-12hr	Q12hr	Q24hr	Y (He, P)
Lamivudine[e]	Renal	1.7-2.5	Q12hr	DI	CrCl 30-49 = 100% and Q24hr 15-29 = 66% and Q24hr 5-14 = 33% and Q24hr <5 = 17% and Q24hr			?
Loracarbef	Renal	0.78-1	Q12hr	I	Q12hr	Q24hr	Q72-120hr	Y (He)
Meropenem	Renal	1-1.4	Q8hr	DI	100% and Q8hr	50-100% and Q12hr	50% and Q24hr	Y (He)
Methicillin	Renal	0.5-1.2	Q4-6hr	I	Q4-6hr	Q6-8hr	Q8-12hr	N (He, P)
Metronidazole	Hepatic (renal)	6-12	Q6-12hr	D	100%	100%	50%	Y (He)
Mezlocillin	Renal (hepatic)	0.5-1	Q4-6hr	I	Q4-6hr	Q6-8hr	Q6-8hr	Y (He) N (P)

e Rate of acetylation of isoniazid.

f For GFR ≥5mL/min, give full dose (150ng adult dose) as first dose; for GFR <5mL/min, give 33% of full dose.

Continued

TABLE 32.1

ANTIMICROBIALS REQUIRING ADJUSTMENT IN RENAL FAILURE—cont'd

Drug	Pharmacokinetics			Adjustments in renal failure				Supplemental dose for dialysis
	Route of excretion[a]	Normal $t_{1/2}$ (hr)	Normal dose interval		Creatinine clearance (mL/min)			
				Method	>50	10–50	<10	
Norfloxacin	Hepatic (renal)	2–4	BID	I	BID	QD–BID	QD	N (He)
Ofloxacin	Renal	5–7.5	BID	I	BID	QD	QOD	Y (He) N (P)
Oxacillin	Renal (liver)	0.3–1.8	Q4–12hr	D	100%	100%	Use lower range of normal dose	N (P)
Penicillin G–potassium/ Na+ (IV)	Renal (hepatic)	0.5–3.4	Q4–6hr	D	100%	75%	20–50%	Y (He) N (P)
Penicillin VK (PO)	Renal (hepatic)	30–40min	Q6hr	I	Q6hr	Q6hr	Q8hr	Y (He) N (P)
Pentamidine	Renal	6.4–9.4	Q24hr	I	Q24hr	Q24–36hr	Q48hr	N (He, P)
Piperacillin	Renal (hepatic)	0.39–1	Q4–6hr	I	Q4–6hr	Q6–8hr	Q12hr	Y (He) N (P)

				DI	100% and Q6-8hr	70% and Q6-8hr	70% and Q8hr	
Piperacillin/ tazobactam	Renal	Piperacillin: 0.39–1 Tazobactam: 0.7–0.9	Q6–8hr		100% and Q6–8hr	70% and Q6–8hr	70% and Q8hr	Y (He) N (P)
Plicamycin	Renal	1	Q24–48hr	D	100%	75%	50%	?
Rifampin	Hepatic (renal)	3–4	Q12–24hr	D	100%	50–100%	50%	N (He, P)
Stavudine	Renal/hepatic	1.1–1.45	Q12hr	DI	100% and Q12hr	50% and Q12–24hr	?	?
Streptomycin sulfate	Renal	2–4.7	Q24hr	I	Q24hr	Q24–72hr	Q72–96hr	Y (He)
Sulfisoxazole	Renal	4–8	Q6hr	I	Q6hr	Q8–12hr	12–24hr	Y (He, P)
Tetracycline	Renal (hepatic)	6–12	Q6hr	I	Q8–12hr	Q12–24hr	AVOID	?
Ticarcillin[c]	Renal	0.9–1.3	Q4–6hr	I	Q4–6hr	Q6–8hr	Q12hr	Y (He) N (P)
Ticarcillin– clavulanate[c]	Renal	Ticarcillin: 0.9–1.3 Clavulanate: 1–1.5	Q4–6hr	I	Q4–6hr	Q6–8hr	Q12hr	Y (He) N (P)
Tobramycin[b,d]	Renal	1.5–3	Q8–12hr	I	Q8–12hr	Q12–18hr	Q24–48hr	Y (He, P)

Continued

TABLE 32.1

ANTIMICROBIALS REQUIRING ADJUSTMENT IN RENAL FAILURE—cont'd

Drug	Route of excretion[a]	Normal $t_{1/2}$ (hr)	Normal dose interval	Method	>50	10–50	<10	Supplemental dose for dialysis
						Adjustments in renal failure — Creatinine clearance (mL/min)		
Valacyclovir	Valacyclovir: Hepatic	Valacyclovir: 2.5–3.6	Q12–24hr	DI	Herpes zoster: 100% and Q8hr	100% and Q12–24hr	50% and Q24hr	Y (He) N (P)
	Acyclovir: Renal	Acyclovir: 2–4			Genital herpes (initial): 100% and Q12hr	100% and Q12–24hr	50% and Q24hr	
					Genital herpes (recurrent): 100% and Q12hr	100% and Q12–24hr	100% and Q24hr	
					Genital herpes (suppressive): 100% and Q24hr	50–100% and Q24hr	50% and Q24hr	
Vancomycin[b]	Renal	2.2–8	Q6–12h	I	Q6–12hr	Q24–48hr	Q48–96hr	Y/N (He)[g] N (P)
Zalcitabine	Renal	1–3	Q8hr	I	Q8hr	Q12hr	Q24hr	?

[g]If using high-flux hemodialysis (polysulfone polyamide and polyacrylonitrile), give supplemental dose after dialysis.

TABLE 32.2

NONANTIMICROBIALS REQUIRING ADJUSTMENT IN RENAL FAILURE

		Pharmacokinetics			Adjustments in renal failure				
						Creatinine clearance (mL/min)			Supplemental dose for dialysis
Drug	Route of excretion[a]	Normal $t_{1/2}$ (hr)	Normal dose interval	Method	>50	10–50	<10	
Acetaminophen	Hepatic	2	Q4hr	I	Q4hr	Q6hr	Q8hr	Y (He)
								N (P)
Acetazolamide	Renal	2.4–5.8	Q6–24hr	I	Q6–8hr	Q12hr	AVOID	N (He, P)
Adriamycin	Renal (hepatic)	16–30	Single dose	D	100%	100%	75%	?
Allopurinol	Renal	1–3	Q8–12hr	D	100%	50%	10–25%	?
Amantadine	Renal	10–14	Q12–24hr	I	Q12–24hr	Q48–72hr	Q168hr (7 days)	N (He, P)
Aminocaproic acid	Renal	1–2	Q4–6hr	D	Reduce dose by 75% in patients with renal disease or oliguria. No specific recommendations available.			Y (He)
Aspirin[b]	Hepatic (renal)	2–19	Q4hr	I	Q4hr	Q4–6hr	AVOID	Y (He)
								Y (P)
Atenolol	Renal (GI)	3.5–7	QD	D	100%	50%	25%	Y (He)
Azathioprine[c]	Hepatic (renal)	0.7–3	QD	D	100%	75%	50%	Y (He)
Bismuth subsalicylate	Hepatic (renal)	Salicylate: 2–5	Q30min–4hr	D	AVOID	AVOID	AVOID	NA
		Bismuth: 21–72 days						

He, hemodialysis; P, peritoneal dialysis; NA, not applicable.

[a]Route in parentheses indicates secondary route of excretion.

[b]With large doses, the $t_{1/2}$ is prolonged up to 30hr.

[c]Azathioprine rapidly converted to mercaptopurine ($t_{1/2}$ = 0.5–4hr).

32

DRUGS IN RENAL FAILURE

Continued

TABLE 32.2
NONANTIMICROBIALS REQUIRING ADJUSTMENT IN RENAL FAILURE—cont'd

Drug	Pharmacokinetics			Adjustments in renal failure					Supplemental dose for dialysis
	Route of excretion[a]	Normal $t_{1/2}$ (hr)	Normal dose interval		Creatinine clearance (mL/min)				
				Method	>50	10-50	<10		
Bretylium	Renal	7-11	Q1min to 6-8hr	D	100%	25-50%	25%		Y (He)
Captopril	Renal (hepatic)	0.98-12.4	Q6-24hr	D	100%	75%	50%		Y (He) N (P)
Carbamazepine	Hepatic (renal)	Initial: 25-65 Subsequent: 8-17	Q6-24hr	D	100%	100%	75% (monitor serum levels)		N (He, P)
Cetirizine	Renal (hepatic)	6.2-9	QD	D	100%	50-100%	50%		N (He)
Chloroquine	Renal (hepatic)	3-5days	Q6hr-7 days	D	100%	100%	50%		?
Cimetidine	Renal (hepatic)	1.4-2	Q6hr	D	100%	75%	50%		N (He, P)
Codeine	Hepatic (renal)	2.5-3.5	Q6-12hr Q4-6hr	D	100%	75%	50%		?
Digoxin[d]	Renal	35-48	Q24hr	D I	100% Q24hr	25-75% Q36hr	10-25% Q48hr		N (He, P)
Diphenhydramine	Hepatic	4-7		I	Q6hr	Q6-12hr	Q12-18hr		?
Disopyramide	Renal (GI)	4-10	Q6hr	I	Q6hr	Q8-12hr	Q24hr		Y (He)

Enalapril	Renal (hepatic)	2-2.7	Q6hr Q8-24hr	D	100%	75-100%	50%	?
Famotidine	Renal (hepatic)	2.5-4	Q8-12hr	D	100%	50%	25%	N (He, P)
				I	Q8-12hr	Q24hr	Q36-48hr	
Fentanyl	Renal (hepatic)	2-4	Q30min-1hr	D	100%	75%	50%	?
Flecainide	Renal/hepatic	8-12	Q8-12hr	D	CrCl <20mL/min: a downward dosing adjustment of 25-50% to be initiated.			N (He, P)
Gabapentin	Renal (hepatic)	5-9	TID	I	TID	BID-QD	QOD	Y (He)
Hydralazine[e]	Hepatic (renal)	2-8	IV: Q4-6hr	I	Normal dosing	Q8hr	Q8-16hr (fast acetylator) Q12-24hr (slow acetylator)	N (He, P)
Insulin (regular)[f]	Hepatic (renal)	5-15min	Variable	D	100%	75%	25-50%	?
Lithium	Renal	18-24	TID-QID	D	100%	50-75%	25-50%	Y (He, P)
Meperidine	Renal (hepatic) (normeperidine: renal)	2.3-4	Q3-4hr	D	100%	75%	50%	?
Methadone	Hepatic (renal)	19-35	Q3-6hr	D	100%	100%	50-75%	?

CrCl, creatinine clearance.

[d] Decrease loading dose by 50% in end-stage renal disease because of decreased volume of distribution.

[e] Dose interval varies for rapid and slow acetylators with normal and impaired renal function.

[f] Renal failure may cause hyposensitivity or hypersensitivity to insulin; adjust to clinical response and blood glucose.

Continued

TABLE 32.2

NONANTIMICROBIALS REQUIRING ADJUSTMENT IN RENAL FAILURE—cont'd

Drug	Pharmacokinetics			Adjustments in renal failure				
						Creatinine clearance (mL/min)		Supplemental dose for dialysis
	Route of excretion[a]	Normal $t_{1/2}$ (hr)	Normal dose interval	Method	>50	10–50	<10	
Methotrexate	Renal	Triphasic, 0.1, 2.3, 27	Single treatment	D	100%	50%	AVOID	Y (He) N (P)
Methyldopa	Hepatic (renal)	1–3	PO: Q6–12hr IV: Q6–8hr	I	Q8hr	Q8–12hr	Q12–24hr	Y (He)
Metoclopramide	Renal	2.5–6	PO: Q6hr IV: Q6–8hr	D	100%	50–75%	25–50%	N (He)
Midazolam	Hepatic (renal)	1–3	Variable	D	100%	100%	50%	?
Morphine	Hepatic (renal)	1–6.2	Variable	D	100%	75%	50%	N (He)
Neostigmine	Hepatic (renal)	0.5–2.1	Single dose	D	100%	50%	25%	?
Phenazopyridine HCl	Hepatic (renal)	?	TID for 3 days	I	Q8–16hr	AVOID	AVOID	NA
Phenobarbital	Hepatic (renal 30%)	65–150	Q8–12hr	I	Q8–12hr	Q8–12hr	Q12–16hr	Y (He, P)
Plicamycin	Renal	1	Q24hr	D	100%	75%	50%	?

Primidone	Hepatic (renal, 20%)	6-12	Q8-12	I	Q8-12hr	Q8-12hr	Q12-24hr	Y (He)
Procainamide	Hepatic (renal)	Procainamide: 1.7-4.7 NAPA: 6-8	PO: Q3-6hr IM: Q4-6hr	I	Normal interval	Q6-12hr	Q8-24hr	Y (He) N (P)
Propylthiouracil	Hepatic (renal)	1.5-5	Q8hr	D	100%	75%	50%	?
Quidinine	Hepatic (renal)	2.5-8	Variable	D	100%	100%	75%	Y (He) N (P)
Ranitidine	Renal (hepatic)	1.8-2.5	Q8-12hr	D	100%	75%	50%	N (He, P)
Spironolactone	Renal (hepatic)	78-84min	Q6-12hr	I	Q6-12hr	Q12-24hr^g	AVOID	?
Terbutaline (IV/PO)	Renal (hepatic)	11-26	Variable	D	100%	50%	AVOID	?
Thiopental	Hepatic (renal)	3-11.5	One-time dose	D	100%	100%	75%	?
Triamterene	Hepatic (renal)	1.5-2.5	Q12-24hr	I	Q12hr	Q12hr^g	AVOID	
Verapamil	Renal (hepatic)	2-8	Variable	D	100%	100%	50-75%	N (He)

^{g}Hyperkalemia common with GFR <30mL/min.

DRUGS IN RENAL FAILURE

TABLE 32.3

DRUGS REQUIRING NO ADJUSTMENT IN RENAL IMPAIRMENT

Acetylcysteine	Caffeine	Cytosine arabinoside	Flumazenil	Mineral oil	Pyrantel pamoate
ACTH	Calcitonin	Dantrolene	Flunisolide	Montelukast	Pyrethrins
Adenosine	Calcitriol	Desferoxamine	Fluticasone propionate	Mupirocin	Pyridostigmine bromide
Adriamycin	Calcium carbonate	Desmopressin acetate	Fosphenytoin	Naloxone	Pyrimethamine
Albumin	Calcium chloride	Dexamethasone	Granisetron	Nedocromil	Salmeterol
Albuterol	Calcium glubionate	Dextroamphetamine	Griseofulvin	Neomycin/polymyxin	Selenium sulfide
Aluminum hydroxide	Calcium gluceptate	Diazepam	Haloperidol	B ± bacitracin	Simethicone
Aluminum hydroxide	Calcium gluconate	Diazoxide[ab]	Heparin	Nifedipine	Streptokinase
with magnesium	Calcium lactate	Dicloxacillin sodium	Hyaluronidase	Nortriptyline	Succinylcholine[d]
hydroxide	Cefoperazone	Digoxin immune Fab	Hydrocortisone	hydrochloride	Sulfacetamide sodium
Aminophylline	Ceftriaxone[a]	Dihydrotachysterol	Hydroxyzine	Nystatin	Surfactant,
Amiodarone	Chlorpheniramine	Diltiazem	Ibuprofen	Omeprazole	pulmonary/beractant
Amitriptyline	maleate	Dimenhydrinate	Imipramine	Oxymetazoline	Surfactant,
Amlodipine	Chlorpromazine	Divalproex sodium	Ipecac	Palivizumab	pulmonary/colfosceril
Amrinone lactate	Cholestyramine	Dobutamine	Ipratropium bromide	Pancreatic enzymes	palmitate

Antipyrine and
  benzocaine
Ascorbic acid
Astemizole
Atropine
Attapulgite
Azelastine
Azithromycin
Beclomethasone
  dipropionate
Benzoyl peroxide
Bethanecol chloride
Bisacodyl
Budesonide
Bumetanide
Bupivacaine
Busulfan

Cisapride
Citrate mixtures
Clemastine
Clindamycin
Clonazepam
Clonidine
Clotrimazole
Cloxacillin
Cortisone acetate
Cromolyn
Cyclopentolate
Cyclopentolate/phenyl-
  ephrine
Cyclosporine or
  cyclosporine
  microemulsion
Cyproheptadine

Docusate sodium
Dopamine
Dornase alpha/DNAse
Doxapram HCl
Doxycycline
Dronabinol
EMLA
Epinephrine HCl
Epinephrine, racemic
Ergocalciferol
Ergotamine
Erythropoietin
Esmolol
Ethosuximide
Filgrastim
Fludrocorticone
  acetate

Itraconazole
Ivermectin
Ketamine
Ketoconazole
Labetalol
Lactulose
Lidocaine
Lindane
Loperamine
Lorazepam
Mebendazole
Metaproterenol
Methimazole
Methsuximide
Methylphenidate HCl
Metolazone
Miconazole

Paromomycin
Pentobarbital
Permethrin
Phenytoin
Pirbuterol acetate
Polyethylene glycol:
  electrolyte solution
Polymyxin B sulfate
  and bacitracin
Polymyxin B sulfate,
  neomycin sulfate,
  hydrocorticone
Prazosin HCl[c]
Prednisolone
Prednisone
Promethazine
Psyllium

Theophylline[e]
Thioridazine
Tolmetin sodium
Tolnaftate
Trazodone
Tretinoin
Triamcinolone
Triethanolamine
  polypeptide oleate
Urokinase
Ursodiol
Valproic acid
Vinblastine
Vincristine
Vitamin E
Zafirlukast
Zileuton

[a]Extra dose for hemodialysis recommended.
[b]Extra dose for peritoneal dialysis recommended.
[c]Patients may respond to low doses.
[d]In end-stage renal failure, acute hyperkalemia may develop.
[e]No adjustments for patients >3mo of age.

32

DRUGS IN RENAL FAILURE

V. REFERENCES

1. Taketomo C, Hodding JH, Kraus DM. *Pediatric drug handbook,* 5th edn. Hudson, OH: Lexi-Comp, Inc; 1998–1999.
2. American Society of Health-System Pharmacists. *American hospital formulary service.* Bethesda, MD: The Society; 1998.
3. Johnson C, Simmons W. Dialysis of drugs. *Pharm Practice News* Dec 1988, pp 30–33.
4. Micromedix, Inc, Vol. 99, 1974-1999. Expires 2/28/99.

INDEX

Page references in *italics* indicate figures; page references followed by *t* indicate
tables.

ALGORITHM FOR TACHYCARDIA WITH POOR PERFUSION

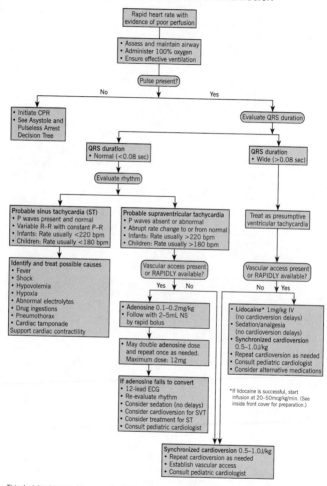

This decision tree provides general guidelines that may not apply to all patients. For all treatments, consider carefully the presence of proper indications and the absence of contraindications.

Adapted from American Heart Association: *Pediatric advanced life support handbook.* Dallas: The Association, 1997.

ALGORITHM FOR PEDIATRIC TACHYCARDIA WITH ADEQUATE PERFUSION

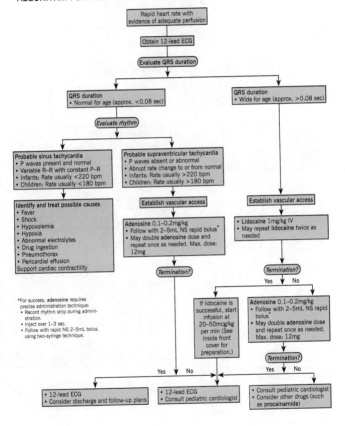

BRADYCARDIA ALGORITHM

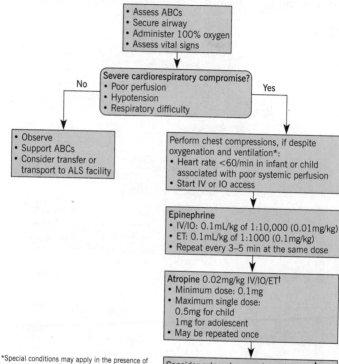

- Assess ABCs
- Secure airway
- Administer 100% oxygen
- Assess vital signs

Severe cardiorespiratory compromise?
- Poor perfusion
- Hypotension
- Respiratory difficulty

No →

- Observe
- Support ABCs
- Consider transfer or transport to ALS facility

Yes →

Perform chest compressions, if despite oxygenation and ventilation*:
- Heart rate <60/min in infant or child associated with poor systemic perfusion
- Start IV or IO access

Epinephrine
- IV/IO: 0.1mL/kg of 1:10,000 (0.01mg/kg)
- ET: 0.1mL/kg of 1:1000 (0.1mg/kg)
- Repeat every 3–5 min at the same dose

Atropine 0.02mg/kg IV/IO/ET†
- Minimum dose: 0.1mg
- Maximum single dose:
  0.5mg for child
  1mg for adolescent
- May be repeated once

Consider external or esophageal pacing‡

If asystole develops, see Asystole/Pulseless Arrest Algorithm

*Special conditions may apply in the presence of severe hypothermia.
†For ET administration, dilute with 3–5mL NS followed by several PPVs.
‡Limited pediatric data.

Adapted from American Heart Association: *Pediatric advanced life support handbook.* Dallas: The Association, 1997.